D1561066

Ambulatory Surgery

Ambulatory Surgery

Bruce David Schirmer, MD
Stephen H. Watts Professor of Surgery
Department of Surgery
University of Virginia Health Sciences Center
Charlottesville, Virginia

David William Rattner, MD
Associate Professor of Surgery
Harvard Medical School
Massachusetts General Hospital
Boston, Massachusetts

W.B. SAUNDERS COMPANY
A Division of Harcourt Brace & Company
Philadelphia London Toronto Montreal Sydney Tokyo

W.B. SAUNDERS COMPANY
A Division of Harcourt Brace & Company

The Curtis Center
Independence Square West
Philadelphia, Pennsylvania 19106

Library of Congress Cataloging-in-Publication Data

Ambulatory surgery / [edited by] Bruce D. Schirmer, David W. Rattner.—1st ed.

p.   cm.

ISBN 0–7216–5889–X

1. Ambulatory surgery.   I. Schirmer, Bruce D.   II. Rattner, David W., MD
  [DNLM: 1. Ambulatory Surgery.   WO 192 A4964 1998]

RD110.A4653 1998   617′.024—dc21

DNLM/DLC   97–41327

AMBULATORY SURGERY   ISBN 0–7216–5889–X

Printed in the United States of America.

Last digit is the print number: 9   8   7   6   5   4   3   2   1

To Geri, Kate Lynn, and Liza,
who have so patiently supported me
during the creation of this work.

To Dr. David Sabiston, my teacher and mentor,
whose surgical scholarship is unmatched
and who provided the inspiration for this text.

Contributors

Frederick W. Ackroyd, M.D.
Associate Professor, Department of
Surgery, Harvard Medical School;
Massachusetts General Hospital, Boston,
Massachusetts
Credentialing Issues

Maria D. Allo, M.D.
Associate Professor of Surgery
(Clinical), Stanford University, Stanford;
Chairperson, Department of Surgery,
Santa Clara Valley Medical Center, San
Jose, California
*Integration of Ambulatory Surgery Into the
Health Care System*

Bruce G. Bateman, M.D.
Associate Professor, University of
Virginia School of Medicine; Director,
Division of Reproductive Endocrinology,
University of Virginia Health Sciences
Center, Charlottesville, Virginia
*Laparoscopic Treatment of Gynecologic
Emergencies*

David J. Bentrem, M.D.
General Surgery Resident, Northwestern
Medical School, Chicago, Illinois
Universal Precautions

Timothy J. Bill, M.D.
Plastic Surgery Resident, Department of
Plastic Surgery, University of Virginia
School of Medicine, Charlottesville,
Virginia
*Preoperative Assessment and Discharge
Assessment Criteria*

Osbert Blow, M.D., Ph.D.
Chief Resident, Department of Surgery,
University of Virginia School of
Medicine, Charlottesville, Virginia
*Special Considerations for Pediatric
Endoscopy*

John W. Braasch, M.D., Ph.D.
Assistant Clinical Professor of Surgery,
Harvard Medical School, Boston; Senior
Consultant in Surgery, Lahey Hitchcock
Clinic, Burlington, Massachusetts
Cholecystectomy: Minilaparotomy

Gene D. Branum, M.D.
Assistant Professor of Surgery, Emory
University School of Medicine; Assistant
Director, Gastrointestinal Surgery,
Emory Clinic; Chief, General Surgery,
Atlanta Veterans Administration Medical
Center; Director, Third Year Surgical
Curriculum, Emory University Hospital,
Atlanta, Georgia
*Laparoscopy for Acute Abdominal Pain and
the Acute Abdomen*

**Ranès C. Chakravorty, M.A.Ed.,
M.B.B.S.**
Professor of Surgery, University of
Virginia School of Medicine,
Charlottesville; Surgeon, Veterans Affairs
Medical Center, Salem, Virginia
Head and Neck

John Morgan Cosgrove, M.D., F.A.C.S.
Assistant Professor of Surgery, Albert
Einstein College of Medicine, Bronx;
Director of Minimally Invasive Surgery,
Long Island Jewish Medical Center, New
Hyde Park, New York
*Special Considerations for Therapeutic Lower
Endoscopy*

James Thomas Cox, M.D.
Staff Anesthesiologist, Memorial
Regional Medical Center, Richmond,
Virginia
Evaluation and Monitoring of the Patient

Mark Dershwitz, M.D., Ph.D.
Associate Professor of Anaesthesia,
Harvard Medical School; Associate
Anesthetist, Massachusetts General
Hospital, Boston, Massachusetts
Agents for General Anesthesia

Don E. Detmer, M.D.
Professor of Surgery, Department of
Surgery, University of Virginia School of
Medicine, Charlottesville; Senior Vice
President, University of Virginia,
Charlottesville, Virginia
Reimbursement Issues

David B. Drake, M.D.
Assistant Professor of Plastic Surgery,
Department of Plastic Surgery,
University of Virginia School of
Medicine, Charlottesville, Virginia
*Universal Precautions; Excisional Biopsy of
Skin Tumors*

William F. Eckhardt III, M.D.
Clinical Assistant Professor of
Anesthesia, University of Arizona School
of Medicine, Tucson; Private
Practitioner, Valley Anesthesiology
Consultants, Ltd., Phoenix, Arizona
Local and Regional Anesthesia

Richard F. Edlich, M.D., Ph.D.
Raymond F. Morgan Professor of Plastic
Surgery and Professor of Biomedical
Engineering, Department of Plastic
Surgery, University of Virginia School of
Medicine, Charlottesville, Virginia
*Preoperative Assessment and Discharge
Assessment Criteria; Universal Precautions;
Surgical Management of Difficult Wounds;
Excisional Biopsy of Skin Tumors*

Aaron S. Fink, M.D.
Professor of Surgery, Emory University
School of Medicine; Chief of Surgery,
Atlanta Veterans Administration Medical
Center, Atlanta, Georgia
*Laparoscopy for Abdominal Pain and the
Acute Abdomen*

Eugene Foley, M.D.
Assistant Professor of Surgery, University
of Virginia School of Medicine,
Charlottesville, Virginia
Hemorrhoids

Shawn Garber, M.D.
Fellow in Laparoscopic Surgery, George
Washington University School of
Medicine, Washington, D.C.
*Special Considerations for Therapeutic Lower
Endoscopy*

Joseph Gerstein, M.D., F.A.C.P.
Assistant Clinical Professor of Medicine,
Harvard Medical School, Boston;
Medical Director, Tufts Health Plan,
Waltham, Massachusetts
Outcome Studies

Jonathan P. Gertler, M.D.
Associate Professor of Surgery, Division
of Vascular Surgery, Harvard Medical
School; Massachusetts General Hospital,
Boston, Massachusetts
Venous Diseases

Arthur I. Gilbert, M.D.
Clinical Associate Professor of Surgery,
University of Miami Medical School;
Hernia Institute of Florida, South
Miami, Florida
Hernias: Traditional Approach

Joel S. Goodwin II, M.D.
Attending Surgeon, Bonner General
Hospital, Sandpoint, Idaho
Hernias: Prosthetic Material Repair

Michael F. Graham, M.D.
Hernia Institute of Florida, South
Miami, Florida
Hernias: Traditional Approach

Charles Harris, M.D.
Community Surgical Group, Fresno,
California
Management of Breast Abnormalities

Kenneth Haspel, M.D.
Instructor in Anaesthesia, Harvard
Medical School; Assistant in Anesthesia,
Massachusetts General Hospital, Boston,
Massachusetts
Evaluation and Monitoring of the Patient

James P. Highland, Ph.D., M.H.S.A.
President, Compass Health Analytics,
Inc., Needham, Massachusetts
Economic Incentives and Cost Effectiveness

Herbert C. Hoover, Jr., M.D.
Professor of Surgery, The Milton S.
Hershey Medical Center, Penn State
University College of Medicine,
Hershey; Chairman, Department of
Surgery, Lehigh Valley Hospital,
Allentown, Pennsylvania
Lymph Node Biopsy

John G. Hunter, M.D., F.A.C.S.
Associate Professor of Surgery, Emory
University School of Medicine; Vice
Chairman of Surgery, Emory University
Hospital, Atlanta, Georgia
The Use of Lasers in Endoscopic Surgery

Judith C. F. Hwang, M.D.
Assistant Clinical Professor of
Anesthesiology, University of California,
Los Angeles; Staff, University of
California, Los Angeles Medical Center,
Los Angeles, California
*Preoperative Assessment and Discharge
Assessment Criteria*

Andrew A. Jeon, M.D., M.B.A.
Instructor in Anesthesia, Harvard
Medical School; Director of Medical
Programs, Harvard Medical
International, Harvard Medical School,
Boston, Massachusetts
*Administration of the Ambulatory Surgery
Unit*

James O. Keck, M.B., B.S.
Senior Associate, University of
Melbourne, Melbourne; Surgeon,
Department of Colorectal Surgery, St.
Vincent's Hospital; Senior Surgeon, Box
Hill Hospital, Melbourne, Australia
Transanal Excision: Traditional Approach

Peter B. Kelsey, M.D.
Massachusetts General Hospital, Boston,
Massachusetts
*Special Considerations for Therapeutic Upper
Endoscopy*

Scott E. Langenburg, M.D.
Resident in the Department of General
Surgery, University of Virginia Health
Sciences Center, Charlottesville, Virginia
Excisional Biopsy of Skin Tumors

Henry L. Laws, M.D.
Clinical Professor of Surgery, The
University of Alabama at Birmingham;
Director of Surgical Education,
Carraway Methodist Medical Center,
Birmingham, Alabama
Laparoscopy for Chronic Abdominal Pain

Robert Marasco, AIA
Marasco & Associates, Inc., Colorado
Springs, Colorado
*Determining the Feasibility of an Ambulatory
Surgery Center*

Eugene D. McGahren III, M.D.
Assistant Professor of Pediatric Surgery
and Pediatrics, Division of Pediatric
Surgery, University of Virginia Health
Sciences Center, Charlottesville, Virginia
*Special Considerations for Outpatient
Pediatric Surgery*

John S. Minasi, M.D.
Assistant Professor of Surgery, General
Surgery Residency Program Director,
University of Virginia School of
Medicine; Director, Surgical Nutrition
Support Service, University of Virginia
Health Sciences Center, Charlottesville,
Virginia
Pilonidal Cysts and Sinuses

Joseph Minasi, M.D.
Director Emeritus, Department of
Anesthesia, On-Site Physician, Cardiac
Rehabilitation Center, South Nassau
Communities Hospital, Oceanside,
New York
Pilonidal Cysts and Sinuses

Marcia Moore, M.D.
Assistant Professor of Surgery,
Department of Surgery, University of
Virginia School of Medicine,
Charlottesville, Virginia
Management of Breast Abnormalities

Raymond F. Morgan, M.D.
Professor and Chairman, Department of
Plastic Surgery, University of Virginia
School of Medicine, Charlottesville,
Virginia
Surgical Management of Difficult Wounds

Nguyen D. Nguyen, M.D.
General Surgery Resident, University of
Virginia School of Medicine,
Charlottesville, Virginia
Surgical Management of Difficult Wounds

Bruce A. Orkin, M.D.
Associate Professor, Director, Division of
Colon and Rectal Surgery, Director,
Colorectal Physiology Laboratory, and
Program Director, The Residency in
Surgery, Department of Surgery, The
George Washington University,
Washington, D.C.
*Transanal Excision: Endoscopic
Microsurgical Technique*

Leslie Ottinger, M.D.
Associate Professor of Surgery, Harvard
Medical School; Visiting Surgeon,
Massachusetts General Hospital, Boston,
Massachusetts
Subcutaneous Nodules

Beverly K. Philip, M.D.
Associate Professor of Anaesthesia,
Harvard Medical School; Director, Day
Surgery Unit, Brigham and Women's
Hospital, Boston, Massachusetts
*Administration of the Ambulatory Surgery
Unit*

John P. Remensnyder, M.D.
Associate Professor of Surgery, Harvard
Medical School; Visiting Surgeon,
Massachusetts General Hospital, Boston,
Massachusetts
Quality Issues in Ambulatory Care

Patricia Roberts, M.D.
Staff Surgeon, Department of Colon
and Rectal Surgery, Lahey Hitchcock
Clinic, Burlington, Massachusetts
Transanal Excision: Traditional Approach

Bradley M. Rodgers, M.D.
Professor and Chief of Pediatric Surgery
and Pediatrics, Division of Pediatric
Surgery, University of Virginia School of
Medicine, Charlottesville, Virginia
*Special Considerations for Pediatric
Endoscopy*

William T. Ross, Jr. M.D., M.B.A.
Professor of Anesthesiology, University
of Virginia School of Medicine; Medical
Director, Virginia Ambulatory Surgery
Center, Charlottesville, Virginia
*The Role of the Medical Director in the
Ambulatory Surgical Center; Evaluation and
Monitoring of the Patient*

Worthington G. Schenk III, M.D.
Associate Professor, Department of
Surgery, University of Virginia School of
Medicine, Charlottesville, Virginia
*Pitfalls in Ambulatory Vascular Access
Surgery*

Bruce David Schirmer, M.D.
Stephen H. Watts Professor of Surgery,
Department of Surgery, University of
Virginia Medical Center, Charlottesville,
Virginia
*History of Ambulatory Surgery; Determining
the Feasibility of An Ambulatory Surgery
Center; Reimbursement Issues; Modern
Technology in the Ambulatory Surgery Unit*

Paul C. Shellito, M.D.
Assistant Professor of Surgery, Harvard
Medical School; Associate Visiting
Surgeon, Massachusetts General
Hospital, Boston, Massachusetts
Perianal Disease

Craig L. Slingluff, Jr., M.D.
Assistant Professor of Surgery, University
of Virginia School of Medicine,
Charlottesville, Virginia
Pigmented Skin Lesions

Stephen D. Small, M.D.
Instructor in Anesthesia, Harvard
Medical School; Department of
Anesthesia, Massachusetts General
Hospital, Boston, Massachusetts
*Special Considerations for Laparoscopic
Surgery*

Nathaniel J. Soper, M.D.
Professor of Surgery, Department of
Surgery, Washington University School
of Medicine; Barnes-Jewish Hospital, St.
Louis, Missouri
Laparoscopic Cholecystectomy

Bobbie Jean Sweitzer, M.D.
Instructor in Anesthesia and Critical
Care, Harvard Medical School; Assistant
in Anaesthesia and Critical Care,
Massachusetts General Hospital, Boston,
Massachusetts
Conscious Sedation

L. William Traverso, M.D.
Section of General, Thoracic and
Vascular Surgery, Virginia Mason
Medical Center, Seattle, Washington
Hernias: Prosthetic Material Repair

Thadeus L. Trus, M.D., F.R.C.S.(C)
Assistant Professor of Surgery, Emory
University; Staff Surgeon/Co-Director,
SICU, Atlanta Veterans Administration
Medical Center, Atlanta, Georgia
The Use of Lasers in Endoscopic Surgery

C. Randle Voyles, M.D.
Clinical Associate Professor of Surgery,
University of Mississippi, Jackson;
Surgical Clinic Associates, P.A., Jackson,
Mississippi
*Special Considerations for Performing
Laparoscopic Surgery: Personnel, Equipment,
and Costs*

John H. T. Waldhausen, M.D.
Assistant Professor of Surgery, University
of Washington School of Medicine;
Attending Surgeon, Children's Hospital
and Medical Center, Seattle, Washington
Pediatric Hernias and Hydroceles

Richard L. Whelan, M.D., F.A.C.S.
Assistant Professor of Surgery, Columbia
University College of Physicians and
Surgeons; Columbia Presbyterian
Medical Center, New York, New York
*Special Considerations for Therapeutic Lower
Endoscopy*

Cameron D. Wright, M.D.
Assistant Professor of Surgery, Harvard
University Medical School; Associate
Visiting Surgeon, General Thoracic
Surgical Unit, Massachusetts General
Hospital, Boston, Massachusetts
Special Considerations for Bronchoscopy

Terrance A. Yemen, M.D.
Associate Professor of Anesthesia,
McGill University School of Medicine;
Chief of Anesthesia, Montreal
Children's Hospital, Montreal, Quebec,
Canada
Managing the Pediatric Outpatient

Introduction

Currently more than half of all surgical procedures are performed on an ambulatory or 23-hour stay basis. The scope and complexity of procedures in the ambulatory surgical setting have increased dramatically over the past two decades. This text is written to provide practicing general surgeons and allied health professionals with a relatively comprehensive reference to the ever-expanding practice of ambulatory surgery.

Although much of the initial increase in volume of ambulatory surgical procedures was driven by economic incentives, favorable experiences on the part of both surgeons and patients now play a major role in this evolutionary process. Innovation in endosurgical and minimal access technology, development of short-acting anesthetic agents, and improvement in postoperative pain control have facilitated the transition of many general surgical procedures from the inpatient to the ambulatory setting.

The dramatic increase in the type and volume of ambulatory general surgery has not been matched with a corresponding production of quality texts dedicated to this field. It is our aim to help fill that void with this work. While the descriptions of many of these procedures may be found in older texts on inpatient procedures, and some found in more recent texts on endoscopic or laparoscopic procedures, this book brings together a relevant body of knowledge about the practical aspects of general surgical procedures now commonly performed on an outpatient basis. The operative descriptive chapters are enhanced by other chapters dealing with the key role of the anesthesiologist in the ambulatory setting. For those interested in providing the total package of ambulatory surgical services to patients, chapters on the economic and administrative aspects of the ambulatory surgical center are also included.

BRUCE DAVID SCHIRMER, MD
DAVID WILLIAM RATTNER, MD

NOTICE

Medicine is an ever-changing field. Standard safety precautions must be followed, but as new research and clinical experience broaden our knowledge, changes in treatment and drug therapy become necessary or appropriate. Readers are advised to check the product information currently provided by the manufacturer of each drug to be administered to verify the recommended dose, the method and duration of administration, and contraindications. It is the responsibility of the treating physician relying on experience and knowledge of the patient to determine dosages and the best treatment for the patient. Neither the Publisher nor the editor assumes any responsibility for any injury and/or damage to persons or property.

THE PUBLISHER

Contents

Introduction

Chapter 1

History of Ambulatory Surgery

Bruce David Schirmer

Ambulatory surgery may be defined as surgical procedures performed outside the realm of an inpatient hospital or associated with no overnight stay or admission to such a hospital. Because surgical operations preceded the establishment of hospitals, the history of ambulatory surgery begins with the history of the earliest surgical procedures themselves. This chapter summarizes the history of the earliest such ambulatory surgical procedures as well as of those performed outside hospitals before the 20th Century. However, the major focus is on the initial rise and acceptance of ambulatory surgery in the 20th Century and on the establishment of the earliest centers dedicated to the performance of ambulatory surgery, its success, and its subsequent proliferation.

PREHOSPITAL SURGERY

Surgical procedures were performed long before recorded history, as is evidenced by skeletal remains of prehistoric man and artifacts found with such skeletons. The practice of trephination is known to have occurred before recorded history, with skulls of primitive man showing evidence of healed wounds. The first recorded practice of surgery was in the kingdom of Babylon, where the code of King Hammurabi (1948–1905 BC) specifically described the payment and punishment for successful and unsuccessful surgical procedures. Punishment for performing an unsuccessful operation (resulting in death of the patient) was amputation of the surgeon's hand.

Ancient Hindu writings document the first written records of hospitals in about the 6th Century BC. King Asoka (273–232 BC) of ancient India authorized the building of a system of hospitals, offering the first opportunity for hospital-based surgery.

SURGERY OF PAST CENTURIES AND CIVILIZATIONS

Greek civilization included significant advances in medical and surgical care, some of which were likely known from earlier Egyptian civilization. Askelepios, the great Greek physician, was deified after his death, and temples known as Askelepieia, or places of care for the sick, were established throughout the Greek empire. Such temples later became the model for the system of hospitals built throughout the Roman Empire. These hospitals were often used to care for the wounded and sick soldiers of the Roman army. Both in Greek and Roman civilization, descriptions of many now commonly performed surgical operations are recorded, many of which were done on an ambulatory basis or in nonhospital settings.

The Christianization of the Roman Empire led to the church being the major institution associated with health care and hospitals in Western Europe for the next 1000 years. However, those hospitals were poorly equipped and often of low quality. In Eastern Europe and under the Moslem empire, hospital development progressed in a more sophisticated and modern manner. Hospitals were established throughout the Moorish empire by the 10th Century, and they contained specialized surgical units where some ambulatory procedures were performed. Western hospitals did not achieve the quality of Islamic hospitals until the Renaissance or thereafter, when royalty and other benefactors began establishing hospitals as centers for the treatment of disease.

Most surgery that was performed until the 19th Century was emergency surgery related to the treatment of injuries or trauma that often was sustained in military conflict. Civilian procedures were generally limited to simple drainage of infections, removal of cysts or superficial tumors, amputations for infection, and other such procedures. It was not until the latter part of the 19th Century, after the invention of anesthesia and the establishment of the practice of antisepsis, that elective surgery became feasible, with a reasonable expectation that the patient would survive the pain and potential morbidity of surgery.

At about this time, the quality of hospitals and hospital care improved dramatically, beginning with the institution of simple yet important measures of proper sanitation, cleanliness, and nutrition for patients. Hospitals became acceptable and then preferred settings for performing surgery. Surgical results were consistently found to be improved for more complicated procedures when they were done in the hospital setting. During the latter part of the 19th Century and the early 20th Century, it became customary for patients undergoing major surgical procedures to have them done in a hospital setting and to be hospitalized postoperatively. Halstead, considered the father of American surgical training, published an article in 1893 that advocated 21 days of bed rest for his patients after inguinal herniorrhaphy.

SURGERY DURING THE 20th CENTURY

Despite the improvement in hospitals, even into the early 20th Century, a significant number of surgical procedures, although more often minor ones, were still performed in settings outside the hospital. Surgeons performed procedures in offices and patient's homes on a routine basis until the start of World War II. After that, however, several factors combined to result in the performance of all but the most minor surgical procedures in a hospital setting. These factors included the increase in surgical specialization and the increased specialization of anesthesiologists, as well as their desire and need to work only in hospital settings. The medical community viewed the hospital, with its potential for quality control and peer review, as the only appropriate place for surgery. This opinion resulted in increased public awareness of this reasoning and the heightened perception that surgery needed to be performed in the hospital setting.

During the first half of the 20th Century, most surgeons thought that patients were best served with prolonged hospitalization and bed rest after major surgery. However, examples of opinions to the contrary date back as far as the start of the century. At the Glasgow Royal Hospital for Sick Children in Scotland, an experience with successfully performing procedures such as cleft palate repair, herniorrhaphy, and orthopedic procedures in children was reported by James Nicoll. Scotland continued to be the nation that most accepted ambulatory pediatric surgery in the first half of the century, with other large experiences being reported during that time as well. Herzfeld of Edinburgh reported in 1938 on a series of more than 1000 successful herniorrhaphies for children using general anesthesia.

During the 1950s, the waiting lists for surgery in the United Kingdom under the socialized British health care system were such that adult patients were waiting more than 2 years for elective herniorrhaphy. This situation led surgeons to extrapolate from the successful experiences of children undergoing pediatric ambulatory surgery and to begin performing ambulatory surgery for adults. The success of these surgeons prompted further discussion of the merits of ambulatory surgery in the United Kingdom, leading to the landmark article by Stallworthy, published in *Lancet* in 1960, which raised the issue of decreasing hospital lengths of stay following surgery and promoted the use of ambulatory surgery and other outpatient care.

In the United States, a duo of gynecologic surgeons, Emil Ries of Chicago and Herman Boldt of New York, were the first advocates of early ambulation following major pelvic surgery. They reported their successful experience with this approach during the first decade of the 20th Century. Most surgeons were slow or reluctant to accept these findings. Surgeons in the United States did not accept or consider ambulatory surgery as a significant part of their practice until after the 1960s, but there were a few notable exceptions. In 1918, Ralph Waters, an anesthesiologist, reported the first successful performance of general anesthesia delivered in an outpatient setting at the Downtown Anesthesia Clinic in Indianapolis, clearly the first freestanding surgicenter in the United States in the 20th Century. The case mix included dental procedures as well as setting of fractures, drainage of abscesses, and other relatively minor procedures done by local surgeons.

MODERN AMBULATORY SURGERY AND THE AMBULATORY SURGERY CENTER

During the 1960s, the first successful units whose sole purpose was the performance of ambulatory surgery were established. The unit given credit as being the first widely publicized such center was opened at the Center for Health Sciences at the University of California at Los Angeles (UCLA) in 1962. Two anesthesiologists, David Cohen and John Dillon, were responsible for the conception and successful initiation of the center. These pioneers thought that safe anesthetic technique could be administered in the ambulatory setting and that the setting was of less importance than the attention to the appropriate screening and selection of patients and the importance of safe anesthetic and surgical technique. Using standards of preanesthetic and postanesthetic care not dissimilar to those in current practice in ambulatory surgery centers, the two physicians established a safe and impressive record of performing general anesthesia for patients undergoing ambulatory surgical procedures.

After the UCLA unit success, other units began to open during the 1960s. A freestanding ambulatory surgical clinic was begun in Vancouver in 1965, where outpatient general and orthopedic surgical procedures were performed. Two years later, a unit for outpatient surgery was opened by the Children's Hospital of Vancouver. The reports and experiences from all these centers continued to be positive ones, with high levels of patient satisfaction.

In 1969, the opening of the Surgicenter in Phoenix, Arizona, marked the beginning of the first highly publicized and highly successful freestanding independent outpatient surgical center for the performance of ambulatory surgery. Founded by two anesthesiologists, Wallace Reed and John Ford, the Surgicenter served as the example of the type of freestanding unit that was to become popular during the subsequent two decades. Reed and Ford were visible promoters of the concept of such centers, and the Surgicenter served as a model for many centers later built by others. Visits to the Surgicenter by planners of such other centers were encouraged by Reed and Ford. The success, acceptance, and promotion of the Surgicenter were key factors in the rapid expansion of outpatient surgical facilities during the 1970s.

In 1972, the U. S. Congress charged the Department of Health, Education, and Welfare to conduct a study on the feasibility of reimbursing freestanding surgical facilities. Although the Surgicenter in Phoenix had succeeded economically, other facilities, notably one established by Charles Hill in Providence, Rhode Island, had failed due to the lack of reimbursement by insurance carriers for services rendered. The government contracted with the Orkand Corporation to perform the study, which showed that outpatient surgery could be performed safely and at a lower cost in freestanding surgical units.

ECONOMIC CONSIDERATIONS AND THE EXPANSION OF AMBULATORY SURGERY

A major factor in the expansion of outpatient surgical centers and facilities in the 1970s was that the sudden onset of an economic recession and restriction of budgets in the early 1970s caused concerns about the increasing costs of health care. The precedent of performing surgical procedures in an office or outpatient setting had, by that time, become established practice in the field of plastic surgery. The cost of cosmetic surgery was usually paid for out-of-pocket by the patient because insurance reimbursement was not possible. Because cosmetic surgery was too expensive when performed in a hospital setting, plastic surgeons performed many minor cosmetic procedures under local anesthesia in an office setting with good safety and results. In the 1970s, practitioners of other disciplines began to examine the potential economic benefits of ambulatory surgery.

During the 1950s and 1960s, economic prosperity and the adoption of Medicare made the health care industry a rapidly expanding and successful field, in which the development of new technology flourished and research and development budgets continuously expanded. Resources for medical research from government funding were readily available. Cost for technologic advances was not regarded with great concern, but the overwhelming consideration was the improvement in delivery of care to patients. In retrospect, this was the golden age of medical research and the health care industry.

The decades from 1950 to 1970 saw, among the advances in surgical care, the successful implementation of cardiopulmonary bypass and great expansion in the field of cardiac surgery, the development of organ transplantation, the development of understanding of shock and its appropriate treatment, and the use of flexible endoscopy for diagnosis and treatment of gastrointestinal disorders. In the field of radiology, highly expensive techniques were developed such as computerized tomography and the common use of ultrasonography in most diagnostic units. The influx of government funding to pay for care for the elderly and poor, via the Medicare and Medicaid programs, further stimulated the health care industry to expand. For example, the performance of hemodialysis, an expensive technique currently covered under government reimbursement, rapidly expanded as an available treatment for patients with renal failure.

The 1970s, however, brought the first concerns that budgets for health care were growing at a rate that threatened to make health care outprice itself before the end of the century. Concerns for providing appropriate and safe delivery of health care services in a more economical manner promoted the concept of the freestanding and outpatient-dedicated surgical care units. Successful centers such as the Surgicenter served as prototypes for the development of ambulatory surgical centers soon to be found in all major cities and affiliated with most major medical centers by the end of the 1980s. These centers were developed according to one of the following three models:

1. Units developed as renovated or converted areas of current inpatient operating units, often with overlapping scheduling, personnel, and facilities with the inpatient unit
2. Units attached to major hospitals but separated physically from the inpatient operating area, with independent scheduling and personnel
3. Freestanding and independent units, totally geographically separate from inpatient surgical facilities

The relative merits and drawbacks of these three types of units are discussed in Section II. The financial advantages in terms of cost of delivery of surgical care favor the independent freestanding unit, which generally provides service at a lower cost because such a unit avoids the increased expenses of the inpatient hospital unit. Patient satisfaction has generally been greater with the latter two models of outpatient units. The first model tends to result in a climate wherein the delay of outpatient cases in favor of inpatient emergencies and the vagaries in inpatient scheduling often result in perceptions by outpatient surgical patients that their procedures are of secondary priority. The choice of model, however, usually depends on the availability of resources and dedicated personnel for such an outpatient facility.

Since the 1970s, the relative benefits to the patient, the high level of patient satisfaction, and the economic savings of ambulatory surgery have been well documented. In 1972, Davis and Detmer published an article documenting the success of an ambulatory surgical unit established at Watts Hospital in Durham, North Carolina. That same year, Cloud and his fellow anesthesiologists at the Surgicenter in Phoenix published an article about the safety and success of pediatric outpatient surgery at their facility. In the 1970s, the medical literature increasingly cited the economic efficiency and patient benefits of ambulatory surgery.

Once the advantages of ambulatory surgery were established for procedures that were generally easily accepted as appropriate for ambulatory care in the 1970s, the focus of the 1980s became the expansion of the numbers and types of procedures that could and should be done in the ambulatory setting. Improvements in anesthetic and surgical techniques, closer attention to pain control, and the increasing acceptance by surgeons and patients of the safety of the ambulatory setting led to a significant increase in the type and number of procedures performed on an ambulatory surgery basis. It was estimated that, even in 1982, 20% of all surgical procedures were done as outpatient procedures. Within the next decade, the number rapidly expanded. By 1995, it was estimated that nearly 60% of all surgical procedures were done on an ambulatory basis, and that figure has not yet peaked.

Introduction of new techniques such as laparoscopy in the areas of general and gynecologic surgery, arthroscopy in orthopedic surgery, lithotripsy and endoscopic surgery in urology, and sinus surgery in otolaryngology has further increased the ability of surgeons to perform many procedures on an ambulatory basis. Much of this technology has only been available or widely used within the past 10 to 15 years; however, its impact has been profound, resulting in a significant decrease in the load of cases scheduled at inpatient facilities and a rapid expansion of the numbers of cases done in ambulatory units.

The development and expansion of ambulatory surgery services at the University of Virginia Health Sciences Center is a typical story for many medical centers. A freestanding ambulatory surgical unit (Virginia Ambulatory Surgery Center) opened its doors in 1984. It was several years before the number of scheduled cases for the four available operating rooms resulted in profitability for the unit. During the mid to late 1980s, the overload of cases scheduled in the limited number of inpatient hospital operating rooms resulted in a restriction of that schedule to inpatient cases only. All ambulatory cases, many of which were still being scheduled for the inpatient operating rooms for the surgeon's rather than the patient's convenience, were required to be scheduled at the ambulatory surgery center. Once surgeon practice patterns changed, the ambulatory center schedule soon became overcrowded, resulting in the need to expand the unit from four to six operating rooms. In addition, the subsequent expansion of the inpatient operating rooms and the diminution of the number of inpatient procedures being performed resulted in a lifting of the restriction of scheduling ambulatory cases for the inpatient rooms.

Currently, not only is the Virginia Ambulatory Surgery Center schedule operating at high efficiency but significant numbers of same-day surgery cases are also performed in the inpatient hospital operating rooms. The inpatient unit has made appropriate provisions in the preoperative and postoperative areas for the special needs of ambulatory surgery patients, resulting in high patient satisfaction in that setting as well.

Selected Readings

1. Cloud DT, Reed WA, Ford JL, Linker LM, Trump DS, Dorman GW. The surgicenter: A fresh concept in outpatient pediatric surgery. J Pediatr Surg 1972;7:206–212.
2. Cohen DD, Dillon JB. Anesthesia for outpatient surgery. JAMA 1966;196:1114–1116.
3. Davis JE. History of major ambulatory surgery. In: Davis JE, ed. Major Ambulatory Surgery. Williams & Wilkins, 1986:3–31.
4. Davis JE, Detmer DE. The ambulatory surgical unit. Ann Surg 1972;175:856–862.
5. Ford JL. Outpatient surgery—present status and future projections. South Med J 1978;71:311–315.
6. Herzfeld G. Hernia in infancy. Am J Surg 1938;39:422–429.
7. Singer HK. Then and now: a historical development of ambulatory surgery. Journal of Post Anesthesia Nursing 1993;8:276–279.
8. Stallworthy JA. Hotels or hospitals. Lancet 1960;1:103–106.
9. Waters RM. The Downtown Anesthesia Clinic. Am J Surg Anesthesia Suppl 1919;33:71–73.

Economics of Ambulatory Surgery

Chapter 2

Economic Incentives and Cost Effectiveness

James P. Highland

Ambulatory surgery in the United States has grown dramatically since the early 1980s. Data from the American Hospital Association indicate that inpatient operations declined in absolute numbers from 15,532,578 procedures in 1982 to 10,552,378 procedures in 1992. At the same time, there was striking growth in the number of outpatient procedures, which increased from 4,061,061 procedures in 1982 to 12,307,594 in 1992, a 203% change. As a result, outpatient procedures increased from 20.7% of community hospital procedures in 1982 to 53.8% of procedures in 1992. Although reliable national data are not available, all evidence suggests that the number of ambulatory surgeries performed outside of hospitals has skyrocketed as well. There are thousands of ambulatory surgery centers, and physician offices are increasingly used for surgery, resulting in dramatic growth in overall ambulatory procedures.

The growth in ambulatory surgery can be attributed to three factors:

1. More surgery is being performed overall.
2. Operations previously performed on an inpatient basis (e.g., hernia repair) are performed on an outpatient basis, but in essentially the same way.
3. New, less invasive surgery technologies (e.g., arthroscopic knee procedures) have been developed, enabling performance on an outpatient basis.

Each of these sources of growth in ambulatory surgery stems from a common set of eco-nomic forces. The forces at work are similar to waves on the ocean—they are visible because they are on the surface, but underlying these visible changes is a rising tide of technologic innovation that can directly or indirectly account for most of the sources of growth in surgery. To sort through these forces, this chapter discusses two key concepts with respect to growth of ambulatory surgery: cost effectiveness and incentives.

"*Cost effectiveness*" is, roughly, the ratio of the "value" of a treatment to its cost, relative to competing alternatives. The highest ratio of value to cost defines the most cost-effective treatment method.

"*Incentives*" are parameters than can be varied to encourage the movement of actual behavior (of physicians and patients) closer to the cost-effective "ideal" when behavior cannot be mandated. Incentives are usually financial rewards or penalties to the physician or patient, the effect of which depends on patient and physician characteristics. Basic preferences (e.g., wealth vs. peace of mind, level of risk aversion, pain tolerance) as well as environmental constraints (e.g., limited income, limited time, family situation) all affect how individuals respond to incentives. First, a careful definition of terms is needed. What exactly does cost effectiveness mean? What are incentives? Second, the perspective taken is critical. Who benefits from the cost-effective measure? To whom do the incentives apply? This chapter also explores the fundamental technologic forces underlying changes in surgery and the factors affecting future growth of ambulatory surgery.

COST EFFECTIVENESS AND AMBULATORY SURGERY

What Does "Cost Effective" Mean?

A loose yet useful definition of "cost effective" is that the ratio of "value" to cost is higher than for competing alternatives. However, it is the difficulty in the definition and measurement of "value" that makes a careful discussion of the term "cost effective" important. Formally, cost effectiveness is one specific type of analysis among a family of analytic tools that are used to evaluate the relative merits of health (and other) programs. The results generated by these evaluation tools are intended to guide resource allocation, so that a given amount of resources is put to its most effective use or, conversely, that a given outcome is achieved with the smallest amount of resources. Cost effectiveness is what economists refer to as a normative concept. That is, it attempts to define what should be, which requires an assessment of value, which, in turn, cannot be divorced from value judgments. The degree of complexity and care involved in the analysis of value distinguishes the various forms of the four basic evaluation tools that are used.

Cost Minimization Analysis (Value Not Measured). When it is known or can be reasonably assumed that the outcomes (or benefits) of two treatments are worthwhile and the same, the only issue that needs to be addressed is the relative cost of the two treatments. The assumption of equivalent outcomes is a strong assumption that should be made only when significant evidence exists to support it. For example, it may be assumed that the outcomes of a hernia procedure performed on an inpatient basis compared with one performed on an outpatient basis are the same; thus, only costs need be compared.

Cost Effectiveness Analysis (Value Is One-Dimensional). In cost effectiveness analysis, costs are compared to some natural measure of outcome, such as years of life gained or number of cancers detected. This natural mea-

sure must be common to the two treatments. The two treatments are usually compared by the ratios of costs and outcomes, such as, cost per year of life gained or cost per cancer detected. The measure chosen should be appropriate and comparable between the treatments. In this type of analysis, the outcome is assumed to have value (e.g., cancers detected) and is compared to the relative cost of achieving the standardized outcome. For cost effectiveness analysis to be useful, there must be only one outcome of interest that is common to the two therapies being compared. For example, if both improved functioning and pain reduction are important outcomes, then cost effectiveness analysis does not allow for assessment of the tradeoffs that different therapies may present relative to these outcomes.

Cost Utility Analysis (Value Is Multidimensional). Simple cost effectiveness measures, such as years of life gained, do not take into account additional dimensions of outcome, such as quality of life. Treatment A may result in 1 year of life gained and treatment B 2 years of life, but treatment B leaves the patient blind. A year of life with blindness may be valued by an individual as equivalent to significantly less than 1 year without such a handicap functioning. Cost utility analysis attempts to refine the measurement of the benefits of the treatment by measuring the relative value to the individual of life under different circumstances by asking questions such as "Given a choice between a full year of life with blindness and some number of months with full functioning, how many months of full functioning would leave you indifferent between the choices?" The outcome measures of this type of analysis are usually expressed as "quality-adjusted life years," or QALYs. If the average answer to this question is 4 months, then 1 year of life with blindness is measured as one third of a QALY. The results of the analysis would then be, for example, that even though treatment B costs less per year of life saved, it costs more per QALY saved because it causes blindness. Or, if 1 year of blindness is equal to 9 months of full functioning, then the result would be that treatment B may cost less per QALY *despite* the fact that it causes blindness. A cost utility analysis allows measurement of such tradeoffs. This type of analysis has become common, and is useful when multiple dimensions of the outcome are relevant.

Cost–Benefit Analysis (Value Is Multidimensional and Measured in Dollars). Cost–benefit analysis takes the refinement of benefit measurement one step further by putting the benefits into dollar terms. To perform a cost–benefit analysis, individuals are asked questions such as, "Relative to the treatment extending your life 1 year, how much more would you be willing to pay for (or how much would you be willing to pay for an insurance policy that covers) a treatment that extends your life 2 years but causes blindness?" The results of this analysis are expressed as a "net benefit" such as "benefits exceed costs by $10,000" (if costs are subtracted from benefits) or cost–benefit ratios such as 0.75 (if costs are divided by benefits). Net benefit or cost–benefit ratios can then be compared between treatments. This approach is particularly useful when the natural units of the alternatives are "apples and oranges," such as when a government must decide whether to put dollars into health care spending or a dam building project.

Cost–Benefit Analysis/Cost Effectiveness Analysis. As discussed, "cost-effective" as an adjective is commonly used in a generic fashion to indicate that something has the best value-to-cost ratio. As a noun, the tools described are collectively referred to in this chapter as CBA/CEA (or cost–benefit analysis/cost effectiveness analysis). Of these tools, the cost–benefit approach is preferred by economists but is not commonly used in health care. In practice, cost effectiveness and cost utility analysis are the most common tools used in the health care field. Performing any of these analyses, or using any of these terms with precision, requires further specificity.

Cost Effective Compared to What?

"Is ambulatory surgery cost effective?" Because cost effectiveness statements are relative, a valid response to this question is "Compared to what?" Ambulatory surgery for a given problem may be more cost effective than the comparable inpatient procedure, but less cost effective than a drug therapy. There must always be at least two alternatives considered. In addition, it is important to be specific in defining the alternatives. It is necessary to specify narrowly which condition and possibly which patient population is being examined. For example, a cost minimization study might conclude that laparoscopic cholecystectomy on an ambulatory basis has 22% lower direct medical costs than the comparable open procedure done on an inpatient basis for otherwise healthy patients younger than age 50 years.

Answering questions with CBA/CEA tools is most straightforward when an alternative treatment "dominates" another (e.g., it is lower cost for the same outcome or it has a better outcome for the same cost). A more difficult (and typical) question arises when both the benefit and the cost are higher (or lower). The heart of the cost effectiveness issue, then, is whether the difference is worth it. For example, if using disposable surgical supplies results in slightly lower infection rates but is more expensive than using reusable supplies, which approach is more cost effective? Either could be, depending on the specific facts of the situation and how the number of "infections avoided" is valued.

Cost Effective for Whom?

It is also important to define the perspective from which cost effectiveness is measured, that is, to define for whom the measure is cost effective. Cost effectiveness can be measured from a number of perspectives, including that of society, the government, a private insurance company, or an individual. This is a crucial issue to keep in mind when discussing cost effectiveness—whose costs and benefits are being measured? If the costs and benefits are measured from the perspective of an insurance company or government insurance program, important costs such as patient and family member time off from work and physician travel time are ignored. In doing a societal cost benefit or cost-effectiveness analysis, all these factors are considered. Even when the societal perspective in the analysis is not being taken, the costs and benefits not considered by an insurance company or other subset of society are still incurred by society for a given

ting of the surgery. This again is a decision for which the likelihood of ambulatory surgery is probably not considered.

3. Whether to seek care. When the patient contemplates seeking care, the prospect of surgery and the difficulty of that surgery may be considerations for some people. Research indicates that this decision is the one most likely to be affected by the deductible and coinsurance level of the patient's insurance policy.

4. Whether to undergo surgery. Patients clearly participate in this decision, along with their families and their physicians. This decision may be constrained by the insurance policy, which may require preapproval for the surgery.

5. The site of the surgery. The patient may have little input into this decision. The insurance policy may require that the procedure be provided on an outpatient basis, in which case neither the physician nor the patient would usually change this decision. If the patient is aware of cost differences between sites, then the patient may take that into consideration. If the insurance policy is flexible, then the patient will, in most cases, follow the physician's plan as to where the surgery is performed. The convenience of the location may be a consideration, for example, the inpatient facility is much closer to the patient's home than the outpatient facility.

All in all, the patient may have little input as to whether surgery is performed on an ambulatory basis. However, the availability of an ambulatory procedure may affect the patient's decision about whether to have surgery or not. If the time lost from work will be less and the direct monetary cost is less, this may influence the patient's decision to undergo the procedure. On the other hand, if the patient does not have help at home and is afraid to recover alone, this may influence the decision not to have surgery. The most important factor in the patient's decision is the technology of the procedure itself that allows it to be performed on an ambulatory basis. For example, because arthroscopic surgery is available for such conditions as cartilage repair of the knee, patients are much more likely to agree to surgery than if the only option was an open knee proce-

dure. Whether an overnight stay is required is of secondary importance. The empiric evidence supports the notion that patients do not have a significant impact on the choice of the setting of their surgery.

Physicians

The physician's decision to perform a procedure in an ambulatory setting depends on a number of patient and clinical considerations, the costs and revenues of the options, and other factors. Which of these factors is important and how strongly they operate depend on the physician's objectives. This is a subject of debate in the health economics profession. Even for a physician solely concerned with maximizing income, the patient's interest must be considered prominently, because professional reputation, referral relationships, and malpractice considerations all financially penalize poor-quality care. There is empiric evidence that physicians respond positively to profit incentives; that is, overall volume declines, other things being equal, when prices decline, and volumes increase when prices increase.[2] In any case, there are several potential factors affecting the physician's decision:

1. Clinical considerations related to the severity of the patient's condition, the need for emergency backup, and the relative capabilities of the facilities and their staffs.

2. The difference in the professional fee per unit of time. Ordinarily, there is no difference in the fee received by the physician based on the site of service, but, if the time required is different, then the physician's effective hourly rate will be different. The time required to travel to and from the facilities and the time required to perform the procedure at each facility thus become important. If a physician can travel 15 minutes each way instead of 30 and can perform three procedures in 3½ hours instead of 4 hours for $1200 in fees, then the difference in the effective hourly rate is $300 versus $240, or $60 per hour.

[2]The debate regarding physicians' response to price changes was particularly heated during the implementation of the Medicare program's RBRVS-based payment system. Surgical fees were lowered across the board; some argued that surgeons would increase volume to make up for the lost income. In fact, volumes have not done so.

These time differences may just as easily favor the inpatient procedure as the outpatient, so it cannot be generalized how this incentive will affect the physician's decision.

3. The difference in facility fee profit. If the physician has no ownership interest in either site of care, then this point is moot. However, if the physician has an ownership interest in the ambulatory surgery center (ASC), there will be a financial incentive to perform the procedure in the ASC if possible, as long as the facility fee received for providing the procedure exceeds the marginal cost of providing the procedure. The decision of the physician to open a surgery center is also one that the physician makes at some point in time.

Incentives as a Tool to Promote Ambulatory Surgery

Insurance plans use three basic incentive tools to encourage physicians and patients to use ambulatory surgery. They are as follow:

1. *Patient cost-sharing incentives.* The patient's cost sharing can be different for certain services if they are performed in an ambulatory setting. For example, the deductible may be waived, or the coinsurance waived or reduced. This presents a financial incentive to the patient to influence the site where care is delivered.

2. *Coverage structures and medical management.* The benefits of the insurance policy may be defined in such a way that some services are only covered if provided in an ambulatory setting. Similarly, they may only be covered in an inpatient setting after review by the plan's utilization management personnel. If these provisions are ignored and the service is provided on an inpatient basis, the insurance company will not pay the provider and will not reimburse the patient. This presents a financial incentive to both the patient and physician to observe the policy's requirements.

3. *Physician payment incentives.* Less common but of increasing importance, the form of the physician's payment can provide an incentive for the site of service. For example, if the physician receives a "capitated" or per person per month payment for services, then a financial incentive exists to provide the care in the least costly setting.

The use of all these incentives has grown along with the growth in ambulatory services. Can it be concluded that the "incentives" are successful in moving patients into the ambulatory setting? Although research is limited, it provides some answers.

Pauly and Erder studied the impact of patient cost-sharing provisions on the probability of having surgery on an ambulatory basis. Using large employer health insurance databases with varying levels of patient cost-sharing differentials for ambulatory surgery (relative to inpatient surgery), the researchers concluded that data did not support the idea that patient cost sharing affected the site where surgery was performed. However, they did find that higher patient cost sharing for surgery, regardless of site, resulted in fewer procedures. These results are consistent with the RAND Health Insurance Experiment (HIE), the largest and most comprehensive examination of the responses to patient cost-sharing provisions. The HIE results suggest strongly that patients' decisions to seek care initially are somewhat responsive to the cost-sharing levels they face, but that once they enter into the medical care system, they are largely unresponsive to cost-sharing incentives.

Less direct evidence is available on the impact of benefit decisions and medical management on use of ambulatory surgery. It is likely that policies that deny coverage if a service is not performed on an ambulatory basis are effective in discouraging use of the inpatient setting for expensive services. More common policies that require review by the plan's utilization review staff (e.g., preadmission certification for hospital admissions) have been studied and have been found to have some impact. For example, Khandker and Manning found that utilization review programs have a one-time effect on inpatient medical expenditures (approximately an 8% reduction). Less pronounced is the impact on outpatient and overall medical expenditures. None of the studies have looked specifically at utilization review policies designed to encourage ambulatory surgery or at the effect of inpatient surgery utilization review policies on the use of outpatient surgery. A "squeeze the balloon" effect is taking place in which use of the more controlled inpatient setting has moved to the outpatient setting. There is no direct evidence on the extent to which this is attributable to the changes in the inpatient surgical utilization versus its being the result of an underlying growth trend in ambulatory surgery due to technologic advances.

Payment incentives for physicians as a means of affecting utilization also have been studied in general but not specifically for ambulatory surgery. Hillman and colleagues found that some payment incentives used by health maintenance organizations (HMOs) that place the physician at financial risk negatively affect the use of both inpatient hospitalization and primary care physician visits. It is not clear whether these effects increase or decrease the use of ambulatory surgery, but it does support the notion that financial incentives affect the behavior of physicians. The payment incentive systems present the physician with an incentive to reduce all services, but there may be a stronger substitution effect from the reduction in hospital use that results in an increase in use of ambulatory surgery. Here, again, research does not directly support whether the incentive has resulted in an increase in use of ambulatory surgery.

In summary, the research evidence does not support the notion that financial incentives designed to encourage use of ambulatory surgery have been responsible for the growth of ambulatory surgery. Evidence on the effect of policies that impact physicians, such as medical management and financial incentives, does not directly address the effect on ambulatory surgery. The more general findings on medical management and payment policies are consistent with their contributing to the growth of ambulatory surgery, although they provide no direct support for it.

Private and public health care insurers are concerned that the rapid growth in ambulatory surgery and outpatient services in general is uncontrolled. For example, many private insurers such as Blue Cross–Blue Shield plans have both heavy utilization review for inpatient services and incentives for hospitals and physicians to control inpatient costs. But there are generally no utilization controls for outpatient services, and only the recent growth in risk-based incentive programs extends to cover outpatient services, including ambulatory surgery. As suggested previously, there has been very rapid growth in these services for all insurers, private and public, a trend of great concern to them. Shifts from the inpatient setting undoubtedly explain some portion of this growth, but it is unclear what portion is attributable to such shifts and what portion is attributable to underlying growth due to technologic advances.

GENERAL ECONOMIC FACTORS AFFECTING SURGERY VOLUME AND MIX

This chapter has reviewed the concepts of cost effectiveness and incentives and discussed the roles they play in decisions about ambulatory surgery made by insurers, physicians, and patients. How does this shed light on the following sources of growth in ambulatory surgery?

- More surgery is being performed overall.
- Surgeries that used to be performed on an inpatient basis (e.g., hernia repair) are being performed on an outpatient basis, but in essentially the same way.
- New, less invasive surgery techniques (e.g., arthroscopic knee procedures) have been developed, enabling their performance on an outpatient basis.

The total number of inpatient operations declined absolutely by 53% between 1982 and 1992, despite population growth. Anecdotal evidence also supports the idea of shifts from the inpatient to the outpatient setting. For example, services such as tonsillectomy, which used to require an inpatient stay, are being done on an outpatient basis. But, research provides only limited support for the idea that insurance plans caused this to happen through explicit policies intended to encourage ambulatory surgery. That is, the shift from inpatient surgery and the general growth in ambulatory surgery were occurring anyway (perhaps to a lesser degree), *even when no direct incentives were used by the insurers.* What else was happening that can explain these changes?

Based on the statistics of hospital surgery growth and the safe assumption that surgery outside the hospital setting has grown rapidly as well, the total number of surgical procedures performed has grown. New techniques have facilitated outpatient operation as well. Arthroscopic meniscectomy and laparoscopic cholecystectomy have not only replaced inpatient open surgical procedures but have also led to a large increase in the volume of knee and biliary surgery being done.

However, questions remain. Why has the overall number of operations per capita increased? Why has surgery shifted from inpatient to outpatient settings? If it is due to greater cost effectiveness, what caused the degree of cost effectiveness to change or what caused the degree of concern about cost effectiveness? What has caused the rapid development of less invasive techniques? To answer these questions, it is necessary to study the fundamental forces driving the dynamics of the health care system.

Forces that at first may not seem to be economically based can, in fact, be analyzed usefully as economic forces, and they may have a larger influence on the growth in ambulatory surgery than direct financial incentives in insurance policies. Changes in technology are thought to be a key driver of the growth. Although possibly not apparent at first, technology change is affected by and leads to powerful economic forces. The technology of production in health care is, in many ways, driven by economics and, in turn, affects the economics of health care. Many economists believe that the following chain of economic events has contributed to the growth in health care technology advances, and that this, in turn, affects costs, utilization, and the site of delivering health care services:

- Health insurance is not taxable as income under federal tax law.
- As a result, people buy more health insurance and higher coverage levels than they would otherwise.
- More highly covered people use more health care services.
- Increased use of services generates profits and incentives for medical technology companies to innovate.

- People want to buy insurance coverage for the new technologies, both because they are valued and because the insurance purchase is tax subsidized.

This dynamic chain can account for the high level of, if not the growth in, overall health care expenditures in the United States. As has been observed by Newhouse, this growth is not necessarily bad and may reflect the purchase of technologies for which individuals are willing to pay. One prominent health economist puts it succinctly, "There hasn't emerged in the market an HMO which advertises '1960s medicine at 1960s prices.'"

Each of the sources of growth in ambulatory surgery can be accounted for by the more fundamental force of technologic change. New and better techniques with the potential to dramatically improve the lives of patients can account for the overall growth of surgery. These techniques have caused the overall number of surgeries performed to increase, as advances in artificial joint placement, corneal lens replacements, and installation of pacemakers make significant improvements in the patient's quality of life. At the same time, the growth in surgery and other medical care techniques and their commensurate costs has led to an increasingly expensive inpatient setting, placing more emphasis on the potential savings of the ambulatory settings. This has accelerated the shift from inpatient surgery to ambulatory surgery. Finally, profit opportunities for techniques that can avoid the use of the inpatient hospital have become greater. The more outpatient-friendly techniques have generally allowed patients to undergo treatment with less time off from work and less pain. This has, in turn, encouraged even greater use of these techniques by those who would not have undergone treatment in the past.

In one sense, the growth in services due to the underlying technologic change is a result of their cost effectiveness; however, these techniques may still cause overall cost to rise. In the example of knee arthroscopy, because arthroscopic repair of the knee is so much less invasive and requires so much less rehabilitation than open knee procedures, the use of the service has increased tremendously. This is cost effective in the sense that many people who would have lived in pain and poor functioning have a relatively attractive recourse to relief. This remedy is worth the extra cost that is reflected in insurance policies. However, the total number of knee operations and the total cost related to this type of surgery have undoubtedly increased. The same can be said for a long list of medical advances, such as cataract removal, lithotripsy, and magnetic resonance imaging.

These developments can be compared with other technologic advances such as those in computer software. Software growth has exploded not just because computers allow things to be done in a different or cheaper way, but because they do the same things faster and better, and they allow new things that were never dreamt of before to be done. As a result, they have value and have become an increasingly large part of the population's collective expenditures. The same could be said of technologic advances in ambulatory surgery.

FUTURE GROWTH OF AMBULATORY SURGERY

What does the underlying engine of technologic growth portend for the future of ambulatory surgery?

The movement of services from inpatient settings to outpatient settings may be approaching a natural limit. There is a large number of services for which inpatient care is the only option. As home care services continue to grow, some additional services may be shifted out of the inpatient setting, but this will be limited by the degree to which patients and families are willing to tolerate this approach.

The aging of the population means that more surgery will be required and that much of this (based on the current composition of surgery) will be ambulatory. Less invasive techniques may reduce the health status of older patients as an impediment to corrective surgical action. As "baby boomers" settle squarely into middle age, many afflictions common to that age group will require ambulatory surgery

and that area of surgery will experience significant growth.

Many of the forces underlying the past growth in ambulatory surgery continue to operate. One critical development, however, is the growth in payment systems for physicians that place them at financial risk for the services provided to patients. Capitated and "fixed price bundles" of services present physicians with different incentives than they have traditionally faced. There is no firm evidence on the impact of such payment policies on ambulatory surgery. These payment incentives will encourage physicians to avoid services that are of only marginal value, which may dampen use of some ambulatory surgical services. On the other hand, when ambulatory surgery can be a cost-effective substitute for more expensive forms of care, incentive payment systems will encourage its growth. An important issue for future research is the relative importance of these counteracting forces on the growth in ambulatory surgery.

Selected Readings

1. American Hospital Association. Hospital Statistics, 1982–1992.
2. Drummond MF, Stoddart GL, Torrance GW. Methods for the Economic Evaluation of Health Care Programmes. Oxford: Oxford Medical, 1987.
3. Ermann D, Gabel J. The changing face of American health care, multihospital systems, emergency centers, and surgery centers. Medical Care 1985;23(5):401–420.
4. Hillman A, Pauly MV, Kerstein JJ. How do financial incentives affect physicians' clinical decisions and the financial performance of health maintenance organizations? N Engl J Med 1989;321(2):86–92.
5. Khandker RK, Manning WG. The impact of utilization review on costs and utilization. In: Zweifel P, Frech HE III, eds. Health Economics Worldwide. Amsterdam: Kluwer Academic, 1992.
6. Manning WG, Newhouse JP, et al. Health insurance and the demand for medical care: evidence from a randomized experiment. American Economic Review 1987;77(3).
7. Mishan EJ. Cost Benefit Analysis. 4th ed. London: Unwin Hyman, 1988.
8. Newhouse JP. An iconoclastic view of healthcare cost containment. Health Affairs 1993;12(suppl):152–171.
9. Pasternak DP, Smith HL, Piland NF. Critical issues surrounding the evolution of ambulatory surgery. Journal of Ambulatory Care Management 1991;14(1):24–33.
10. Pauly MV, Erder H. Insurance incentives for ambulatory surgery. Health Services Res 1993;27:814–839.

Determining the Feasibility of an Ambulatory Surgery Center

Robert Marasco • Bruce David Schirmer

Ambulatory surgical facilities proliferated rapidly in the 1970s and 1980s when the concept of ambulatory surgery became popular and when the clear benefits to the patient and high levels of patient satisfaction fueled the performance of many procedures from the inpatient to the outpatient setting. In this climate, many facilities were successful because of the changing concept of public opinion and opinion of the surgical community regarding ambulatory surgery, making increasing availability of surgical procedures for such facilities likely to guarantee success. In addition, little competition from other ambulatory facilities was usually present. Therefore, most facilities, even if not optimally designed or planned, were successful because of this evolution of ambulatory surgery.

Currently, the situation is considerably different for persons interested in building an ambulatory surgery facility. Profit margins are lower. Reimbursement increases have slowed. Professional fees have often decreased. In such a climate, the success of an ambulatory surgery center is far from guaranteed.

This chapter focuses on the needs assessment and financial feasibility analysis indicated before initiating construction of an ambulatory surgery facility. The basis of this chapter is the personal experience of the first author (Robert Marasco) in medical design (26 years) and design of ambulatory surgery centers (18 years, with involvement in the design of 120 centers).

FACILITY TYPES

There are three basic types of ambulatory surgery facilities:

1. Hospital-based unit
2. Hospital satellite unit
3. Freestanding unit

The first type of unit is basically administered and run by the hospital, often by converting operating room and surrounding facilities previously used for inpatient surgery to an outpatient function. In terms of physical plant, the ambulatory unit is often indistinguishable from the inpatient facility. In this hospital-based unit scheduling and administration are intermixed with inpatient surgery, and, usually, the operating room manager is oriented toward the inpatient facility. As such, scheduling conflicts and emergencies created by the inpatient unit often adversely affect the efficiency of the outpatient unit, hence negating one of the potential advantages of this unit.

The hospital satellite unit is similarly administered by the hospital and attached to it, but the actual facility is separate from the inpatient operating room facilities. This arrangement offers access to more sophisticated equipment and techniques by users and patients of the ambulatory unit, because such equipment can be used in conjunction with the hospital. This arrangement often requires patient transportation to a site outside the ambulatory unit, however, which can be more time consuming, expensive, and inconvenient for the patient. The other potential disadvantages of this arrangement are that the administration may still function with a "hospital" mentality, basing decisions on the traditional inpatient operating room model rather than the more efficient outpatient-type model. Finally, access to parking may be a problem if the unit is attached to the hospital and hospital parking is at a premium.

Because most new ambulatory units, particularly those being contemplated for construction or being financed by physicians, are likely to be freestanding units, the remainder of this chapter and the needs assessment focus largely on the assessment of the feasibility of a freestanding unit.

PROJECT ANALYSIS: INFORMATION GATHERING

The initial process in determining the feasibility for an ambulatory surgical facility is to determine who will use the facility. The surgeons involved must have a sincere and dedicated commitment to the facility, because bringing the project to fruition takes a great deal of effort. They must believe it will benefit the medical community and the community at large in the area.

The focus and aim of the facility should be defined. The freestanding facility may be constructed as an extension of the practice of a single physician or of a group of physicians. Alternatively, a group of interested parties may work together to initiate the project. Defining clearly and concisely who is involved in the project from the outset is critically important. It is also important to know which other surgeons or procedure-performing physicians (e.g., gastroenterologists) are likely to be recruited to participate in the workings of the facility.

The optimal function of the ambulatory surgery center, from the practicing surgeon's point of view, is to be an extension of the surgeon's practice. Therefore, physical continuity with an office facility essentially sets up a "center" for the treatment of the patient. An orthopedic surgeon, for example, by constructing an office complex adjacent to the ambulatory facility and a rehabilitation complex similarly adjacent, develops a relatively comprehensive center for treatment of the orthopedic patient's common outpatient problems. Such reasoning by the surgeons wishing to build such a facility is sound in that cooperation among a smaller number of participants is more likely to be successful than is bringing many diverse and otherwise previously unrelated practices together under one roof.

Hospital involvement is usually not helpful for the freestanding facility. Hospital administration often is counterproductive to the orientation of the ambulatory center. The physicians involved in the project should be responsible and able to select the medical director of their choice, usually one of their members, who has the authority to hire and fire personnel. This authority should not be given to the hospital. Nor should the hospital appoint the manager of the facility, because the ambulatory center should avoid having a manager with an "inpatient" facility mindset. The need for more surgical beds in an inpatient hospital facility should not initiate the investigation to form an ambulatory center. Sometimes, however, a hospital with too many beds can benefit from conversion of the space to an ambulatory facility. This then follows the hospital-based model.

The founders of the ambulatory center must determine which type of facility to build based on accreditation. The most stringent accreditation guidelines are put forth from the federal system for certification for Medicare reimbursement. Recently, the Joint Commission on Accreditation of Healthcare Organizations (JCAHO) has instituted guidelines for outpatient facilities as well. Less stringent guidelines are those of the Accreditation Association for Ambulatory Health Care, Inc. (AAAHC). Reimbursement by payors depends on accreditation status.

Competition from other ambulatory surgical centers must be considered. Although competition is less likely if projections of cases and revenues are based on the current practices of participating surgeons, it is relevant if the plan for the facility includes potential expansion and involvement of other surgeons. The likelihood of surgeons converting increasing percentages of their caseloads to the ambulatory setting must be conservatively assessed as well.

Site location is also an important initial piece of information. Consultation with groups of physicians planning an ambulatory center has often shown that choice of site may not be optimal. Factors to consider in choosing a site should include proximity to the practice facility, ability for expansion, and accessibility. It is recommended that the site be chosen carefully, with a mind toward potential expansion. This also discourages initial overbuilding when the project is on the least sound fiscal footing.

CASE ANALYSIS

Needs assessment begins with a conservative estimate of the volume of operations likely to be done. The initial step in determining future revenue is to generate a case analysis based on current volume of cases performed by the surgeons who will be using the facility. Table 3–1 is a sample caseload analysis for five physicians. In this analysis, each physician was asked to classify the number of cases performed in the past year for the various Medicare groupings based on Current Procedural Terminology (CPT) code category. These would be only those procedures that would be performed in the projected ambulatory surgery center in the future. It is also crucial to give an accurate assessment of the numbers of procedures reimbursed by third-party payers versus Medicare. In general, third-party reimbursement has been 130% to 140% of Medicare reimbursement for ambulatory procedures.

The projected caseload in Table 3–1 is discounted by 15%, providing for the potential for a decrease in case volume or decreased ability to collect revenues. This is in keeping with the philosophy of making the projected financial analysis of the facility on a very con-

Table 3–1. Caseload Analysis

	Medicare Groupings											
1998	***I***	***II***	***III***	***IV***	***V***	***VI***	***VII***	***VIII***	***IX***	**Total**	**% Medicare**	**% Third-Party Payer**
Physician 1	160	94	96	213	26	18	46	0	0	653	12%	88%
Physician 2	0	23	60	18	53	23	0	0	0	177	15%	85%
Physician 3	0	0	0	45	24	19	0	230	0	318	80%	20%
Physician 4	0	18	87	88	65	40	39	0	0	337	20%	80%
Physician 5	180	80	270	190	50	14	54	0	0	838	16%	84%
Total	340	215	513	554	218	114	139	230	0	2323		
Discount 15%	51	32	77	83	33	17	21	35	0	348		
Total anticipated caseload	289	183	436	471	185	97	118	196	0	1975	24%	76%
Future anticipated caseload												
1999										2073*		
2000										2177		
2001										2286		
2002										2400		
2003										2520		
2004										2646		

*Assume 5% increase per year.

Modified from Marasco R, Marasco J. Ambulatory surgery centers. Creating success in a future of change. Presented at American Association of Ambulatory Surgery Centers 18th Annual Meeting. San Diego, February 20–22, 1997.

servative basis. This caseload component of the cash flow analysis is used in the final equation given in subsequent discussion.

FACILITY COMPONENTS AND FUNCTIONAL DESIGN

It might seem that considering project facility design should follow determination of the feasibility of an ambulatory surgery center and not precede it, but an accurate assessment of the financial feasibility of the center cannot be done without a relatively accurate projection of the facility to be built. The aim and purpose of the facility should be kept in mind as this process occurs. Fiscal prudence is indicated; often, the surgeon is tempted to design and build a facility that is excessive in terms of size. Allowing room for future expansion is more prudent.

The composition of the facility is dictated by several factors. The first is the projected number of cases to be managed. The other important influence is the facility requirements of the local health codes and those of the insurance accreditation organizations. Fire code regulations must also be considered.

States differ in their requirements for the elements of an ambulatory surgery center. Therefore, it is important for the planners of a center to familiarize themselves, *at the time of the feasibility planning stage,* with the local requirements. Certain requirements are always true for national certification organizations such as Medicare. In the following discussion, these criteria are used as the default reference criteria for a facility. However, the details of certain requirements, such as whether the facility must have a staff locker room that could be unisex or a locker room for each gender, vary from state to state.

Operating Rooms

The first consideration should be given to the number of operating rooms to be constructed. In most cases, surgeons want to build facilities with multiple operating rooms, especially if they are thinking in an inpatient mode, in which turnover times may be 45 minutes. There is an inherent inefficiency in that system that virtually requires the overlapping use of two operating rooms to generate any efficiency in the surgeon's time. However, in the well-functioning ambulatory surgery unit, a 10-minute turnover time is not uncommon, with some achieving less routinely. This allows a greater number of procedures to be done each day per operating room.

Although case type dictates length of operating room time, it is a conservative estimate that, given the efficiency of rapid turnover, eight cases can be done in an average workday in an ambulatory facility operating room. If the operating room is operating for 5 days per week for 50 weeks per year at 75% efficiency, this represents a total of 1500 cases per year. Based on such a calculation, surgeons must carefully consider how many operating rooms are necessary for a facility. Often, the answer is only one or two. This is an important consideration, because the cost of building and equipping the operating room is considerably higher per square foot than any other area of the facility. Building excessive operating room space only increases the initial outlay of expenses with no return.

The operating room calculation points out the general fact that, when considering facilities, it is better to be leaner and more efficient. This is the appropriate approach from the business sense of operating the unit.

Figure 3–1 gives an example of an operating room analysis that takes into account several facts:

1. Average duration of an outpatient procedure by the surgeon. It is important to give accurate and honest estimates based on operative records.

2. An estimated turnover time of 10 minutes, which is realistic in an efficient unit.

3. Prep time of 30 minutes per patient before each procedure.

4. A recovery time of 60 minutes per case.

It is calculated in Figure 3–1 that the operating room, at 70% efficiency, would be used to perform 1575 cases per year. This is similar to the estimate of 1500 cases that was not based on specific numbers.

Figure 3–1 also shows that, for this particular

OPERATING ROOM ANALYSIS
(Sample)

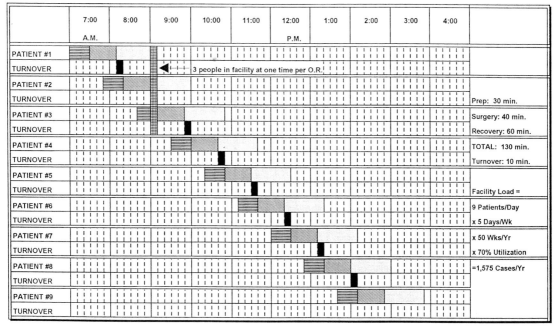

LEGEND

Prep:
Surgery:
Recovery:
Turnover:

Figure 3–1. An example of an operating room analysis for daily schedule capability. Based on an average time per procedure, and fixed turnover, recovery, and prep times, the estimated number of cases performed in an ambulatory surgery operating room for the day is calculated. (From Marasco R, Marasco J. Ambulatory surgery centers. Creating success in a future of change. Presented at American Association of Ambulatory Surgery Centers 18th Annual Meeting. San Diego, February 20–22, 1997.)

operating room in this facility, an expected number of patients in the facility at any one time is three. Accurate estimates of maximum numbers of patients is important to provide adequate prep and recovery space as well as other space requirements, such as parking.

The actual space required for the operating room must be considered. Federal law requires that an operating room be 270 square feet of free floor space (no cabinet-covered floor). Most general surgery procedures can be done in rooms of this size or only slightly larger. Any room larger than 400 square feet is probably too large for the needs of most general surgeons, although certain subspecialties in which large pieces of equipment are used may require such a large room. A 270-square-foot room is almost too big for efficiency in performing endoscopic procedures, for which ef-

ficiency in reaching equipment in cabinets during the procedures can be impeded by a large room.

The most common error that the first author has encountered in the projected plans of surgeons designing ambulatory facilities is in planning too many and oversized operating rooms. Again, efficiency should be the watchword, assuming the space is adequate to perform the intended procedures.

Table 3–2 lists recommended space requirements for two types of ambulatory units: a single specialty facility attached to a practice and a two operating room multispecialty freestanding facility. In this table, a generous estimate of 350 to 400 square feet for operating rooms is used to account for a higher end expense in building for the projected cost analysis.

Table 3–2. Surgery Area Space Program

	Single Specialty Attached to Practice		Multispecialty Freestanding	
A. Vestibule	80 to 120 SF	_____ SF	80 to 120 SF	_____ SF
B. Waiting		_____ SF		_____ SF
1. Seats	No. of ORs @ 18 SF/seat	_____ SF	No. of ORs @ 18 SF/seat	_____ SF
2. Nourishment/TV	1 @ 15 SF =	_____ SF	1 @ 15 SF =	_____ SF
C. Waiting room toilet	1 @ 55 SF =	_____ SF	1 @ 55 SF =	_____ SF
D. Business Area		_____ SF		_____ SF
1. Positions				
Reception/scheduler	60 SF/person	_____ SF	60 SF/person	_____ SF
Transcription	40 SF/person	_____ SF	40 SF/person	_____ SF
Billing/collection	40 SF/person	_____ SF	40 SF/person	_____ SF
2. Files	40 SF/OR	_____ SF	40 SF/OR	_____ SF
3. Work/computer	30 to 50 SF	_____ SF	30 to 50 SF	_____ SF
E. Family room	1/OR @ 80 SF	_____ SF	1/OR @ 80 SF	_____ SF
F. Patient dressing		_____ SF		_____ SF
1. Toilet/dressing (1 per OR)	@ 55 SF =	_____ SF	@ 55 SF =	_____ SF
2. Patient lockers/gowns (3 per OR)	@ 55 SF =	_____ SF	@ 55 SF =	_____ SF
G. Control station	80 to 120 SF	_____ SF	100 to 150 SF	_____ SF
H. Prep/recovery		_____ SF		_____ SF
1. Curtained stations	@ 80 SF =	_____ SF	@ 80 SF =	_____ SF
2. Enclosed stations	@ 100 SF =	_____ SF	@ 100 SF =	_____ SF
3. Recovery lounge (3 per OR)	@ 65 SF =	_____ SF	@ 65 SF =	_____ SF
I. Operating rooms		_____ SF		_____ SF
1. Two rooms	350 to 400 SF		350 to 400 SF	
J. Soiled utility	60 to 80 SF	_____ SF	80 to 120 SF	_____ SF
K. Clean utility/sterilization	60 to 80 SF	_____ SF	80 to 120 SF	_____ SF
L. Sterile storage	60 to 80 SF	_____ SF	80 to 150 SF	_____ SF
M. Scrub sink	1/OR @ 10 SF		1/OR @ 10 SF	

Waiting Room

Federal law for Medicare reimbursement requires that the facility have a waiting room. The size is not specified and can be tailored to patient volume. However, we recommend that the waiting room be one area, if any, where extra expense is incurred. It is the first area that the patient sees, and first impressions are important. Furthermore, it is the area where family members wait throughout the procedure, so comfort is crucial. Provision of a nourishment station (coffee, juice) is appreciated by family members. It must be within control of the receptionist to monitor its use.

If a facility is large enough, a "quiet" and a "noisy" area of the waiting room can be designed. The latter can house a television set, with programming controlled again by the receptionist. Television, if used correctly, can be a calming influence for children awaiting surgery. The provision of seats and a movie such as "Cinderella" likely produces a quieter preoperative condition for the young child than a set of "action" toys.

The number of seats in the waiting room is determined by the number of patients anticipated to be within the facility at any one time, with an incremental additional estimate, based on the practice, to avoid overcrowding. For example, the waiting room for a surgeon performing pediatric cases needs to be larger, assuming the parents will bring other children along.

Table 3–2. Surgery Area Space Program *Continued*

	Single Specialty Attached to Practice		Multispecialty Freestanding	
N. Clean storage	30 to 50 SF	_____ SF	40 to 80 SF	_____ SF
O. Soiled holding	30 to 50 SF	_____ SF	40 to 80 SF	_____ SF
P. Anesthesia/work storage	40 to 80 SF	_____ SF	40 to 80 SF	_____ SF
Q. Staff dressing		_____ SF		_____ SF
1. Male dressing	80 to 120 SF _____ SF		100 to 150 SF _____ SF	
2. Female dressing	100 to 150 SF _____ SF		120 to 180 SF _____ SF	
3. Toilet with shower	2 @ 65 SF = _____ SF		2 @ 65 SF = _____ SF	
4. Break room	80 to 100 SF _____ SF		100 to 120 SF _____ SF	
R. General storage	80 to 180 SF	_____ SF	100 to 250 SF	_____ SF
S. Equipment storage	60 to 120 SF	_____ SF	100 to 250 SF	_____ SF
T. Janitor's closet	20 to 30 SF	_____ SF	20 to 30 SF	_____ SF
U. Gas storage	30 to 50 SF	_____ SF	30 to 50 SF	_____ SF
V. UPS room	30 to 50 SF	_____ SF	30 to 50 SF	_____ SF
W. Mechanical space	80 to 100 SF	_____ SF	80 to 120 SF	_____ SF
X. Miscellaneous areas				
1. Laser room	80 to 120 SF	_____ SF	80 to 120 SF	_____ SF
2. Dark room	30 SF	_____ SF	30 SF	_____ SF
3. Director's office	80 to 120 SF	_____ SF	80 to 120 SF	_____ SF
Y. Endoscopy suite				
1. Procedure room	260 SF	_____ SF	260 SF	_____ SF
2. Prep/recovery with toilet	110 SF	_____ SF	110 SF	_____ SF
3. Control station	60 to 80 SF	_____ SF	60 to 80 SF	_____ SF
4. Utility	135 SF	_____ SF	135 SD	_____ SF
5. Storage	40 SF	_____ SF	40 SF	_____ SF
Total net area	Sum of A through Y	_____ SF	Sum of A through Y	_____ SF
40% Circulation	40% of total net	_____ SF	40% to total net	_____ SF
Total gross area	Total net + circulation	_____ SF	Total net + circulation	_____ SF

SF = square feet; OR = operating room.
Modified from Marasco R, Marasco J. Ambulatory surgery centers. Creating success in a future of change. Presented at American Association of Ambulatory Surgery Centers 18th Annual Meeting. San Diego, February 20–22, 1997.

A separate toilet for the waiting room is desirable. It should *not* open directly into the waiting room; despite the sound-proofing, the illusion of little privacy from such a design makes those waiting in the room loathe to use it.

Business Area

Accreditation requires that a business area exist within the ambulatory facility. This may be only a desk that can be incorporated into the receptionist area. There needs to be some area where medical records are kept. These records do not need to be all-inclusive for patients but should represent an important

summary of their medical problems and be readily available. Large numbers of records from past cases should be stored in the practice offices.

Table 3–2 lists additional space for a work station and computer for the facility, which is a realistic and important addition for automated billing. This enables the receptionist to perform other secretarial duties if needed.

Family Room

A family room is not an insurance or health code requirement; however, it makes excellent business sense. Having a place within the facility where the family of the patient in surgery can wait and be educated about the procedure, in particular what to expect postoperatively, can be anxiety-relieving for the family and save many needless phone calls by panic-stricken relatives who are unfamiliar with the expected postoperative events. This is efficiently done, from the family's point of view, during the otherwise anxious waiting time during the procedure. Some facilities have even set up a room for family viewing, via videotelescopic transmission or even direct vision, of the operation. A trained nurse assistant must be present to explain the procedure to the family under such circumstances. This has proven surprisingly popular with families. Explanation of a procedure and viewing it make the family feel involved, more knowledgeable, and less likely to have questions postoperatively. However, such a tactic can succeed only if the surgeon feels comfortable with the arrangement.

Patient Dressing Area

A patient dressing area is a Medicare requirement. The dressing area often by state law also requires a toilet. Here, the combination of using the patient toilet with the dressing room is desirable. It meets several requirements. It fulfills the requirement for handicapped toilets, which must be extra large to conform with standards. By slightly enlarging the handicapped toilet area, the planners can design the dressing room to be a part of it.

The facility must have provisions for patients' clothing. Lockers are one solution. Patients should be discouraged from bringing any valuables with them. The number of toilets and changing rooms and the number of lockers are derived directly from the operating room case analysis (for Figure 3–1, it was three patients per operating room).

Control Station

The manager of the facility is best given a small but centrally located control station. This should have visual access to the prep and recovery areas. It should be close to both the operating rooms as well as the reception area.

Size should be small because, ideally, the manager is out working within the facility much of the day.

Prep and Recovery Area

It is strongly recommended that the areas for prep and recovery be overlapping for flexibility of use. In the early part of the day, there is a greater demand for prep; in the later part of the day, there is a greater demand for recovery. Locating these areas separately is inefficient and wastes space.

The number of prep and recovery spaces needed is again based on the case analysis for each operating room (see Fig. 3–1). In calculating the number of recovery spaces, consideration should be given to procedures with the shortest operating time and the longest recovery. For example, pediatric hernia repairs have long recovery times relative to procedure times. Consideration of the case mix and of the potential for such cases determine the required number of prep and recovery spaces needed for the facility.

Prep area requirements are less of a concern than recovery area requirements, where patients are in a variety of states. Basically, there are three types of patients to be provided for in recovery:

1. Those who are not ambulatory and not alert
2. Those who are not ambulatory but are alert
3. Those who are awake and ambulatory

Patients in the first two categories require gurneys or stretchers for recovery. Patients in the last category can recover nicely in recliner chairs. Once again, the case mix in terms of types of cases performed determines how many patients in each of these groups should be anticipated for the facility.

Table 3–2 lists space requirements for the different types of recovery stations. An enclosed station is probably desirable for all facilities, because the potential for a patient with significant postoperative pain, nausea, or other problems should be anticipated. Such patients recover best in a glass-enclosed area, relatively away from other patients in terms of sound, but accessible to visual observation by staff. The enclosed room is also useful for preparing the particularly anxious patient pre-operatively. Rules for an enclosed recovery station are that the bed must have a 3-foot clearance on each side and at one end. Adding room for an 18-inch shelf at the head of the bed produces a space requirement of approximately 100 square feet for such a station.

Curtained recovery stations are more efficient in terms of space use, but they are less private. Here, curtains are used instead of walls, with a decrease in the lateral space required on each bedside, resulting in an estimated 80 square feet per recovery space.

Recovery lounges or recliners are listed in Table 3–2 as requiring approximately 65 square feet per recliner.

Storage and Utility Areas

Table 3–2 lists estimates for the space needed for the storage and utility components of the center. A clean utility and sterilization area is an important component. It should be designed so that there is a unidirectional flow of instruments from the operating room to the sterile storage area. Clean storage for linen and other supplies is a legal requirement and can be small but must be appropriately designated. A designated area is needed for soiled utility as well.

Law requires that there be a janitor's closet and that it be so designated. Some states require one janitor's closet in the clean and one in the unclean areas of the facility.

Other areas that must be provided for include equipment storage. No laws regulate size, but recommendations are given in Table 3–2.

Staff Dressing Area

Medicare certification requires that the facility have a dressing area for staff. Local requirements vary as to the specifications of the dressing area. Some states require separate areas for each gender. Some states require toilets in the dressing areas, and others require showers as well. The main concern in the location of

the dressing area is that it be placed so as to allow separation of the unclean from the clean area of the facility. Medicare certifiers are very concerned about clean and dirty areas and their relative separation. Once staff have changed clothes and placed on shoe covers, caps, and so on, they should not need to traverse the area of the facility that is designated for supply delivery, waiting, and so forth. Similarly, consideration of these criteria is important in placing the staff lounge, if one is included in the design.

Miscellaneous Areas

Other miscellaneous areas that should be at least considered as part of a multispecialty facility are listed in Table 3–2. These include space provisions for gas cannister storage, a room for receiving delivered packages, and space for storing ancillary equipment such as a laser machine. A dark room, if necessary, must be included in the space allocation.

All ambulatory facilities must have emergency generator capacity that may be part of the mechanical storage area. Heating and air conditioning equipment also requires mechanical space.

Endoscopy Rooms

Space recommendations for dedicated endoscopy rooms are listed in Table 3–2. Because of the nature of the procedures and the equipment involved, these dimensions are smaller in size than those for the operating rooms. There is still need for storage, utility, recovery, and prep areas, and a control station is still desirable.

Hallways

Federal regulations require that any hallway through which a patient is transported on a stretcher be 8 feet wide.

Circulation Space

Table 3–2 includes a 40% additional space estimate for "circulation space." The planner is cautioned not to diminish this percentage, because it is necessary to allow space for reasonable traffic patterns and flow within the building and to prevent an overcrowded feeling.

FACILITY EQUIPMENT CONSIDERATIONS

The ambulatory surgery center has certain equipment requirements by law. Again, these may vary by locality. It is imperative that the planning team be aware of these requirements.

All facilities have the legal requirement to supply emergency generator power for at least 30 minutes. This is often accomplished through the use of a system of batteries to generate power in smaller facilities. Some commercially produced systems smoothly introduce power in the event of a blackout. Such systems prevent damage to microscopes and other sensitive equipment that can be harmed by power surges. The number of outlets that are needed to hook into such a system can be limited by design, reducing the cost of the system.

All facilities must be constructed with the provision of fire walls around the facility. These walls must meet certain heat retardant standards designed to last 1 hour. This requirement is particularly important when an ambulatory surgery facility is being added on to an existing building.

Provision for gas lines and suction lines must be made in the design of the facility. These can be less extensive and costly than those used for standard inpatient operating suites.

It is probably helpful to enlist an anesthesiologist when planning space considerations for the anesthesia and monitoring equipment. This can impact room design.

INSPECTIONS AND CERTIFICATION

Design of the facility should always be geared toward the expected certification of the facility. Fulfillment of requirements for in-

surance approval accreditation is paramount to securing maximal reimbursement fees for the facility. Accreditation is required because insurance companies are concerned that they will pay a facility fee for a procedure that should not be done in that facility and therefore be held liable. Medicare requirements are generally more stringent than AAAHC or JCAHO requirements. Based on patient case mix, this may necessitate meeting Medicare requirements. If the Medicare component of the practice is minimal, the additional requirements imposed for such accreditation may not be financially worthwhile. In general, it is not likely that a facility will meet Medicare requirements unless it is at least 1100 to 1200 square feet in size. Many ambulatory facilities are not currently Medicare certified.

As discussed, it is also important to be sure that the design will be approved by state inspectors before building begins.

Inspection of the facility is done by two individuals or groups. The first is the fire marshall, who is largely interested in the appropriately designed and constructed fire wall and that codes are met for exits, hallways, and so forth.

The second inspection is by the state Department of Health designee. This person is often a nurse who is concerned about the need for a facility procedure manual and the fact that described protocols in the manual be known by personnel working in the facility. The state inspector is also concerned about sterile, clean, and unclean areas and traffic flow between them. Each state's Department of Health does the certification for Medicare accreditation. Some states also require state certification in addition to federal certification. In some states, a certificate of need for the facility is still required for an ambulatory surgery facility.

LAND REQUIREMENT

The land requirements for the facility are related to the building size itself in terms of minimal requirements. Land is probably one of the cheapest components of the startup cost equation, and the purchase of additional land for future potential expansion should be considered if it is available and reasonably priced.

Table 3–3 shows the space requirements for parking and "green area" (50% of the total space for building and parking) required for meeting most building codes. The specifics of the local building code in terms of easements, offsets from property lines, building height, and external design restrictions should all be known during the planning stage.

DEVELOPMENT OF A 5-YEAR CASH FLOW ANALYSIS

The 5-year cash flow analysis determines the financial feasibility of the proposed project. Once the space requirements, land requirements, and other aspects of the requirements for the building itself have been determined, an estimation of the remaining expenses can be calculated and balanced against expected revenue.

Revenue

In Table 3–1, a case analysis was performed to determine the anticipated number and type of cases to be performed in the facility. Using those data, Table 3–4 gives the average Medicare reimbursement (figures accurate prior to October 1996) for the various levels of the cases. By determining the percentage of Medicare versus third-party payer cases for each level, an average reimbursement fee for each level is determined. This average is then multiplied by the number of cases at that level

Table 3–4. Revenue Levels

Group	Medicare Fee* 20%–80% of Practice	Estimated Third-Party Carriers 20%–80% of Practice	Average
I	$312.00	**	Average of Medicare fee and 3rd party carriers
II	$419.00		Average of Medicare fee and 3rd party carriers
III	$479.00		Average of Medicare fee and 3rd party carriers
IV	$591.00		Average of Medicare fee and 3rd party carriers
V	$674.00		Average of Medicare fee and 3rd party carriers
VI	$785.00 ($635.00 + $150.00)		Average of Medicare fee and 3rd party carriers
VII	$935.00		Average of Medicare fee and 3rd party carriers
VIII	$923.00 ($773.00 + $150.00)		Average of Medicare fee and 3rd party carriers
IX	$1150.000		Average of Medicare fee and 3rd party carriers

*Changed by HCFA Oct. 1, 1996.
**Could be 25%–50% over Medicare payment.
Modified from Marasco R, Marasco J. Ambulatory surgery centers. Creating success in a future of change. Presented at American Association of Ambulatory Surgery Centers 18th Annual Meeting. San Diego, February 20–22, 1997.

to give a subtotal of income per category. Addition of the income subtotals for the categories produces a sum of the expected annual revenues for the facility for the first year of operation.

Table 3–5 summarizes this process in the top portion of the table. The projected 5-year revenue from the facility is then calculated based on the revenue for the first year. Conservative growth figures in numbers of cases of 3% to 10% are given as examples. This figure should be modified if additional surgeons are likely to be added to the user list. A conservatively low figure of 3% to 5% annual facility fee increases is used in the calculation based on increases in the past decade; however, such increases may be accurate based on current budget-cutting trends in health care.

Rent

A major expense of the project is the cost of purchasing or leasing the site. Table 3–6 gives an example of the formula that is used to calculate costs per square foot if the building is to be owned by the users. The top section of

Table 3–3. Surgery Area Land Requirement*

1. Building footprint from space program
2. Parking 4 Stalls per preoperative/postoperative station 350 SF/stall
Subtotal
3. Green area (1 + 2) × 0.5
Total land area

*Does not include practice area.
SF = square feet.
Modified from Marasco R, Marasco J. Ambulatory surgery centers. Creating success in a future of change. Presented at American Association of Ambulatory Surgery Centers 18th Annual Meeting. San Diego, February 20–22, 1997.

Table 3–5. Projected Unit Revenues

Year	Group	No. of Cases	Unit Revenue	Revenue per Year
1998	I	From caseload study	From revenue chart	No. of cases × unit revenue
	II	From caseload study	From revenue chart	No. of cases × unit revenue
	III	From caseload study	From revenue chart	No. of cases × unit revenue
	IV	From caseload study	From revenue chart	No. of cases × unit revenue
	V	From caseload study	From revenue chart	No. of cases × unit revenue
	VI	From caseload study	From revenue chart	No. of cases × unit revenue
	VII	From caseload study	From revenue chart	No. of cases × unit revenue
	VIII	From caseload study	From revenue chart	No. of cases × unit revenue
	Miscellaneous	From caseload study	From revenue chart	No. of cases × unit revenue
	Total	Total no. of cases	Total revenue divided by cases	Total $ amount of revenue
1999 _____ Surgeons		Increase by 3%–10%	Increase by 3%–5%	No. of cases × unit revenue
2000 _____ Surgeons		Increase by 3%–10%	Increase by 3%–5%	No. of cases × unit revenue
2001 _____ Surgeons		Increase by 3%–10%	Increase by 3%–5%	No. of cases × unit revenue
2002 _____ Surgeons		Increase by 3%–10%	Increase by 3%–5%	No. of cases × unit revenue
2003 _____ Surgeons		Increase by 3%–10%	Increase by 3%–5%	No. of cases × unit revenue
2004 _____ Surgeons		Increase by 3%–10%	Increase by 3%–5%	No. of cases × unit revenue

Modified from Marasco R, Marasco J. Ambulatory surgery centers. Creating success in a future of change. Presented at American Association of Ambulatory Surgery Centers 18th Annual Meeting. San Diego, February 20–22, 1997.

Table 3–6. Estimated Economic Pro Forma (Ownership)

	Surgery Area
I. Project description	
A. Building area (See Table 3–2)	
B. Site area (See Table 3–3)	
1. Land area	
II. Project cost	
A. Land value (consult local realtor)	
B. Construction cost	
1. Building cost—$100.00 to $150.00/SF	
2. Site work—$2.50 to $3.00/SF of land	
C. Architect's fee—10%–12% of B	
D. Contingency/Miscellaneous—6%–8% of B	
Subtotal	Sum of A through D
E. Finance fees—3%–4% of subtotal	
Total project cost	Add A, B, C, D, and E
III. Project financing	
A. Long-term loan—75%–80% of total project cost	
B. Land equity (Land value if land is owned free and clear)	
Subtotal	Add A and B
C. Cash equity	Total project cost minus subtotal
Total project financing	Add A, B, and C
IV. Annual gross cost	
A. Debt service	Loan amount × 0.09655
B. Fixed, operating, and tax expenses	$5.00 to $7.00/SF
C. Return on investment	10% of IIIC (cash equity)
Net annual cost	Add A, B, and C

SF = square feet.
Modified from Marasco R, Marasco J. Ambulatory surgery centers. Creating success in a future of change. Presented at American Association of Ambulatory Surgery Centers 18th Annual Meeting. San Diego, February 20–22, 1997.

the table simply describes the building and land areas. Section II details the project cost, which includes the purchase price of the land, construction costs, architect's fees, and contingency fees for errors in construction, revisions, penalties, and so on, which may occur during construction. A generous allowance of 6% to 8% of building costs is used to estimate the latter. Site work for the land usually costs approximately $3 per square foot of land. Actual construction costs per square foot vary by region (e.g., costs in West Coast and northeast cities are more than in the southeast). These costs should be estimated as lower than the costs per square foot to build a hospital but higher than the costs per square foot to build an office facility. Addition of a 3% to 4% estimate for finance fees gives a total project cost.

The total project cost in section II of Table 3–6 is probably not as important as the figure in section IIIA. This is the percentage of the total project cost that can be secured through a loan. The larger this amount, then the lower the actual cash equity required for the project. Success in obtaining a loan for the project is greatly enhanced by having a well-conceived financial plan such as the cash flow analysis described here. The bank financial officer is most concerned about the likelihood of the project generating revenue to repay the loan.

Section IV in Table 3–6 shows the annual costs for owning and operating the facility in terms of the building itself. These include repayment of the building and construction loan, fixed expenses including taxes, and a 10% return on the equity invested to begin the project. The latter is a realistic business consideration, because the money so invested would otherwise be expected to earn interest through a different investment vehicle.

Equipment

Table 3–7 is a rough calculation of start-up equipment costs for each operating room, including completely furnishing the room. This is estimated at a very conservatively high figure of $250,000 to $350,000 per operating room. Additional money for the purchase of highly expensive equipment such as a laser should also be calculated if necessary. See

Table 3–7. Equipment

I. Assume equipment cost to include the following:
 ($250,000 to $350,000 per operating room)
 ($125,000 to $150,000/spec. procedure room)
  1. Autoclave
  2. Prep recovery bed
  3. Operating room table
  4. Operating room light
  5. Microscope
  6. Other equipment
II. Assume equipment is paid for with borrowed money
 7%–10% for 5 years = loan constant of:
III. Therefore, equipment cost/year =
 Equipment cost × loan constant

Modified from Marasco R, Marasco J. Ambulatory surgery centers. Creating success in a future of change. Presented at American Association of Ambulatory Surgery Centers 18th Annual Meeting. San Diego, February 20–22, 1997.

Chapter 12 for further details on some of the costs of basic equipment to furnish a general surgery operating room.

Using the estimated figures given, the equipment costs are calculated based on repayment of a 7% to 10% loan obtained for a 5-year period. The loan constant (for example, 0.2491 for a 9% 5-year loan) is multiplied by the equipment cost to give the annual cost of equipment per year.

Staff

Staff salaries are a very high proportion of the operating budget of any ambulatory surgery facility (see Chapter 4). Table 3–8 is a formula for calculating the estimated annual expenses for staff salaries based on the number of operating rooms. The number of personnel needed to staff the facility is given at the bottom of the table, based on number of operating rooms. For example, a two-operating room facility requires one director, two registered nurses, four technicians, and two other personnel (secretarial and other support). The average salaries per hour are given for these personnel. In the upper portion of the table, estimates of the average overall hourly facility salary for the personnel are multiplied by the number of hours per case (here given as 6 to 10, but a more conservative estimate is 12) and by the total number of cases. To this number, an additional 20% (25% is not unrealistic) in fringe benefits is added.

Table 3–8. Staff

Year	Average Salary/ Hour	Number of Cases	Total Hours	Salary	Fringe 20%–25%	Total
1998	$12.00 to $16.00/ hour	Take from caseload (Table 3–1)	6–10 hours per case	Salary/hour × total hours	Salary × 20%	Salary plus fringe
1999	Increase by 5%/year	Take from caseload	6–10 hours per case	Salary/hour × total hours	Salary × 20%	Salary plus fringe
2000	Increase by 5%/year	Take from caseload	6–10 hours per case	Salary/hour × total hours	Salary × 20%	Salary plus fringe
2001	Increase by 5%/year	Take from caseload	6–10 hours per case	Salary/hour × total hours	Salary × 20%	Salary plus fringe
2002	Increase by 5%/year	Take from caseload	6–10 hours per case	Salary/hour × total hours	Salary × 20%	Salary plus fringe
2003	Increase by 5%/year	Take from caseload	6–10 hours per case	Salary/hour × total hours	Salary × 20%	Salary plus fringe
2004	Increase by 5%/year	Take from caseload	6–10 hours per case	Salary/hour × total hours	Salary × 20%	Salary plus fringe

	1996 Salary Levels		
Position	Hourly Salary*	Number of Positions† 1 OR/2 OR/3 OR/4 OR	
Director	$20.00 to $24.00	1 / 1 / 1 / 1	
Registered nurse	$16.00 to $20.00	1 / 2 / 3 / 5	
Technician	$10.00 to $14.00	2 / 4 / 6 / 8	
Other	$6.00 to $10.00	1 / 2 / 2 / 2	
Total			
Avg/Hour			

*Increase by 3%–5% per year.
†Number of staff per case is based on 6–10 hours per case.
Modified from Marasco R, Marasco J. Ambulatory surgery centers. Creating success in a future of change. Presented at American Association of Ambulatory Surgery Centers 18th Annual Meeting. San Diego, February 20–22, 1997.

This gives the annual staff salary plus fringe benefits cost in the far right-hand column. Increases in salary by 5% per year are used to project expenses for the subsequent years beyond year 1.

Supplies

Supplies are another major component of the annual operating budget of the ambulatory surgery facility, exceeded only annually by salary expenses for many centers. Table 3–9 calculates the estimated supply costs annually for a facility, based on a figure of $150 to $250 of costs in supplies per case. Clearly, this figure can vary widely among general surgeons. If laparoscopic cases are prevalent, costs for disposable supplies can be considerably higher and must be factored into the equation at this point. The figures used are for more traditional cases such as biopsies or open herniorrhaphies. Supply costs are also projected to

increase, and a 3% to 5% rate is used for calculating expenses in subsequent years.

CASH FLOW ANALYSIS CHART

Table 3–10 combines all the information derived from the previous tables into the final cash flow analysis chart. Summary figures for rent, equipment, staff, and supplies are combined with a "miscellaneous" cost (10% to 20% of variable cost categories of equipment, staff, and supplies) to cover any unexpected costs, miscalculations of expenses, unexpected price increases, and so forth. Such a margin of safety is viewed as appropriately conservative in estimating expenses. An additional amount for "start-up costs" for the first year is added, based on facility size.

The total expense figure is subtracted from the revenue figure to give the profit or loss for the first year. Subsequent years are calculated to determine the yearly profit or loss, which

Table 3–9. Supplies

Year	Average Supply/Case	Number of Cases	Total
1998	$150 to $250/case	From caseload study	Average supply × no. of cases
1999	Increase previous year by 3%–5%	From caseload study	Average supply × no. of cases
2000	Increase previous year by 3%–5%	From caseload study	Average supply × no. of cases
2001	Increase previous year by 3%–5%	From caseload study	Average supply × no. of cases
2002	Increase previous year by 3%–5%	From caseload study	Average supply × no. of cases
2003	Increase previous year by 3%–5%	From caseload study	Average supply × no. of cases
2004	Increase previous year by 3%–5%	From caseload study	Average supply × no. of cases

Modified from Marasco R, Marasco J. Ambulatory surgery centers. Creating success in a future of change. Presented at American Association of Ambulatory Surgery Centers 18th Annual Meeting. San Diego, February 20–22, 1997.

is added to or subtracted from the previous year's figure to give an accrued profit or loss for all subsequent years.

This cash flow analysis yields a reasonable conservative estimate of the potential of the facility to generate a profit. If the proposed user group derives a very positive bottom line, then the project should be undertaken. We *recommend that the 5-year cash flow analysis be performed before architects and other expensive con-sultants are hired.* The consulting firm of the first author (R. M.) performs an initial consultation visit with a relatively low charge plus expenses to generate such a cash flow analysis for groups potentially interested in constructing an ambulatory surgery or other medical facility. This avoids high initial consulting expenses for a project that is doomed to financial failure. It also greatly facilitates procurement of the appropriate loans for the project.

Table 3–10. 5-Year Cash Flow Analysis

Year	Revenue	Expenses					Yearly Profit (Loss)	Accrued Profit (Loss)
		Rent	Equipment	Staff	Supply	Miscellaneous		
1998	No. of cases × facility fee per case	Building rent	Equipment lease	Staff salaries and fringe benefits	Cost of supplies per case × no. of cases	10%–20% of building, equipment, staff, and supplies*	Total revenue less expenses	Same as this year's profit or loss
1999	No. of cases × facility fee per case	Building rent	Equipment lease	Staff salaries and fringe benefits	Cost of supplies per case × no. of cases	10%–20% of building, equipment, staff, and supplies*	Total revenue less expenses	Last year's profit or loss + this year's profit or loss
2000	No. of cases × facility fee per case	Building rent	Equipment lease	Staff salaries and fringe benefits	Cost of supplies per case × no. of cases	10%–20% of building, equipment, staff, and supplies*	Total revenue less expenses	Last 2 years' profit or loss + this year's profit or loss
2001	No. of cases × facility fee per case	Building rent	Equipment lease	Staff salaries and fringe benefits	Cost of supplies per case × no. of cases	10%–20% of building, equipment, staff, and supplies*	Total revenue less expenses	Last 3 years' profit or loss + this year's profit or loss
2002	No. of cases × facility fee per case	Building rent	Equipment lease	Staff salaries and fringe benefits	Cost of supplies per case × no. of cases	10%–20% of building, equipment, staff, and supplies*	Total revenue less expenses	Last 4 years' profit or loss + this year's profit or loss

Average:

*Plus start-up costs: 1 OR = $40,000, 2 OR = $60,000, 3 OR = $80,000, 4 OR = $100,000.
OR = operating room.
Modified from Marasco R, Marasco J. Ambulatory surgery centers. Creating success in a future of change. Presented at American Association of Ambulatory Surgery Centers 18th Annual Meeting. San Diego, February 20–22, 1997.

If a net loss is estimated from the 5-year analysis, then some key aspects of the project must be reconsidered. Can the facility be made smaller? Alternatively, can other surgeons be reliably brought into the project, thus increasing caseload? Can a plan be devised whereby hospital-assisted financing is possible? If the latter is contemplated, the users must be careful not to undermine the goal of the facility as an ambulatory surgery center. In any case, the individuals determining the feasibility of an ambulatory surgery center are appropriately cautioned of the potential financial consequences of proceeding under the original plan and design.

Selected Readings

1. Davis JE. The major ambulatory surgical center and how it is developed. Surg Clin North Am 1987:67:671–692.
2. Marasco R, Marasco J. Ambulatory surgery centers. Creating success in a future of change. Presented at American Association of Ambulatory Surgery Centers 18th Annual Meeting. San Diego, February 20–22, 1997.

Chapter 4

Reimbursement Issues

Bruce David Schirmer • Don E. Detmer

Because reimbursement for services rendered is the major source of income for ambulatory surgery facilities of all types, reimbursement issues have been and will likely remain of great importance. The entire formula of reimbursement for services is being modified by the movement toward capitated forms of payment for health care. This chapter addresses the issues of reimbursement as they have evolved for ambulatory surgery, with emphasis on current issues.

OBTAINING INSURANCE REIMBURSEMENT

Ambulatory surgery initially was not accepted by third party insurance payers in certain locations. A freestanding surgicenter begun in Providence, RI, in the late 1960s by Charles Hill was unsuccessful because insurance companies in the area would not reimburse the center for facility fees for procedures. This was not a uniform problem, however, and other early surgicenters such as the one established in Phoenix by Reed and Ford and the one established in Durham by Davis and Detmer were successful at obtaining third party payment for services. Because those centers foresaw the importance of gaining such acceptance, they included it as part of the initial plan of organization.

In 1972, the Orkand study (Orkand Corp.), commissioned by the U.S. government, found that ambulatory surgery could be performed as safely as inpatient surgery for designated procedures and at a lower cost in freestanding surgicenters. Since that time, surgicenters and other providers of ambulatory surgical services have been accepted by insurance carriers.

BUDGET CONSIDERATIONS

The budget of a freestanding ambulatory surgical center depends on its receipt of anticipated reimbursements to meet expenditures. Even small cuts in reimbursement rates can significantly affect the profit margin and viability of some centers, depending on a variety of factors including inherent financial solvency, projected profit margin, and volume of procedures.

A freestanding outpatient surgical unit often operates on a budget that relies on net charges to compose more than 98% of the net revenue. Less than 2% is composed of interest and miscellaneous income. Disposition of revenue generally includes salaries and supplies as the two largest items. These typically range from 35% to 40% and from 20% to 25%, respectively, of expenses. Rent, interest on loans, maintenance, and utilities are variable expenses based on the situation of the individual unit, but they should optimally be kept to as low a percentage of the operating budget as possible. Collection expenses may be as much as 8% of the budget. The greater the net surplus each year, the greater the financial cushion for purchasing major new equipment, expanding, or enduring episodes of decreased revenue. A net surplus of more than 10% is a reasonable benchmark in the current climate of financial uncertainty.

As a general rule, an ambulatory surgery center should perform approximately four or more procedures per operating room per day to maintain an adequately profitable caseload. This formula is based on previous payment schedules. Limitations in future payments may require increasing caseloads per operating room per day to ensure profitability.

Fee reimbursement for typical general surgery cases currently is on the order of $450 to $600. For example, at an ambulatory surgical facility with which we are familiar, the facility fee for an inguinal hernia repair is approximately $1400, and reimbursement from third party payers is approximately $600.

Traditionally, the freestanding ambulatory surgical center has received facility fee reimbursement on a basis different from that of the hospital-based ambulatory surgical unit. Medicare and other major insurers have reimbursed freestanding units on a prospective basis for the procedures performed, whereas hospital units have been reimbursed on a cost basis for procedures performed, with the rationale being that overhead and overall costs for the hospital units are higher to support the more expensive technology and personnel. This payment plan has generally worked in favor of the hospital-based units, which usually receive higher fees on an identical per-case basis. Comparison between reimbursement fees for a freestanding ambulatory surgical center in Charlottesville, VA, versus an inpatient facility shows that the freestanding center is reimbursed at a 30% to 50% lower facility or room fee for many similar procedures. Overall, the costs of the freestanding facility are approximately 60% of those of the inpatient unit, allowing for this discrepancy while maintaining financial solvency.

INCENTIVES PROMOTING AMBULATORY SURGERY

Once insurance carriers realized the potential savings of ambulatory surgery over performance of the same procedure in the inpatient setting, incentives were incorporated into policies to encourage patients to choose an ambulatory setting for their operation. During the past decade, when such incentives became commonplace, the volume of ambulatory surgery and the percentage of surgical procedures performed on an ambulatory surgical basis increased dramatically. However, although it has been inferred that the changes in insurance reimbursement have been an important factor in this change, there remains some question as to what extent these incentives have had in affecting patient choice of the outpatient setting.

The rationale for insurance companies to encourage surgical procedures to be done in the outpatient setting is stimulated by the fact that surgery itself accounts for an estimated 50% to 60% of all hospital expenditures, and more than 20% of all health care expenditures. The shift to an outpatient setting, with its resultant cost savings of one or more inpatient hospital days per procedure, results in a tremendous cost savings. In the past decade, the percentage of all surgical procedures done on an ambulatory basis has increased from roughly 30% to 35% to more than 50%, a nearly 67% increase. Considering that more than 2 million operations are performed in general community hospitals annually, where much of the shift from inpatient to outpatient procedures would be expected to occur, the conservative estimate in hospital charge savings for this shift of 400,000 procedures at 1 day per procedure and $500 per day (again a conservative estimate) is $200 million. This does not account for increases in ambulatory procedures in tertiary or large secondary care facilities.

Several studies have specifically looked at the hospital charge differences for performing procedures on an ambulatory versus traditional inpatient setting. Most of these have involved the comparison of a laparoscopic procedure with the similar procedure performed by celiotomy. Because of their advanced technologic nature, laparoscopic procedures have been associated with higher costs because of their more expensive equipment requirements. Even so, one study showed an average $2000 savings per case when hospital charges for laparoscopic cholecystectomy were compared with those for open cholecystectomy. Many other laparoscopic procedures have been shown to be cost effective as well when hospital charges were compared with those for a similar open procedure. However, if the open procedure such as inguinal herniorrhaphy was traditionally done in an outpatient setting, then the laparoscopic method was uniformly more costly.

Hospital charges may not accurately reflect the actual resources expended by the hospital to provide the service. Critics have said that savings such as those calculated previously far exceed the actual savings in resources expended. However, studies done to address this concern have shown that the actual costs per patient of providing the surgical procedure in an ambulatory surgical setting was less, chiefly because costly overhead and expenses from high-technology equipment and personnel are not necessary for the ambulatory procedure.

The switch to performing ambulatory surgery has been stimulated by several influences. Demand by patients to have the procedure performed on an outpatient basis has not always been driven by reimbursement issues alone. First, the perceived lesser nature and thereby lesser risk and danger of an ambulatory procedure to the patient is a compelling influence, no matter how subtle it is made to appear in the explanation of the procedure by the surgeon. Second, patients generally perceive that ambulatory surgery is less of a burden on their time and their family's time, although some of the burden of postoperative care comes to rest with the family in the aftermath of ambulatory surgery. Avoiding the necessity of having a family member stay overnight near the hospital or return the next day to the hospital is an incentive for patients.

Physician preference for ambulatory surgery may often influence patient choice as well. It is generally thought that ambulatory procedures are favored by the surgeon because of their efficient nature, thereby saving the surgeon time. Physician counseling is important in the patient's choice of ambulatory surgery, particularly as it relates to being sensitive to financial requests of patients who are faced with increased financial burden from not having a procedure done on an ambulatory basis. It has been the personal experience of one of the authors (BDS) that, often, the most common reason for a patient to request that a laparoscopic cholecystectomy be performed on a same-day basis rather than a 24-hour overnight basis is insurance copayment or coverage. Sur-

geon compliance with such a request is essential for its performance in such a time frame.

Improvements in the anesthetic and perioperative care of ambulatory surgical patients have also contributed to the popularity of ambulatory surgery. Newer anesthetic agents that produce less nausea, such as propofol, are more widely used. Significantly more attention is being given during the procedure to the potential of rapidly reversing the anesthetic effects in the recovery room. Improvements in the use of regional anesthesia and pain control have also facilitated ambulatory surgery. Finally, simply the increase in clinical experience by the anesthesiologist, the nursing staff, and the surgeon of managing the ambulatory surgical patient has improved results with ambulatory surgery.

Over the past 2 decades, technologic and technical developments in the practice of surgery have made possible ambulatory procedures that had been impossible. Most notably in the field of general surgery is the development of laparoscopic surgery. Currently, cholecystectomies, enteral feeding access, enterolysis of adhesions, and other procedures previously requiring hospitalization for more than 24 hours when done via laparotomy are routinely done on an ambulatory basis or are done with a less than 24-hour stay. Even more complicated procedures such as Nissen fundoplication and adrenalectomy have been reported as being successfully performed with less than 24-hour stays. Inguinal hernias, traditionally an ambulatory procedure, have remained so with a laparoscopic approach.

EFFECTIVENESS OF FINANCIAL INCENTIVES

Several studies have been done to look at the question of whether a lower insurance copayment or deductible for having a procedure done as an outpatient does indeed influence patient choice of an ambulatory procedure. Studies by Davis and Russell in 1972 and later by Gold in 1984 found outpatient hospital services were sensitive to market price. Gold showed a substitution effect between inpatien' and outpatient services. In a more recent stu' done by Pauly and Erder, however, thes' studies are criticized for study design, with the former study being based on data from a state and the latter being based on a geographic area, not the individual patient, as the unit of analysis. Pauly and Erder's study showed instead that, when financial incentives were used by an insurance company to influence the patient's choice of having a surgical procedure as an inpatient or an outpatient, lower out-of-pocket expenses for the patient did not directly influence the choice of the ambulatory setting. Higher out-of-pocket expenses, regardless of the site of surgery chosen, however, did adversely influence the rate of surgery in the patients studied. This study points out the fact that the initial patient decision to proceed with an operation is perhaps the pivotal one in dictating the volume of surgery performed, whether on an inpatient or outpatient basis. Negative financial incentives, by this study, clearly affected patient use of services and resources.

This study also points out that, if the patient's decision to have surgery is influenced by some of the factors listed (e.g., improved technology, less fear of a long hospital stay, perceived notion of greater safety) and ambulatory surgery is chosen, then an increase in total volume of ambulatory surgery and increased expenses as a result of this surgery actually have the opposite effect desired by some third party payers.

The incentives that insurance companies have instituted to influence the patient to seek ambulatory surgery have included a coverage of only a portion of the surgical fee for an inpatient procedure (often as low as 80%), but a 100% coverage for an outpatient procedure. Other companies have adopted the policy of completely denying coverage for certain procedures if they are not performed as an ambulatory procedure.

The emergence of the diagnosis-related group (DRG) concept in the mid-1980s also stimulated increases in outpatient procedures over inpatient ones. Because the hospital received a fixed prospective fee for the patient's major diagnosis or problem under the DRG system, the cost of surgery, if done on an inpatient basis, was deducted from that fee for that admission. Performing the procedure on an outpatient basis avoided the prospective payment system, because Medicare and most other insurers that have not incorporated the patient in a capitated plan still reimburse outpatient procedures in a retrospective, cost-based manner. The reforms in Medicare that are being formulated will likely address the payment of outpatient procedures in a less costly, more prospective manner.

The percentage of surgery done on an outpatient basis has increased dramatically in the past 20 years, but whether this has always meant a dramatic savings to payers is unclear. Whereas, in most cases, ambulatory surgery costs less than inpatient surgery for the identical procedure, it is also true that the same improvements in technology and perioperative management that have made ambulatory surgery feasible and popular, may have also increased the total number of operative procedures performed. From the insurance payer's perspective, a cost savings of 25% for a procedure done on an outpatient basis is positive, resulting in lower payments for the identical services. However, if the number of such procedures done on an outpatient basis is greater than 25% more than was done on an outpatient basis, the total cost of the service for the payer increases. Such a pattern would then likely result in lower reimbursement fees for the procedure on a prospective basis by the payer.

The total increase in the number of outpatient surgical procedures, together with the associated increased cost, has led providers to institute discounted fee plans for certain procedures performed in higher volume. They have also sought to limit the volume of procedures through increasingly stringent utilization review and utilization management models. However, these measures have often not been particularly successful.

PREPAID AND CAPITATED CARE SYSTEMS

The popularity of prepaid insurance plans has increased sharply in the 1990s. The exact percentage of the population currently enrolled in health maintenance organizations and preferred provider organizations is unknown, but coverage by such organizations substantially exceeds the majority of the population in certain urban areas. Over 40% of employer-sponsored health plans are now prepaid in design. Through their regulations and structure, these plans assist the payer in shifting surgical procedures to the outpatient setting.

While the payers are benefitting from the use of an HMO-type model to curb health care costs and cut expenditures for surgical procedures, they are also shifting the financial risk from themselves to the providers when a capitated reimbursement system is used. Under such a system, the provider group receives a fixed fee per patient, regardless of expenses incurred for medical care by that patient. In a price-focused competitive market, there is inherent incentive to limit surgical procedures, eliminate all but necessary ones, and perform as many of them as possible in as low cost a setting as possible (e.g., the ambulatory surgical center). For the freestanding surgicenter, this means accepting a certain upfront fee for coverage of a fixed number of patients, then providing the services required. Because of the local market dominance by HMOs, the surgicenter may face certain bankruptcy if it does not participate in such a plan. The center must then refocus its attention on providing services with as little cost incurred as possible to maintain a margin of profit adequate to allow continued smooth operation. As a group, the payers are at a great advantage in this situation, and only through the dominance of several large HMOs and payer groups has this become possible.

Additional measures that payers of capitated plans have begun to institute to limit the cost of ambulatory surgery, thereby further placing financial pressure on the ambulatory surgery center, include combining into a single charge the professional and facility fees for certain procedures. Total reimbursement reduction is inherent in such "bundling" of these charges. By doing this, the payers limit the decrease at any one time to either the professional staff or the facility, thereby seemingly lessening the increased financial burden on both.

Adoption of a prospective payment system by payers for all procedures, regardless of site, works to the advantage of the freestanding center if costs are lower; however, payers have not been willing to increase the reimbursement fees to freestanding facilities, even if they were willing to cut reimbursement to hospital-based facilities. The move toward a managed care system inherently prepays the cost of the anticipated procedures in advance, with the facility then assuming the burden of providing the services required of the patient population within that budget. Although this may seem to work in favor of the freestanding facility, the hospital-based facility may have some financial advantages in its greater potential to absorb short-term losses and greater ability to negotiate for low-cost buying opportunities for supplies and equipment.

SUMMARY

Financing and reimbursement are of paramount importance to the ambulatory surgery center, because profit margins are generally thin and facility fee reimbursement has made up virtually all of the operating budget in the past. Ambulatory surgery has been in a favorable position during the past 20 years in that insurance payers have realized that there is a cost savings for performing surgery on an ambulatory basis rather than on an inpatient hospital basis. However, reimbursement, although adequate, has not been excessive for freestanding units, and has usually been lower on a fee-per-case basis than reimbursement for hospital-based units. Incentives by insurance companies to influence patients to undergo their operations in an ambulatory setting have been questionably successful, but probably have had an influence on increasing the popularity of ambulatory surgery. Other factors, such as improved technology, patient acceptance and perception, and physician counseling, may have had even greater influences on this trend. Whereas ambulatory surgery saves money for the insurance payers when analyzed on a per-case basis, the overall increase in numbers of ambulatory cases has, in many cases, more than negated such savings, and the increased volume of ambulatory surgery is a target for cost-cutting measures by the payers, just as inpatient procedures were previously. Including ambulatory surgery in a prospective, prepaid health plan system has placed the burden of operating in a highly cost-efficient manner on the ambulatory surgery center. The challenge of the modern ambulatory surgery center is to provide such cost-efficient services while maintaining high quality and attractiveness of services to maintain surgeon and patient user volume.

Selected Readings

1. Detmer DE, Gelijns AC. Ambulatory surgery. A more cost-effective treatment strategy? Arch Surg 1994; 129:123–127.
2. Roos NP, Freeman JL. Potential for inpatient–outpatient substitution with diagnosis-related groups. Health Care Finance Rev 1989;10:31–38.
3. Pauly MV, Erder MH. Insurance incentives for ambulatory surgery. Health Services Res 1993;27:814–839.
4. Shelver SR, Moss MT. Operating room budget factors: a pocket guide to OR finance. Nursing Economics 1994;12:146–152.
5. Davis JE. Ambulatory surgery . . . how far can we go? Med Clin North Am 1993;77:365–375.
6. Gold M. The demand for hospital outpatient services. Health Services Res 1984;19:383–412.
7. Wilson TD. Global fees for managed care in ambulatory surgery. J Clin Anesth 1995;7:578–580.

Chapter 5

Integration of Ambulatory Surgery Into the Health Care System

Maria D. Allo

EVOLUTION OF THE AMBULATORY SURGERY UNIT

More than half of all surgical operations are performed in the ambulatory setting. The first ambulatory surgery units opened 30 years ago and were hospital based. The concept of performing a major operation in an ambulatory setting under general anesthesia was considered a radical departure from the "usual standard of care." Nonetheless, with careful patient selection, meticulous preoperative evaluation, and surgical and anesthetic controls imposed to guarantee patient safety, the feasibility of the concept was established. Subsequently, freestanding "surgicenters" evolved, thus demonstrating that many major procedures could be done safely and at lower cost in facilities entirely separate from inpatient hospitals.

Ambulatory surgery centers may be hospital based, hospital affiliated, or freestanding. Originally, most ambulatory units were hospital operating rooms where both inpatient and outpatient operations were performed within the same venue. In this model, there is usually a designated area within the hospital where outpatients can register and be prepared for operation, and then be received postoperatively and readied for discharge. Many hospitals found this to be the simplest, most economical way to transition from an entirely inpatient surgical service to one that allowed for major ambulatory surgery. This had a major advantage in that there was minimal capital investment required to create the unit. Except for construction of the "ambulatory surgery unit," which could usually be done by remodeling any underutilized existing space, no building costs were incurred by the hospital; consequently, there was minimal risk of financial loss to the hospital if the ambulatory surgery program was unsuccessful. Many organizations have begun their ambulatory surgery programs using this type of facility only to make the transition to either a hospital-based satellite facility or an autonomous ambulatory surgery unit within the hospital once the initial program proves successful. Currently, the hospital unit that integrates inpatients and outpatients is obsolete; these units cannot compete either from the standpoint of economics or that of "user-friendliness." The fixed costs of an inpatient operating room are generally higher than those of an ambulatory surgical facility. Furthermore, many states have requirements and standards applicable to all users of an inpatient facility, regardless of the magnitude of the operation, that may be in excess of what is appropriate to the ambulatory case.

The hospital-based but autonomous unit has its own dedicated operating suites and recovery and intake areas that are located within the hospital but are separate from the inpatient operating rooms. This arrangement permits significant cost savings and tends to be preferred by patients and staff. Cost savings related to having a dedicated staff dealing with a single level of service and acuity and working in a dedicated space have been realized in most places where inpatient and outpatient functions have been separated. Attention can be focused on the outpatients rather than, for example, having a single nurse assigned to both "heavy" patients (such as one awakening after thoracotomy) and "light" patients (such as one recovering after a breast biopsy). Intuitively, the nurse's focus of attention is on the patient who has undergone the more extensive operation. In a facility that separates inpatients and outpatients, outpatients receive appropriate and undivided attention from their caretakers. In an area with inpatients and outpatients, outpatients may be subjected to cancellations or delays caused by emergencies or inpatient procedures that are more complex than anticipated. This does not happen in a separated outpatient facility where the focus is on expediting the care of the outpatient and providing a comfortable and convenient environment. One significant drawback to building outpatient operating rooms within a hospital is the cost; many states have code requirements for hospital operating rooms that do not account for whether they are being used exclusively for ambulatory surgery. In some jurisdictions, standard building codes apply whether the ambulatory unit is within the physical confines of the hospital or is a geographically separate ambulatory surgery center. Thus, a hospital satellite unit may not circumvent code requirements that escalate construction costs. Decisions need to be made regarding the types of procedures to be done in the ambulatory unit, whether the unit will be administered separately from the hospital inpatient operating room management, and how the hospital services will interface with the ambulatory unit.

Freestanding surgicenters have maximal flexibility in their design, location, and scope of services. They may serve a single specialty or multiple specialties, and they may be multifunctional—for example, the building may house office space, clinical examination rooms, procedure rooms, and full-scale operating areas. They are not constrained by the preexisting goals and mission of a larger par-

ent institution. The freestanding surgicenter must employ, regulate, and control both the professional and business staffs of the facility. Credentialling and quality assurance activities should be carried out in a manner that is independent of parties having a fiduciary or proprietary relationship with the facility. The construction and start-up require considerable capital investment, and it may be years before a profit is realized.

STARTING AN AMBULATORY SURGERY UNIT

Cost drives the decision of whether to build a new facility or whether to renovate existing space. The age and condition of the existing facility and the extent of renovation required to meet code requirements and space needs are key factors in determining the cost of renovation. If the decision is made to proceed with renovation, it is important to determine the relationship of the space to be renovated within the existing structure. This includes determination of what, if any, of the existing functions will remain as shared space, where the renovation is to be located within the existing unit, and how the renovated space will affect the overall organization and circulation within the existing structure. Cost estimates should account for revenue loss related to disruption or relocation of existing operations within the facility. They should also allow for unexpected problems that can escalate construction cost, such as removal of asbestos or hidden structural obstacles. Usually, freestanding facilities have lower construction costs per square foot than hospitals, but they lack the advantage of being able to share some of the conveyances of a large hospital. Nonetheless, new construction is a tabula rasa that offers flexibility in layout and design.

The construction of any new facility begins with a planning and programming phase. Again, space and money are the primary issues that define whether the unit is to be built based on the ideal, the purely functional, or something in between. In terms of space, the functional objectives of the facility must be defined; in terms of money, it is necessary to formulate a budget for design, construction, capital equipment, and interior furnishings. The minimum space required is based on anticipated workload requirements. Space needs depend on how many operations are to be performed, the time required for each operation, and the efficiency of turnover between cases. The usual minimal space allowance per operating room is 250 square feet. Most typical inpatient operating rooms are based on a 400 net square foot size. However, many modern procedures routinely done as outpatient operations (e.g., video-assisted laparoscopic procedures or some laser endoscopic procedures) have equipment needs that necessitate a larger work area. Simple procedure rooms (such as might be used for endoscopy or simple local procedures) may be 200 to 300 square feet. The added flexibility of larger operating rooms must be balanced against the significantly higher initial construction cost.

Subsequent modifications of room size are often impossible or prohibitively expensive so that actual operating room space ought not be the place to compromise on space planning. Operating rooms have infrastructure needs and code requirements that differ substantially from those of a waiting area or storage space. For this reason, making one of these areas smaller or even eliminating it altogether may not generate cost savings that would allow the addition of comparable space to an operating room. Based on a 5- or 6-day week, 8-hour operating day schedule, an ambulatory surgical operating room can usually accommodate approximately 1500 cases per year, depending on the complexity of the operations and the efficiency of the facility. Many subtle variables affect the efficiency of a room so that the number of procedures actually performed may vary significantly from day to day, depending on how the room is used. In addition to the actual operating rooms, space must be allocated for reception, toilets, waiting areas, dressing areas, storage of equipment, business functions, anesthesia and nursing work areas, and utility rooms (see Chapter 3).

Once the needed spaces have been designated, crucial adjacencies and traffic patterns must be considered because these may identify space needs that were not previously allocated. The space required for the listed functions constitutes the net area. In addition, space for

circulation must be allocated. The circulation space is the space required to house the ventilation, electrical, mechanical, and structural systems that make the rest of the space functional. This is usually calculated to be approximately 40% of the total net area. The net area plus the circulation space determines the gross area.

When a freestanding facility is being built, it is also necessary to consider the costs of the land on which the building is to be constructed, including space for parking stalls. The latter varies in cost, depending on whether the parking area is a vertical structure or multiple stalls on the grounds. The cost of landscaping should also be included in the budget. Once this preliminary planning is done, floor plans and models can be constructed. This not only allows visualization of the imagined product (and the first opportunity for modifications) but also permits better estimation of the design and construction costs.

As the plans become further developed, fixed equipment, mounted fixtures, cabinetry, and other built-in needs can be incorporated into the plans. At this time, it is important to decide which items are to be permanently located in the operating rooms. Besides influencing cost, these decisions profoundly influence flexibility, need for storage space, and other seemingly less-related issues such as traffic patterns and materials management. The importance of flexibility cannot be overemphasized. Every detail of every function at every level of the unit must be programmed according to its physical location within the unit, its effect on overall flow through the unit, and the features that are pertinent to each of the areas within the unit. For example, for the reception area, the amount of seating that will likely be needed for patients and family members must be considered. However, because this is the area of first impression, it must also be comfortable and have an ambiance appropriate to the facility. Adjacencies to rest rooms, telephones, and refreshments for family members waiting for patients are important considerations. It is desirable to have an area designated for physicians to talk with family members privately and out of hearing distance of other waiting persons. Some facilities have "mini offices" or play areas incorporated into the reception and waiting areas; others have begun to provide beepers so that family members can go about other business while their loved ones undergo their procedures.

Once the design decisions are resolved, construction can begin. The construction costs include not only labor and materials but also ancillary costs of building inspections, permits, compliance with regulatory agency standards, and inflation adjustments that occur during the time of actual construction.

PHILOSOPHICAL CONSIDERATIONS

Both traditional hospital-based operating rooms and outpatient surgical suites, whether freestanding or part of a hospital system, must be designed to accommodate changing needs over a 20- to 30-year span. They must be versatile enough to adapt to new and changing technologic advances. Ambulatory care facilities differ from inpatient facilities because provider and patient expectations are different. Sick inpatients are much less aware of the ambiance of the operating suite than are outpatients, who are taking time out for a procedure but do not perceive themselves as being ill. For outpatients, privacy, flow and efficiency, and comfortable, aesthetically pleasing environments are important components that contribute to their impression of the health care experience.

For the provider, the outpatient surgical suite is an extension of the clinic or office. User friendliness is measured by the ease with which administrative functions can be done and the efficiency of the actual operative process. As procedures of increasing complexity are done in the outpatient venue, the challenge is to maintain the amenities that attract patients and providers to this venue. The future may take either of two directions: (1) closer integration with the inpatient facility and increased regulation and restriction as to which sorts of procedures may be done in each setting, or (2) expansion of services in surgicenters to include procedures that require overnight monitoring or short postoperative stays in a recovery facility. If the latter becomes the trend, the differentiation between the small, low-acuity community-based hospital surgical service and the surgicenter–recovery facility will become less well defined.

ORGANIZATIONAL CONSIDERATIONS

In the present climate of health care alliances, mergers, and managed care, it is difficult to precisely define the best organizational model. Flexibility, in a setting committed to efficient, service-oriented, clinically excellent care, regardless of ownership, will probably determine the ultimate success of a unit. Measurement instruments in the areas of utilization management and review, outcome measurement, and practice standards will be important both as internal indicators of the quality of care being delivered and as marketing tools. To perform these functions, a well-designed information system is essential. This system not only must capture patient demographic information and billing and financial data and track patients through the facility but also must interface with ancillary service data systems including laboratory, radiology, materials management, and ideally even individual surgeon's offices. As outpatient procedures become increasingly complex, ambulatory operating rooms are more and more coming to resemble inpatient operating rooms. The challenge to be faced will be one of increasing the complexity of the procedures being done in outpatient facilities while maintaining an atmosphere of patient safety, cost efficiency, and user-friendliness.

Selected Readings

1. Berkoff MJ, Pangrazio JR. Planning and designing ambulatory surgical facilities. In Davis JE, ed. Major Ambulatory Surgery, Baltimore: Williams & Wilkins, 1986:73–88.
2. Davis JE. The major ambulatory surgical center and how it is developed. Surg Clin North Am 1987;67(4):671–692.
3. Grubb RD, Ondov G. Planning Ambulatory Surgery Facilities. St. Louis: CV Mosby Company, 1979.
4. Knauer-Stengel CS, Allo MD. Critical issues in the planning of surgical suites. In Malangoni M, ed. Critical Issues in Operating Room Management. Philadelphia: Lippincott-Raven, 1997:1–32.

Standards for the Ambulatory Surgery Center

Chapter 6

Quality Issues in Ambulatory Care

John P. Remensnyder

The central issue of providing quality medical care has built momentum over the years until, at the present time, those who take care of patients are riding the crest of what is known in some circles as the "quality movement." What has spurred this movement? What is the definition of quality medical care? And, what forms to assure quality care have developed? These are all crucial questions to be answered in order to penetrate the confusing thicket of modern concepts of quality in medicine.

The simple act of a physician taking care of a sick person has progressed to the current complex of provision of medical care by physicians, nurses, hospitals, managed care plans, insurance schemes, and government regulation. Even as medical care delivery has become more complicated, several forces have focused on the quality of care delivered. Third party payers insist that hospitals and doctors reduce costs substantially while they also market the quality of their managed care plan to prospective buyers. Meanwhile, a growing realization on the part of the public at large that the results of medical care are not uniformly excellent or of high quality has led to demands for ever ascending levels of quality in the medical care received. An increasingly sophisticated lay public has come to realize that a reliance on technologic advances in medical care has not been followed in all cases by an improvement in the quality of care rendered. These factors are real and constitute a force to be reckoned with. At the same time, it is not clear what the phrase "quality health care" means for each factor. Such definition is essential if there is to be any precision in discussions of quality issues in medicine. Several definitions of quality health care have been put forth in recent years, and several of these are considered.

In 1974, The Institute of Medicine, which is a part of the National Academy of Science, grappled with the emerging issues of assessing and assuring quality in medical care, and it defined quality health care as that which is "... effective in bettering the health status and satisfaction of a population, within the resources that society and individuals have chosen to spend for that care." As comprehensive as this definition is, it omits any mention of goals and aspirations for quality care of a given population.

The American Medical Association in 1986 issued a report that listed eight features that should be part of goals in achieving quality health care. They are to (1) produce optimal improvement in a patient's health, (2) emphasize health promotion and disease prevention, (3) be provided in a timely fashion, (4) be predicated on informed consent, (5) be based on accepted medical principles, (6) use empathy in providing care, (7) use technology appropriately and efficiently, and (8) be documented to allow for professional review. These features clearly reflect an individual physician's optimal practices while omitting organizational considerations in providing quality medical care.

In 1983, Palmer described five critical factors to be at the base of quality care provided by both individuals and organizations. "Effectiveness" is the power of a particular procedure or treatment to improve health status. "Efficiency" is the delivery of the maximum number of compatible units of health care for a given number of health resources used. "Accessibility" is the ease with which health care can be reached in the face of financial, organizational, cultural, and emotional barriers. "Acceptability" is the degree to which health care satisfies patients. "Provider competence" is the ability to use the best available knowledge and judgment to provide health and satisfaction of patients, with the provider being either an individual or an entire health care delivery system.

One of the many federal agencies involved with health care regulation and provision, the Office of Technology Assessment (OTA), put forth a succinct definition of quality health care in 1988, stating ". . . the quality of health care is the degree to which the process of care increases the probability of outcomes desired by patients and decreases the probability of undesired outcomes, given the state of medical knowledge." Based on the goals and aims of an individual patient, the OTA laid emphasis on the outcome of medical care, a critical element in the contemporary health care environment.

Each of the definitions given captures important facets of quality in health care. In a laudable and largely successful effort to blend various elements into a unified definition of quality health care, Benson and Townes, drawing heavily on the concepts of The Institute of Medicine and Palmer, put forth a concept of quality medical care as ". . . that which *works*, that is *cost effective*, that is delivered by *appropriate providers*, that extends care to *all who need it when they want it*, and that *satisfies* the full set of the customer's requirements." This definition, which is brief yet comprehensive, is the basis for the following discussion of quality issues in the provision of care in the ambulatory surgical setting.

QUALITY ASSURANCE AND QUALITY IMPROVEMENT

In modern health care, the drive for quality has taken many forms, the two outstanding ones being quality assurance and quality improvement. Quality assurance is most often known by its initials QA, whereas quality improvement is known by several initial combinations: QI, CQI (continuous quality improvement), and TQM (total quality management). Initially separate, these two forces have become increasingly intertwined in the continuous effort to raise the quality of medical care, hence the combination QA/QI is encountered with greater frequency.

Quality Assurance

The definition of quality assurance lies largely within programmatic boundaries. Simply put, quality assurance refers to those activities of a clinical unit or health care organization that are designed to assess and monitor the quality of care provided by that group; the results of the assessment and monitoring process are then used to change existing practices or institute new methods to assure or improve high quality care in that unit or organization. A critical aspect of this program is that the results must be communicated widely and effectively within the organization to achieve the results desired.

Quality assurance has a distinguished lineage. More than a century and a half ago, Florence Nightingale carefully collected data that documented the wounded and ill British soldiers admitted to field hospitals during the Crimean War, nearly half of whom died. Her quantitation rang alarms in the halls of the British military establishment, which subsequently took steps to improve hygiene and medical and nursing care. Her later work, quantitatively assessing mortality rates in London hospitals, led to serious inquiries regarding the effect of hospital care on mortality rates.

Ernest Amory Codman at the Massachusetts General Hospital during the years preceding World War I developed a method of assessing the end results of treatments using carefully kept records and continuous appraisal of patient outcomes. He emphasized ". . . the end result idea . . . which was merely the common sense notion that every hospital should follow every patient it treats, long enough to determine whether or not the treatment has been successful, and then inquire 'if not, why not' with a view to preventing similar failures in the future."

Efforts at quality assurance first became institutionalized on December 20, 1917, when the American College of Surgeons (ACS) established the Hospital Standardization Program. Concerned about the deplorable standards of care in many American hospitals, the ACS put forth a single-page statement of minimum requirements for hospitals to meet in order to provide quality medical care. Beginning inspections the following year, the ACS found that only 13% of hospitals surveyed met the minimum standards. From this dramatic beginning, the Hospital Standardization Program grew to be the keystone of the overarching functions of evaluating and assuring quality care in this country.

In 1951, the Joint Commission on Accreditation of Hospitals (JCAH) was formed through the conjoined efforts of the ACS, the American College of Physicians, the American Medical Association, the American Hospital Association, and the Canadian Medical Association. The Canadian organization withdrew in 1959, opening the door for the American Dental Association to join in sponsorship in 1980. In 1952, the JCAH began its formal hospital accreditation program, which superseded the ACS Hospital Standardization Program. By 1989, the accreditation process had been extended to a wide spectrum of health care facilities, thus necessitating a name change to the Joint Commission on Accreditation of Healthcare Organizations (JCAHO).

Initially, the JCAH relied on existing hospital statistics, data, and systems upon which to base its assessments. Quality assurance was clearly identified by the JCAH as the responsibility of the medical staff of hospitals and other health care institutions. There was little structured quality assurance effort until the early 1970s, at which time the JCAH acted in response to growing legislative and regulatory efforts to review and judge quality of medical care. Formal assessment processes and standards were devised to identify quality assurance during hospital surveys. Since that time, the form of quality assurance has undergone at least four metamorphoses. The first phase emphasized focused medical care studies by conducting chart audits and reviews of specific medical and surgical conditions, seeking general problems emerging from specific reviews. The second phase occupied the first half of the decade of the 1980s and stressed problem seeking in the broadest sense. The JCAH relaxed restrictions on the methodology of problem finding but required an examination of the broad systematic aspect of delivery of health care within medical institutions. Organizational commitment to the quality assurance process was fundamental to this process. Phase 3 followed during the next 5 to 7 years, returning to an emphasis on structural analysis with rigorously defined monitoring and assessment activities with its associated Ten-Step Process and the requirement for the development of clinical indicators of important aspects of medical care. The emphasis still was on the conduct of medical care with relatively little concern for the organizational aspects of hospitals. The fourth phase, which was heralded by the JCAHO Agenda for Change and which is currently in place, embodies a radical shift from traditional quality assurance activities to the rapid assimilation of industry-based concepts of quality improvement, which emphasize that the individual practitioner does not so much cause problems of medical care as do deficiencies in systems throughout the health care organization in question. Although much of the traditional monitoring and evaluation processes remain, the accreditation process currently relies heavily on evidence of organizational commitment to traditional industrial concepts of CQI and TQM. In the evolution of QA/QI under the aegis of the JCAHO, there has been little formal attention to QA/QI in the ambulatory care setting until recently. Standards for the evaluation and accreditation of ambulatory care facilities by the JCAHO are being revised in the face of accrediting activities by a variety of governmental and nongovernmental agencies.

Quality Improvement

The basic concepts of quality improvement are based on the theories of W. Edwards Deming and Joseph Juran who introduced quality improvement theory and methods into the post-World War II Japanese automobile industry and are generally credited as being responsible for the Japanese processes and products becoming preeminent in the industrial field. Quality improvement relegates classic quality control to a minor role in achievement of industrial excellence while centering on the description, measurement, and constant improvement of all key and critical processes. Constant seeking to improve all aspects of the industrial process is the hallmark of the successful application of quality improvement.

Defining quality improvement in a single statement is difficult because quality improvement embodies attitude, method, and assumption. The attitude is one of proactive striving to avoid errors and constantly improve the processes at hand by the methods of systems analysis, measurement, and institution of action. Quality improvement assumes that it is not individuals who are at the root of most quality problems, but rather systems and processes. Industrial concepts of quality improvement are directly transferrable to health care systems because health care organizations have operational defects just as do industrial organizations. For example, hospitals have many process areas amenable to quality improvement including clinical care, governance, management, and support procedures. Hospitals share several characteristics of quality improvement in common with industry: the leadership of organizations drive the QI process, customer–supplier relationships become understood, QI concentrates on variations in normal processes and seeks to control such variations, all organizational personnel are involved in the process of examining processes, and formal problem-solving methods and statistical tools are used.

Deming compiled a succinct set of principles regarding quality improvement that has come to be known as "Deming's 14 Points," which can be applied to improve delivery of quality health care (Table 6–1). These critical points have been used in appropriately altered forms in virtually every attempt to introduce quality improvement thinking and methods into health care organizations and accrediting agencies such as the JCAHO.

Quantitative tools underlie much of the methodology of quality improvement. The

Table 6–1. Deming's Fourteen Points

1. Create constancy of purpose toward improvement of product and service.
2. Adopt the new philosophy of continuous improvement.
3. Cease dependence on inspection to achieve quality.
4. End the practice of awarding business on the basis of price tag.
5. Improve constantly and forever the system of production and service.
6. Institute training on the job.
7. Institute leadership to insist on quality improvement.
8. Drive out fear and foster trust within the organization.
9. Break down barriers between departments.
10. Eliminate slogans, exhortations, and targets for the work force.
11. Eliminate numerical quotas and management by objective.
12. Remove barriers to pride of workmanship.
13. Institute a vigorous program of education and self-improvement.
14. Put everyone in the organization to work to accomplish the transformation

Adapted from Out of the Crisis by W. Edwards Deming by permission of MIT and The W. Edwards Deming Institute. Published by MIT, Center for Advanced Educational Services, Cambridge, MA 02139. Copyright 1986 by the W. Edwards Deming Institute.

seven methods of quantification that are generally part of the quality improvement process are listed in Table 6–2. The "tools" listed in Table 6–2 are familiar because they appear in medical journal articles and presentations of clinical and basic research data. In their simplest forms, they can be deceptively useful in dissecting problems and identifying opportunities for improvement in the processes and systems of health care organizations.

The current accreditation process of the JCAHO includes five important areas of quality improvement emphasis, which are designed to more fully incorporate principles and tech-

Table 6–2. Quantitative Tools of Quality Improvement

Cause and effect charts—are otherwise known as "fishbone" or Ishikawa charts.
Pareto diagrams—are rank-ordered histograms used to identify the important causes of problems as opposed to the many others.
Flow charts—help to identify opportunities for improvement and problems needing solution.
Control charts—show variations in a process and show which variations need corrective action.
Run charts—are similar to control charts but are designed to show performance over time and identify trends.
Histograms—of the traditional variety measure the rate and frequency of an occurrence.
Scatter diagrams—graphically show a relation between two variables.

niques that will assure continuous improvement in performance and quality: (1) leadership responsibility for quality improvement, (2) techniques of quality improvement, (3) education and training, (4) communication and collaboration, and (5) evaluation of effectiveness of quality improvement activities.

Interrelation of Quality Assurance and Quality Improvement

The older concepts and processes of quality assurance are rapidly merging with the theory and practice of quality improvement in the management and accreditation of health care organizations. Table 6–3 demonstrates the evolution of this process.

The relation between quality assurance and quality improvement is best described as a sequential one: quality assurance triggers quality improvement. At this time of transition in the assessment of quality, traditional quality assurance analyses and activities are well established in hospitals, outpatient centers, and other health care organizations. Problems identified by the quality assurance process are then subjected to quality improvement procedures and techniques to achieve not only specific problem resolution but also identify ways to improve overall functioning. Current experiences with the use of quality assurance and quality improvement in quality assessment in the hospital settings vary among institutions, lending further credence to the contention that the current quality assessment climate is one of transition.

There appear to be at least four approaches to the use of quality assurance and quality improvement in individual hospitals. First,

Table 6–3. Evolution of Quality Assessment in Health Care Organizations

Chart and incidents review using traditional mortality and morbidity reviews

Clinical practices studies using specific time intervals and retrospective audits

Standard-based ongoing monitoring and evaluation using traditional quality assurance approach

Organization-wide program of process and systems analysis and continual improvement using total quality management approach

some health care givers do not perceive the two to be integrated at all, believing that quality assurance is the more important of the two and that it should take precedence over any form of quality improvement, which is completely separate. Second, certain institutions have adopted the tools of quality improvement to help facilitate the quality assurance process. Third, other institutions understand that, even though quality assurance is essential to the monitoring and evaluation process, it is used to identify quality improvement opportunities, at which point quality improvement teams, using quality improvement tools, are formed to investigate and solve problems identified in the original quality assurance process. Fourth, some hospitals have completely integrated the two, with traditional quality assurance being absorbed as the initial segment of a comprehensive CQI or TQM program.

Regardless of the stage of integration of quality assurance and quality improvement at any given hospital, major currents are flowing in the direction of more complete blending and integration of the two. In this evolving blend, one important change already underway is the changing character of the monitoring tools used to evaluate important aspects of practice. Increasingly, monitors are converted from their current high specificity to instruments that measure entire processes and outcomes of those processes as defined in the broadest sense. Outcome evaluation increasingly is being recognized as a crucial part of the quality assessment process.

OUTCOMES IN QUALITY ASSESSMENT

The analysis and definition of the outcomes of medical care plans, procedures, techniques, and systems represent a key feature of contemporary and future attempts to assess quality in the delivery of health care. Together with the "quality movement," the "outcomes movement" has assumed a life and momentum of its own. Ellwood has proposed a broadly based, straightforward, and highly pragmatic definition of the modern outcome analytic process as ". . . a technology of patient experience designed to help patients, payers, and providers make rational medical care–related choices based on better insight into the effect of these choices on the patient's life." Ellwood describes the five main components of outcomes management as (1) a heavy reliance on standards and guidelines developed by professionals to guide therapeutic choices made by physicians, (2) a dependence on a regular and systematic quantification of patients' well being and functioning, (3) the availability of the aggregation of clinical and outcome data to physicians as large unified databases, (4) the easy availability of the appropriate sections of the databases to physicians and health care organizations as they make clinical and other forms of decisions, and (5) the importance of the patients' perception and assessment as an important aspect of quality of care outcomes.

Endpoints in outcomes evaluation continually shift and proliferate while new forms of data sources and measurement methods emerge. A consideration of the current spectrum of outcome endpoints provides a view of the broadening character of the "outcomes movement." Traditional endpoints in analyzing outcomes have been mortality, morbidity, and charges. These endpoints still serve as the important beginnings for any comprehensive analysis of outcomes of patient care; however, collection of data based on the experience of a single practitioner or institution is becoming increasingly supplanted by the use of state-wide, national, and provider databases. Beyond the three endpoints stated, more reliance will be placed on conditions of survival measures in assessing outcome. Queries in this area will seek to determine whether patients surviving a treatment course are disease-free, palliated of their condition, or incompletely treated. Administrative and organizational endpoints assume increased importance in this field. Virtually every step in organizational processes (e.g., the admitting process, discharge procedures, patient education) has an outcome that can be measured using traditional methods as well as quality improvement techniques and managed care data. Costs—not simply financial charges—are a key area of outcomes evaluation. Cost–benefit analyses of critical processes and their outcome will subject such areas as clinical expertise, organizational resources, personnel practices, finan-

cial structure, and physical plant to intense scrutiny. Finally, patient preference and satisfaction has become progressively identified as one of the most important measurable outcomes of quality health care, an area in which surveys and questionnaires, as well as individual experiential data, will be used.

Outcomes management and QA/QI in determining quality in health care delivery and its associated organizations become increasingly joined as quality assessment progresses and matures. An appreciation of this phenomenon helps in understanding the present status of the accreditation process, especially the growing efforts to judge and accredit ambulatory care facilities and ambulatory surgical centers in particular.

QUALITY ISSUES AND THE AMBULATORY SURGICAL CENTER

Before considering the specifics of quality assessment and accreditation of ambulatory surgical centers (ASCs), it is necessary to gain an overview of the process as it is currently being performed in inpatient facilities. At the moment, the full force of quality assessment requirements and accreditation demands has not been directed at ambulatory facilities, so it is crucial to examine the procedures of inpatient quality determination and accreditation because what is being done today in this area will determine how the process will be shaped tomorrow in reference to ambulatory care and surgical centers.

Generic Accreditation and Quality Concerns

Fundamental to the Agenda for Change of the JCAHO is the concept that, in response to the rapidly changing health care and cost environment, hospitals and other medical facilities will no longer be permitted to simply point to quality improvement processes that they have in place but will be required to demonstrate such improvement in quality care by means of clinical outcome assessment systems. Previously, indicators have stressed structures and processes; currently, it is necessary to develop standards against which to measure outcomes to gain an assessment of quality and appropriateness of care. The JCAHO stresses the following six key elements in determination of quality care:

1. Quality must be emphasized as a central priority of the health care organization in question, not only in its mission and vision statements but also in the day-to-day care and other activities.
2. The leaders of the institution must be knowledgeable and actively involved in the pursuit of quality.
3. The central focus must be on processes that lead to a determination of outcomes that will be used in evaluating quality levels.
4. Reliable and appropriate statistical methods must be used.
5. A spirit of cooperation will characterize the health care organization dedicated to quality.
6. Likewise, mutual respect and support among the people and units reflect a barrier-free organization.

The JCAHO summarizes its current efforts, stating, ". . . [the] manual is being issued at a time when the health care field is redesigning its performance-improvement mechanisms to incorporate concepts and methods developed by other fields. Such concepts and methods include total quality management (TQM), continuous quality improvement (CQI), and systems thinking. The health care field is also incorporating into its performance-improvement mechanisms concepts and methods developed by the health service research community, such as reference databases, clinical practice guidelines or parameters, functional status, and quality-of-life measures."

Unique Features of Ambulatory Surgical Centers in Quality Assessment Accreditation

Ambulatory surgical care is delivered in at least four settings: (1) clinics and private offices, (2) freestanding ASCs (either single specialty or multispecialty), (3) hospital-based ASCs, and (4) as integrated hospital-based ambulatory surgery. Costs are least at clinics and most at integrated hospital-based settings. The chance for ensuring quality, however, is lowest at the office and highest in the fully integrated ambulatory surgical environment. This highlights the fact that only recently have full accreditation procedures been developed for ambulatory care facilities, especially since traditional QA techniques were not easily applicable to the ambulatory care and ASCs.

Determination and assurance of quality in the ambulatory surgical experience, regardless of the setting, may be confounded by several factors unique to ambulatory care. Outcomes are often difficult to define. For example, adverse events or complications may occur unreported at home after discharge from the ASC and may even be treated at another facility or provider. Furthermore, there is less control over the patient and postoperative care because the patient leaves the ASC directly from the recovery area and the surgeon therefore has to rely on the effectiveness of the patient education process at discharge and the reliability of the patient to carry out instructions for postoperative care. Coordination of care among several providers in the ambulatory setting may be difficult to achieve unless the ASC is part of a tightly integrated organization in possession of a superior information management system. Patient rapport with the surgeon may not be as secure as that developed in the inpatient circumstance because of duration of contact and intensity of the clinical encounter. All of these factors may result in failure of compliance and follow-up—both being critical factors in determining outcomes and assessing the quality level of care.

Elements involved in quality assessment of the ASC are somewhat different compared with those of inpatient facilities. Quality care elements or important aspects of care from a quality assurance standpoint include both clinical and organizational factors. Clinical elements are summarized in Table 6–4 and organizational elements are tabulated in Table 6–5. Two important sources amplify and provide extended discussions of quality factors in the ASC: the publication by the ACS Board of Governors' Committee on Ambulatory Surgical Care titled "Guidelines for Optimal Office-

Table 6–4. Clinical Elements of Quality Assessment in Ambulatory Surgical Centers

Patients' rights
Preadmission evaluation and testing
Preoperative laboratory testing
Preoperative patient and family education
Operating room
Anesthesia procedures
Monitoring techniques (intraoperative)
Recovery process and monitoring
Discharge process
Postoperative patient and family education
Ambulatory surgery center follow-up process
Qualifications of professionals (surgeons, anesthesiologists,
    nurses, ancillary personnel)
  Credentialing
  Continuing education
  Performance evaluations
  Competence assessment
Emergency procedures and equipment
Pathology and clinical laboratory services
Radiology services

Table 6–6. JCAHO 10 Steps of the Monitoring and Evaluation Process

Steps

1:	Assign responsibility
2:	Delineate scope of care and service
3:	Identify important aspects of care and service
4:	Identify indicators
5:	Establish means to trigger evaluation
6:	Collect and organize data
7:	Initiate evaluation
8:	Take actions to improve care and service
9:	Assess the effectiveness of actions and ensure that improvement is maintained
10:	Communicate results to relevant individuals and groups

Based Surgery" and the "Ambulatory Health Care Manual" of the JCAHO.

The JCAHO has recently promulgated indicators for areas of anesthesia, obstetrics, cardiovascular disease, oncology, and trauma. The intended use of these indicators is to provide health care organizations common indicators for the assessment process against which to judge performance and quality. This will confer a greater degree of uniformity in the evaluation process. In the use of such indicators in the assessment process, or, as more traditionally viewed, the monitoring and evaluation process, the JCAHO has for some time recom-

Table 6–5. Organizational Elements of Quality Assessment in Ambulatory Surgical Centers

Governing body and leadership
Administration and organization
Patient information system
  Medical record
  Office record
  Information transfer to other facilities
Admission process
Scheduling process
Physical plant
Equipment and supplies
  Product evaluation
  Safe Medical Devices Act
  Maintenance and inspection
Decontamination and sterilization
Infection control
Safety—patients and personnel
Efficiency evaluation
Financial procedures

mended the use of a so-called Ten-Step Process, which is detailed in Table 6–6. Even though this process continues to undergo slow change, the process is soundly based and useful. In addition, the Ten-Step Process contains a feedback loop, demonstrating yet another interaction between quality assurance and quality improvement, that is, after the completion of the 10 steps, information communicated to individuals and groups may identify problems that necessitate further data collection, thereby serving to reinitiate step 6, which then continues back again through steps 7 through 10. The process, whereby problems identified in the traditional quality assurance process using the ten steps serve to identify opportunities to set in motion quality improvement analyses and procedures, clearly describes the intimate and increasingly inextricable relation between the two qualities: assurance and improvement.

THE FUTURE OF QUALITY ISSUES IN AMBULATORY SURGICAL CENTERS

Attempts to describe the future of any endeavor are risky at best, but, in striving to provide the best quality care for patients, it is imperative to continually make improvements. Benson and Townes point out several factors in ambulatory care and surgery that will soon have a profound effect on quality assessment and accreditation. With managed care and gatekeepers dominating the field, there will be substantial compensation changes for all physicians and surgeons. Ambulatory reimbursement schemes will move toward a diagnosis-related group style or capitated form. Information and communication technology will become essential for proper clinical and organizational function. With the ultimate creation of national databases for ambulatory care statistics, quality in the broadest sense will become evermore important. Certainly, the value of QA/QI will become more greatly accepted by individual practitioners as well as by health care and managed care organizations. Given such acceptance, the increasing sophistication of quality technology, and the growing importance of outcomes analysis and management, it is almost inevitable that some sort of clearly defined national quality leadership will emerge. With these changes, the seismic landscape of the quality and outcomes movements is likely to undergo major and minor tremors for years to come.

Selected Readings

1. AMA Council on Medical Services. Quality of care. Conn Med 1986;50:832–834.
2. Benson DS, Townes PG Jr. Excellence in Ambulatory Care. San Francisco: Jossey-Bass, 1990:56.
3. Deming WE. Out of the Crisis. Cambridge, MA: MIT Press, 1986.
4. Ellwood PM. Shattuck Lecture. Outcomes management: a technology of patient experience. N Engl J Med 1988;318:1549–1556.
5. Institute of Medicine. Advancing the Quality of Health Care: Key Issues and Fundamental Principles. Washington, DC: National Academy of Sciences, 1974.
6. Joint Commission on Accreditation of Healthcare Organizations. 1995 Accreditation Manual for Hospitals. Oakbrook Terrace, IL: Joint Commission on Accreditation of Healthcare Organizations, 1994.
7. Joint Commission on Accreditation of Healthcare Organizations. Ambulatory Health Care Manual. Oakbrook Terrace, IL: Joint Commission on Accreditation of Healthcare Organizations, 1994.
8. Palmer RH. Ambulatory Health Care Evaluation: Principles and Practices. Chicago: American Hospital Association, 1983:15.
9. US Congress Office of Technology Assessment. The Quality of Medical Care: Information for Consumers. Washington, DC: US Government Printing Office; June 1988; OTA-H-386.

Credentialing Issues

Frederick W. Ackroyd

Life is short and art is long; the time and instant of treatment precarious, and the crisis grievous. It is necessary for the physician not only to provide the needed treatment but to provide for the patient himself and for those beside him and to provide for his outside affairs.

HIPPOCRATES, 5TH CENTURY BC

Throughout the ages, the need for accountability of physicians and surgeons produced codes of conduct designed to ensure competence and ethical practice and assign responsibility for adverse outcomes. Society has, through legislation, regulation, and licensure, defined the education, training, and experience, as well as the professional ethics, expected of its surgeons to ensure their competence and social responsibility. The process of credentialing has traditionally been seen as a means of certifying a person's claim to competence for the privilege of performing surgery.

Avery Codman in his "End Results Hospital" in the 1920s, Frederick Taylor at the Hawthorne Research Laboratories of the General Electric Corporation, and Juran and Demming in the industrial engineering setting have all attempted to define the ingredients of quality performance and its impact on the outcomes. Credentialing is an exercise to help ensure quality performance in an appropriate and ethical manner by practitioners of surgery. To restore public trust in the profession, it has become necessary to strengthen controls and accountability of what goes on between doctors and patients. Thus, quality assurance activities and regulation of the medical profession have grown. The introduction of a large number of middle-level quality assurance and qual-

ity improvement monitors and utilization review managers has introduced a costly layer of bureaucracy without necessarily demonstrating a noticeable improvement in quality.

CREDENTIALING AND QUALITY ASSURANCE

Quality in health care is an elusive concept. Most people know it when they see it, but it is hard to document and define. Avis Donabedian at the University of Michigan described three components of quality in healthcare: structure, process, and outcome.

Structural components of health care quality include the physical plant as well as a well-integrated staff and strong trustee leadership working in an organization that is reflective of the mission of the organization. The financial structure should create incentives that are socially redeeming in terms of patient care but should also include fiscal responsibility and survival of the institution.

The day-to-day care of patients depends on coordinated activities by physicians and hospital staff in many different departments. The success with which this is achieved is a measure of the commitment to excellence of the organization and the quality of the process. Hospital staffs develop programs of continuing quality improvement and quality assurance, which include morbidity and mortality meetings, the setting of guidelines and critical pathways to help achieve consensus in the management of patients, and the measurement of conformance of surgeons to the standards that are mutually arrived at as criteria for staff membership.

The development of quality indicators and the awareness of complications ensure that outcomes are measured so that the welfare of patients is documented, their health is maintained, and they are satisfied with their care. There is a growing tendency to separate evaluation of adverse events—those relating to negligence, incompetence, or lapses of judgment—from those deriving from systems problems. Professional competency issues can be dealt with in credentialing, mentoring, proctoring, and continuing remedial educational activities at the staff level. Process and systems issues must be addressed at hospital-wide levels to enhance organizational improvement.

The medical profession no longer is the only one monitoring the quality of care. The federal government, the Office of Consumer Affairs of the state, the Board of Registration in Medicine, third party payers, the general public in the form of consumer advocates, and the legal profession in the form of the plaintiffs' bar are all overseeing the activities of practitioners in the care of patients. The quid pro quo for tort reform to obtain relief from increasing malpractice insurance rates was an aggressive program of quality assurance, which includes strict quality control of surgical privileges and establishing whether the skills and competence were in place to ensure the best outcome that could be expected under the given circumstances. The matter is perceived as a problem of trust and lack of confidence in the medical profession due to increasing awareness of the occurrence of adverse events, occasionally resulting from physician neglect and incompetence or poor judgment, and the failure of the medical profession to weed out and correct malfeasance and incompetence in its ranks.

ESTABLISHING THE CREDENTIALING PROCESS

Whenever people are entrusted with the welfare and physical well being of others (e.g., a ship captain, an airline pilot, a surgeon), society sets standards that must be met to protect the interests of persons using the services. All models of this process share the concept of education, training, and experience, coupled with maturity, good judgment, integrity, and reliability to carry out the appropriate function.

When a health care institution is established to care for people by physicians, nurses, and other staff, the trustees or governing body first must determine the mission, goals, and objectives of the organization. They ensure that the facilities and personnel are adequate and appropriate to carry out that mission. They establish an organizational structure and adopt bylaws, which specify functional relationships among the various components of the organization. They ensure that the quality of care is evaluated and that problems are appropriately identified and corrected. The medical staff must be carefully screened for appointment and reappointment, and a rigorous standard of performance must be exacted or the hospital will fail to fulfill its primary mission, the provision of high-quality patient care.

Credentialing is the process of setting performance standards and then awarding the right to care for patients on the basis of these standards. The social agenda of persons who set the standards often dictates the outcome of the process. Depending on the social goals of those entrusted with setting the priorities for the process, credentialing can achieve many different outcomes. It is a form of social engineering and has both risks and benefits.

Criteria could be established that would achieve certain goals, such as providing high-quality care or selecting only those surgeons who are minimal users of resources, which is attractive to insurance companies. Setting criteria that selected only surgeons whose patients had no complications or few deaths might result in selecting surgeons who did simpler procedures on healthier patients and declined to care for high-risk patients with complicated problems.

Regrettably, credentialing is sometimes used to get rid of employees who are troublesome for a variety of reasons, some economic, some administrative and departmental, some psychological and social. Avery Codman, who pioneered the "end results concept" of quality control in the 1920s, was not reappointed to

Table 7–1. Criteria in the Credentialing Process

Certification: a written confirmation that the surgeon has
  satisfactorily completed courses of study (e.g., medical
  school, residency, American Board of Surgery, specialty
  certificates)
State licensure
Competence: peer review and recommendations and
  evaluation to ensure a level of skill and ability necessary to
  satisfactorily carry out procedures in the care of patients
Mentoring: supervision, usually on an individual basis, such as
  by the training program director who recommends the
  surgeon for privileges
Proctoring: the observation and evaluation of the
  performance of a trainee as part of the credentialing
  process to establish the qualifications of the operator
Personal interview
National Physician Data Bank report
Malpractice carrier—claim and judgment review
Narcotics and controlled substances license
Peer evaluation
Ethics review
Professional performance
Felonies or criminal proceedings
Psychological evaluation
Absence of substance abuse
General health
Continuing medical education participation
Record keeping
Conformance with bylaws
Successful completion of American Board of Surgery
  examination
Morbidity and mortality review cases reviewed
Participation in departmental activities
Contribution to scientific journals
Contributions to resident and medical student teaching
Participation in medical school and hospital committee work
Community service outside the hospital
Free service in clinic for indigent patients

the surgical staff of his own hospital when he questioned the surgical methods and outcomes assessment of patients by the senior surgical staff.

To guarantee integrity, the credentialing process must be open and shared, and the criteria for appointment must be mutually agreed upon (such as Joint Commission on Accreditation of Healthcare Organizations [JCAHO] guidelines) to best serve the rights and interests of all concerned. Elements for consideration in the credentialing process are listed in Table 7–1.

CREDENTIALING A SURGEON— THE PROCESS

The governing body of the hospital (in most cases the trustees), directs the chairman of the department to set up criteria in consultation with its section chiefs and direct the quality assurance committees to review the individual surgeon's performance in each of the areas stipulated, by prior consensus, for evaluation. Hospital privileges are granted by the board of trustees based on the recommendation of the department chairman and must be earned by satisfactory performance in all areas.

Care and sensitivity must be exercised to avoid conflict of interest in recruitment of staff and granting privileges across disciplines. Many procedures are being done by physicians, gastroenterologists, interventional radiologists, as well as surgeons, and the criteria for privileges must be essentially the same, assuming similar education, training, experience, and competence of the candidates.

When the credentialing process reveals questions about an individual surgeon's capabilities, physical capacity, or performance, the matter should be discussed with the individual by the chairman of the department of surgery. If the surgeon disagrees, an appeal mechanism, including a hearing by a committee of peers and limited due process, should be considered to protect the rights of the individual and the integrity of the credentialing process. The determination of this committee, as well as the recommendation of the chairman, should be referred to the trustees for final action.

The mechanisms for defining which procedures or types of patients alluded to in the surgeons' request for privileges can be either a list of specific procedures for which the surgeon is certified or can be a general grouping of patients or procedures such as pediatric surgery, endoscopy, orthopedic arthroscopy, cosmetic procedures (e.g., face-lifts, breast augmentation, breast reduction), or hand surgery (e.g., for carpal tunnel). Whereas large groupings of procedures are too general, particularly in an age of specialization and technically demanding procedures, the individual procedure list approach may be too specific. If a particular procedure was not included in the itemized list and an adverse event or poor outcome occurred, the hospital and the surgeon might be left open to legal challenge after the event. Volume of cases, particularly for complex procedures, may determine maintenance of skills necessary to provide for patient safety. Considerations such as average length of stay for different diagnoses, consumption of hospital resources for each diagnosis, and number of complications occurring in relation to the number of major cases are all criteria that may be carefully considered in reappointment.

When a new procedure is introduced, such as laparoscopic hernia repair, it must first be determined that the procedure is reasonable and efficacious. Any practice that might be construed as experimental requires review by the institutional review board. Surgeons who have not been trained in the new procedure or technique must take postgraduate didactic courses and have hands-on mentoring to develop the skills necessary to do the procedures safely.

FUTURE CONCERNS

In the future, there will be improved patient care information systems with better databases. They will span the state and federal payers for health care [i.e., Medicare, Medicaid, and other third party payers such as indemnity plans, managed care plans, and health maintenance organizations (HMOs)]. This means that there will be economic credentialing as these enormous databases are developed across different hospitals by the managed care insurance companies to keep score of the use of resources by surgeons. Medicare, Medicaid, managed care, and indemnity insurance companies will provide documentation in great detail of the financial aspects of health care, and physicians will be judged by their consumption of resources as well as by outcomes and patient satisfaction. As capitation arrangements for risk sharing become more widespread in health plans, economic credentialing may be used by physician groups to evaluate surgeons for reappointment on the basis of their ability to conserve resources as well. The lack of stratification of patients for complexity of the surgical procedure and severity of illness often makes these raw data misleading and invalid to determine surgeon skill and competence.

Legal issues surrounding "any willing provider" legislation will arise when surgeons are denied access to patients as certain insurance plans perceive them to be less thrifty in their use of medical resources than their peers. This legislation originally guaranteed that patient choice of physicians would not be limited by insurers except on the basis of legitimate considerations of quality and cost. The ability of the insurance companies to bargain with surgeons would be greatly impaired by "any willing provider" legislation. The corollary to this is that surgeons will be recruited only when willing to give discounts to insurance companies in return for patients and to be thrifty in allowing access to care and use of resources for those patients who are referred to them.

The documentation of length of stay for different diagnoses, the use of hospital resources per diagnosis, and use of the practitioner data bank will provide ample means to evaluate surgeons in the future, more on an economic basis than on quality of care. It will remain for the surgical profession to develop valid indicators of quality of care to substantiate the profession's claim as the advocate for the patient in this tug-of-war for resources. In future use of resources, the surgeon must be sensitive to third party payer attention to the bottom line, malpractice exposure for adverse outcomes, and the consumer advocate watchdog approach to quality of care and denial of access.

CONCLUSIONS

Credentialing is an effort to ensure the quality of surgical care for patients. It dates back to earliest recorded time in its pure form and is designed to protect patients. It can be misused and, depending on the social agenda of those carrying it out, may achieve a number of different social goals, some not necessarily related to quality of patient care. It must be carried out with sensitivity and integrity, or credibility will be lost, which was one of its original purposes.

The replacement of professionalism and ethically driven behavior with algorithms and continual quality improvement activities seems to be the direction of medicine for the 1990s.

It is expensive, and it remains to be seen if it will improve quality of care and outcomes.

Selected Readings

1. Danabedian A. The quality of care. How can it be assessed? JAMA 1988;260:1743–1748.
2. Dent T. Credentialing and proceedings for endoscopy and lap surgery. Surg Clin North Am 1992;72(5):1003–1009.
3. Dent TL. Training, credentialling, and granting of privileges in laparoscopic cholecystectomy. Am J Surg 199;161:399–403.
4. Greene FL. Training, credentialling, and privileging for minimally invasive surgery. Probl Gen Surg 1991;8:502–506.
5. Joint Commission on Accreditation of Healthcare Organizations. 1995 Accreditation Manual for Hospitals. Oakbrook Terrace, IL: Joint Commission on Accreditation of Healthcare Organizations, 1994.
6. Lyons AS, Petrucelli RJ. Medicine, an illustrated history. New York: Harry N Abrams, 1987.
7. Society of American Gastrointestinal Endoscopic Surgeons. Granting of privileges for gastrointestinal endoscopy by surgeons. Los Angeles: Society of American Gastrointestinal Endoscopic Surgeons, 1989.
8. Society of American Gastrointestinal Endoscopic Surgeons. Granting of privileges for laparoscopic (peritoneoscopic) general surgery. Los Angeles: Society of American Gastrointestinal Endoscopic Surgeons, 1992.

8

Outcome Studies

Joseph Gerstein

TERMINOLOGY

Various descriptive terms have been applied to the performance of surgical procedures on nonhospitalized patients. The degree of complexity and the likelihood of complications of such out-of-hospital procedures range from the trivial to the considerable. Clearly, no fair comparison of the results of series of procedures can be made without some agreement on the terminology describing the intensity level of care delivered in the settings in which surgery is undertaken.

The term "ambulatory surgery" was originally developed to signify those procedures performed in a hospital operating theater on inpatients, usually under general or regional anesthesia, who were then discharged the same day. Because of economic considerations (related to nonremuneration of cosmetic procedures by third party payers), relatively aggressive ambulatory anesthesia and plastic surgery have been practiced since clinical ambulatory surgery was in its infancy. Conversely, there have been physicians who persisted in performing relatively minor procedures in the hospital setting.

"Outpatient surgery" originally referred to the types of minor surgery then performed in an office or emergency room setting, such as the lancing of boils, suture of simple lacerations, and small skin biopsies, usually under local anesthesia. There have always been some exceptions to this terminology, such as procedures done in dental surgery offices in which third molar extractions were done routinely using intravenous or inhalational anesthesia.

"Ambulatory surgery" in this chapter indicates only the category of procedures that require anesthesia and postoperative observation. Herniorrhaphies under local anesthesia, for example, fit into this category of ambulatory surgery.

It is not always possible in the literature to distinguish the "hospital integrated" ambulatory surgical unit from the "hospital-dedicated" ambulatory surgical unit. In the former arrangement, the regular hospital operating suite is used by the ambulatory surgery unit. Patients are processed separately, but the presence of the regular anesthesiologists and operating room staff allows more aggressive case selection and more facile postoperative admission to the hospital, if necessary, which affects any comparison between ambulatory and inpatient settings for surgery.

The hospital-dedicated ambulatory surgical unit consists of a separate facility on hospital grounds exclusively dedicated to ambulatory surgery. The patient is admitted to, operated on, and discharged from this unit. It is similar to a freestanding unit, but its proximity to the hospital gives it significant advantages in case of an emergency or the necessity of overnight stay in a hospital bed.

The freestanding ambulatory surgery center (FASC) may be adjacent to a hospital or be some distance away. The greater the distance, the more reluctant surgeons and anesthesiologists are to undertake surgery on high-risk patients, despite the presence of transfer agreements. Such a facility may be owned by a hospital, by private entrepreneurs (including physicians), by for-profit chains, or by health insurers or health maintenance organizations (HMOs). In some cases, surgeons are equity holders, potentially raising issues of propriety in terms of the most appropriate locus for surgery on a given patient. Freestanding ambulatory facilities may be able to accommodate surgeons in other ways, such as offering more convenient scheduling, especially "block" scheduling, which might be difficult to duplicate in a hospital operating suite. Except for some special guidelines, FASCs were specifically excluded from the stringent self-referral proscriptions of the "Stark" legislation in 1994, a clear indication that the U. S. Congress perceived this type of entity to be efficient and inexpensive, relative to other forms of physician-owned clinical enterprises.

"Outcome studies" usually measure the effect of a given treatment in terms of degree of success in relieving some symptom or physical manifestation of a disease process. This success is conditioned by how little damage was done to the patient in the process of treatment and the immediate recovery process (i.e., complication rate or "morbidity and mortality"). Studies in the ambulatory surgery arena usually focus on additional parameters, such as cost and patient and family satisfaction.

"Cost outcomes" in ambulatory surgery are usually assessed by comparing the costs of the same procedure performed in the inpatient or the ambulatory setting and sometimes by assessing the total societal cost, usually quantified by assessing the amount of time that the patient spent in recuperation from the procedure before return to remunerative work plus the time expended by nonprofessional caretakers until the patient recovers.

"Complication rates" in ambulatory surgery have historically been assessed by the same criteria that are used in judging inpatient procedures: recurrences, wound infections, wound dehiscences, damage to collateral tissues and organs, urinary retention, cardiac and pulmonary events, anesthetic accidents, and so on. However, collection of these data is sometimes hindered by the absence of the direct observation of the ambulatory surgery patient for much of the postsurgical period.

Until the publication of an extensive study of the potential for late (up to 1 month) major morbidity and mortality subsequent to ambulatory surgery by the Mayo Medical School, useful, statistically valid information about this crucial "late" phase of ambulatory surgery was almost nonexistent. In this study of almost 40,000 adult patients who underwent 45,000 ambulatory procedures and anesthetics, the follow-up rates for 72 hours and 30 days were 99.94% and 95.9%, respectively. No patient died of a medical complication within 1 week of surgery. Only 13% of the serious cardiovascular or pulmonary events occurred within 8 hours of surgery, 48% in the next 40 hours, and 39% in the next 28 days. Five patients had pulmonary embolism, a rate of approximately 1/10,000, which is quite acceptable, even if all of them were due directly to the ambulatory surgery, which is not necessarily the case. When compared with the results of community prevalence studies of these same types of events (e.g., pulmonary embolus, cardiac events), the rates in the postambulatory surgery patients were in the same general range, indicating that, although much of the major morbidity was late, much of it was probably unrelated to the ambulatory surgery per se and that ambulatory surgery, at least in a major medical center, is reasonably safe.

One of the early reasons for the performance of ambulatory surgery was the expectation that the likelihood of wound infection with a resistant organism would be significantly diminished in that setting. No real evidence that such was the case ever emerged. A review of the literature on postoperative infections after outpatient surgery found that from 20% to 70% of postoperative surgical site infections do not become apparent until after the patient's discharge, resulting in serious under-reporting of true rates. New national guidelines for valid postdischarge surveillance for potential nosocomial infections are probably needed.

Another parameter frequently reported in the "morbidity" section of ambulatory surgery studies is the number or percentage of patients that required hospitalization directly from the ambulatory facility. Except when previously arranged home care becomes unavailable, such a result indicates some level of morbidity beyond what was expected. It might be as trivial as persistent nausea or as serious as a major cardiac event.

One additional set of complications is unique to the ambulatory surgical situation:

the necessity for postoperative hospital admission and hospitalization from home because of physiologic or pathologic dysfunctions or intractable pain. These parameters are reported in almost all reports of series of ambulatory surgical procedures.

Both of these numbers are affected by the discharge criteria that are in use at the individual facility. If criteria for discharge include the patient's ability to drink fluid and hold it down or the need for the patient to void, then the frequency of hospitalization from the facility will be fairly high and will tend to vitiate cost effectiveness of the organization. Again, with the gain in confidence that comes from experience, the criteria for discharge from the FASC will become more liberal (see Chapter 9).

SURGICAL SKILLS

There is a "learning curve" for surgeons trying to assimilate a new technology. A recently published multicenter trial of laparoscopic inguinal herniorrhaphy demonstrated clearly that the recurrence rate was related to a given surgeon's experience. Likewise, the occurrence of neuralgia seemed to decrease progressively as the number of cases performed increased, a clear indication of a learning curve.

Residents are learning these avant garde procedures during their training, but surgeons in practice must depend on in-service training, which may vary in quality and offer limited hands-on experience. An example of the deficiencies in training that can accrue in this environment and then manifest as increased patient morbidity is documented in a study of urologists who attended a laparoscopy training course and whose clinical practice was followed subsequently. Surgeons who performed clinical procedures without additional training were 3.39 times more likely to have at least one significant complication compared with their colleagues who sought additional training. At the end of 12 months, those who had only attended one training course, who were in solo practice, or who performed laparoscopic surgery with a different assistants were even more likely to have had a complication as compared with those who attended the course with a partner, were in group practice, or operated with the same, regular assistant. This study graphically demonstrates that the numbers that are published in a journal by a surgeon with special skills, training, and experience may be an order of magnitude better than those that can be achieved, at least initially, by the relatively inexperienced surgeon of average skills.

PATIENT SELECTION

Every surgeon would, ideally, like to operate on patients who are completely healthy, except for the condition provoking the surgery. This criterion is probably met in many patients who undergo ambulatory surgery. The data of any report of outcomes or complication rates of ambulatory surgery depend somewhat on the basic medical condition of such patients.

The medical status of the patients allowed to undergo a given procedure is dependent on a number of factors: the distance of the FASC from its affiliated hospital, the experience of the surgeon and anesthesiologist, the stage of sophistication of the facility with the given procedure, and the confidence level of the surgeon and anesthesiologist. There is room for much subjectivity here. Often, the threshold for selection of medically compromised patients decreases as confidence and competence progress during a series of procedures. For example, in the series of ambulatory transurethral prostatectomies reported by Klimberg and colleagues, operative candidates showed a progressive increase in the estimated size of their prostate glands and of the severity and complexity of their medical conditions as well as their age as the series progressed. Even so, the number of patients being transferred to the hospital after surgery decreased progressively.

The proper selection of patients is crucial to the success of an ambulatory surgical program. If the selection process is too conservative, the ambulatory site will not operate up to capacity and probably will not prosper; if it is too liberal, patients will be put at unnecessary risk and excessive transfers to the hospital will distort the valuable functionality of the ambulatory facility and escalate cost. The preoperative evaluation and screening of the potential ambulatory surgery candidate is discussed in Chapter 9.

THE SOCIAL SETTING OF SURGERY

The nature of the health insurance system in the United States has led to a bias on the part of the public (and physicians) toward having procedures of all kinds performed in a hospital. This was true even in the case of young children, who, as patients, are likely to find the hospital an alien and frightening environment.

Rhode Island Memorial Hospital in Pawtucket has capitalized on the concept of minimizing the imagery of illness by creating a unit for its short-stay patients that deemphasizes the stigma of illness in the environment. Patients admitted to this unit drive up to a separate entrance covered by a canopy. Their car is parked by an attendant. The wing of the hospital in which this unit is located has been completely refurbished and has the appearance of a moderately expensive hotel. No hospital paraphernalia are in view. The rooms are richly paneled, and all equipment, such as oxygen flowmeters and suction bottles, is recessed behind cabinetry. Colors are bright and tasteful. Furniture does not appear to be institutional. This ward connects directly to the operating suite, but via a separate entrance and separate holding room. At no time do patients from this area intermingle with sicker hospital patients. Average length of stay for a total abdominal hysterectomy (non-oncologic) is 2.2 days. The nurses and the patients are oriented to expeditious care and rapid mobilization. Although this does not represent ambulatory surgery per se, because most patients remained in the unit more than 24 hours, the general approach of deemphasizing the illness role and enhancing patients' expectations of speedy discharge is equally applicable to the true ambulatory setting.

For many years, the policy of many medical insurers was to compensate physicians for procedures only when patients were hospitalized. They thought that, in this way, the necessity for hospitalization would act as some sort of severity screen, relieving them of paying for simple discretionary procedures. However, this attitude led to some perverse practices, such as admitting patients to the hospital for procedures as trivial as a barium enema.

In Europe, until recently, there was little incentive for hospitals or physicians to use outpatient facilities for surgical procedures. Although there may be some differences in definition of categories, it appears that ambulatory surgery accounts for approximately 25% of surgery in the Netherlands and only 5% in France. Most European systems of hospital compensation did not account for the "efficiency trap," which penalizes a hospital for a greater flow of patients, thus providing disincentive to "clean up" extensive waiting lists. Consequently, there are extensive waiting lists for all sorts of elective and even some urgent procedures. Only in the last few years has there been any movement toward the sort of ambulatory surgery revolution that has occurred in the United States.

The National Health Service in the United Kingdom is bringing more and more general practitioners under a capitation system (i.e., fund holding) and is giving hospitals incentive to reduce waiting lists by allowing them to keep some of the savings generated by more efficient operation. The ready cash that these capitated physicians can direct to facilities that accommodate their patients more expeditiously will likely drive the system toward a more efficient mode of surgical health care delivery.

Approximately 50% of surgery in the United States was performed in the ambulatory setting in 1991, and this percentage appears to be heading toward approximately 65% by the end of 1995. The Health Care Financing Administration has been moving toward a prospective payment system for hospital outpatient surgery. However, Medicare has continued to pay hospitals considerably more than FASCs. Over time, it is likely that such payments will shrink toward the standard freestanding fee, and the number of procedures denoted as appropriate for ambulatory surgery will gradually increase.

HISTORICAL FACTORS

During the 1950s, a perception emerged that bed rest was not necessarily a panacea for convalescing patients. A greater appreciation of the role of stasis in the production of postoperative pulmonary embolism and an awareness of the deconditioning effects of the 6-week bed rest regimen for acute myocardial infarction patients led to a gradual but progressive reduction in the emphasis on the role of bed rest in most treatment regimens. A shorter stay and earlier mobilization gradually became the rule after myocardial infarction and, subsequently, for many other conditions.

The work of some early pioneers then started a revolution in surgery. In 1955, Farquarson reported a series of herniorrhaphies performed in an outpatient setting under local anesthesia. Results seemed comparable to the standard approach, thus reducing the legitimate concern that early activity would result in breakdown of the repair. In 1968, Chiang and coworkers reported a series of 40,000 tonsillectomies performed on an outpatient basis in Los Angeles without a single death and with only a handful of complications. These dramatic papers did much to galvanize others to reorient their surgical activities to the ambulatory setting. What was the motivation to perform these procedures in the ambulatory setting at a time when, it would appear, there was little economic incentive to do so? Chiang and coworkers clarify this enigma by stating, "In this modern age there is an increasing shortage of hospital beds. . . ."

Currently, there is an excess of beds, even an excess of hospitals. Even so, and because of the *perception* that ambulatory surgery is less expensive than inpatient surgery, there appears to be an inexorable movement toward the ambulatory setting for surgery. Additionally, there is a thrust toward experimentation with techniques and equipment to enable patients to undergo surgery for certain conditions in the ambulatory setting that otherwise would have to be performed in the inpatient setting. This may have the perverse effect of increasing the frequency of procedures because of the perceived simplicity and safety of the new approach. This has already been shown to have occurred in the instance of laparoscopic cholecystectomy.

Finally, the interface between ambulatory and inpatient hospital surgery is further blurred when a variety of hospital facilities receive and hold a postsurgical patient from an ambulatory surgery area for periods of up to 48 hours (even 72 hours) without actually necessitating admission to the hospital as an inpatient. This is achieved at some institutions by extending the hours of the recovery area and at others by admitting the patient to an "observation area," which is not considered inpatient territory (even though sometimes the patient shares a room with an inpatient). Again, this "Alice-in-Wonderland" type of "distinction without a difference" is generally engendered by arcane insurance company reimbursement schemes rather than any rational concept of distinction between an inpatient and an outpatient. Therefore, the percentage of postoperative patients reported in various categories of postoperative observation in surgical reports discussed in this chapter cannot be definitively standardized and remains somewhat idiosyncratic to the facility in which the primary procedure was performed.

STUDIES COMPARING INPATIENT SURGERY AND AMBULATORY SURGERY

There is a dearth of well-controlled, randomized studies comparing inpatient and ambulatory surgery (except in the anesthesia arena, where such abound). In general, studies comparing the two settings of surgery attempt to measure several parameters such as mortality, morbidity, outcome, convenience, patient satisfaction, and cost. Cost turns out to be an arcane issue and the least accessible.

The Data

Most papers fall into three categories: the contemporaneous, nonrandom comparison group, the noncontemporaneous comparison group, and the evolving comparison group. This latter approach starts with a small group of relatively low-risk patients with a given clinical condition who are the subjects of a somewhat innovative approach to surgery in the ambulatory setting. As time goes on and more experience is gained by the surgeon and the team, the threshold for patient selection changes and patients at progressively higher levels of risk are allowed into the ambulatory setting. Although such poorly controlled studies are not pristine in the statistical sense, much can be learned from them, assuming patient morbidity turns out to be low.

Most of these scientific papers in the "ambulatory surgery" database reflect the search for the most propitious type of anesthesia to use in the ambulatory surgical environment. Minimizing the occurrence of postoperative nausea and vomiting (PONV), cognitive impairment, and disequilibrium is absolutely crucial to the success of that ambulatory center. Therefore, literally hundreds of reasonably controlled and randomized trials have been done in ambulatory centers to establish which combination of anesthetic drugs and which sequence of administration is most effective in producing good analgesia and amnesia. Many of these studies are funded by the manufacturers of anesthetic and antiemetic medications. Additionally, new ideas concerning such issues as how long a patient should forego fluids before anesthesia and whether endotracheal intubation is necessary during anesthesia (versus the laryngeal mask) have been worked out effectively using careful protocols. (See Section 5, Anesthesia for Ambulatory Surgery.)

Cost Issues

It would seem that at least the comparative cost of the procedure in an inpatient setting can be discerned and compared with the costs accumulated by patients in the outpatient setting, but even this apparently simple issue is often obscured by complex hospital pricing policies and by the fact that prices may vary dramatically depending on who is the payer. Additionally, Medicare fees, which could offer a benchmark, are not always reasonable, and some well-established ambulatory procedures are still judged by Medicare to be inappropriate for that environment and are therefore not remunerated in the outpatient setting.

Randomized Trials

Berk and Chalmers found only 4 of 134 relevant papers prior to 1986 provided enough data on cost and efficacy to allow statistically valid conclusions concerning the benefits or detriments of ambulatory versus in-hospital surgery for a given condition. Two studies demonstrated that the potential savings would come at the cost of a slightly poorer clinical outcome; two showed ambulatory care to be as effective as inpatient care and less costly.

Adler and colleagues in 1978 compared a short-stay (2 days) group of patients treated surgically for varicose veins with a group that remained 6 to 7 days in the hospital. Although not strictly a study of "ambulatory surgery," it did validate in a solid, if primitive, way that the quality of the short-stay group's result was equal to that of the long-stay group and that costs (accounted for stringently) were significantly less in the former. Patients, retrospectively assessed, were agreeable to either approach.

Also in 1978, Ruckley and coworkers studied varicose vein and hernia repairs, but compared ambulatory surgery to inpatient treatment. Again, consumer acceptability and clinical outcome were comparable and cost was significantly higher in the inpatient group.

Pineault and colleagues published in 1985 a randomized clinical trial of 1-day surgery. The authors assigned 182 patients about to undergo tubal ligation, hernia repair, or meniscectomy to either 1-day surgery or inpatient surgery. A significant number of patients in the ambulatory surgery group said they wished they had more time to recuperate in the hospital. Clinical outcomes were equivalent in all three groups. Costs were significantly lower for ambulatory tubal ligation and herniorrhaphy and significantly higher for ambulatory meniscectomy. The structuring of the costs of procedures in different areas and the establishment of a day rate based on the global budget, which was the practice in Montreal at the time of this study, is somewhat murky. Also, no numbers were given for the dwell time in hospital of the inpatients, so it is not known whether lackadaisical bed use might have produced excessive inpatient costs. The major conclusion to be drawn from this study is that the clinical outcomes were equivalent.

Nonrandomized Trials

Cataract surgery patients were characteristically treated with "kid gloves" prior to the ambulatory surgery era. The necessity for this approach was thought to be the fragility of the eye structures subsequent to surgical manipulation. Therefore, it was with some temerity that ophthalmologists began to remove cataracts in an ambulatory setting. Because of the huge cost impact of this most common of operations on elderly persons, Medicare scrutinized it closely and, in 1983, proscribed inpatient cataract surgery in patients unless they had significant and serious comorbidity.

A review of extensive subsequent experience with cataract surgery demonstrated that there were no statistical differences between the inpatient and ambulatory groups for visual acuity. There was a slight predominance ($P = 0.03$) of cystoid macular edema in the inpatient cohort, but, after correction for complicating illness, this disappeared. No significant differences in rates for other operative and postoperative complications were identified. No cost or patient satisfaction analyses were done.

The data on "time out of work" as reported in studies are collected in such nonstandard formats that it is almost impossible to assess the comparability of such data. The demographics of the study population would have tremendous influence on this variable. If blue-collar workers predominate in the study population, especially if Workmen's Compensation cases abound as would be possible in series of herniorrhaphies or lumbar disc herniations, only a carefully randomized study would have internal consistency. Unless the demographics of the groups are delineated in exquisite detail, comparison between studies is unlikely to have any real relevance.

Trials of Standard Inpatient Surgical Techniques in the Ambulatory Setting

Transurethral resection of the prostate (TURP) began to supplant suprapubic prostatectomy as the standard treatment for benign prostatic hypertrophy (BPH) about 25 years ago. At that time, 5 days in the hospital was standard after TURP. Recently, with the pressures of managed care, some urologists have been willing to send patients with minimal bleeding home with an indwelling catheter in

place on the second or third hospital day. Klimberg and coworkers proposed that TURP be performed on suitable candidates in an ambulatory setting and reported on the results in 125 patients.

This report is typical of the genre and therefore is discussed in detail. Perhaps 400,000 transurethral resections of the prostate are done annually in the United States; therefore, a substantially less expensive approach, using standard technical methodology, would be extremely helpful in reducing medical costs. Because of the perception that TURP would likely remain an inpatient procedure and that only a totally new approach to the problem might allow an ambulatory setting to be used, several alternative methodologies have been proposed, namely laser-assisted TURP, high-intensity focused ultrasound via the rectum, and transurethral incision of the prostate (TUIP). Another approach, the transurethral balloon distention of the prostate, had limited duration of efficacy and has mostly been abandoned. These other procedures provoke less bleeding than TURP and are therefore better adapted to the ambulatory setting. They do have the shortcoming of failing to detect cancer or intraepithelial hyperplasia of the prostate because they do not salvage the obstructing tissue for histologic analysis. In addition to standard data, authors often accumulate information on postvoid residual and maximum urinary flow rate, as well as the standard symptom score before and after surgery. Klimberg and his colleagues appear to have developed a meticulous technique with the standard method so as to perform it safely in the ambulatory setting. This may mean that new techniques need not be learned nor new equipment purchased by urologists or FASCs, a major saving on a national level.

Five of Klimberg and colleagues' patients (4%) required hospital admission. All were transferred from the recovery room, none from home. None of the last 75 patients required transfer to the hospital, indicating improved results with time, which is typical in such series. Sixty more patients, not included in the study but reported in an addendum, have subsequently undergone TURP without another transfer to the hospital. Whereas, initially, men in the recovery area with some persistent bleeding were automatically transferred to the hospital, subsequently, these men were placed on irrigation at home under the scrutiny of a home-care agency.

In the first 18 months of this protocol, 57% of TURPs were performed on an ambulatory basis. In the last 6 months, the percentage was 90%. This suggests there was the typical "learning curve" plus a progressive comfort with the setting, which allows gradual expansion of the spectrum of patients who are judged eligible for the procedure to include older patients and those with larger prostate glands and higher grades of comorbid conditions.

Another procedure that involves slight modification of a standard approach rather than a total technologic refoundation was reported by Tyagi and associates who call it "subxiphoid 'minimal stress triangle' microceliotomy." Using endoscopic tools and a 5- to 10-cm muscle-sparing incision, the investigators performed cholecystectomy in an ambulatory setting on 73% of a series of 142 consecutive patients. Twenty-seven percent of patients had been admitted to the hospital for acute conditions before the surgery. The procedure in only one patient had to be converted to the standard open cholecystectomy approach. Morbidity was modest. Twenty-seven patients (19%) required postoperative hospitalization for management of associated medical conditions; 94% of those scheduled for ambulatory surgery were discharged within 23 hours. Duration of surgery was comparable to that of open cholecystectomy. Whether this technique can be mastered by other surgeons without extensive training or whether there will be any impetus to learn it in the face of almost universal use of the laparoscopic approach by surgeons currently is a pertinent question. In the third world, this microceliotomy technique would represent an important advance, because it would obviate the capital investment necessary for laparoscopic surgery.

NEW SURGICAL TECHNOLOGY IN THE AMBULATORY SETTING AND ITS EFFECT ON CASE SELECTION

Urologic Surgery

The difficulty of predicting which man will benefit from a surgical procedure to relieve presumed obstruction of the prostate might be expected to restrain the frequency of procedures designed to relieve obstruction. This is especially true with the availability of drugs that have some efficacy in reducing the cardinal symptoms of BPH. Even state-of-the-art preoperative testing for a variety of parameters of the voiding function of men with BPH does not have much utility in predicting who will benefit from prostatic surgery and who will retain the exact symptoms for which they had the surgery. In such a setting, minimizing the trauma and complexity of a procedure as perceived by surgeons, primary care physicians, and patients is likely to increase the frequency with which it is performed significantly. Thus, the apparent cost savings produced by moving a procedure from the inpatient to the ambulatory setting can, at the societal level, evaporate rapidly, and total costs might even escalate.

Biliary Surgery

The guidelines generated by the 1992 Consensus Conference of the National Institutes of Health recommend against surgical removal of asymptomatic gallstones except in the case of calcification of the wall of the gallbladder and a few other exotic situations. Other authorities add the presence of very large gallstones to the list of indications, because of the presumed 2% potential for development of biliary cancer. However, it seems likely that many asymptomatic gallstones are being removed, that the threshold for what constitutes a gallbladder disease symptom has been significantly lowered, or that patients with minimal symptoms have become emboldened to have a laparoscopic cholecystectomy, whereas, in the era of open cholecystectomy, such patients decided to avoid surgery. Some or all of these factors probably account for the dramatic increase in the rate of cholecystectomy since the laparoscopic procedure was introduced. It remains to be seen whether the rate of cholecystectomy will decline toward the rate of the past few years before the availability of laparoscopic cholecystectomy, suggesting that the "overhang" of minimally symptomatic patients has been cleared up, or whether it will persist, suggesting that the threshold for surgery has been reset permanently at a lower level of symptomatology or that, national norms notwithstanding, open season has been declared on asymptomatic gallstones.

Medicare authorities initially decided not to pay for laparoscopic cholecystectomy done in an ambulatory setting. The system of evaluation, based on the percentage of procedures being done on Medicare patients in FASCs rather than in the hospital, is bound to be biased toward the *status quo*, because it is always retrospective and thereby affected by the failure of Medicare to pay for the procedure in this setting—a typical bureaucratic Catch 22.

Lumbar Disc Surgery

The status of percutaneous lumbar disc surgery is in flux. A number of techniques, including laser, have become popular and there is a vast body of literature that consists mainly of retrospective, uncontrolled clinical studies, technical articles, and case reports.

The two major approaches being used appear to be selective removal of nucleus pulposus and intradiscal decompression. Both procedures can be accomplished by a variety of instruments and with seemingly good initial results. However, recurrence rate is higher than with the inpatient laminectomy. More importantly, nonstandardization of patient selection criteria and follow-up that is often biased (evaluation by the operator) and of short duration have led to a situation characterized by one physician as "the rape of the spine." Another posits that "each year tens of thousands of persons with backache are misled into considering these procedures (percutaneous microdiscectomy and chemonucleolysis) as 'advances.'"

Because there is less reluctance of patients to undergo a relatively brief outpatient procedure with a minimum recuperation time than a more intensive inpatient procedure, there is a danger that these percutaneous approaches may become fairly routine before they have even achieved solid evidence of long-term efficacy.

Follow-up indicates that there is almost no differential long-term outcome in the level of pain or neurologic deficit between series of patients who underwent conservative treatment or surgery for herniated lumbar disc disease. Surgically treated cases were relieved of pain somewhat more quickly, however. Perhaps, therefore, patients could return to work somewhat sooner, but this has not been investigated directly. This category does not include patients with rapidly deteriorating neurologic status or bladder and bowel compromise.

Patients who undergo standard laminectomy in the hospital setting can almost always be discharged on the second day, occasionally on the first. This is the definitive procedure, although recurrence is fairly common, even in this situation, and patient selection must be scrupulous. Recuperation time before return to work is likely longer than with the less invasive procedures.

On the other hand, rapid return to work is a bona fide objective, too. Again, societal cost has not been carefully studied in the case of minimally invasive lumbar disc surgery. The avoidance of a long period out of work for a significant number of patients may more than compensate for the costs of a somewhat higher recurrence rate that may require additional treatment, to say nothing of several months without pain versus several months with significant pain. Clearly, if selection criteria are too liberal or are slackly applied to ambulatory procedures, no amount of differential savings between the two approaches will compensate for the many "extra" procedures that might have to be done.

Hernioplasty

Hernioplasty is an area roiled with controversy. There appears to be no standard, well-accepted method of approaching hernias surgically in the ambulatory setting. The laparoscopic approach is popular and appears to be relatively effective but requires general anesthesia. There are advocates of extraperitoneal and intraperitoneal methods. The traditional open approach can use local anesthesia, which is less complicated and less traumatic to the patient and has the additional virtue of eliminating an anesthesiology charge. Recurrence rate, cost, and duration of disability therefore become the critical evaluative issues (see Chapters 23 and 24).

There is still controversy about many issues in the herniorrhaphy debate. Several reviews have reached similar conclusions: local anesthesia has advantages over general or regional anesthesia; patients prefer the laparoscopic approach and recuperate sooner; recurrence rate appears higher with the laparoscopic procedure, but this may relate to the fact that the laparoscopic technique is more demanding and therefore the learning curve may be longer; randomized, controlled multicenter trials comparing a variety of techniques are in order.

A fair evaluation of the comparative cost of these procedures is not a simple proposition. The open procedure, especially under local anesthesia, is "cheaper" in terms of out-of-pocket cost to patient, employer, or insurer. However, the patient's longer "down-time" subsequent to the open procedure has a cost. Sometimes this is clear, such as when there is continued salary paid for sick leave. Sometimes it is obscure, such as when people who are ordinarily "at home" are limited in their activities for a considerable period of time. This cost issue is germane because 700,000 hernia repairs are done annually in the United States with a 5% to 10% recurrence rate.

Hysterectomy

The Lancet recently published a commentary entitled "Shifting Indications for Hysterectomy." The author noted that the indications for hysterectomy have narrowed in recent decades. Such factors as the gender of the gynecologist and the interval since graduation from medical school were found to have an influence on frequency with which hysterectomy is performed. Hysteroscopic endometrial ablation has obviated the need for some procedures. The efficacy of conization for treatment of carcinoma in situ of the cervix has eliminated the need for other hysterectomies. Chronic pelvic pain (sometimes referred to as "pain of uterine origin") still accounts for a small but significant number of hysterectomies in almost all series reported. Again, as morbidity of surgery diminishes, the potential for

symptoms of less clinical significance to enable patients to become surgical candidates is enhanced. The Lancet commentary asserts that asymptomatic fibroids of even moderate size need not be removed unless they are actively degenerating.

Two recent studies evaluated the role of vaginal hysterectomy for benign gynecologic conditions whether assisted by laparoscope (laparascopically assisted vaginal hysterectomy [LAVH]) or not. Summit and colleagues concluded, after a randomized comparison of the two procedures, that the major difference between the two groups was that the LAVH procedures were almost twice as expensive as the standard vaginal hysterectomy ($7905 vs. $4891), partly because operating time was much longer (120 vs. 65 minutes). A total of 96% of the patients in this study were discharged within 12 hours of surgery. Only one patient (LAVH group) had to be admitted from home to the hospital for pain control. Again, the apparent perversity of the Medicare fee scheme is demonstrated with this procedure. Ambulatory fee scale for vaginal hysterectomy is level 4: $558, whereas in-hospital treatment under DRG 353 pays a hospital approximately $10,000. The surgeon's fee for procedure is identical in either locale: $905.

Kovac did an extensive study to rationalize the guidelines for determining the type of hysterectomy appropriate for benign disease. Vaginal hysterectomy alone was feasible in 548 of 617 patients. Sixty-three additional cases could be done via the vaginal route with the aid of the laparoscope working above (LAVH). His study demonstrated that the traditional indications for avoiding the vaginal route and opting for total abdominal hysterectomy are too conservative. Incidentally, postoperative complication rate was much lower in vaginal hysterectomy. In the United States, it appears that three times as many total abdominal hysterectomies are performed as vaginal hysterectomies. According to Kovac's study, this ratio could be at least reversed without any real detriment to patients and with savings of millions of dollars nationally. Surgeons who are not particularly skilled in the technique of vaginal hysterectomy might have a difficult time in the early procedures and would presumably see a temporarily higher rate of patient morbidity.

CONCLUSIONS

Because the frequency and scope of ambulatory surgery are expanding rapidly, what it costs and how it is reimbursed become weighty issues for the medical profession, the hospital and surgicenter, industries, and society. Most comparative studies reviewed in this chapter make some attempt at an assessment of the economic impact of a given procedure performed in different settings or under different circumstances, but these analyses are usually primitive and simplistic. Society has to make a fundamental decision whether to consider or ignore the cost to the individual or to the employer of nonproductive recuperative time as a factor in the cost–benefit equation when evaluating a procedure or a site of procedure. Alternatively, should only the cash outlay for the procedure be assessed? Also, should the integrity and even the survival of the community and teaching hospitals, which are potentially compromised when many procedures are removed from their bailiwick, be considered when calculating what a given procedure is worth? Complicating this issue is the problem of establishing the proper indications for surgery.

In 1986, Berk and Chalmers found "only 4 of 134 relevant papers . . . that we analyzed provided enough data on both cost and efficacy to allow statistically valid conclusions." In the ensuing 10 years, not much has changed in this regard. However, there is a body of knowledge gradually accumulating that hopefully will define more clearly the costs of and quality of surgery done in various locales. The trend seems to be accelerating.

Selected Readings

1. Adler MW, Waller JJ, Creese A. Randomised controlled trial of early discharge for inguinal hernia and varicose veins. J Epidemiol Community Health 1978;32:136–142.
2. Berk AA, Chalmers TC. Cost and efficacy of the substi-

tution of ambulatory for inpatient care. N Engl J Med 1986;304:393–397.
3. Chiang TM, Sukis AE, Ross DE. Tonsillectomy performed on an outpatient basis. Arch Otolaryngol 1968;83:308–310.
4. Detmer DE, Gelijns AC. Ambulatory surgery: a more cost-effective treatment strategy? Arch Surg 1994;129:123–127.
5. Farquarson EL. Early ambulation with special reference to herniorrhaphy as an outpatient procedure. Lancet 1955;ii:517.
6. Fitzgibbons RJ Jr, Camps J, Cornet DA, et al. Laparoscopic inguinal herniorrhaphy. Ann Surg 1995;221:3–13.
7. Grimes DA. Shifting indications for hysterectomy: nature, nurture, or neither? Lancet 1994;344:1651–1652.
8. Hadler NM. Surgery for herniated lumbar disc: a review. ACP Journal Club. 1994;Jan/Feb:15.43.
9. Hitchcock M, Ogg TW. Antiemetics in laparoscopic surgery (letter). Br J Anaesth 1994;72:608. Reply: Raphael JH, Norton AC. 1994;72:608–609.
10. Holland GN, Earl DT, Wheeler NC. Results of inpatient and outpatient cataract surgery. Ophthalmology 1992;99:845–852.
11. Hoffman RM, Wheeler KJ, Deyo RA. Surgery for herniated lumbar disc: a literature synthesis. J Gen Intern Med 1993;8:487–496.
12. Klimberg IW, Locke DR, Leonard E. Outpatient transurethral resection of the prostate in a urological ambulatory surgery center. J Urol 1994;151:1547–1549.
13. Kovac SR. Guidelines to determine the route of hysterectomy. Obstet Gynecol 1995;85:18–22.
14. MacLean LD. The repair of inguinal hernias (editorial). Ann Surg 1995;221:1–2.
15. Pineault R, Contandriopoulos A, Valois M. Randomized clinical trial of one-day medical care: patient satisfaction. Med Care 1985;23:171–182.
16. Rhodes RS. Ambulatory surgery and the societal cost of surgery. Surgery 1994;116:938–940.
17. Robertson JT. Rape of the spine. Surg Neurol 1994;39:5–12.
18. Ruckley CV, Cuthbertson C, Fenwick N. Day care after operations for hernia or varicose veins: a controlled trial. Br J Surg 1978;65:456–459.
19. Schumpelick V, Treutner K, Arit G. Inguinal hernia repair in adults. Lancet 1994;344:375–379.
20. See WA, Cooper CS, Fisher RJ. Predictors of laparoscopic complications after formal training in laparoscopic surgery. JAMA 1993;270:2689–2692.
21. Steiner CA, Bass EB, Talamini MA, et al. Surgical rates and operative mortality for open and laparoscopic cholecystectomy in Maryland. N Engl J Med 1994;380:403–408.
22. Summit RL Jr, Stovall TG, Lipscomb GH, et al. Randomized comparison of laparoscopy-assisted vaginal hysterectomy with standard vaginal hysterectomy in an outpatient setting. Obstet Gynecol 1992;80:895–901.
23. Stuart AE. Taking the tension out of hernia repair (editorial). Lancet 1994;343:748.
24. Tyagi NS, Meredith MC, Lumb JC, et al. A new minimally invasive technique for cholecystectomy: subxiphoid "minimal stress triangle" microceliotomy. Ann Surg 1994;220:617–625.
25. Warner MA, Shields SE, Chute CG. Major morbidity and mortality within 1 month of ambulatory surgery and anesthesia. JAMA 1993;270:1437–1441.

Preoperative Assessment and Discharge Assessment Criteria

Judith C. F. Hwang • Timothy J. Bill • Richard F. Edlich

One of the earliest settings for outpatient surgery was the Downtown Anesthesia Clinic in Sioux City, IA, which opened in 1916. In 1962, a formal ambulatory surgery program was started at the University of California at Los Angeles by two anesthesiologists. Since then, surgery has evolved to where a majority of patients are being operated on in the ambulatory setting. Although much of this growth has been fueled by economic demands, a large number of patients undergoing a variety of procedures benefit from having surgery on an outpatient basis. By not staying in the hospital, they can sleep in their own bed the night before and after surgery, thus avoiding the unfamiliar surroundings of a hospital and the associated anxiety and risk of nosocomial infections. Moreover, advances in techniques, such as laparoscopic procedures for general surgical patients, continue to increase the percentage of patients being operated on in an ambulatory setting. From the anesthesiologist's viewpoint, the ambulatory surgery patient population is changing as well.

PATIENT SELECTION

The American Society of Anesthesiologists (ASA) ranks patient physical status on a grade of 1 to 4 (Table 9–1). Initially, ambulatory surgery was restricted to "healthy" patients with ASA physical status 1 or 2. Today, ASA physical status 3 patients are not unusual in

the outpatient setting if their systemic disease is medically stable. Therefore, careful patient selection for ambulatory surgery is critical. The appropriateness of a patient for outpatient surgery must account for the patient's medical condition, the proposed surgical procedure and anesthetic technique, and the anesthesiologist's experience. Patients who have complex medical problems, which may be exacerbated after surgery and anesthesia, should not be operated on in an ambulatory care setting. Patients who are unable to adhere to postoperative instructions, make transportation arrangements, or have responsible adult care at home or at an aftercare facility should also not be considered for ambulatory surgery.

Details of postoperative assessment of adults from the anesthesiologist's point of view are given in Chapter 19.

Age

Extremes of age were previously considered to be a contraindication to ambulatory surgery. In a retrospective study of more than 1500 patients anesthetized for ambulatory surgery, Meridy was unable to demonstrate an age-related effect on the duration of recovery or the incidence of postoperative complications. Other investigators agree that there is probably no upper limit of age for patients undergoing simple outpatient procedures, particularly under local anesthesia or moni-

Table 9–1. American Society of Anesthesiologists Physical Status Classification

Classification	Description
Class 1	A healthy patient
Class 2	A patient with mild systemic disease
Class 3	A patient with severe systemic disease that is not incapacitating
Class 4	A patient with incapacitating systemic disease that is a constant threat to life
Class 5	A moribund patient not expected to survive for 24 hours with or without operation
Emergency (E)	The suffix E is used to denote the presumed poorer physical status of any patient in one of the above categories who is operated on as an emergency.

tored anesthesia care, as long as the patient's functional status is good.

In the pediatric age group, there are still some restrictions on outpatient surgery. It is widely acknowledged that former premature infants who are younger than 44 to 60 weeks postconceptual age or children with a history of apneic spells, significant bronchopulmonary dysplasia, or a family history of sudden infant death syndrome should be observed in the hospital after surgery. Healthy term infants may undergo elective surgery in an ambulatory setting if they are monitored for a prolonged period in the postanesthesia care unit and remain problem free.

Essential Hypertension

Patients with poorly controlled hypertension present multiple potential problems to the anesthesiologist, including the presence of end-organ disease, such as left ventricular hypertrophy, congestive heart failure, cardiac diastolic dysfunction, coronary artery disease, and renal insufficiency. In the patient who remains hypertensive before the induction of anesthesia, the incidence of hypotension and evidence of myocardial ischemia on the electrocardiogram during the maintenance of anesthesia is increased. Ideally, the poorly controlled hypertensive patient should be rendered normotensive before elective surgery. The well-controlled hypertensive patient is a reasonable candidate for elective surgery on an ambulatory basis.

Cardiac Disease

Given the prevalence of coronary artery disease in the general population, many patients with this condition are considered for ambulatory surgery. A careful history is needed to identify the high-risk patient who is not a candidate for outpatient surgery. Patients with stable angina or who have previously undergone coronary bypass or angioplasty and who have good functional status may be considered for ambulatory surgery. Patients with a history of congestive heart failure should be evaluated to determine the cause and the degree of treatment success for this condition. Depending on the patient's ventricular function and the proposed surgery and anesthetic technique, a decision can be made to proceed on an ambulatory basis.

In the pediatric population, a child with a previously diagnosed cardiac murmur or disease can undergo surgery on an ambulatory basis if the condition is stable. Antibiotic prophylaxis should be considered to prevent subacute bacterial endocarditis. Appropriateness of a child with a heart murmur that is first identified during the preanesthetic evaluation is an area of controversy. Some researchers believe that, if the child is stable, growing well, and has no symptoms, ambulatory surgery can be performed with a follow-up evaluation of the murmur. Others believe that evaluation to determine the cause must be done before surgery (see Chapter 17).

Pulmonary Disease

Patients with asthma or chronic obstructive pulmonary disease may be candidates for ambulatory surgery if the disease is well controlled and there is not significant functional limitation. Medications, particularly the nebulized β-agonists, should be continued through the morning of surgery.

Upper Respiratory Infection

Whether to proceed with elective surgery in patients with an upper respiratory infection remains controversial. This issue arises most frequently in the pediatric population when children requiring otolaryngologic procedures often have chronic respiratory infections and may be scheduled for surgery on multiple occasions. Cohen and Cameron suggest that children with a recent upper respiratory infection may have airway hyperactivity for several weeks after the acute episode and may have a higher incidence of respiratory complications with general anesthesia, especially if intubation is required. If the child is thought to be at baseline or if the patient only has rhinorrhea, which is thought to be vasomotor or allergic rhinorrhea without associated problems, most anesthesiologists would proceed with anesthesia and surgery (see Chapter 17).

Diabetes Mellitus

Diabetes mellitus is a chronic systemic disease characterized by a disturbance in the metabolism of glucose and associated with coronary artery disease, cerebrovascular disease, renal insufficiency, autonomic neuropathy, gastroparesis, and peripheral neuropathy. Ideally, patients with diabetes mellitus undergoing ambulatory surgery would be scheduled for their procedure as early in the day as possible, with the morning dose of insulin being withheld. However, if a decision is made to use an insulin infusion for brittle diabetes, the patient is not a candidate for ambulatory surgery, because prolonged fasting would be required. Procedures using local anesthetics in patients with brittle diabetes are appropriate in the ambulatory setting.

Severe Obesity

Patients with severe obesity have a higher incidence of coexisting diseases, such as hypertension, diabetes mellitus, congestive heart failure, restrictive lung disease, and sleep apnea. They may have difficult airways to manage during mask ventilation as well as during intubation. If severely obese patients do not have significant concurrent disease and have an adequate airway, they may be considered as candidates for ambulatory surgery.

Drug Abuse

Abuse of alcohol and illicit drugs increases the risk of acute and untoward responses to anesthesia. Patients with a history of drug abuse require a careful history and a high index of suspicion. They should be counseled that any sign of recent use will result in cancellation of elective surgery. Cocaine used acutely causes sympathetic nervous system stimulation; manifestations include hypertension, cardiac dysrhythmias, and ischemia, possibly by coronary artery vasospasm in patients without prior abnormalities.

Malignant Hyperthermia

With the development and availability of nontriggering intravenous anesthetic agents suitable for ambulatory surgery, patients with the potential for malignant hyperthermia are being safely anesthetized for outpatient surgery. However, the anesthesiologists must be ready to handle a malignant hyperthermia emergency with the immediate availability of dantrolene and be familiar with the malignant hyperthermia treatment protocol. Some institutions prefer to have patients susceptible to malignant hyperthermia stay overnight for observation.

PROCEDURE SELECTION

Initially, only short procedures were done on an ambulatory basis. With the development of shorter-acting anesthetic agents, duration in and of itself is no longer a limiting factor for outpatient surgery. The length of the procedure becomes an important factor primarily when it is a reflection of the difficulty of surgery and its potential for physiologic compromise both intraoperatively and postoperatively. Although all ambulatory surgery centers should be able to cope with any eventuality, patients who may experience massive fluid shifts, have a large amount of blood loss, or require invasive monitoring should be scheduled for inpatient management. Other factors to be considered are whether the surgery is associated with the risk of airway obstruction and whether the surgery will compromise early postoperative ambulation. These recommendations, however, are only guidelines as emphasized by the frequent performance as outpatient procedures of (1) tonsillectomy and adenoidectomy, which may be accompanied by postoperative hemorrhage, and of (2) laparoscopy, which invades the peritoneal cavity.

PREOPERATIVE TESTING

Routine preoperative testing is an inefficient and costly method for identifying asymptomatic disease. Numerous studies have found that nonselective testing has a poor yield in detecting disease that would impact on anesthesia or surgery. Although laboratory tests can help to optimize a patient's preoperative condition once a disease is diagnosed, the tests possess some inherent shortcomings: (1) they frequently fail to uncover pathologic conditions, (2) the abnormalities that they sometimes discover do not necessarily improve the patient care or outcome, (3) they are inefficient in screening for asymptomatic diseases, which are not identifiable through a careful history and physical examination, (4) abnormalities that are discovered through laboratory screening are often not appropriately followed up, leading to increased medicolegal risk, and (5) false-positive results on laboratory screening often lead to increased patient anxiety, increased operating room delays and costs, and may lead to more invasive diagnostic tests and therapies that can actually injure patients.

The best ways to screen for disease are obtaining the history and performing physical examination. Preoperative laboratory testing should then be ordered based on the patient's history. According to recommendations by the University Hospital Consortium: (1) all patients older than age 60 years and all other patients with a specific clinical indication noted on the medical record should have a preoperative chest x-ray; (2) all men aged 40 years and older, women aged 50 years and older, and all other patients with a specific clinical indication noted on the medical record should have a preoperative electrocardiogram; (3) complete blood counts, serum chemistries, and urinalysis should be obtained

when specific clinical indications determine the need for these tests; and (4) platelet counts and prothrombin and partial thromboplastin times should be obtained when the clinical history or specific clinical indications determine the need for these tests. Various standard-setting organizations have developed recommendations for preoperative evaluation of the surgical patient that are different from those of the University Hospital Consortium (Table 9–2).

Healthy children older than 1 year of age undergoing surgical procedures without significant potential for blood loss do not require any blood tests unless clinically indicated. Most clinicians would determine that serum or urine human chorionic gonadotropin tests are needed if the last menstrual period or contraceptive use is questionable.

MECHANISMS FOR PREOPERATIVE EVALUATION

The goals of preoperative assessment are to optimize perioperative management and outcome by evaluating the patient's condition, to reduce patient anxiety, and to obtain informed consent. Currently, patients are screened in a variety of ways. Depending on the system used by the anesthesiologists and the surgeons, a patient can be (1) seen during a facility visit before the day of surgery, (2) seen in an office visit before the day of surgery, (3) interviewed by telephone before surgery with no visit, (4) asked to fill out a written questionnaire, (5) asked to fill out a computer-aided survey (HealthQuiz), and (6) seen the morning of surgery. Adequate preoperative screening allows surgery to proceed as scheduled.

The greatest advantage of a facility visit is that it allows adequate time for a thorough preoperative evaluation to be performed and for consultations to be obtained as indicated. At the same time, patients can familiarize themselves with the hospital or facility. An office visit allows the same thorough preoperative assessment and is less of a scheduling hardship for the anesthesiologist. Telephone interviews are convenient for the patients who are ASA physical status 1 or 2. Written questionnaires have the same limitations as tele-

Table 9–2. Tests Recommended by Various Organizations in Asymptomatic Preoperative Patients

Test	Organization		
	ACP	ACS	ASA
Chest x-ray	Patients with specific indications	All patients	Preanesthetic laboratory and clinical diagnostic testing is often essential; however, no routine* laboratory or diagnostic screening† test is necessary for the preanesthetic evaluation of patients. Appropriate indications for ordering tests include the identification of specific clinical indicators or risk factors (e.g., age, preexisting disease, magnitude of the surgical procedure).
ECG	Men >40 years old, postmenopausal women, patients with specific clinical indications	All patients	
CBC	Patients with specific clinical indications and for institutionalized elderly persons, immigrants, and candidates for procedures with expected substantial blood loss	All patients	
Electrolytes	Patients with specific clinical indications	All patients	
BUN/Cr	Patients with specific clinical indications	All patients	
Glucose	Patients with specific clinical indications	All patients	
PT/PTT	Patients with clinical evidence of a coagulation disorder	All patients	
Platelets	No recommendation	All patients	
Urinalysis	No recommendation	All patients	
Occult fecal blood test	No recommendation	All patients	

*Routine refers to a policy of performing a test or tests without regard to clinical indications in an individual patient.

†Screening means efforts to detect disease in unselected populations of asymptomatic patients.

ACP = American College of Physicians; ACS = American College of Surgeons; ASA = American Society of Anesthesiologists; ECG = electrocardiogram; CBC = complete blood count; BUN/Cr = blood urea nitrogen/serum creatinine; PT/PTT = prothrombin time/partial thromboplastin time.

phone interviews unless they are used in conjunction with a visit, which allows further workup to be pursued as indicated. A recently developed device, HealthQuiz, poses questions to patients and then provides recommendations to the physician for preoperative testing. Finally, the morning-of-operation visit relies on the surgeon to do a complete and thorough preoperative evaluation with appropriate referral to the anesthesiologist if problems arise. Often, the result is that unnecessary "routine" preoperative testing is done at great cost to avoid postponement or cancellation of surgery.

USE OF PRIOR DIAGNOSTIC TEST RESULTS

Given the various mechanisms by which a patient is preoperatively evaluated, laboratory tests may not be obtained the day before surgery. There have been few studies that examine the longevity of diagnostic test results. Recommendations by the University Hospital Consortium regarding the use of prior results are: (1) a chest x-ray showing normal results

that was performed within 1 year of surgery can be used if there has been no intervening clinical event, (2) an electrocardiogram showing normal results that was performed within 6 months of surgery can be used if there has been no intervening clinical event, and (3) blood tests performed within 6 weeks of surgery that show normal results can be used if there has been no intervening clinical event. In one of the few studies that examine the longevity of diagnostic test results, Macpherson and colleagues indicate that, if the previous results are normal and there has been no change in the patient's clinical condition, test results from up to 4 months before the operation could be used without repeat testing. Most guidelines for outpatient surgery require a hemoglobin determination within 30 days of surgery.

RECOVERY AND DISCHARGE

Because more extensive operations requiring longer duration of anesthesia are being performed on an outpatient basis, the assessment of recovery from anesthesia is increasingly significant. The timing of patient discharge following day surgery has major implications for the safety and well being of the patient and for the cost effectiveness of care. Premature release of patients who later experience postoperative complications requiring unanticipated admission to the hospital or an emergency care unit should occur as seldom as possible, preferably not at all.

Definition of the Stages of Recovery

Recovery occurs in three stages. Early recovery refers to emergence from general and local anesthetic and sedative drugs. The patient regains consciousness, airway reflexes, and motor activity. Intermediate recovery refers to "home readiness" and discharge from the surgical facility. The patient regains coordination and has demonstrated the ability to tolerate oral intake, to ambulate, and to void. The latter is particularly important if the patient has had a urologic or gynecologic procedure or has had spinal or epidural anesthesia. Late recovery refers to the period at home during which the patient gradually resumes normal daily activities and recovers fine psychomotor skills.

According to the Joint Commission on Accreditation of Healthcare Organizations, which established Standards of Care in January 1990, a licensed independent practitioner is responsible for the discharge decision. If that person is not personally present, that person's name is still recorded on the medical record. Discharge criteria must be approved by the medical staff and rigorously enforced. A physician must be immediately available in the facility to provide emergency care. Written instructions need to be provided for follow-up care, and these are reviewed with the patient or responsible companion. Patients must be accompanied by a responsible adult. The Accreditation Association for Ambulatory Health Care standards go further in requiring that the patient be seen by the surgeon, anesthesiologist, or dentist before discharge and that the physician available for emergency care is qualified in resuscitative techniques. Table 9–3 lists the

Table 9–3. Clinical Discharge Criteria After Ambulatory Surgery

The patient's vital signs must be stable for at least 1 hour. Blood pressure should be stable ± 20 mm Hg, consistent with age and preanesthetic level.

The patient must have no evidence of respiratory depression such as tachypnea, bradypnea, stridor, obstructed respirations, new onset snoring, retractions, or croupy cough.

The patient must be oriented to person, place, and time; and must be able to dress without dizziness, ambulate without assistance, maintain orally administered fluids, and void. Each should be consistent with age, development, and preanesthetic skill of the patient.

The patient must **not** have more than minimal nausea and vomiting, excessive pain, or excessive bleeding.

After spinal or epidural anesthesia, the patient must have return of sensation before discharge.

After a peripheral nerve block or an axillary block, the patient may not have complete return of sensation before discharge. However, patients must be instructed to monitor circulation, sensation, and swelling, and to protect the affected limb.

The patient must be discharged by the person who gave the anesthesia or by that person's designee.

Patients must have a vested adult to escort them home and stay with them.

Written instructions should be given to the patient for the postoperative period at home, and a contact place and person needs to be reinforced.

The patient should have no new signs or symptoms that may threaten a safe recovery. For example, there should be no evidence of swelling or impaired circulation in an extremity covered by a cast and good circulation and sensation should have returned to an extremity operated on with the use of a tourniquet.

Ideally, the patient will be within 1 hour traveling time from the hospital and have reliable transportation.

clinical discharge criteria for a patient following ambulatory surgery.

Postanesthesia Discharge Scoring Systems

With a system known as the Post-Anesthesia Recovery score (PAR), 0, 1, or 2 points are given for each of five categories (similar to the Apgar score)—activity, respirations, circulation, consciousness, and color. A score of 10 indicates complete recovery from anesthesia, whereas a score of 0 indicates no recovery. A score of less than 7 is not satisfactory for discharge to the floor. Adapting this scoring system for ambulatory surgery requires the use of this system during early recovery as a determinant of the patient's readiness to go to an area designated for intermediate recovery. The PAR cannot be used as the sole determi-

Table 9–4. Postanesthesia Discharge
Scoring System*

Vital signs
   2 = within 20% of preoperative value
   1 = 20%–40% within preoperative value
   0 = >40% preoperative value
Activity and mental status
   2 = oriented × 3 and has a steady gait
   1 = oriented × 3 or has a steady gait
   0 = neither
Pain, nausea, or vomiting
   2 = minimal
   1 = moderate
   0 = severe
Surgical bleeding
   2 = minimal
   1 = moderate
   0 = severe
Intake and output
   2 = has had PO fluid and has voided
   1 = has had PO fluid or has voided
   0 = neither

*Maximum total score is 10; patients scoring ≥9 are considered fit for discharge. Patients are oriented sufficiently to know their name, location, and what time it is.
PO = oral administration.

nant of discharge from the ambulatory surgery unit because it does not take into account the outpatient's need to be able to tolerate oral intake, void, or ambulate.

A simple cumulative index, the Post-Anesthesia Discharge Scoring System (PADS), has been developed by Chung and coworkers to measure the home readiness of ambulatory surgical patients. The PADS is based on several main criteria: (1) vital signs (blood pressure, heart rate, respiratory rate, temperature), (2) ambulation and mental status, (3) pain or nausea and vomiting, (4) surgical bleeding, and (5) intake and output (Table 9–4).

There are many reasons for unanticipated hospital admissions. The patient may have sustained complications due to surgical intervention (e.g., bleeding, uterine perforation). In addition, the patient may have experienced medical complications due to a preexisting disease. The side effects of anesthesia, such as nausea and vomiting, somnolence, and aspiration, are important considerations. The social aspects of patient care cannot be overlooked. When a patient requests to be hospitalized after surgery, it is prudent to comply with the request rather than giving the patient the perception of abandonment, an indication for litigation. The outpatient surgical treatment center must continually record the rate and cause of unanticipated hospital admissions on a monthly basis. When sufficient data are collected, it can be annualized allowing for comparison of intrainstitutional rates from one year to the next. Ideally, it is helpful to compare the results with those of a similar ambulatory care facility. It is often more important to analyze the specific factor that led to unplanned admissions in a given patient or group of patients rather than to look at the overall frequency of admissions within an institution or between facilities. Health care providers must strive to improve the outcomes of the ambulatory care facility, particularly as more complex and new surgical procedures are undertaken in older, sicker patients.

Selected Readings

1. American Society of Anesthesiologists. The ASA Directory of Members 1994. American Society of Anesthesiologists, Park Ridge, IL: 1994:775.
2. American Society of Anesthesiologists. New classification of physical status. Anesthesiology 1963;24:111.
3. Berry FA. Miscellaneous potholes. In: Berry FA, ed. Anesthetic Management of Difficult and Routine Pediatric Patients. 2nd ed. New York: Churchill Livingstone, 1990:411–432.
4. Chung F, Chang VW, Ong D. PADS—a discriminative discharge index for ambulatory surgery (abstr). Anesthesiology 1991;75:A1105.
5. Cohen MM, Cameron CB. Should you cancel the operation when the child has an upper respiratory tract infection? Anesth Analg 1991;72:346–359.
6. Eiseman B. Necessary preoperative tests. In: Wilmore DW, Brennan MF, et al (eds). Medicine: Care of the Surgical Patient, American College of Surgeons. Vol 2. New York, Scientific American, 1989:1.
7. Joint Commission on Accreditation of Healthcare Organizations. Accreditation Manual for Hospitals 1990. Hospital-Sponsored Ambulatory Care Services. SA 1.3.2.1–1.3.2.3, 1989.
8. Macpherson DS, Snow R, Lofgren RP. Preoperative screening: value of previous tests. Ann Intern Med 1990;113:969–973.
9. Meridy HW. Criteria for selection of ambulatory surgical patients and guidelines for anesthetic management. A retrospective study of 1,553 cases. Anesth Analg 1982;61:921–926.
10. Sox HC Jr, ed. Common Diagnostic Tests: Use and Interpretation. Philadelphia: American College of Physicians, 1990.
11. University Hospital Consortium Technology Advancement Center. Recommendations. In: Technology Assessment: Routine Preoperative Diagnostic Evaluations. Oak Brook, IL: University Hospital Consortium, 1994:3.

10

Universal Precautions

Richard F. Edlich • David J. Bentrem • David B. Drake

In 1983, the Centers for Disease Control (CDC) published a report "Guidelines for Isolation Precautions in Hospitals" that had a special section entitled "Blood and Body Fluid Precautions." The CDC recommended blood and body fluid precautions for a patient known or suspected to be infected with blood-borne pathogens. Four years later (August 1987), it recommended that blood and body fluid precautions be consistently used regardless of the blood-borne infectious status of the patient. This expansion of blood and body fluid precautions to all patients is referred to as "universal blood and body fluid precautions" or "universal precautions."

The universal precautions were developed to prevent the spread of blood-borne pathogens, which included primarily viruses and retroviruses. The hallmark feature of retroviruses is that they use a process called reverse transcription to synthesize a DNA copy of an RNA strand during their replication (a reversal of the ordinary flow of genetic information—from DNA to RNA to protein). The most common blood-borne viruses are hepatitis B, C, and D, and the retroviruses are the human immunodeficiency virus (HIV) and the human T-cell lymphotrophic virus type-I (HTLV-I) and type-II (HTLV-II).

Hepatitis B virus (HBV) has been estimated to infect 12,000 health care workers annually who have occupational contact with blood. HBV causes approximately 3000 cases of acute hepatitis B annually; approximately 500 persons so infected are hospitalized, and 200 die.

Deaths are caused by either acute hepatitis or the complications of chronic HBV infection, including hepatoma, cirrhosis, and chronic hepatitis. Despite these complications of HBV infection, fewer than one half of the health care workers at risk for occupational HBV infection have received the hepatitis B vaccine.

Whereas HBV infection is an established occupational hazard for workers exposed to blood, those individuals infected with HBV can, in turn, infect their patients. Since the early 1970s, there have been reports of 20 clusters in which a total of 300 patients were infected by HBV-infected health care workers. In 12 of these clusters, the infected workers did not wear gloves, and several who were infected had skin lesions that may have facilitated transmission.

A review of these clusters identified two important risk factors that contribute to the transmission of HBV from the health care workers. First, the potential exists for contamination of the surgical wound or traumatized tissue with HBV from the worker when there is a major break in universal precautions (e.g., by not wearing gloves during invasive procedures or from inadvertent injury to the infected worker during the invasive procedure [e.g., needle sticks]). Second, 17 of the 20 workers whose hepatitis B and antigen (HBeAg) status was determined, were HBeAg positive. Because the presence of HBeAg in the serum is associated with higher levels of circulating virus, these infected individuals are especially prone to transmit the infection. The risk of infection of the patient after percutaneous exposure to HBeAg-positive blood is approximately 30%.

This research was supported by a generous gift from Beth Ross, Orlando, Florida.

Seven of the workers who were in the clusters were allowed to perform invasive procedures after adhering to appropriate modification in their technique and practices (e.g., wearing double gloves and restricting certain high-risk procedures). No further transmission to patients was observed in the records of five workers; thus, infected workers who adhere to universal precautions and who perform certain exposure-prone procedures present a small risk to patients.

When diagnostic tests became available for hepatitis A and B, it was apparent that the major proportion of post-transfusion hepatitis was due to an unknown agent, subsequently shown to be an RNA flavovirus, named hepatitis C virus (HCV). It is a blood-borne virus transmittable by blood transfusions and other parenteral routes. There is some evidence that HCV may be vertically transmitted from infected mothers to their children. A small proportion of cases occur through household contact with infected patients; sexual transmission is also believed to occur. The overall risk of HCV transmission from a single needle stick accident from an infected patient is estimated to be 3% to 10%.

Seroconversion does not occur for weeks to months after infection so that the period of infectivity is long before seropositivity is established. Approximately 5% to 10% of patients with HCV infection become chronic carriers, with a small proportion of these cases progressing to chronic active hepatitis and cirrhosis. Approximately half of the cases of HCV infection progress to chronic liver disease and some 20% of these to cirrhosis. Because the serologic test for HCV cannot distinguish between present and past infection, all anti-HCV–positive patients must be presumed to be infectious.

Hepatitis D virus (HDV), also called delta virus, causes infection only in the presence of active HBV infection. Transmission usually occurs through blood contacts, especially among intravenous drug users and hemophiliacs. The mortality rate associated with acute HDV infection is higher than with other forms of viral hepatitis, varying from 2% to 20%. A test for detection of IgM anti-HDV is commercially available.

The risk of HIV transmission to a health care worker after percutaneous exposure to HIV is considerably less than the risk of HBV transmission after percutaneous exposure to HBeAg-positive blood (0.3%–30%). Consequently, the risk of transmission of HIV from an infected health care worker is proportionally lower than the risk of HBV transmission from an HBeAg-positive health care worker during a similar procedure. However, health care workers are much more complacent about contracting hepatitis than HIV because HIV infection is lifelong and remains transmissible throughout the period of infection. Progression of HIV infection to symptomatic illness can be expected in most patients in a period of years.

Hepatitis B virus is transmitted much more readily than HIV. When it was realized that the recognizably ill HIV-infected patients represented only a small fraction of the patient population, the CDC applied its precautions for prevention of HIV transmission in health care settings to all patients at all times in all health situations and called them universal precautions.

The HTLV-I was the first pathogenic retrovirus identified in humans. The major modes of HTLV-I transmission include perinatal, which occurs predominantly postnatally through breast feeding, parenterally through blood transfusion or exposure to needles or syringes contaminated with blood, or sexually. HTLV-I infection is endemic primarily in the Caribbean, some areas of Africa, southwestern Japan, and Italy. In the United States, HLTV-I infection has been identified primarily in intravenous drug users. HTLV-I infection is associated with adult T-cell leukemia and lymphoma and HTLV-I–associated myelopathy and tropical spastic paraparesis. Certain screening tests have been licensed by the Food and Drug Administration to detect HTLV-I antibodies in human serum. In the absence of a vaccine, there is sufficient epidemiologic information to bring the infections under control.

Because HTLV-I infection is not transmitted by casual contact, health care workers in the ambulatory surgery department should be concerned about percutaneous exposure to HTLV-I–contaminated needles. One health care worker was inadvertently inoculated with blood from a T-cell leukemia and lymphoma adult patient in Japan and subsequently underwent seroconversion. Of the 31 other laboratory personnel and workers exposed to HTLV-I via puncture wounds, no other seroconversion has been reported.

Human T-cell lymphotrophic virus type II is so closely related to HTLV-I that there is extensive serologic cross-reactivity among proteins from HTLV-I and HTLV-II. There is no specific information regarding the seroepidemiology or the modes of transmission of HTLV-II. However, there is evidence that some of the HTLV-I seropositivity in the United States may be caused by HTLV-II, especially in intravenous drug users.

Only a few cases of disease have been associated with HTLV-II infection. This retrovirus was first isolated from a patient with a rare T-lymphocytic hairy cell leukemia. Another case of HTLV-II infection was identified in a patient who had the more common B-lymphocytic form of hairy cell leukemia and who also had a T-suppressor lymphoproliferative disease. An additional 21 cases of hairy cell leukemia had no serologic evidence of HTLV-II infection. Consequently, the disease association of HTLV-II is unclear; the lifetime risk of disease among infected persons is also uncertain.

HEALTH CARE WORKER SURVEILLANCE

The current assessment of the risk of infected health care workers to transmit HIV or HBV during exposure-prone procedures indicates that these workers should know their HIV and HBV antibody status. Health care workers who are infected with HIV or HBV (and are HBeAg positive) should not perform exposure-prone procedures unless they have counsel from an expert review panel that has the following participants: (1) the worker's personal physician, (2) an infectious disease specialist, (3) a surgeon who performs similar exposure-prone procedures, and (4) a state and local health official. If the review panel advises any special circumstances for the health care worker to perform these procedures, then the health care worker may continue to perform these procedures. Prospective patients should be notified of the

seropositivity of the health care worker before undergoing the exposure-prone procedure. Mandatory testing of these workers for HIV antibody, HBsAg, or HBeAg is not recommended. The current assessment of the risk that infected health care workers will transmit HIV or HBV to patients during exposure-prone procedures does not support the diversion of resources that would be required to implement mandatory testing programs. Compliance by health care workers with recommendations can be increased through education, training, and appropriate confidentiality safeguards.

PATIENT TESTING

Personnel in some hospitals have advocated serologic testing of patients in units in which health care workers may be exposed to large amounts of patients' blood. Specific patients in whom serologic testing is advocated are those undergoing major operative procedures and those treated in critical care units for conditions involving uncontrolled bleeding. When deemed appropriate, testing of individual patients may be performed on agreement between the patient and physician. The seropositive patient must be counseled by properly trained persons. Confidentiality safeguards must be in place to limit knowledge of the test results to those directly involved in the care of infected patients.

EXPOSURE-PRONE PROCEDURES

Certain invasive surgical and dental procedures have been implicated in the transmission of HBV infection from infected health care workers to patients despite adherence to universal precautions, and these should be considered to be exposure prone. Characteristics of exposure-prone procedures include a highly confined or poorly visualized anatomic site that may require digital palpation of a needle tip. This circumstance is often encountered in cardiothoracic, colorectal, obstetric-gynecologic, and oral surgery.

Wright and coworkers reported that the

majority (67%) of the sharp injuries to the surgeons was due to a needle stick and usually occurred during suturing. These sharp injuries caused bleeding in 85% of incidences, suggesting the possibility of disease transmission. Similarly, Tokars and colleagues observed that 77% of the injuries were due to needle punctures to surgeons and commonly affected the nondominant hand (63%), especially the distal index finger. The risk of injury (adjusted by confounding variables by logistic regression) was higher during vaginal hysterectomy.

MANAGEMENT OF HEALTH CARE WORKERS AFTER OCCUPATIONAL EXPOSURE

Employers should make available to workers a system for promptly initiating evaluation, counseling, and follow-up after a reported occupational exposure that may place the worker at risk of acquiring infection. If an exposure occurs, the circumstances should be recorded in the worker's confidential medical record. Both the exposed worker and the source individual should be evaluated to determine the possible need for the exposed worker to receive prophylaxis against hepatitis B. In addition, the source individual should be informed of the incident and, if consent is obtained, tested for serologic evidence of HIV infection. If consent cannot be obtained (e.g., if the patient is unconscious), policy should be developed for testing source individuals in compliance with applicable state and local laws.

Confidentiality of the names of the source individual and the health care worker should be maintained at all times. If the source individual has acquired immunodeficiency syndrome (AIDS), is known to be HIV seropositive, or refuses testing, the health care worker should be evaluated clinically and serologically for evidence of HIV infection as soon as possible after exposure and, if seronegative, should be retested periodically for a minimum of 6 months after exposure to determine whether HIV infection has occurred. If the source individual is HIV seronegative and has no clinical manifestations of AIDS or HIV infection, no further HIV follow-up of the exposed worker is necessary.

UNIVERSAL PRECAUTIONS

The fundamental basis for universal precautions is the interposition of barriers between patient body fluids and the health care worker. In the ambulatory admission suite and the recovery room of the ambulatory surgery center, personnel protective equipment for the health care worker is recommended and related to the task or activity as listed in Table 10–1. In the operating room, gloves provide a barrier to infection that is too easily breached by needles and sharp surgical instruments. Once breached, a glove is no longer an effective barrier to infection, necessitating a change of gloves as soon as practical after the breach is visually detected. The most common method of protecting the surgeon against

Table 10–1. Examples of Recommended Personal Protective Equipment for Worker Protection Against HIV and HBV Transmission in Prehospital Ambulatory Surgical Care Setting

Task or Activity	Disposable Gloves	Gown	Mask	Protective Eyewear
Bleeding control with minimal bleeding	Yes	No	No	No
Blood drawing	At certain times	No	No	No
Starting an intravenous line	Yes	No	No	No
Oral and nasal suctioning, manually cleaning airway	Yes	No	No, unless splashing is likely	No, unless splashing is likely
Handling and cleaning instruments with microbial contamination	Yes	No, unless soiling is likely	No	No
Measuring blood pressure	No	No	No	No
Measuring temperature	No	No	No	No
Giving an injection	No	No	No	No

glove puncture is by use of the double-glove system. The concept of the double-glove technique became popular during performance of the total hip arthroplasty. In a prospective study at the Medical College of Georgia, McCue and associates reported that changing the outer glove at appropriate times during the procedure was an effective way to minimize contamination during the operative procedure. They reported that the gloves that most frequently were contaminated were the ones used exclusively for draping. Of the 275 gloves tested, there were 35 holes in the outer gloves and only 12 in the inner gloves.

In a later study, Matta and coworkers reported that wearing double gloves confers some protection for the surgeon against contamination of the surgeon's skin with the patient's tissue and fluids. In their study, 77 (11%) of the outer gloves were punctured; 15 of the 77 inner gloves were punctured. These results indicated that double gloving maintained a barrier between the wearer and the patient in four out of five cases.

In light of the continuing reports suggesting the inadequacy of the single-glove technique as a surgical barrier, Cohn and Seifer performed a prospective study measuring the presence of visible blood on the hands of surgeons wearing either single or double gloves during 45 consecutive major obstetric and gynecologic operations. Single-gloved hands revealed the presence of blood in 38% of cases, whereas visible blood was noted in only 2% of double-gloved hands. In addition to reducing the risk of contaminating surgeons, double gloving has also been shown to reduce the risk of HBV transmission from surgeon to patient.

The success of the double-gloving technique in preventing needle perforation has been attributed to the increased resistance of the doubled glove to needle penetration. This hypothesis has been confirmed by our quantitative measurements of the needle penetration force and work required for taper point needles to penetrate either a single-glove or double-glove system. For the double-glove systems, the mean penetration force and the penetration work for the taper point needle to perforate the system were approximately twofold greater than those for the single glove.

Some surgeons have reservations about double gloving because of their concerns regarding their previous experiences of reduced dexterity and decreased sensation when using doubled gloves. These perceptions were not supported by Webb and Pentlow in their comparison of double gloving versus single gloving with regard to its effects on tactile discrimination and dexterity in 17 surgeons. Double gloving did not alter two-point discrimination or their ability to tie knots.

GLOVE PUNCTURE INDICATION SYSTEMS

Most glove breaches are unnoticed for some time after perforation. Results of one study showed that glove damage goes unnoticed in as many as 58% of cases. Failure to detect the breached glove has led to development of a colored glove hole detection system as well as an electronic puncture detection system. The colored glove hole detection system is the Biogel Reveal system (Regent Hospital Products, Greenville, SC), which is a double-glove system with a special inner and outer glove. Each component of this glove system has several important unique features.

The inner and outer gloves are manufactured without the chemical accelerators mercaptobenzothiazole and thiurams, which are responsible for allergic reactions (e.g., chronic urticaria of the hands) as well as generalized cutaneous symptoms and anaphylactic reactions. In their place, dithiocarbamate is used as an accelerator because carbamates are thought to sensitize the skin to a lesser extent than other accelerators. The Biogel latex gloves typically contain less than 0.1% residual carbamate; this level of carbamate is 15 times less than the amount of carbamate that the Food and Drug Administration allows in food contact materials.

Besides using minimal amounts of accelerators, the glove manufacturing process includes several processing steps (rinsing and leaching procedures) designed to remove residual accelerators as well as latex proteins. The latter have been incriminated as other causal factors of allergic reactions. The extractable latex proteins in these gloves are virtually undetectable

(>8 μg/g of glove), thereby considerably reducing the risk of sensitization.

The Biogel outer glove and the inner glove have a hydrogel polymer lining that has important clinical implications. The outer glove has the lining only on its inner surface, whereas the inner glove has the lining on its inner and outer surfaces. Hydrogels have been used to make contact lenses in the United States and have undergone extensive clinical testing for safety. The hydrogel polymer lining facilitates donning with both dry and wet hands without the presence of cornstarch powders, eliminating glove-powder complications. This lining also provides a barrier for the wearer against direct skin-to-latex contact, which is especially important in individuals with sensitivities to latex proteins or accelerators.

The Biogel Reveal system is a complete puncture detection system. The inner glove, which is a half size smaller than the outer glove, is colored with a green dye. When the outer glove is punctured, leakage of fluids through the needle puncture hole causes the inner glove to develop a dark patch around the punctured hole, signaling the presence of a needle puncture hole, an indication for glove removal and the donning of a new intact glove system. This color change is an optical effect and does not involve release of dye or any other material. Both the outer and inner gloves have beaded cuffs to prevent glove roll down.

The recent increase in concern over microbial contamination in operating rooms has prompted the development of several electronic hole detection monitors that warn the operating team member when a surgical glove has a hole. The Barrier Integrity Monitor (BIM) (InCoMed, Inc., San Diego, CA) and the Surgic Alert Monitor (SAM) (Novatech Medical Products, Inc., Houston, TX) are two of the newest hole detection systems. The SAM uses several favorable design features. The SAM console is four times smaller than the BIM control unit and attaches to the user's scrub suit. Because all team members have their own device, there is no limit to the number of personnel being monitored by the SAM system. Hospital personnel do not have to stand on conductive mats to complete the electrical circuit in the SAM system, a design feature that allows for increased mobility in the operating room. The SAM device sounds two distinctly different alarms, one for glove hydration and another to signal the presence of a hole. In contrast, the BIM is only able to monitor one parameter. The BIM alarm is the same for both hydration and hole detection. In rapidly hydrating gloves, the BIM sounds excessive false alarms indicating a hole when none is present, causing hospital personnel to change gloves unnecessarily. The SAM does not sound any false alarms. In the case of gloves hydrating rapidly, within less than 20 minutes, the SAM device always sounds the "end-of-use" hydration warning, but occasionally fails to signal the "end-of-use" alarm in the presence of a hole.

Both the BIM and SAM systems performed better when used with a glove that resists hydration. The role of hydration in glove performance is unclear and may have potential deleterious effects. Hydration may affect the elastic properties of a glove so that the glove no longer fits snugly and uniformly. The glove may also become more susceptible to needle penetration. The current of electrocoagulation devices may damage the hydrated glove, predisposing it to the formation of holes. The validity of these hypotheses must be tested in well-controlled, experimental studies that can be replicated in any research laboratory.

OTHER PROTECTIVE CLOTHING CONSIDERATIONS

Although the presence of powder on surgical gloves did not influence the duration of hydration time, powdered gloves have been shown to act as foreign bodies, which predispose the patient to infection by damaging local tissue defenses. With the advent of a wide variety of powder-free gloves, the surgeon no longer must resort to the use of powdered gloves during surgery.

Leakage of blood onto the surgeon's hands can also occur at the gown sleeve–glove junction. This exposure to blood can be prevented by a modification in the design of the surgical gloves. In abdominal procedures in which the abdomen is filled with fluid, an elbow-length glove could prevent this exposure to blood.

Health care workers with exudative lesions or weeping dermatitis should refrain from all direct patient care and from handling patient care equipment. The operating room personnel should adhere to appropriate hand washing before donning surgical gloves. Hands should always be washed after the gloves are removed, even if gloves appear to be intact. When surgical procedures involve splash, splatter, or generation of blood and body fluids, conjunctival, nasal, and oral mucosa should be protected from blood splatter or aerosolization. A variety of devices have been designed to protect all three sites simultaneously and include full-face shields and disposable masks with upper eye shields. Disposable or reusable operating gowns that resist wetting should be worn during the operative procedures. The most recent Occupational Safety and Health Administration (OSHA) memorandum indicates that protective gowns should be fluid proof or fluid resistant. In Smith and Nichols' study of the barrier efficiency of surgical gowns, they reported that disposable and reusable gowns currently available exhibit varying resistance to blood strike through. Only those gowns with impervious plastic reinforcement offered complete protection.

SPECIAL CIRCUMSTANCES

In addition to universal precautions recommended for all patients, certain additional precautions for the care of HIV-infected patients undergoing major surgical operations have been proposed by personnel in some hospitals. For example, surgical procedures on an HIV-infected patient should be altered so that hand-to-hand passage of sharp instruments would be eliminated. Stapling instruments rather than hand suturing equipment should be used to perform tissue approximation. Electrosurgical devices rather than scalpels should be used as cutting instruments. Gowns that prevent blood strike through are mandatory.

Proper handling of needles and other contaminated sharp objects and the appropriate disposal of used sharp needles is essential. Jagger and coworkers found that one third of the venipuncture needle injuries occurred during recapping of needles. More injuries occurred during the disposal process than while the devices were in use. Consequently, recapping of needles should be avoided. Needle and sharps disposal containers should be placed as near to the areas of use as possible. Needle disposal containers must be rigid, impervious to accidental extrusion of their contents, and clearly labeled. Desirable design features include ease of insertion of a fairly large needle syringe unit, resistance to accidental removal of its contents, and an indication of depth of its contents.

All instruments, materials, and devices must be sterile. Sterilization is a strictly defined process and must be monitored for compliance with standards.

Selected Readings

1. Cohn GM, Seifer DB. Blood exposure in single versus double gloving during pelvic surgery. Am J Obstet Gynecol 1990;162:715–717.
2. Cox MJ, Bromberg WJ, Zura RD, Foresman PA, Morgan RF, Edlich RF. New advances in electronic devices for hole detection. J Appl Biomat 1994;5:257–264.
3. Jagger J, Hunt EH, Brand-Einaggar J, Pearson RD. Rates of needle stick injury caused by various devices in a university hospital. N Engl J Med 1988;319:284–288.
4. Manson TT, Bromberg WG, Thacker JG, McGregor W, Morgan RF, Edlich RF. A new glove puncture detection system. J Emerg Med 1995;13:357–364.
5. Matta H, Thompson AM, Rainey JB. Does wearing two pairs of gloves protect operating theatre staff from skin contamination? BMJ 1988;297:597–598.
6. McCue SF, Berg EW, Saunders EA. Efficacy of double-gloving as a barrier to microbial contamination during total joint arthroplasty. J Bone Joint Surg [Am] 1981;63:811–813.
7. Smith JW, Nichols RL. Barrier efficiency of surgical gowns. Are we really protected from our patients' pathogens? Arch Surg 1991;126:756–763.
8. Tokars JI, Bell DM, Culver DH, et al. Percutaneous injuries during surgical procedures. JAMA 1992;257:2899–2904.
9. Webb JM, Pentlow BD. Double gloving and surgical technique. Ann R Coll Surg Engl 1993;75:291–292.
10. Wright JG, McGeer AJ, Chyatte D, Ransohoff DF. Mechanisms of glove tears and sharp injuries among surgical personnel. JAMA 1991;296:1668–1671.

Components of the Ambulatory Surgery Center

11

The Role of the Medical Director in the Ambulatory Surgical Center

William T. Ross, Jr.

The successful coordination of the work of a modern ambulatory surgical center is complex and requires several disciplines to work well together. The central goal is *"the provision of effective care of patients"* in a framework that recognizes and manages the competing nature of the following:

Health care professionals

Ancillary health care workers

Systems to provide supplies

Scheduling

Maintenance

Systems to manage and account for disbursements and receipts

Systems to analyze and describe the results of the work of the organization

Cutting edge technology

Established technology

Costs, charges, and prices

Purchasers of health care services

Regulators and regulations

In this chapter, some topics are discussed from the perspective of a physician medical director. It should be noted that health care delivery, documentation, costs, and reimbursement are in a state of active change.

ADMINISTRATION

The work of an ambulatory surgery center requires the coordination of a number of ad-

ministrative functions. The necessary administrative structure depends greatly on the way a particular surgery center is organized and its relation to other entities. An independent freestanding surgery center must provide all administrative functions, whereas a center that is a unit within an existing inpatient hospital has access to many existing administrative capabilities. Hospital-affiliated centers then may function with less apparent overhead when, in fact, the necessary administrative functions are made available to the surgery center by the parent organization. Such shifts of support services, early in the existence of a start-up surgical center, may be made without assignment of costs of such services to the budget of the center. However, it is typical for such support services costs to be added into the costs of business at some point after the start-up period. Such adjustments are correct and proper, but, if not clearly understood, may be of great concern for the staff. In the long run, it may be prudent for the center to identify such issues at the outset and to budget and operate accordingly.

Outpatient and inpatient operations are different enough that management conflicts can arise and may jeopardize the success of the ambulatory surgical center. For example, the more costly anesthetic agents, from which rapid recovery is predictable, are recognized as facilitating the steady and predictable flow of patients through the postoperative spaces of the ambulatory surgery center. They contribute to the ability to maintain the steady flow of patients that is seen as effective and efficient by those who use the facility. On the other hand, for inpatient surgery, the patients' beds are held available while the patient is cared for in surgical and postanesthesia suites. The result is a difference in the concern for the details of recovery from anesthesia. The inpatient bias often is toward the less costly anesthetic agents rather than on the speed and quality of recovery from the operation and anesthesia. Similar considerations have favored the development and advancement of a wide variety of endoscopic surgical procedures and have resulted in placing newer (and often "better") equipment in ambulatory surgery centers.

Supplies and equipment are one of the major items in the budget of an ambulatory surgery center. It is essential that the purchase of these items be coordinated within the administrative structure of the center. When this occurs, prices are virtually always subject to negotiation downward and suppliers are willing to work with the facility to provide the timely arrival of smaller shipments. This helps the center maintain a smaller, less costly inventory and does not require as much valuable storage space. Surgical facilities must be able to monitor and negotiate all areas of cost to their enterprise. Price increases go unnoticed unless someone is responsible for monitoring them. All but the smallest facilities find that this monitoring more than pays the salary of an individual assigned to this job.

The staffing requirements of an ambulatory surgery center require provision for a range of functions (Table 11–1). Such requirements are most extensive for an autonomous freestanding center and may be less so for centers that are administratively a part of a larger parent organization in which such functions may be derived from the parent organization.

Many of the tasks listed in Table 11–1 overlap with others in the list. Some of these tasks may be performed by one individual. On the other hand, operation of larger or growing facilities may require a larger staff. Personnel issues related to hiring, salaries, evaluation, suitability for continued employment, reassignment, and remediation occupy significant portions of senior administrative time and effort.

When good employees are identified, they can be encouraged to further improve and be rewarded by a personnel system that recognizes good performance and encourages (and permits) self-improvement through continuing education. Such opportunities should be made available with *strong* educational offerings to staff members who are so inclined. These individuals typically bring more back to the center than they cost in the course of continuing their education and they tend to become the most loyal employees.

MEDICAL PRACTICE WITHIN THE SURGERY CENTER

The medical director should be able to set priorities and establish a mission for the center. This important task needs to be developed in concert with the governing body and senior administrative personnel. It provides foresight for the goals of the center and is most effective when published as a written statement. Its implementation requires intimate knowledge of

Table 11–1. Staffing Requirements

Medical Direction	Administrative	Nursing
Policies	Reception	Operating room
Practice guidelines	Clerical/billing	Nurses
Practitioner credentialling	Scheduling	Licensed practical nurses
Risk management	Administrative support	Technicians
	Financial management	Preoperative
	Personnel/hiring and evaluation	Postanesthesia
	Maintenance	Teaching
	Quality improvement	Attendants
		Anesthesia support
		Central sterile supply

the way in which groups of people function well together and especially of essential elements in the safe and effective delivery of the perioperative experience for patients. One individual cannot perform all the tasks necessary to manage the facility. The medical director must be able to enlist the aid of personnel who can effectively contribute to the operation of the center.

SCHEDULING AND PERIOPERATIVE CARE OF PATIENTS

Patients are typically seen in a surgical clinic or surgeon's office where the need for surgery is determined. After a discussion of treatment options, the patient and physician may decide to schedule the procedure at the ambulatory surgical center. Once the patient is booked for a date and time, the center has effectively entered into a contract with the patient and surgeon, and will probably be involved in securing anesthesia services for the surgical encounter. All involved parties have important expectations. Most such expectations are handled implicitly. The way in which the work of the center is perceived and evaluated is heavily colored by the manner in which the expectations of the various parties to the perioperative encounter are met. When expectations are recognized and managed well, the center is seen as supportive, friendly, and efficient.

If the nature of the practice at the ambulatory surgical center allows the surgeon and surgical staff to adequately evaluate patients at the time the decision for surgery is made, preoperative testing can be handled there without a requirement for another (or multiple) appointment(s) for further preoperative evaluation. The center should take an active role in coordinating the preoperative evaluation (including evaluation for anesthesia) and scheduling the patient so there is adequate time for arrival, "day of surgery" preoperative evaluation, changing of clothes, preparation, insertion of an intravenous line, premedication, and similar tasks. Consistent with good, safe medical practice, the goal is to recognize that the patient's time is valuable and to set

up the visit to the ambulatory surgical center with this in mind.

Consistently applied, these considerations may be extended to the whole of the visit to the surgical center, giving the patient a sense of comfort because needs were addressed, or better, anticipated. The staff of the center must be honest about pain, tubes, and needles, and they must be well informed so they can convincingly, yet kindly, discuss the questions that repeatedly arise. Having their needs satisfactorily addressed in a caring manner is particularly reassuring to patients. The nursing staff should be encouraged to ask questions of concern regarding the patient's comfort (e.g., "I see you're shivering. Would a warm blanket help?") and to provide prompt solutions when necessary (e.g., delivering a warmed blanket immediately from the adjacent well-stocked blanket warmer).

HISTORY AND PHYSICAL EXAMINATION

The best single diagnostic tool for assessing a patient's suitability for anesthesia and surgery is an appropriate history and physical examination. In the day-to-day operation of an ambulatory surgical center, there are times when the definition of "appropriate" must be clear to all involved in caring for patients. It is very important that the center establish clear policies for the care of its patients.

FACILITY POLICIES

It has been established that institutions are responsible for the quality of care they provide, including those elements that are delivered by practitioners who are not employees of the facility. The policies with respect to patient evaluation need to be set with broad acceptance by all who work at the center. Exceptions to well-designed policies should rarely be necessary. Exceptions tend to be viewed as a precedent for continuing deviation from the policy. For this reason, it is important that policies be constructed so they function well in the everyday work of the surgical center.

Policies should not be written if they cannot be used.

ANESTHESIA SERVICES

Providers of anesthesia services in the ambulatory surgical center play an important role in accomplishing the work of the center. The medical director must evaluate these practitioners, be they anesthesiologists or certified registered nurse anesthetists (CRNAs). The lines of responsibility for CRNAs depend on the law in the jurisdiction in which they are working, on liability carrier requirements (or preferences), and on local practice patterns. All persons who provide anesthesia care in a busy ambulatory surgical practice must be able to rapidly and accurately assess patients and make clinical judgments about the match of proposed anesthetic care to each patient.

The medical director has to assume a major role in providing an environment in which anesthesia personnel can work safely and effectively, and the medical director should be sufficiently knowledgeable about the anesthetic care of patients to support the clinical concerns of the anesthesia providers. For example, the choice may arise whether to stage patients in the preoperative area on stretchers or in chairs. If chairs are used, would they tilt so that feet could be elevated? Some further questions might be as follows:

Will intravenous lines be started in the preoperative area or in the operating room?

How will the patients who faint be treated?

Will premedication be administered in the preoperative area?

During surgery, will the patient be on a stretcher or on an operating table that remains in the operating room?

Many questions of this sort are most easily answered when immediately followed by a second question: "Who will provide this element of care to the patient?" The answers to such questions have implications related to staffing patterns, equipment requirements, assignment of tasks, patient satisfaction, facility effectiveness, and patient safety.

The American Society of Anesthesiologists and other organizations have provided guidelines for the perioperative care of patients. For monitoring for general and regional anesthesia, continuous monitoring of blood pressure, electrocardiogram, respiration, and pulse oximetry are required. In addition, temperature monitoring should be available and end tidal CO_2 must be assessed when endotracheal intubation is used. Most anesthesia practitioners monitor end tidal CO_2 and volatile anesthetic concentration during all general anesthetics. S-T segment analysis of the electrocardiogram is being used increasingly in anesthetic management during the perioperative care of inpatients. As the characteristics of surgical outpatients approach those of the population in general, a trend toward the use of S-T segment monitoring in outpatients may be expected.

PREOPERATIVE CARE

Patients' perceptions of their care are strongly influenced by their reception during the preoperative phase of their visit to the ambulatory surgery facility. Time spent waiting without acknowledgment that the patient's time is valuable is a frequent source of patient dissatisfaction. When the schedule falls behind, patients should be informed that their appointment has been delayed and be offered a rescheduled time when appropriate. A sensitive preoperative nurse is more effective, projects more authority, and can provide more information when delivering such messages.

INTRAOPERATIVE CARE

In recent years, there has been a great deal of discussion about the qualifications of operating room personnel. In the 1980s, the use of an all-registered nurse (RN) staff was in vogue. It has been demonstrated, however, that licensed practical nurses (LPNs) and operating room technicians work well when sound nursing direction and support are provided. Such employees are less expensive, more focused, and have fewer pressures to perform tasks other than their surgical support function. Their availability in conjunction with adequate RN staff is an effective way to contain personnel costs and maintain a very capable staff. The facility operating room staff must work closely and continually with operating surgeons to know in advance what instruments and supplies the surgeon will require for each case. This is particularly true in the freestanding facilities where equipment cannot be borrowed from other departments. Planning ahead for equipment purchases often permits a facility purchasing agent to obtain more favorable pricing for high cost items and results in substantial savings.

The availability and use of good lighting and magnification intraoperatively have made an enormous improvement in the application of many surgical techniques. This lighting commonly includes overhead lights, headlights, lighted retractors, microscopes, and compound lens binocular loupes. The exact devices purchased depend on the procedure, the surgeon, and the budget. Because of the general recognition of the importance of these devices, they are available from a variety of sources. There are many opportunities to find good value from various suppliers. The medical director should become acquainted with the issues involved in the acquisition of the more expensive equipment items and promote the search for good value that will meet or exceed the purely medical requirements.

Over the past 15 years, there have been striking developments in all types of endoscopic surgery. The techniques and equipment have undergone rapid refinement. The continuous availability of new and better endoscopes, trocars, introducers, and instruments has made the timing of purchases difficult and has kept prices relatively high. As this field matures, opportunities will appear for facilities to better plan purchases while maintaining a high level of current sophistication in procedures. This rapid development of endoscopic surgery has had an interesting effect on the care of patients. In the first analysis, procedures once performed only in an inpatient hospital are now routinely done in an outpatient setting. Even in situations in which it is judged possible to perform a particular procedure for a particular patient only on an inpatient basis, consideration will have been given to performing the proposed surgery in the outpatient setting. As criteria, protocols, and

follow-up care evolve, more surgery will be performed on an outpatient basis. All persons involved in patient care need to recognize that the economic advantage occurring with surgery performed without hospital admission will be moderated by costs that are incurred by patient recovery in a nonhospital site.

POSTSURGICAL AND POSTANESTHESIA CARE

Care of the patient in the immediate postoperative period is provided in a postanesthesia care unit (PACU). Even though the emergence from anesthesia is a phase of care that demands special vigilance, attention to a range of issues related to the particular surgical procedure must also be addressed. In the outpatient setting, the PACU can conveniently be divided into an acute or first phase PACU and a step-down or second phase PACU. Particularly in the first phase, there needs to be some separation of patients from one another because early PACU care may involve coughing, retching, a need for active airway management, removal of packs or drains, and wound care.

PREPARATION FOR DISCHARGE

Once patients are comfortable and ready to sit, they may be moved to the second phase PACU where they can be joined by family or a friend. It is good to use this opportunity for an accompanying adult to help with the care of the patient. He or she may assist with dressing and should be present when postoperative instructions are given. In this way, the accompanying adult becomes involved in providing help to the patient and can have any lingering questions answered. It is important to provide written instructions to patients and their escorts explaining the range of expected events as well as unexpected events and guidelines for how to handle them. Telephone numbers along with instructions are provided regarding how to contact the surgeon (or designee) if necessary.

It generally is best if the staff of the surgical center provides instruction regarding the procedure for making an appointment for a return visit rather than making the appointment for the patient.

FOLLOW-UP

In the usual circumstances, patients follow up with their surgeons concerning the surgical procedure itself. To satisfy institutional needs to document outcomes of care, the surgical facility will conduct at least some follow-up of those for whom it has provided care. This can take the form of a postoperative telephone call or a follow-up questionnaire. These instruments seem to be received well when they are brief and require only "yes" or "no" answers. This should not prevent patients from amplifying a response, and space should be provided on questionnaires for their comments. Even when patients have negative comments, most respond to this search for information in a positive and constructive manner. Facilities can also improve their outcome evaluation by querying physicians concerning infections and unexpected visits, among other things.

SUMMARY

Medical direction of an ambulatory surgical facility should be provided by a physician who is committed to the goals and mission of the facility. Such an individual will probably conduct a large part of his or her practice within the facility and must certainly be aware of day-to-day operations. The medical director will have the opportunity to be involved in medical, physical plant, fiscal, personnel, supply, quality assurance, risk management, and accreditation areas. This person needs to be able to work well with and leverage the skills of administrative as well as medical personnel.

Selected Readings

1. Finkler S. The distinction between cost and charges. Ann Intern Med 1992;96:102–109.
2. Macurio A, Dunn B, Vitez TS, McDonald T. Where are the costs in perioperative care? Anesthesiology 1995; 83:1138–1144.
3. Ross WT. General Management Issues in Perioperative Medicine. In: Stone DJ, ed. Perioperative Medicine. Philadelphia: WB Saunders, 1997.
4. University Hospital Consortium. Technology Assessment: Routine Perioperative Diagnostic Evaluations. Oak Brook, IL, 1994.
5. Grigsby EJ, Cucchiara RF: Operating Room Management. In: Miller RD, ed. Anesthesia. 4th ed. New York: Churchill Livingstone, 1994.

12

Modern Technology in the Ambulatory Surgery Unit

Bruce David Schirmer

The explosion in medical technology predated the explosion in popularity of ambulatory surgery by at least a decade. The rapid increase in national spending on health care also preceded the need to furnish and equip ambulatory surgery centers. Therefore, when ambulatory surgery was emerging, an array of high technology equipment and the tendency to invest significantly in new technology were present. In the 1980s, however, most ambulatory surgery units required less expensive equipment and technologic methods than hospital operating suites. This was due, in part, to the more basic types of operations done on an ambulatory basis at that time. Also, certain techniques such as laparoscopy, either were not in use or were in considerably less demand than they are currently. All disciplines, from anesthesiology to the various surgical subspecialties and general surgery, have seen a dramatic increase in the types of new technologic methods and equipment that have become desirable, if not standard, for the inpatient operating room. Some of these methods have become either standard or highly desirable for the ambulatory surgery operating room as well.

Each ambulatory surgical unit must judge its mission, projected type and number of cases, and surgeon and patient populations to appropriately form a plan for the equipment needed in the unit. This is clearly a dynamic process, and competition for business and profitability has narrowed the margin between financial success and failure for many ambulatory units. Appropriate purchase and maintenance of equipment can often make the difference between success and failure. Similarly, whereas new techniques can potentially attract more patients and a higher volume of cases, these potential benefits must be weighed against the risks of the financial burden of investing in such technologic advances.

This chapter discusses the equipment needed to furnish and equip a modern ambulatory surgical unit designed for use by general surgeons. This is somewhat unrealistic, because at most ambulatory units, the majority of procedures (cases) are done by surgical subspecialists. In general, it is estimated that general surgical procedures account for approximately 20% to 25% of the caseload in most freestanding ambulatory surgicenters. This chapter, however, focuses on the general surgeon's performance of ambulatory surgery.

COST OF TECHNOLOGY

The cost of equipment in an ambulatory surgical unit is a major portion of the operating budget. The need for nonreusable supplies is an ongoing major element of the budget. However, the purchase of new major equipment items is often calculated into the annual budget, and it is in the consideration of such equipment that the balance between technologic improvements, user (surgeon) request, frequency of use, and budget capacity usually dictates whether the additional cost of further technologic developments is appropriate for the ambulatory surgical unit. In the following discussion, an attempt to give current best estimated costs has been made. Such figures are estimates only, because the price of technologic developments is as dynamic as technology itself. Other factors such as market demand and availability are also factors in the acquisition and price of new equipment.

Basic Equipment

Basic equipment required to furnish an operating room for general surgical ambulatory surgery, without specialized technology, is listed in Table 12–1. Estimated cost of purchase of each individual item is also listed. Variability in cost may be considerable for some items based on market conditions. The most expensive items are the anesthesia machine and monitors and the operating room lights.

Technologic features can be considered for several of the items listed in Table 12–1. The "standard" operating room table is somewhat variable in its capacity. Better-quality tables are hydraulically operated for shifting positions

Table 12–1. Equipment Needed to Furnish a Standard Ambulatory General Surgery Operating Room (Within Room)

Item	Cost Each	Total Cost
OR bed	$6,500	$6,500
OR lights (2)	$20,000	$40,000
OR tables (back) (2)	$325	$650
Prep table	$300	$300
Warming cabinet	$4,400	$4,400
OR stools (2)	$625	$1,250
Mayo stand (2)	$375	$750
IV poles (2)	$200	$400
Kick buckets (2)	$100	$200
Ring stands (2)	$400	$800
Anesthesia machine	$30,000	$30,000
Anesthesia monitors	$17,000	$17,000
Anesthesia drug cart	$750	$750
Anesthesia chair	$125	$125
Electrosurgical unit	$8,000	$8,000
Patient roller	$175	$175
Stirrups (pair)	$1,900	$1,900
Headlight	$1,800	$1,800
Basic instrument set	$4,500	$4,500
Total		$119,525

OR = operating room; IV, intravenous.

and heights. The weight capacity for such tables is usually limited to 400 pounds; special design and higher capacity hydraulics increase the bed capacity to 600 pounds or more. Another factor to consider when purchasing operating room tables is whether they allow the use of fluoroscopy.

There is wide variability in the type of anesthesia monitoring devices that may be purchased for the operating room. The monitoring items normally include CO_2 rascals in the modern operating room. Monitors to digitally assess electrocardiographic patterns and changes intraoperatively are becoming increasingly popular, but these are not included in Table 12–1. Technologic aspects of anesthesia equipment is an area of constant advancement, making reassessment of equipment purchases necessary every few years, not only for replacement but also for improvement in capability.

Operating room lights, the largest expense in furnishing an individual operating room, are a major consideration to surgeons in terms of their working conditions. The lights must be mounted so as to allow full range of positioning for illumination not only of the abdomen or chest when the patient is supine but also of the buttocks in cases of rectal surgery when the patient is in lithotomy position. Illumination power with appropriate focusing of the light beam is a major consideration in choosing any particular type of operating light. Quality and price vary.

The price of surgical instruments has decreased in recent years, with increasing competition among instrument companies for a somewhat fixed market. Buying "package" deals, buying in quantity, or buying as part of a consortium are all approaches to limiting the cost of acquiring new surgical instruments.

Table 12–2 lists equipment that is necessary for the functioning of an ambulatory surgical suite. Such equipment may be and usually is shared between two or sometimes more operating rooms. Items such as scrub sinks, autoclaves, and refrigerators must be readily available to a limited number of rooms and should be duplicated in several locations in a multiroom facility. The design and location of such equipment must fit with the traffic pat-

Table 12–2. Equipment Needed to Furnish One General Surgery Ambulatory Surgical Operating Suite (In Substerile or Outside Room)

Item	Cost Each	Total Cost
Washer/decontaminator	$34,000	$34,000
Prevacuum autoclave	$23,200	$23,200
Washer sterilizer autoclave	$3,400	$3,400
Ultrasonic cleaner	$400	$400
Scrub sinks (2)	$8,000	$16,000
Refrigerators (2)	$100	$200
Total		$77,200

tern and sterile–substerile and nonsterile areas of the operating facility.

Maintenance of major equipment items, especially technologically sophisticated machinery such as laparoscopic or endoscopic equipment, is a major concern for the ambulatory surgical unit and its ability to stay within a projected budget. The training of nursing personnel in the appropriate care and handling of equipment is essential to its maintenance. In some cases, this may require that dedicated teams of nurses be assigned to manage the care of certain equipment items, often related to the types of procedures in which they are primarily asked to participate. Ignorance of the care and function of equipment by the nursing team leads not only to intraoperative problems and inefficiencies but also to significantly higher breakage and replacement costs. The inadvertent disposal of a laparoscopic camera within its disposable camera cover and the failure to clean the channels of a flexible endoscope after use, resulting in a costly repair bill, are incidents that I have experienced that emphasize this point. Within ambulatory surgical units that are freestanding or smaller in size there is less likelihood of inexperienced personnel being asked to care for equipment, whereas in a large operating facility, where ambulatory surgery is done as part of the surgical caseload, such incidents are more likely.

Specialty Items of Equipment

Within the spectrum of general surgical practice, there are numerous areas that require specialized equipment.

The pediatric surgeon requires an entirely different set of instruments and equipment than the adult general surgeon. It is therefore advisable to equip one operating room (or more, based on caseload) within the ambulatory center for use primarily by the pediatric surgeon. Even though major equipment items such as those listed in Tables 12–1 and 12–2 do not change, the supplies and instruments for each case are clearly different for the pediatric population. The same is true for the anesthesiologist, for whom equipment and supplies appropriate to the child must be readily available. Special consideration must also be given to room temperature and measures to maintain the infant's or child's body temperature during procedures. The room must be equipped with appropriate-sized catheters, tubes, sutures, and monitoring equipment. Pediatric endoscopic equipment must be available (see Chapter 45).

Ambulatory vascular procedures, such as creation of Cimino shunts, arteriovenous access procedures, placement of Permcaths, and so forth, all require the necessary specialized vascular instruments. Vascular trays can be made up and can be available for these procedures. The only other major technologic items for such procedures include the fluoroscope (preferably) or portable x-ray machines (less preferable) and Doppler ultrasound. Fluoroscopy is valuable in any catheter insertion procedure, while also being helpful for analyzing the anatomy of fistulas and their intraoperative problems and management. Doppler technology is a quick and easy method of confirming and quantitating blood flow after vascular procedures. Simple confirmation of flow is shown by the use of a small portable unit for Doppler sound alone, whereas quantitative measurements of flow require a small transducer as part of a standard ultrasound machine with color flow and Doppler capabilities.

Colorectal surgery requires specialized instrumentation. The ready availability of both rigid proctoscopic and flexible sigmoidoscopic equipment is a prerequisite for the safe conduct of such surgery. Stirrups and spreader bars are required for many procedures. Prone positioning of the patient is also required at times, and the availablity of the appropriate cushions and supports, as well as the capacity of the operating table to accommodate these needs, is necessary. Perianal retractors are essential for proper exposure during rectal surgery. Dedicated instrument pans containing such reusable instruments are essential. The colorectal surgeon also usually benefits from use of a headlight for additional illumination during procedures such as transanal excision of lesions. Headlights are also useful in a variety of other surgical procedures, particularly those involving work within deeper body cavities besides the anus (Fig. 12–1). Further details of the techniques and equipment specific to colorectal ambulatory procedures are discussed in Chapters 37, 38, and 40. Minimally invasive management of midrectal tumors has also been developed using transanal microsurgical technology (see Chapter 41). This specialized equipment is appropriate for the ambulatory setting, but its cost and limited application have made it beyond the scope of equipment used in most ambulatory surgical operating rooms.

Lasers

Perineal warts (condylomata acuminata) are a problem treated by the colorectal and general surgeon in the ambulatory setting. Although various methods are used to treat this condition, a common one is the CO_2 laser (Fig. 12–2). A CO_2 laser is also useful for gynecologic procedures, and plastic surgeons have indications for its use. The laser unit costs approximately $80,000. Special safety equip-

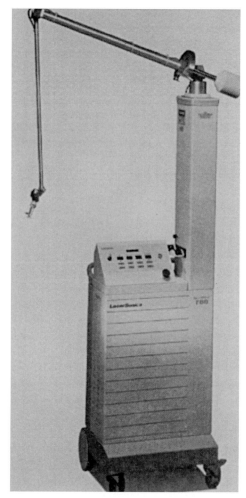

Figure 12–2. A portable CO_2 laser unit suitable for use in destruction of skin lesions and other general surgical uses. (Courtesy of Laserscope.)

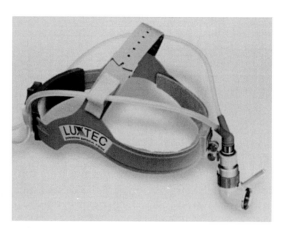

Figure 12–1. A typical headlight used during a variety of general surgical procedures, but particularly in procedures involving deep orifices or recesses where overhead lighting is insufficient. (Courtesy of Luxtec Corp.)

ment, eye protection, smoke evacuator (cost $2300), and appropriately trained assisting personnel are necessary for the initiation of an experience in CO_2 laser procedures. A dedicated room specially equipped to handle laser therapy is recommended as the optimal way to meet the safety and equipment requirements of this technologic method. Endoscopic procedures can use laser technology for procedures such as tumor ablation and destruction of lesions. These procedures generally use an Nd-YAG type laser, which again is a very expensive piece of equipment for the ambulatory unit. Caseload would need to be sufficient to warrant its purchase. Further details regarding lasers and their use in endoscopic surgery are given in Chapter 46.

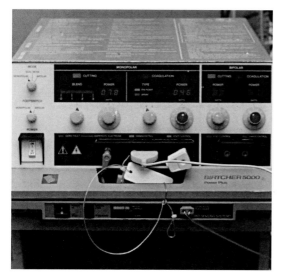

Figure 12–3. An electrocautery unit with the capacity to generate energy in a cutting or coagulating mode for monopolar or bipolar applications.

Cautery and Energy Sources for Hemostasis

A major item in all operating rooms is the electrocautery unit. Monopolar electrocautery, with its capacity for both cutting and coagulating energy forms, is the standard for energy-produced hemostasis in the current ambulatory general surgery operating room (Fig. 12–3). Cautery unit prices are listed in Table 12–1, with electrosurgical units currently costing about $8000. Bipolar cautery units confer some advantages in terms of limiting the capacity for burn injuries away from the operative site. Pricing for such units can be higher than for monopolar units. Individual surgeon preference and the type of procedures being performed often dictate which of the two energy modes are most appropriate.

An alternative means of hemostasis being increasingly used by general surgeons, particularly in the performance of laparoscopic surgery, is that of ultrasonic energy for hemostasis of vessels. The "harmonic scalpel" is an instrument that has achieved recent popularity among laparoscopic general surgeons for its ability, through high-frequency ultrasonic energy, to coapt blood vessels of up to 3 mm in size and thereby allow vascular division without the more time-consuming process of clipping and cutting or ligating and cutting (Fig. 12–4). Even though most general surgeons purchase such a unit (base price approximately $20,000) for advanced laparoscopic operations, it has similar capabilities for use during celiotomies.

Imaging Equipment

The degree and amount of radiology equipment needed in an ambulatory surgical unit depend on caseload and type of procedure. A standard portable x-ray machine and the capacity to develop and process plain radiographs is essential for the safe conduct of many ambulatory procedures. Fluoroscopy is also very useful in assisting with orthopedic procedures, endoscopic procedures, and laparoscopic procedures such as laparoscopic cholecystectomy. Cholecystectomy probably should not be done unless fluoroscopy is avail-

Figure 12–4. The "harmonic scalpel" system. The ultrasonic energy-generating unit is pictured at left, along with its controlling foot pedal. The laparoscopic probe attached to the standard handle is shown below right. The three close-up views depict the flat, side (very flat), and sharp surfaces of the probe, which are used for coapting (flat) and cutting (sharp) applications. (Courtesy of Ethicon Endosurgery, Inc.)

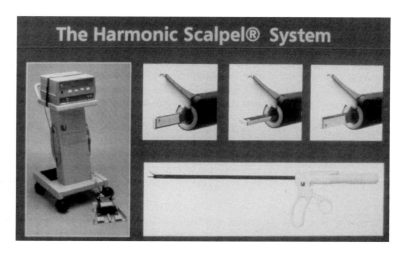

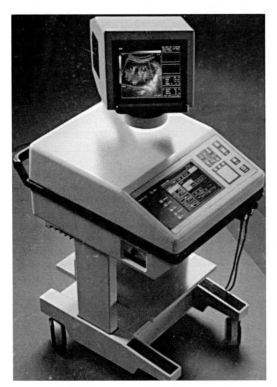

Figure 12–5. Ultrasound unit featuring the main energy-generating unit and computer components, with attached monitor above. The unit is portable. Different probes may be inserted on the right front side of the machine, depending on the application desired. (Courtesy of B&K Medical, Inc.)

able, because the potential need for cholangiography is always present and the potential for bile duct exploration is not insignificant. Whereas the former can be accomplished with static radiographs, the latter is much more difficult laparoscopically without fluoroscopy and would require choledochoscopy. The cost of a portable x-ray machine is approximately $40,000. The cost of a C-arm for fluoroscopy is approximately $150,000. The fluoroscopy machine often has the capacity for obtaining plain radiographs as well.

Ultrasound

The general surgeon in the United States has only recently embraced the use of ultrasound as being a valuable tool in daily surgical practice. General surgeons in Europe and Japan have relied on diagnostic and therapeutic ultrasound for many years: in Germany, a surgeon must demonstrate proficiency with ultrasound to be board certified. General surgeons in the United States have begun to routinely use ultrasound in the office diagnosis and treatment of breast disease. They are more commonly performing their own intraoperative assessments of solid organs. Laparoscopic ultrasound probes have given the laparoscopic surgeon the capacity to evaluate solid organs intraoperatively as well; otherwise, the surgeon would be unable to evaluate these organs by palpation during staging laparoscopy for oncologic or other purposes. Vascular surgery, however, is one area of general surgery in which the surgeon has typically used ultrasound and ultrasonographic Doppler techniques in the past to evaluate peripheral pulses and perfusion, and to diagnose peripheral vascular disease and carotid arterial disease.

A complete ultrasound machine with several probes for intraoperative, small parts, breast, laparoscopic, and vascular ultrasound (Figs. 12–5 through 12–7) is an expensive proposition for the ambulatory surgery center. A price tag of $125,000 to $140,000 is a reasonable current estimate for such an assembly of ultrasonographic equipment. This price is clearly

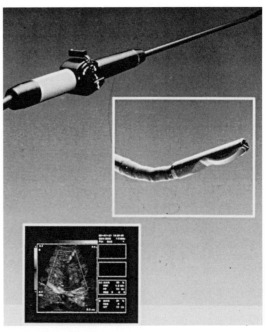

Figure 12–6. View of the laparoscopic ultrasound probe, which has a flexible tip (similar to a standard bronchoscope) allowing maximal tissue contact by the probe during laparoscopic procedures. (Courtesy of B&K Medical, Inc.)

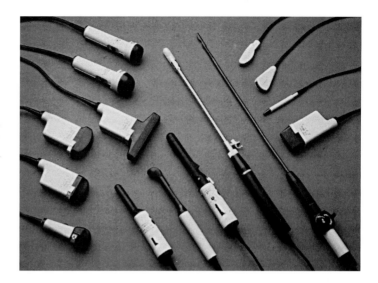

Figure 12–7. Various types of ultrasound probes include abdominal, intraoperative, vascular, endorectal, small parts, and laparoscopic. (Courtesy of B&K Medical, Inc.)

beyond the realm of many freestanding centers of modest size to consider. As general surgical operations become increasingly technologically oriented, however, ultrasound may become a necessity for their performance. Volume of cases and types of users will be important factors to assess for the purchase of any such technologically advanced equipment by an ambulatory unit.

LAPAROSCOPY

Videotelescopic Equipment

Laparoscopic procedures, performed by not only general surgeons but also gynecologists and urologists, require the items listed in Table 12–3 as major videotelescopic items. Figure 12–8 shows a model operating room maximally equipped for videotelescopic surgery, with two monitors and all necessary major

equipment items. The insufflator should have sufficiently high flow to allow performance of more advanced cases, for which extracorporeal suturing and frequent passage of different instruments make ongoing carbon dioxide losses from the pneumoperitoneum a potential problem. Telescopes of different viewing angles can be purchased, but it has been my experience

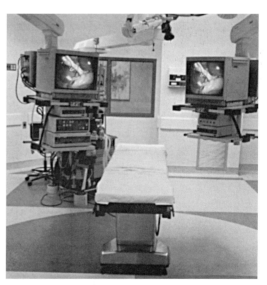

Figure 12–8. The videotelescopic operating room. The room is equipped with dual ceiling-suspended monitors as well as shelves beneath the monitors for the major components of the videotelescopic system. Note the additional camera in the center for recording the view of the operative field outside the body. Such a system is adaptable for telesurgical transmission of the operative procedure to a distant site, once the transmission capacity of the video image and external camera image is established. (Courtesy of Stryker, Inc.)

Table 12–3. Equipment Needed for Videotelescopic (Laparoscopic) Surgery

Item	Cost
Camera	$15,000
Light source	$5,000
Insufflator	$6,000
Printer	$4,000
Telescope	$1,800
Basic instrument set	$10,000
Total	$41,800

that the 30° telescope offers considerable viewing advantages over its 0° counterpart. This is especially true when working in either end of the peritoneal cavity: the esophageal hiatal area or the pelvis. It also confers advantages during laparoscopic cholecystectomy in severely obese patients, allowing a better viewing angle of the infundibular area of the gallbladder over the obese omentum. At my institution, the telescope has usually been the component of the videoendoscopic system with the shortest half-life and is responsible for the greatest loss of light transmission after a period of time. Nevertheless, with care, such telescopes should last for several years. Video monitors are of variable quality, but most provide sufficient resolution for a very clear image on the screen. It is important to match the resolution of the monitor, telescope, and camera so that one component does not significantly limit the image quality.

The cameras used for laparoscopy have several different features and consequently vary in price. The standard one-chip camera has been the mainstay of most laparoscopic surgeons. However, some have found the additional image and color enhancement of the three-chip camera to be worth the approximate doubling in cost of purchase. Finally, even more expensive are systems that allow a three-dimensional view for the laparoscopic surgeon, either through a system of rapidly alternating images from a bifocal image system in the specially designed telescope or through the use of special glasses to be worn by the surgeon that convert the image to three dimensions. The camera is the single most expensive item in the videotelescopic system.

Additions to the basic videotelescopic system, based on surgeon demand, include some form of photographic system that can provide digital images of intraoperative findings. This is in addition to the usual documentation capacity of video. Finally, screen splitters are available for those procedures requiring intraabdominal endoscopy and laparoscopy at the same time. Such procedures are currently relatively uncommon; therefore, the need for such a piece of equipment, particularly in the ambulatory setting, is small.

Portability of the videotelescopic system is

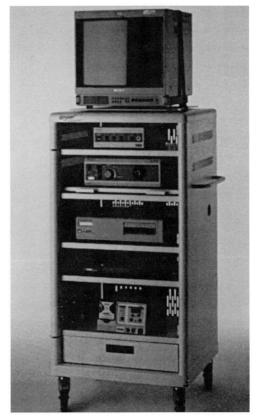

Figure 12–9. The portable cart allows the entire videotelescopic set of equipment to be rolled from one operating room to another. (Courtesy of Stryker, Inc.)

possible through the use of specially designed carts that allow all the major components of the system to be rolled from one operating room to another (Fig. 12–9). This provides maximum flexibility in terms of case scheduling and room use.

Another technologic innovation that may be considered part of the videotelescopic system is a mechanical arm to hold the telescope. Such arms can be a simple apparatus that holds the telescope and camera unit in one position and that must be manually adjusted to view different fields. Such a piece of equipment is of some value only when assisting personnel for the surgeon are in short supply. The need for constant readjustment of the camera, along with the potential to perform insertion and withdrawal of instruments outside the viewing field, is a distinct disadvantage of this system. A far more sophisticated piece of equipment is the recently developed voice-controlled telescope holder, wherein the

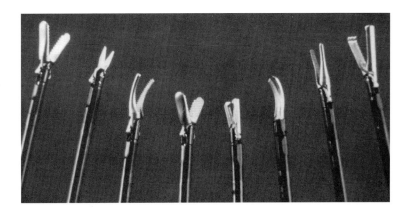

Figure 12–10. Working ends of some basic laparoscopic instruments used for most general surgical procedures. (Courtesy of Ethicon Endosurgery, Inc.)

sound of the surgeon's voice activates the mechanical arm to change position. Although expensive, this technique offers tremendous advantages to the surgeon who would otherwise have inadequately trained personnel assist with camera-holding. Proper camera operation makes a considerable difference in the duration and safety of a laparoscopic operation.

Laparoscopic Instruments

Laparoscopic instruments can be classified as basic multipurpose type instruments as well as specialized instruments. Included in the basic instruments are atraumatic and toothed grasping forceps, scissors, aspiration needles, biopsy forceps, needle holders, dissecting forceps, knot pushers, and retractors (Fig. 12–10). With the exception of scissors, none of these instruments is usually connected to an energy source for cutting or coagulation. Many laparoscopic operations require vascular division, and, for this, the most commonly used device for small to medium-sized blood vessels is a clip applier. Even though reusable single-capacity clip appliers are available, most sur-

geons prefer the convenience and speed of an automatic multiclip applier, which is a disposable instrument (Fig. 12–11).

A suction–irrigation type instrument is used for many laparoscopy operations, and the design of these suction–irrigators varies (Fig. 12–12). All supply the basic functions of suctioning and irrigating, but the mechanisms of control, force, and volume of capacity, lumen size of the tube, and whether they are equipped to be modified with cautery-instrumented tips varies among manufacturers and models.

Instruments that are designed to be used with monopolar electrocautery are most commonly used by general surgeons for performing basic laparoscopic operations. These instruments are often made in conjunction with a suction–irrigation device as the handle of the instrument; interchangeable distal shafts allow exchange of instrument tips for different tasks. A hook-type cautery instrument is commonly used to dissect the triangle of Calot structures during laparoscopic cholecystectomy. Spatula-type tips are also commonly used by general surgeons (Fig. 12–13).

Most general surgeons use energy to facili-

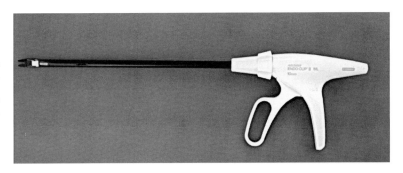

Figure 12–11. Disposable laparoscopic clip applier. (Copyright © 1997 United States Surgical Corp. All rights reserved. Reprinted with permission of United States Surgical Corp.)

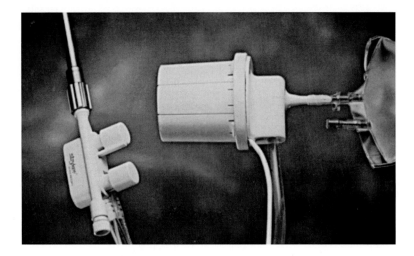

Figure 12–12. Laparoscopic suction–irrigator system. The handle, at left, has buttons for thumb-pressure control of both suction and irrigation. At right is shown the end of the unit that connects to the irrigation bag. (Courtesy of Stryker, Inc.)

tate dissection and hemostasis during laparoscopic operations. Monopolar electrocautery is the most common energy source used, but surgeons also use bipolar cautery based on personal preference and availability. See Chapter 26 for information regarding the safe use of electrocautery during laparoscopic surgery. Alternative energy sources to electrocautery used in laparoscopic surgery include laser energy (see Chapter 46).

Specialized laparoscopic instruments are available for specific applications, examples of which include bowel clamps and curved retractors for the esophagus. Many of the specialized laparoscopic instruments are disposable, including intestinal staplers, hernia staplers, and retractors. Intestinal staplers of all types used for open intestinal surgery, including longitudinal intestinal and transverse occlusive type staplers as well as circular staplers, are available on long handles or in airtight casing for laparoscopic use (Fig. 12–14). Such staplers

allow total intracorporeal laparoscopic gastrointestinal anastomoses to be performed with relative expediency and excellent safety. Longitudinal staplers with low-height staples capable of ligating and dividing major vascular structures are used for laparoscopic appendectomy, colectomy, splenectomy, and other operations for which division of vascular pedicles is necessary (Fig. 12–15).

Staplers for laparoscopic herniorrhaphy are also available for securing the mesh to the abdominal wall. Staple cartridges are manufactured with differing staple heights for moderate or deeper penetration into tissues (Fig. 12–16).

Other examples of disposable laparoscopic instruments that facilitate the difficult technical aspects of advanced laparoscopic procedures include suturing devices that automatically pass the needle back and forth between two needle-grasping arms, speeding the creation of a running suture line (Fig. 12–17).

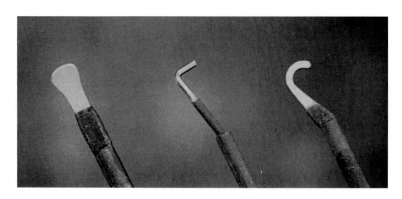

Figure 12–13. Working tips of interchangeable shafts that can be inserted into the handle of the laparoscopic electrocautery instrument, attached usually to a source of monopolar cautery energy. (Courtesy of Stryker, Inc.)

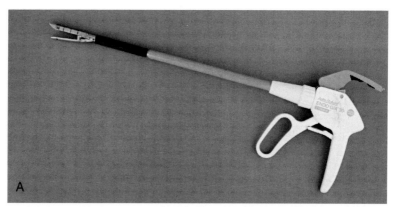

Figure 12–14. (A) Endoscopic linear 30-mm stapler (Endo GIA) used for creating an intracorporeal gastrointestinal anastomosis or dividing the gastrointestinal tract. **(B)** Close-up view of the working end of the Endo GIA. Note the relatively dark (in this case blue) cartridge for staples of height appropriate for gastrointestinal anastomosis and division. **(C)** A 60-mm Endo TA type laparoscopic stapler, fired by a compressed gas cartridge and used for closing defects in the gastrointestinal tract. **(D)** Close-up view of the working end of the 60-mm Endo TA. **(E)** The laparoscopic circular Stealth stapler, manufactured to maintain the air-tight seal during laparoscopic use and used to create circular gastrointestinal anastomoses. (**A** through **D**, Copyright © 1997 United States Surgical Corp. All rights reserved. Reprinted with permission of United States Surgical Corp. **E,** Courtesy of Ethicon Endosurgery, Inc.)

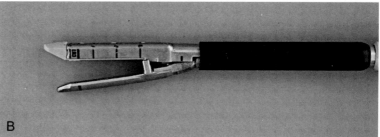

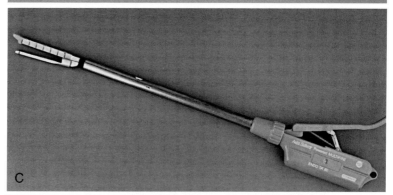

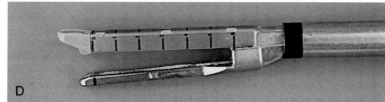

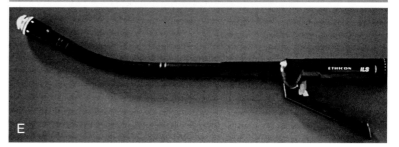

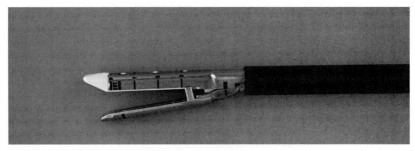

Figure 12–15. A 30-mm Endo GIA stapler using a vascular staple load. Note the white cartridge designating this staple load as having a shorter staple height appropriate for use in dividing vascularized tissue such as the mesoappendix. (Copyright 1997 United States Surgical Corp. All rights reserved. Reprinted with permission of United States Surgical Corp.)

Reusable Versus Disposable

Considerable controversy and debate arise when discussing the use of reusable versus disposable instruments of laparoscopic surgery. The largest instrument manufacturers for laparoscopic surgery have emphasized the disposable instrument line. Competition has resulted in a dynamic situation with respect to laparoscopic instrumentation, resulting in constant improvements and refinements. This has, in some ways, given the advantage to disposable instruments, in that new and better models seem to be available on an annual basis. Another argument for using disposable instrumentation is that multiple procedures can be performed sequentially, without the need to await instrument processing and sterilization between cases. Disposable instrumentation limits the potential for disease transmission. In addition, the cost of personnel required to clean and sterilize reusable instruments must be factored into the total equation when comparing costs of reusable versus disposable instrumentation.

Arguments for using reusable instruments

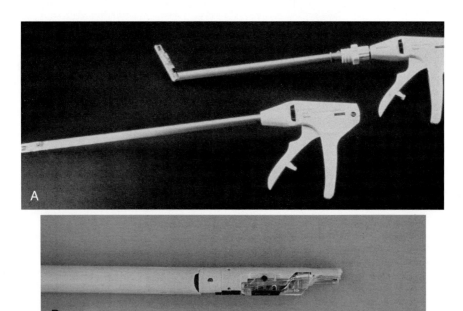

Figure 12–16. A, Laparoscopic hernia stapler used to affix mesh to the inguinal structures during laparoscopic herniorrhaphy. There are different staple heights for the tissue being stapled: shorter for more dense tissue such as Cooper's ligament and longer heights for muscle. **B,** Close-up view of the working end of the laparoscopic hernia stapler. Each staple cartridge holds 10 staples. (Copyright 1997 United States Surgical Corp. All rights reserved. Reprinted with permission of United States Surgical Corp.)

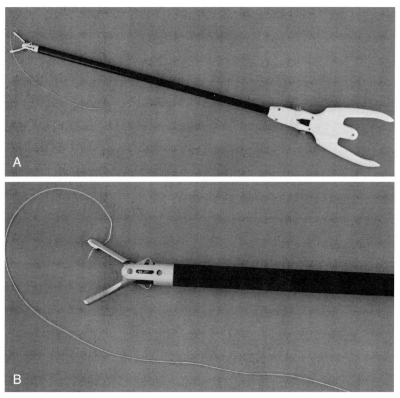

Figure 12–17. A, The Endostitch device, used to facilitate laparoscopic intracorporeal suturing. By toggling the handle back and forth, the surgeon can pass the needle through tissue to the opposite jaw of the working end, which then secures the needle for suturing back in the opposite direction. **B,** Close-up view of the working end of the Endostitch, showing the two sides of the suturing device, each capable of holding the needle and passing it back to the other side where it is again secured within the holder. (Copyright 1997 United States Surgical Corp. All rights reserved. Reprinted with permission of United States Surgical Corp.)

have been documented in several studies that show that the cost of a given procedure can be significantly decreased by such an approach. Even though a reusable instrument costs considerably more than a disposable one, the large number of reuses makes it clearly much less expensive in the long run. One careful study of factors amenable to the laparoscopic surgeon to limit the cost of any one laparoscopic procedure showed that use of reusable instruments and decreasing the duration of operation through mastery of the laparoscopic skills necessary to perform the procedure were the two major factors in cost that could be influenced by the surgeon. Most ambulatory laparoscopic procedures are amenable to the substitution of reusable instruments for some of the currently used disposable instruments, assuming local conditions for resterilization and safety are satisfactory.

Microlaparoscopy

Recently, the manufacturers of laparoscopic instruments have developed a line of extremely delicate instruments for use through 2-mm trocars (Fig. 12–18). Experience with these instruments is limited, and there are few reports with significant data regarding their efficacy. However, this instrumentation has been successfully used with significant experience by gynecologists for pain mapping. The small size of the instrumentation allows laparoscopy to be performed under local anesthesia using low insufflation pressures. General surgeons have reported successful use of this instrumentation for diagnostic procedures for trauma and oncology and for therapeutic procedures including cholecystectomy and feeding jejunostomy. Substitution of 2-mm trocars for larger ports has been successfully done for

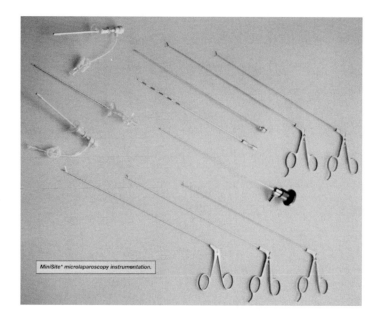

MiniSite* microlaparoscopy instrumentation.

Figure 12–18. View of a set of microlaparoscopy instruments. Notice the instrument shaft diameters (2 mm) are comparable in size to the Veress needle in the mid upper left portion of the figure. (From Laparoscopy in Focus, Vol. 4, No. 1, p. 4, United States Surgical Corp. Copyright © 1997 United States Surgical Corp. All rights reserved. Reprinted with the permission of United States Surgical Corp.)

more involved therapeutic procedures such as Nissen fundoplication, adrenalectomy, and splenectomy. In the latter procedures, general anesthesia is still required.

The general goal of such instrumentation is to limit the trocar size to 2 mm for all but one larger port, which is needed for instrumentation and organ extraction. Similarly, complete use of 2-mm instruments and telescopes is the goal for diagnostic laparoscopy. Durability of this instrumentation must be confirmed, as must its applicability in the obese patient. However, the trend toward developing narrower and less invasive instrumentation that can be used through increasingly smaller trocars is clearly present with this innovation.

NEW TECHNOLOGY

The 21st century will not have arrived before substantial operating room technologic innovations have made their way onto the scene. The era of the computerized operating room is beginning, in which there is less dependence on human skill and greater reliance on computerization, and reliably reproducible robotic-controlled movements by mechanized assisting surgical machines will be the state-of-the-art. As discussed, voice-controlled laparoscopic camera operating machines are already being used. Similarly, three-dimensional video-

telescopic systems are becoming more commonly used in laparoscopic operating rooms.

Robotic arms that reproduce intracorporeally what the directing human hand does extracorporeally may become available in the next few years as the newest wrinkle in advanced minimally invasive technology. It is not inconceivable to suggest that the surgery of the future may be greatly influenced or performed by computer-driven mechanical devices, removing the surgeon from the need to even be physically next to the patient for some procedures. The increasing feasibility of teleconferencing makes the potential for telesurgery or telesurgical consultation a hotly debated topic. The most controversial areas of debate regard the basic issues of establishing medicolegal liability and credentialing and of licensing domains regulating such innovations.

The computerized, digitized operating room equipped with three-dimensional video equipment and telemonitoring capability is still a thing of the future and has little practical impact on the current practice of ambulatory general surgery. The development of such sophisticated technology does suggest, however, that its availability may play an important role in the future distribution of cases in ambulatory surgery centers. The freestanding ambulatory surgicenter may compete extremely well in the future in an environment of cost containment and financial austerity. However, if technologic advances, which are inherently expensive, allow certain ambulatory procedures to be advantageously done in a more minimally invasive manner, then it may only be large institutions that can afford such innovations and in turn may then be able to selectively attract patients for such procedures. The balance of cost containment versus improved expensive techniques with subsequent demand to their access by the media-informed patient may play an interesting role in the evolving use of ambulatory surgery facilities and in the purchase of equipment to furnish those operating rooms in the future.

Selected Readings

1. Apelgren KN, Blank ML, Slomski CA, Hadjis NS. Reusable instruments are more cost-effective than disposable instruments for laparoscopic cholecystectomy. Surg Endosc 1994;8:32–34.
2. Begin E, Gagner M, Hurteau F, De Santis S, Pomp A. A robotic camera for laparoscopic surgery: conception and experimental results. Surg Laparosc Endosc 1995;5:6–11.
3. Berci G, Paz-Partlow M. Video imaging. In: MacFadyen BV Jr, Ponsky JL, eds. Operative Laparoscopy and Thoracoscopy. Philadelphia: Lippincott-Raven, 1996: 57–78.
4. Deloitte & Touche. Economic impact of laparoscopic surgery. Boston, MA. August 1993.
5. Hunter J. Laser or electrocautery for laparoscopy? Am J Surg 1991;161:345–349.
6. Melzer A. Endoscopic instruments—conventional and intelligent. In: Toouli J, Gossot D, Hunter J, eds. Endosurgery. New York: Churchill Livingstone, 1996:69–98.
7. Rattner DW, Dawson SL. The operating room of the future. In: Brooks DC, ed. Current Review of Laparoscopy. 2d ed. Philadelphia: Current Medicine, 1995: 186–195.
8. Sackier JM, Wang Y. Robotically assisted laparoscopic surgery—from concept to development. Surg Endosc 1994;8:63–66.
9. Satava RM. Robotics, telepresence and virtual reality: a critical analysis of the future of surgery. Minimally Invasive Therapy 1992;1:357–363.
10. Unger SW, Unger HM, Bass RT. AESOP robotic arm. Surg Endosc 1994;8:1131.
11. Voyles CR, Tucker RD. Education and engineering solutions for potential problems with laparoscopic monopolar electrosurgery. Am J Surg 1992;164:57–62.

13

Administration of the Ambulatory Surgery Unit

Andrew A. Jeon • Beverly K. Philip

Effective administration is crucial to fulfillment of the most commonly expected goal of the ambulatory surgery unit (ASU), that is, the provision of high-quality, cost-effective care delivered efficiently in an environment that is patient- and physician-oriented. Frequently, the same level of attention to detail in planning the physical design and patient flow issues of the ASU is not extended to the creation of an administrative structure that will be held accountable for the success of the unit. Regardless of whether ambulatory surgery is conducted in the inpatient operating room, a separate suite in the hospital, or a freestanding facility, an administrative structure designed to support the mission of ambulatory surgery must be created to optimize overall success. With the advent of a prospective ambulatory procedure payment system from the Health Care Financing Administration (HCFA), an increasingly cost-conscious payer system, and more stringent accreditation and regulatory requirements, the collection of skills necessary to maintain ASUs as viable entities will be great.

ADMINISTRATIVE STRUCTURE

An organizational structure that is easily understood and that clearly delineates lines of responsibility and accountability is essential to the efficient functioning of an ASU. Job descriptions should clearly state the scope of responsibilities, reporting relationships, and ideal personal characteristics for all positions.

Director

The designation of one individual to be accountable for all operational aspects of the ASU is essential. No business would tolerate the diffuse responsibility for the extensive resources represented by an ASU to the extent that this situation exists in many hospital-based facilities today. Freestanding for-profit units are typically structured more closely to a business model. The director should be a nurse or physician with an extensive understanding of the operating room environment. The director should have a demonstrated record of working well with physicians and nurses, possess excellent managerial skills, and be service-oriented in philosophy. The director's primary responsibility is to ensure programmatic cohesiveness with close attention paid to morale, teamwork, staff retention, and development. Besides fiduciary accountability, the director must develop performance evaluation tools that monitor all aspects of the care delivered in the ASU. The director is responsible for the physical facility, equipment, supplies, and all ancillary and administrative services. The appropriate resources must be made available to the director to carry out this mission. Depending on the setting of the ASU, this individual should report to the director of the operating room or the board that manages the freestanding unit. One example of a typical organization chart is shown in Figure 13–1. The director should be visible and available at all times to uphold policies, resolve disputes, and facilitate interdisciplinary cooperation.

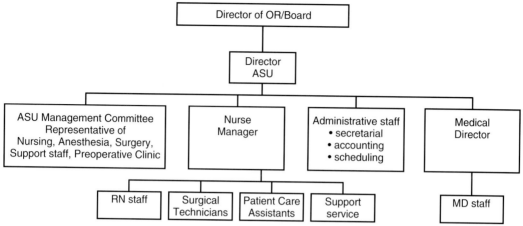

Figure 13–1. Organization chart delineating reporting relationships for ambulatory surgery unit.

Many successful ASUs have established a multidisciplinary committee to assist in the management of the unit. Committee membership may include the medical director, staff surgeons, anesthesiologists, and nurses, as well as representatives from administration. The scope of input may range from decisions on purchasing new equipment to staffing, hours of operation, and appropriate policies and procedures. This participative process supports the open communication and interdisciplinary cooperation that typifies the culture in many ASUs and minimizes the sometimes contentious relationships that evolve between medical and administrative staffs. The committee structure also maximizes opportunities for innovation and responsiveness to changes in the external environment, which must be accommodated for continued successful operations.

Medical Director

The role of the medical director is addressed in Chapter 11 and should be considered an integral component of the administrative structure. The medical director should be a respected clinician and possess a service orientation similar to that described for the director of the ASU. In many units, the director and medical director may be the same individual. In this case, the director should not be expected to be a full-time clinical practitioner and should be provided adequate time for performance of management functions.

Nurse Manager

It is important that a nurse manager be identified as accountable for nursing practice and staffing in the ASU. The nurse manager is responsible for the recruitment and retention of a critically important component of the ASU staff. The ideal nurse manager is respected by both physicians and nurses, is enthusiastic, patient oriented, and willing to "dig in" if the need arises. Such a person sets an example for the ideal set of professional skills and behaviors of the nursing staffs observed in well-run ASUs.

STAFF SELECTION

Surgical

The surgeon is a primary customer for ambulatory surgery services and the source of patients. To attract and keep these primary customers satisfied, the ambulatory surgery facility might begin by ascertaining what factors are important to these customers. An organization must identify the wants and needs of the target market, and then adapt the services it provides to meet these identified needs. One such marketing questionnaire was conducted by MacDowell and Perry. Based on interviews with key members of the administration and surgical staff, the authors selected several attributes as potentially important in determining surgeon satisfaction and, by implication, willingness to use the ASU. These were presented to the surgeons as a return-mail questionnaire. The results of this survey are shown in Table 13–1. The quality of anesthesia services was rated highest, 3.96 ± 0.19 on a 4-point scale. The quality of the surgical suites and equipment together rated next highest, and then the quality of nursing staff. Patient preference also rated highly, as the fourth factor. The authors also compared the responses of low-volume surgeons and high-volume surgeons, and the ranking of the four major areas of desirable attributes was the same.

However, surgeons must be evaluated as consumers of expensive resources as well as providers of patients. This evaluation can influence the selection of surgeons for participation in cost-conscious ASUs. Surgeons' consumed resources include operating room time and surgical supplies. How the surgeon interacts with other facility personnel is also important because smooth interactions facilitate the surgical process. Evaluations of surgeons' resource consumption can rank surgeons within their group of colleagues. Such comparisons can be used to identify and minimize outlying practice patterns and as a possible basis for acceptance or selection for staff positions in ambulatory surgical facilities or economic credentialing.

Anesthesia

Selection of anesthesia personnel must take into account the specific needs of the ambulatory surgical unit. The presence of physician anesthesiologists provides the administrator and surgeon with individuals who can be responsible for adverse outcomes and who can provide leadership in formulating anesthesia policies. The anesthesiologist is often a daily constant presence. When surgeon-directed nurse anesthesia is used, these responsibilities may fall on the surgeon. Whomever the anesthesia providers are, they must have both the professional skills and the can-do attitude to enhance the facility's goals. Knowledge of the new anesthetic agents and techniques must be incorporated into a base of strong fundamental techniques. In addition, the anesthesia care givers must have a commitment to cost effectiveness, both in their own practice and as leaders to others.

Nursing

The concept of ambulatory surgery nursing involves more than the operative procedure. It includes a philosophy of patient care that considers the patient to be a functioning whole. Ambulatory surgical nursing care must be provided through all phases of the perioperative experience.

In addition to possessing the skill complement expected of every operating room nurse, the nurse in an ASU must possess additional competencies if the unit is to operate at its most effective level. Cross-training is critical to providing the flexibility required to serve the varied operational and functional needs of a busy ASU. Not only must expertise be developed in a number of surgical specialties, but it must also be expanded to include proficiency in preoperative patient preparation, postoperative recovery care, and discharge of the patient. A willingness to take on new responsibilities as the need arises is necessary for the viability of the ASU in a rapidly changing

Table 13–1. Surgeon's Responses to Questions Measuring the Influence of Selected Characteristics on Satellite Surgicenter Use*

Characteristics	Mean	SD	N
Quality of anesthesia services	3.96	.19	27
Quality of surgical suites	3.73	.60	26
Modernness of the equipment	3.70	.61	27
Quality of nursing staff	3.63	.74	27
Reputation of the facility	3.56	.64	27
Patient preference	3.43	.69	28
Travel time from home	3.22	.80	27
Travel time from office	3.22	.80	27
Modernness of the facility	3.15	.77	27
Quality of laboratory services	2.77	.91	26
Parking	2.78	.70	27
Interior appearance	2.78	.64	27
Promptness in test reporting	2.83	.87	24
Communication with administration	2.81	.96	27
Voice in policy making	2.56	1.05	27
Exterior appearance	2.11	.75	27

*Rating based on 4-point scale: 1 = no influence, 2 = slight influence, 3 = moderate influence, 4 = considerable influence. N varies because not all surgeons responded to all questions.

From MacDowell NM, Perry R. Factors influencing physician choice of an outpatient surgery and testing facility. J Health Care Marketing 1990;67–74.

environment. One example is the acquisition of skills to monitor patients during conscious sedation. Enthusiasm to do things outside of one's traditional "job description" is essential, not only for the nursing staff but also for all members of a successful ASU.

Nurses who are to be selected for positions in an ambulatory surgical facility must have specific qualities: a holistic approach to patient care, good communication skills, and strong professional pride. Williams describes a similar, detailed approach to selecting those individuals who will enhance the functioning of the facility (see Ancillary Personnel). Once the appropriate nurses are selected, they should be given specific didactic workshops to enhance those skills that are especially required in ambulatory surgery nursing. Topics for these workshops include the history and philosophy of ambulatory surgery, holistic medical and surgical approaches, communications and conflict resolution skills, and interdisciplinary cooperation. Practical training includes work with preceptors and individual involvement and responsibility as team members.

Ancillary Personnel

Registration and clerical personnel are often the first representatives of the facility who the customer sees. Therefore, the selection of these personnel is of particular importance.

Williams has emphasized that the employees of the ASU are responsible for the success of the facility by enacting its mission on a practical and daily basis. All staff must be "above average" and provide exceptional service to the customers, physician, and patient. Staff members must not only be technically competent in their field but also have the appropriate personality and attitude. During the hiring process, it is important to provide potential employees with enough information about the facility's goals so that they can decide whether they are able to commit to these goals. An employee's job description must include not only technical competency but also personality attributes. Once personnel have been hired, they must be given appropriate orientation to

the facility's policies, procedures, and routines.

One potentially problematic issue is maintaining proper staffing levels, despite lack of control of the actual facility utilization. To minimize the expenses associated with overstaffing, many facilities make significant use of part-time and on-call personnel to supplement their base of full-time individuals. Another facet of the efficient use of staffing involves cross-training, both within the person's technical field (e.g., preoperative and intraoperative nursing) and beyond the job description and outside that field. Levels of staffing may be used to extend productivity, using practical nurses and physician assistants under professional direction.

Staffing efficiency also includes retention of these selected and trained employees. Job satisfaction is essential to provide exceptional service. One factor that enhances employee satisfaction in ambulatory surgery facilities is the opportunity for more control of the work environment, due to the small size of the organization and better access to management. Another factor that enhances employee satisfaction is the opportunity for ongoing internal and external education programs as well as the opportunity for advancement.

Evaluating the numbers of staff needed must be done within the framework of staffing efficiency. Calculations for a freestanding ambulatory surgery center can serve as a benchmark. One full-time employee (FTE) represents 173 hours worked during a month, or 2080 hours worked a year. An efficiently managed surgery center with a volume of 3000 mixed surgical subspecialty cases per year requires an average of 13.5 to 14 FTEs. If calculated as work hours per case, an average of 9.5 work hours are needed. It is important to include only those hours actually worked in calculations of FTEs or work hours, and not the numbers of employees generating the hours, nor vacation or other leave time. Efficiency can also be calculated as the dollars of salary and benefits as a percentage of total revenue dollars. A ratio of 24% to 28% of revenue is expected. When comparing facilities, actual case mix is an important factor for all these methods.

SCHEDULING

Surgical scheduling impacts heavily on the efficient use of personnel and supplies in the ambulatory surgical unit. Scheduling is influenced by a number of variables: surgeon preference, case volume, type of patient, and type of unit. Surgeon preference for scheduling pattern includes preassigned block time as well as an add-on case availability. Patient factors are age and illness severity of the population served. A self-contained unit is easier to schedule than a shared hospital operating facility. All scheduling problems are compounded if the facility is mixing complex inpatient surgical procedures with the ambulatory surgical cases.

There are two basic methods of scheduling. One method is first-come, first-served case booking, based on operating time available. Advantages of this method are greater room flexibility, increased available time, and the perceived equitability of this system. However, first-come, first-served scheduling is associated with major drawbacks, which are gaps between cases, leading to poor room utilization as well as nurse and technician staffing problems due to the varying kinds of cases scheduled. The second method of scheduling is block scheduling in which a surgeon or surgical specialty is assigned dedicated time. Advantages of this method are better room utilization and avoidance of surgeon-related delays when surgeons follow themselves directly, as well as simplified staffing patterns and more efficient use of equipment and supplies. Disadvantages of this system are unused time within blocks and accommodation of additional cases. Overall, the block time system is superior, and its disadvantages can be minimized by releasing blocks a set time before the date of surgery. The gaps can then be filled from a waiting list or on a first-come, first-served basis. Other combination methods, which dedicate some of the rooms for block time scheduling, also work.

Either method of scheduling can be done by hand or, increasingly, using computerized systems that integrate multiple aspects of patient care and operating room management. Industrial engineering methods have been applied to analyze patient flow through the ambulatory surgical process. This computerized patient tracking system has resulted in enhanced methods of patient processing, internal communication, and documentation.

Implementation of an efficient schedule requires avoidance of delays to patient flow. Preoperative delays can be minimized by thorough patient evaluation before the day of surgery. Written questionnaires filled out by the patients supplementing the surgical history and physical examination should be received and reviewed by the ambulatory surgical facility with enough time to resolve questions. Complete instructions that cover in detail all phases of the operative experience must be provided to the patient in advance of the surgery. Many facilities finish these preparations with a telephone call to the patient (usually by a member of the nursing staff) that confirms medical data, clarifies preoperative teaching, and answers questions.

The healthy patient should have the option to visit the ambulatory facility before the day of surgery for the preoperative evaluation and education. Twersky and colleagues evaluated the effect of the timing of the preanesthesia interview on patient anxiety and satisfaction. Patients received a structured in-depth anesthesia interview either in advance or on the day of operation. The authors found that there was no difference in patient anxiety or satisfaction with the ambulatory surgical experience based on the timing. However, this study does not address the effects of seeing patients "on the conveyor belt." A focused preoperative interview with a discussion obtaining informed consent is still required.

Intraoperative delays may be due to equipment failure or unavailability or inadequate supplies, and can often be resolved by improved scheduling of the equipment and personnel as well as increased preprocedure testing. A system should be in place to monitor and reduce these occurrences. Intraoperative delays due to surgical or anesthetic complications do occur, but they should be monitored to detect and address any patterns. A review of historic performance of critical parameters on a quarterly or semiannual basis directs attention to problem areas and enhances productivity through a process of continuous improvement.

Scheduling of postoperative care also im-

BRIGHAM AND WOMEN'S HOSPITAL
A Teaching Affiliate of Harvard Medical School
75 Francis Street, Boston, Massachusetts 02115

2 NCR Form
Use ball point pen (press hard)

Intravenous Conscious Sedation Record   Date: ____/____/____

Procedure:

Procedure Status:
☐ Pre-Scheduled   ☐ Emergency   ☐ Urgent

Patient Identification:
☐ Bracelet   ☐ Verbal

Patient Status:
☐ In-patient   ☐ Out-patient   ☐ Emergency Dept.

Addressograph

Procedure Location:
Building _____ Floor _____ Room _____

Recovery Location:
Building _____ Floor _____ Room _____

Age

Sex
☐ M   ☐ F

Height

Weight
                                                                                Kg

☐ Signed Consent

NPO since: ___/___/___ ____ AM PM

Allergies/Adverse Reactions:

Diagnosis:

Pertinent Medical History:

Equipment Safety Check:
☐ Stethoscope   ☐ Cardiac Monitor   ☐ Defibrillator   ☐ O_2 Supplies   ☐ Ambu and Airways
☐ Vital Sign Monitor   ☐ Pulse Oximeter   ☐ Emergency Cart   ☐ Suction Supplies   ☐ Antagonist

Pre-Sedation Assessment: _____ AM/PM

Temp _____ HR _____ Cardiac Rhythm ASA ≥ 3 _____ Resp _____ BP _____ mmHg

O_2 Sat _____ % on ☐ Room Air or _____ O_2 L/min via _____ ASA   1   2   3   4   5

Sedation Scale: _____   Pain Scale: _____

Intravenous:
Type: _____ Size: _____ Site: _____

Airway Assessment:
☐ Teeth   ☐ Dentures   ☐ Partial Plate   ☐ Natural Airway   ☐ NP/OP Airway   ☐ Intubated   ☐ Tracheostomy

Procedure Time   Start _____ AM/PM   Stop _____ AM/PM

Sedation Time   Start _____ AM/PM   Stop _____ AM/PM

TIME	OBSERVATIONS	B.P.	H.R.	R.R.	O_2 SAT.	DRUG, DOSE, ROUTE	TIME GIVEN	GIVEN BY

Time			Total	N/A	Yes	No	Post Sedation Assessment
Intake							Vital signs stable
							Oxygen saturation stable
							Swallow, cough, gag reflexes present to baseline
Output							Alert or appropriate to baseline
							Able to sit/walk appropriate to baseline or procedure
							Minimal nausea or dizziness

Procedure Site: _____ ☐ N/A

| | | | | | | | Hydration adequate |

Dressings: _____   Other: _____

| | | | | | | | Dressing and/or procedure site checked if applicable |
| | | | | | | | **Assessment Prior to Discharge/Transfer** |

Drains: _____   Tubes: _____

							Patient and/or family given written discharge instructions
							Patient and/or family questions answered
							Patient and/or family verbalizes their understanding of instructions
							Discharge order written

Signature Initials	Signatures	Physician Clinical ID#	Disposition: ☐ Discharge to Home ☐ Admit ☐ Transfer to _____
	Operators		Comments: _____
	Operator		_____
	Monitor		_____
	Monitor	R.N.	_____
		R.N.	Time _____ AM/PM Signed _____ , R.N.

Page _____ of _____ Pages

Figure 13–2. Intravenous Conscious Sedation Record used at Brigham and Women's Hospital, Boston, MA.

pacts on efficiency by affecting procedural efficiency as well as patient satisfaction. Adequate facilities and staffing for postoperative care prevents operating room delays and prolonged turnover. Many facilities use a flexible, two-stage recovery process, in which somnolent patients are cared for in a more intensely staffed area and more awake patients can be cared for with more extended staffing. Patients can be admitted to the extended care area directly from the operating room if appropriate. The family often joins the patient in this second-stage area.

POLICIES AND PROCEDURES

A comprehensive list of policies and procedures must be available to ensure compliance with regulatory agencies and facilitate smooth day-to-day function of the unit. Clearly written practical policies must be established for all operational aspects of the ASU to avoid delays and cancellations. Policies should be flexible enough to allow practical implementation and to accommodate changes in the practice environment. According to Nean, policies should include aspects of the following:

Medical staff credentialing

Required committees

Quality assurance programs; safety and risk management plans

Infection control measures

Emergency transfer or admission arrangements

Consultant use and criteria for selection

Job descriptions

Medical and surgical staff privileges

Anesthesia services

Pathology services

Radiology services

Medical direction

Hours of operation

Scheduling procedures

Preadmission criteria

Preoperative and postoperative contact with patients

Distribution of clothing and valuables

Responsible person requirements

Acceptable procedures and anesthetic agents

Laboratory requirements

In-service education plans

A number of practice policies are required by various credentialing organizations including the Joint Commission on Accreditation of Healthcare Organizations, the Accreditation Association for Ambulatory Health Care, and the Association of Operating Room Nurses. Some state medical registration boards have additional requirements. The use of standardized forms and records facilitates compliance with policies and enhances quality outcomes measurement (Fig. 13–2).

CONCLUSIONS

The necessity for greater efficiencies and effectiveness of ASU operations will increase as the health care industry responds to a myriad of pressures exerted by cost control, governmental regulations, overcapacity, and emerging technologies. This goal will be achieved through sound fiscal management by a minimally bureaucratic administrative infrastructure supported by interdisciplinary cooperation among health care providers. Communication and collaboration between administrative and clinical staffs will be a key component to the attainment of mutual objectives while the highest standards of patient care are maintained.

Suggested Readings

1. Berryman JM. Development and organization of outpatient surgery units: the hospital's perspective. Urol Clin North Am 1987;14:1–9.
2. Brannan P. Selecting and educating perioperative nurses for an ambulatory surgery setting. Association of Operating Room Nurses Journal 1986;4:307–310.
3. Journal of Ambulatory Care Management, Aspen Publishers, Inc.
4. MacDowell NM, Perry R. Factors influencing physi-

cian choice of an outpatient surgery and testing facility. J Health Care Marketing 1990;10:67–74.

5. Nathanson SN. Managing resources effectively in a hospital-based ambulatory surgery program. J Ambulatory Care Management 1988;11:63–71.

6. Philip BK. Cost effective choices for ambulatory general anesthesia. J Clin Anesth 1995;7:606–613.

7. Twersky RS, Lebovits AH, Lewis M, et al. Early anesthesia evaluation of the ambulatory surgical patient: does it really help? J Clin Anesth 1992;4:204–207.

8. Wetchler BV, ed: Anesthesia for Ambulatory Surgery. 2d ed. Philadelphia, JB Lippincott, 1991.

9. White P, ed: Outpatient Anesthesia. New York: Churchill Livingstone, 1990.

10. Williams RC. Selecting the right staff for your center. MGM J 1989;36:46–51.

11. Zerbe TR. Engineering methods in an ambulatory surgery clinic: a case study in computerized patient tracking. J Ambulatory Care Management 1989;12:48–60.

Anesthesia for Ambulatory Surgery

14

Agents for General Anesthesia

Mark Dershwitz

The state of general anesthesia is one characterized by a loss of consciousness and a lack of reaction to noxious stimuli. A decrease in skeletal muscle tone is produced by some general anesthetics. Thus, when an adequate depth of general anesthesia is induced and a painful stimulus is applied to the patient, the patient should not move, manifest alterations in vital signs consistent with pain such as tachycardia or hypertension, or have any recollection of the experience.

The anesthesiologist caring for the patient undergoing outpatient surgery under general anesthesia has a substantial list of goals for such a patient in comparison to that for the inpatient. At the end of most inpatient surgical procedures, the patient should be awake, breathing spontaneously, extubated, and able to follow commands. The patient is usually transported to the postanesthesia care unit (PACU) and then to a hospital room and placed in bed. In addition to these rather simple goals, the outpatient surgical patient must, within a reasonably short time after arriving in the PACU, eat and drink without vomiting, urinate, dress and walk with little or no assistance, be given orally administered pain medications, and be able to comprehend and remember instructions. For the outpatient to attain these goals within a reasonably short time, the anesthesiologist must plan the anesthetic carefully so that the patient is unresponsive to noxious stimuli during the procedure yet emerges from the anesthetic with minimal residual effect. In most cases, the anesthesiologist administers a combination of intravenous and inhaled agents that render the patient unconscious and immobile during surgery, yet

permit rapid recovery and discharge from the hospital.

PHARMACOLOGY OF INTRAVENOUS AGENTS

Pharmacokinetic Principles

The most common way to describe the time course of a drug is to specify its half-life, defined as the time required for the blood concentration of the drug to decline by 50%. Figure 14–1 depicts the behavior of a drug with a half-life of 1 hour. This approach works well for drugs that follow one-compartment pharmacokinetics; however, most agents used in anesthesia require a three-compartment model to adequately represent their time course. The three compartments may be viewed as the central compartment, a compartment composed of tissues with high blood flow, and a compartment composed of tissues with low blood flow. Figure 14–2 shows the decline in the blood concentration of a drug whose behavior is approximated by a three-compartment model and is similar to that of the opioids used in anesthesia.

The concentration of such a drug at a given time, t, may then be described by the following equation:

$$\text{Concentration} = Ae^{-\alpha t} + Be^{-\beta t} + Ce^{-\gamma t}$$

where α, β, and γ are the rate constants for the three phases of the disappearance curve, and A, B, and C are the fractional coefficients describing the relative importance of each of

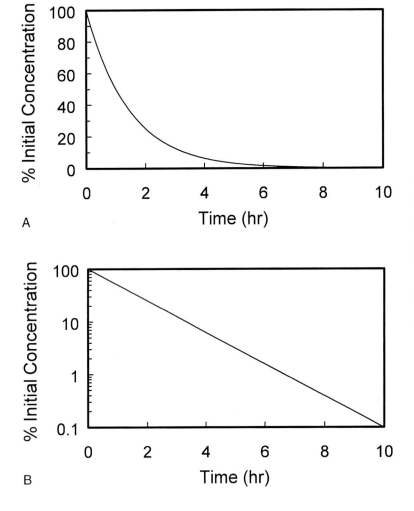

Figure 14–1. (A) The time course of the decline in the blood concentration of a medication having a half-life of 1 hour. This medication can be represented by a single exponential decay, indicating that it may be described by a one-compartment model. **(B)** The same time course as in view *A* with the y-axis drawn with a logarithmic scale. A single exponential decay is apparent because the time course is represented by a single straight line.

the three phases. A rate constant is related to the half-life of the phase by the following equation:

$$t_{1/2_\gamma} = \frac{\ln 2}{\gamma}$$

The other half-lives, $t_{1/2\alpha}$ and $t_{1/2\beta}$, may be similarly calculated.

The value $t_{1/2\gamma}$, often called the terminal half-life, has been used to compare medications in terms of their durations of action. When considering the intravenous medications used in anesthesia, the value of $t_{1/2\gamma}$ often correlates poorly with the clinical duration of a drug (see the first equation and Fig. 14–2). If a drug has a very long terminal half-life (i.e., a very small value for γ) but a very small value for C (indicating that the third phase of the

decay curve occurs at blood concentrations of less than those that cause a significant pharmacologic effect), the terminal half-life is unimportant in describing the clinically apparent time course of the drug. Thiopental is a good example of this principle.

Because of the inadequacy of the terminal half-life in describing the clinical duration of a drug, a new parameter has been introduced to describe more accurately how long the effect of a drug will last: context-sensitive half-time. The context-sensitive half-time is defined as the time required for the drug concentration in the central compartment to decrease by half after an infusion of specified duration. Thus, the duration of the drug is described in the context of how it was administered. For agents administered by intravenous infusion, the context-sensitive half-time increases with

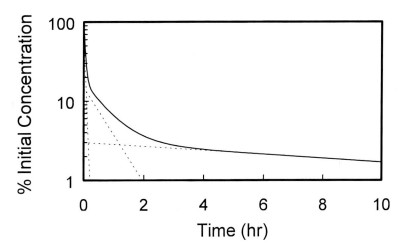

Figure 14–2. The time course of the decline in the blood concentration of a medication described by a three-compartment model. The triexponential decay is apparent because the time course curve is the sum of the three phases represented by each of the dashed lines. The half-lives of the three phases of the curve are 2 minutes, 30 minutes, and 12 hours.

an increase in infusion duration. Applied to anesthetic agents, this means that a longer infusion requires a longer recovery time.

Agents for Induction and Maintenance

Barbiturates

The barbiturates, particularly thiopental, have been used for more than a half century to induce anesthesia by the intravenous route. Intravenous induction (in contrast to inhalational induction) is fast and well tolerated by patients. When an adequate dose is administered, sleep occurs within one arm-to-brain circulation time, or within 15 to 30 seconds in most patients.

Thiopental is prepared as a 2.5% solution. It is highly alkaline with a pH of 10 to 11 and is quite irritating to tissues if an intended intravenous injection extravasates. Thiopental is thought to act via interaction with the neurotransmitter γ-aminobutyric acid (GABA), the primary inhibitory transmitter in the human brain. Thiopental appears to bind to GABA receptors and increase the effect of GABA at its receptors.

The central nervous system (CNS) is profoundly depressed by thiopental. In a dose-dependent fashion, brain metabolic activity (i.e., oxygen consumption) and the electroencephalogram are depressed. Cerebral blood flow and intracranial pressure are also decreased. At lower sedative (i.e., subanesthetic)

doses, thiopental causes hyperalgesia, an increase in the perception of pain. Thiopental causes dilation of capacitance vessels and decreased cardiac contractility. The overall cardiovascular effect is usually hypotension, decreased cardiac output, and reflex tachycardia. These effects are exaggerated in patients with hypovolemia or congestive failure. Ventilatory depression also results after thiopental administration. Induction of general anesthesia usually results in apnea, and a decreased ventilatory response to hypercarbia or hypoxia persists well after the time of awakening.

The toxicity of thiopental is, in most cases, an extension of its pharmacologic effects: cardiorespiratory depression and drowsiness. Most patients experience some degree of "hangover," often manifested as drowsiness, inability to concentrate, and nausea, after thiopental administration. The duration of the hangover depends on the total dose of thiopental administered. Thiopental may cause severe illness or death if given to patients with acute intermittent porphyria, coproporphyria, or variegate porphyria.

After a single intravenous injection of thiopental, the blood concentration declines rapidly as the drug is redistributed; that is, the central compartment concentration declines while the concentration in other tissues increases. The short duration of thiopental is, therefore, due to this process of redistribution and not to metabolism or elimination. Typically, a patient would be expected to regain consciousness approximately 5 minutes after a dose of thiopental adequate to induce general anesthesia. However, when given by repeated injections to maintain general anesthesia, the duration of effect after each dose is longer than after the prior dose because of the accumulation of thiopental in peripheral tissues. The context-sensitive half-time of thiopental is shown in Figure 14–3. For intravenous infusions of 1 hour or less, the time required for the central compartment concentration to decrease by 50% exceeds the duration of the infusion; therefore, thiopental is a poor choice for continuous infusions when rapid awakening is desired.

Thiopental remains an extremely popular induction agent. Its advantages include a proven track record and low cost. The typical induction dose is approximately 4 mg/kg in healthy, unpremedicated patients and is less in elderly patients and in patients given other CNS depressants before surgery. In the outpatient practice of many anesthesiologists, use of thiopental is being supplanted by propofol because of the superior recovery profile of the latter drug.

Methohexital is another barbiturate often used to induce or maintain anesthesia. It is more potent than thiopental, and an equivalent induction dose is approximately 1.5 mg/kg. Its duration of action is less than that of thiopental, and Figure 14–3 shows that the context-sensitive half-time of methohexital is much less than that of thiopental, regardless of infusion duration. Methohexital may be given by continuous infusion to maintain general anesthesia while permitting the patient to awaken and recover within a reasonably short time. In comparison with thiopental, its disad-

vantages include more pain on injection and involuntary movements and hiccoughing under anesthesia.

Propofol

Propofol is the newest intravenous anesthetic available in the United States. Its popularity is increasing because it results in more rapid recovery with fewer postoperative adverse effects. Propofol is insoluble in water and is prepared as an emulsion formulation of propofol in a mixture of soybean oil, glycerol, and lecithin. Even though lecithin, a phospholipid, is derived from eggs, persons with an allergy to egg protein are not at increased risk of a hypersensitivity reaction to propofol.

The mechanism of action of propofol appears to be similar to that of thiopental. The CNS and ventilatory effects of propofol are qualitatively similar to those of thiopental, except propofol is not associated with hyperalgesia in subanesthetic doses. In comparison with thiopental, propofol causes a greater decrease in blood pressure and less change in heart rate, possibly by interfering with the barostatic reflex.

Like thiopental, the adverse effects of propofol are generally extensions of its pharmacologic effects. In addition, propofol frequently causes pain on injection, which may be minimized by using a large vein, a slower rate of injection, and adding lidocaine to the propofol emulsion. It is not irritating to tissue if it extravasates. The incidence of postoperative nausea and vomiting is low after administration of propofol; in fact, propofol appears to

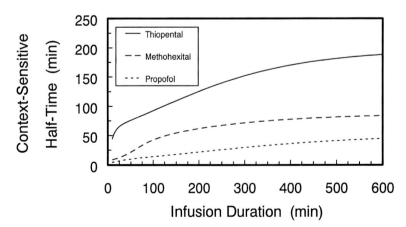

Figure 14–3. The context-sensitive half-times of thiopental, methohexital, and propofol. Propofol blood concentrations decay much more quickly than those of the other two agents regardless of the duration of the infusion. (Data from Hughes MA, Glass PSA, Jacobs JR. Context-sensitive half-time in multicompartment pharmacokinetic models for intravenous anesthetic drugs. Anesthesiology 1992; 76(3):334.)

have intrinsic antiemetic activity because the administration of propofol in subhypnotic doses may relieve nausea resulting from diverse stimuli.

The major advantage of propofol is its superior recovery characteristics compared with other intravenous anesthetics. Patients awaken more quickly whether propofol is given by bolus injection or continuous infusion. Figure 14–3 depicts the very short context-sensitive half-time of propofol. In addition, psychomotor impairment is shorter after administration of propofol, and patients have a greater sense of well-being, perhaps due to an intrinsic euphoric effect of the drug.

The usual induction dose of propofol is approximately 2.5 mg/kg, and general anesthesia may be maintained by continuous infusions of 100 to 200 µg/kg/min. Propofol is also used for producing conscious sedation by infusion at 25 to 50 µg/kg/min (see Chapter 15). The required infusion rates are decreased by the prior or concomitant administration of opioids, benzodiazepines, nitrous oxide, or volatile anesthetics.

Etomidate

Etomidate has several characteristics that differentiate it from other intravenous anesthetics. Its major advantage is its minimal effect on the cardiovascular system. After the usual induction dose (0.3 mg/kg), there is usually little or no change in heart rate, blood pressure, cardiac output, or vascular resistance. Among intravenous or inhalational anesthetics, this lack of cardiovascular effects is unique.

Etomidate also produces a number of troubling adverse effects that make it less desirable for use in outpatients. The incidence of postoperative nausea and vomiting is higher after administration of etomidate than after any other agent in current use. It often causes pain on injection, involuntary movements, and hiccoughs. In addition, etomidate inhibits the synthesis of cortisol. The clinical significance of this effect in outpatients undergoing short procedures is controversial.

Ketamine

Ketamine is the only induction agent suitable for use by intramuscular route. Its mechanism differs from the other agents in that ketamine is an antagonist at the N-methyl-D-aspartate receptor. The anesthetic state induced by ketamine is called dissociative anesthesia; it does not resemble normal sleep but patients appear to be dissociated from their environment. For example, under ketamine anesthesia, the patient may vocalize, have eyes open, and make ocular tracking movements. Patients are, however, anesthetized because they do not respond to noxious stimuli or have recall of events that occurred during the influence of the anesthetic. Ketamine causes profound analgesia that persists well into the postoperative period. Ketamine anesthesia is often accompanied by vivid dreams or hallucinations that may be perceived as unpleasant.

In contrast to other intravenous anesthetics, ketamine causes increased cerebral metabolism, cerebral blood flow, and intracranial pressure. It is thus relatively contraindicated in persons with intracranial conditions. Ketamine also stimulates the cardiovascular system and is associated with increased blood pressure, heart rate, and cardiac output. Ketamine produces minimal ventilatory depression and may not ablate airway reflexes. It also causes significant bronchodilation.

Ketamine has a longer duration of action than other induction agents. The usual intravenous induction dose is approximately 2 mg/kg, and unconsciousness lasts 10 to 15 minutes after this dose. Recovery, including emergence delirium and hallucinations, takes longer than after administration of other agents. The unpleasant emergence phenomena can often be prevented or mitigated by the concurrent administration of a benzodiazepine. Many anesthesiologists have found that low intravenous doses of ketamine (0.5 to 1 mg/kg) along with propofol, a benzodiazepine, or both produces acceptable recovery after short procedures.

The primary benefit of ketamine in outpatients is that it may be given intramuscularly to induce general anesthesia; two to four times the intravenous dose is required. Lower intramuscular doses may be used for sedation. Intramuscular ketamine may thus be useful in the patient with poor venous access or in the uncooperative patient in whom an intramuscular injection will be less traumatic than physical restraint for the placement of an intravenous catheter.

Opioids

Opioids are given during general anesthesia because of their analgesic activity. This class of agents contains both naturally occurring (e.g., morphine, codeine) and synthetic (e.g., fentanyl, alfentanil) compounds. All bind to specific receptors (primarily in the CNS) to produce a similar constellation of effects: analgesia, sedation, ventilatory depression, decreased gastrointestinal (GI) motility, increased GI sphincter tone, tolerance, and physical dependence. They differ in terms of their pharmacokinetic parameters and specific adverse effects.

Morphine

Morphine is the prototypical opioid to which all others are compared. A dose of 10 mg is the standard reference used when describing the potencies of other opioids. When morphine is injected intravenously, there is an almost immediate release of histamine from mast cells, resulting in peripheral vasodilation, flushing, and a decrease in blood pressure. The patient may describe a feeling of warmth. Soon afterward, the patient also begins to feel drowsy, and pain (if present) is perceived as less unpleasant. The patient's pupils constrict and the ventilatory rate decreases. Morphine has little direct effect on the heart; however, there may be a reflex increase in heart rate and cardiac output. The peripheral vasodilation often results in orthostatic hypotension.

Patients receiving chronic therapy with an opioid become tolerant to its effects. When such a patient is to undergo surgery, amounts well in excess of the patient's maintenance dose may be necessary to achieve adequate analgesia in the perioperative period.

Even after intravenous administration of morphine, the onset of analgesia is comparatively slow, requiring 15 to 30 minutes to peak. The duration of analgesia depends on the dose given, but is usually approximately 2 to 4 hours. Some studies suggest that morphine may delay the time to discharge in outpatients.

Meperidine

Meperidine became a popular agent in anesthesia because of its more rapid onset in comparison to morphine, having a time to peak effect of approximately 5 to 10 minutes. Its duration of action is also shorter, approximately 1.5 to 3 hours. An 80-mg dose of meperidine is approximately equivalent to 10 mg of morphine.

Histamine release is less pronounced than after administration of morphine. Meperidine is unique among opioids in having a potentially catastrophic interaction with monoamine oxidase inhibitors (MAOI). The patient on chronic MAOI therapy given meperidine may manifest a hypermetabolic state characterized by hyperthermia and seizures. For reasons that are poorly understood, meperidine is uniquely effective in stopping postoperative shivering. A small dose (25 mg intravenously) may be used for this purpose.

Fentanyl

Fentanyl is the first in a class of opioids having much greater lipid solubility in comparison with older agents. It therefore has a more rapid onset of action (time to peak effect approximately 3 to 5 minutes) and a shorter duration of action due to redistribution of the drug out of the central compartment. A dose of 100 µg is approximately equivalent to 10 mg of morphine, and its duration of action is approximately 30 to 60 minutes.

Fentanyl and its derivatives do not cause histamine release. They may produce skeletal muscle rigidity, especially when given in larger doses by rapid intravenous injection. This rigidity is most apparent in the muscles of the chest wall, head, and neck, and the patient may be unable to ventilate or be ventilated. The rigidity is reversed by depolarizing or nondepolarizing muscle relaxants (see Pharmacology of Muscle Relaxants).

Fentanyl is usually given by intermittent bolus injection. Because its effects are terminated primarily by redistribution, subsequent doses may last longer than earlier ones. When given repeatedly over a period of several hours, fentanyl may accumulate and behave as a drug with a long duration. This effect is due to the long elimination half-life of fentanyl(3 to 5 hours), which is usually not relevant in shorter outpatient procedures.

Alfentanil

Alfentanil has a shorter duration than fentanyl because of more rapid redistribution and elimination. It is less potent than fentanyl; a dose of 750 μg is approximately equivalent to 10 mg of morphine. After intravenous administration of alfentanil, its peak effect occurs in 1 to 2 minutes and its duration is 10 to 15 minutes.

Alfentanil is most commonly given by continuous infusion after a loading dose. Infusion rates of 1 to 2 μg/kg/min may be used during general anesthesia, and rates of 0.25 to 0.5 μg/kg/min may be used for conscious sedation.

The context-sensitive half-time for alfentanil is shown in Figure 14–4. For infusions of less than 2 hours duration, alfentanil is longer-acting than fentanyl. The context-sensitive half-time of alfentanil plateaus at 60 minutes; however, regardless of the length of the infusion, the time for the blood concentration to decrease by 50% is not more than 1 hour.

Sufentanil

Sufentanil is shorter acting than alfentanil. For infusions of less than 10 hours' duration, it is shorter acting than alfentanil (see Fig. 14–4). For example, after a 1-hour infusion, the time required for the blood opioid concentration to decrease by 50% is approximately 18 and 34 minutes, respectively, for sufentanil and alfentanil. Sufentanil is approximately 10 times as potent as fentanyl; a 10-μg dose of sufentanil is approximately equivalent to 10 mg of morphine.

Remifentanil

Remifentanil is the newest intravenous opioid. It is an ester that is rapidly metabolized by tissue esterases. It is therefore usually given as a loading dose followed by a continuous infusion. As shown in Figure 14–4, its context-sensitive half-time plateaus at approximately 3.5 minutes; patients emerge rapidly from anesthesia independently of the duration of the infusion. Recovery does not depend on the infusion rate used to maintain anesthesia, the cumulative dose of remifentanil given, or the length of the procedure. The actual dose does not need to be adjusted for gender or the presence of hepatic or renal dysfunction. Its potency is approximately the same as that of fentanyl. For general anesthesia, a bolus dose of 1 μg/kg is usually given, and infusion rates of 0.5 to 2 μg/kg/min are adequate for most procedures.

Remifentanil is the first extremely short-acting opioid. It is theoretically appropriate for use when rapid emergence is desirable. If a patient is expected to have substantial postoperative pain and the rapid disappearance of analgesia is a significant disadvantage, alternative analgesics or analgesic modalities should be administered before emergence. In all likelihood, the use of remifentanil will, in large part, depend on its price.

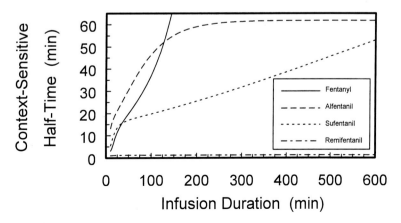

Figure 14–4. The context-sensitive half-time of the opioids. For infusions of clinically relevant durations, the blood concentrations of sufentanil decay much more quickly than those of fentanyl or alfentanil. Note the extremely short context-sensitive half-time of remifentanil, which is independent of infusion duration. (Data from Hughes MA, Glass PSA, Jacobs JR. Context-sensitive half-time in multicompartment pharmacokinetic models for intravenous anesthetic drugs. Anesthesiology 1992;76-(3):334.)

Naloxone

Naloxone is a competitive antagonist at opioid receptors and is therefore able to reverse opioid-induced effects. In the outpatient setting, naloxone is most commonly used at the end of a procedure to speed the rate of recovery. Thus, naloxone administration antagonizes opioid-induced ventilatory depression and sedation, increasing the patient's minute ventilation and level of consciousness. In a patient expected to have postoperative pain, naloxone administration may also increase the severity of the pain. When naloxone is given, it is therefore important to titrate the dose carefully to achieve the desired degree of ventilation and arousal without causing excessive pain. Giving intravenous doses of 40 μg and waiting a minute between doses to assess the effect is a reasonable regimen. It is also important to remember that naloxone is of shorter duration than the opioids (except remifentanil) it may be used to antagonize; once the effect of naloxone has diminished, a repeat dose may be necessary.

PHARMACOLOGY OF INHALATIONAL AGENTS

Although induction of general anesthesia is usually accomplished via intravenous injection, maintenance of general anesthesia is still most commonly achieved by having the patient inhale a gas. The exact mechanism of action of the anesthetic gases remains obscure; however, they may act by altering the lipid domain of transmembrane proteins such as ion channels.

Principles of Uptake and Distribution

The rate at which an inhalational anesthetic agent approaches a steady-state concentration in the body (i.e., the ratio of the concentration of the agent in the body to its concentration in the mixture of gases inspired by the patient) is related to the rate at which the agent reaches a steady-state concentration in alveolar gas. This rate controls the speed of onset of the anesthetic effect and is dependent upon several factors:

1. Inspired concentration of the anesthetic agent. The higher the concentration of the anesthetic agent in the mixture of inspired gases, the more rapid the onset of the anesthetic effect.

2. Alveolar ventilation. The higher the rate of alveolar ventilation, the more rapid the onset of the anesthetic effect.

3. Fresh gas flow. The higher the flow rate of fresh gas from the anesthesia machine (usually oxygen and nitrous oxide), the more rapid the onset of the anesthetic effect.

4. Solubility. As tissue solubility of the anesthetic agent decreases, the onset of the anesthetic effect becomes more rapid.

5. Cardiac output. As cardiac output increases, the onset of the anesthetic effect decreases; an increase in cardiac output increases the removal of anesthetic gas from the lung, thus delaying the attainment of a steady-state alveolar concentration.

6. Functional residual capacity (FRC). The lower the value for FRC (as might occur as a result of ascites, pregnancy, obesity, or restrictive lung disease), the more rapid the onset of the anesthetic effect; the anesthetic gas needs to mix with a lower volume of lung gas as the FRC decreases.

In practice, a steady-state concentration of anesthetic gas is rarely achieved because of the time required to do so. Figure 14–5 shows the ratio of alveolar to inspired concentrations of the inhalational anesthetics, thus demonstrating the speed of onset of the anesthetic effect. All of the factors listed (except the inspired concentration of the anesthetic agent) that increase the rate of onset of an inhalational agent also increase the rate of offset (i.e., awakening).

Pharmacodynamic Principles

The potencies of the inhalational anesthetics may be related by comparing their values for minimum alveolar concentration (MAC). MAC is defined as the alveolar concentration of the gas at which 50% of individuals will not move in response to a skin incision. It has been observed that the greater the tissue solubility of an agent, the lower its value for MAC;

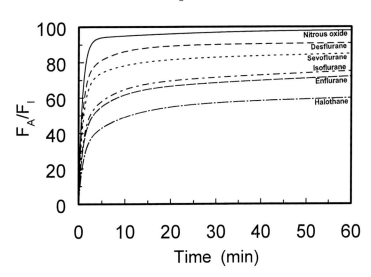

Figure 14–5. The ratio of the alveolar to inspired concentrations of the inhalational anesthetics as a function of the duration of administration. The speed at which the alveolar concentration approaches the inspired concentration determines the rapidity of wash-in and wash-out of the inhalational agent. The relative speed for these agents may thus be described: nitrous oxide > desflurane > sevoflurane > isoflurane > enflurane > halothane. (Data from Eger EI. A mathematical model of uptake and distribution. In: Papper EM, Kitz RJ, eds. Uptake and distribution of anesthetic agents. New York: McGraw Hill, 1963.)

the least soluble volatile agent, desflurane, has a higher value for MAC than the most soluble agent, halothane. When two inhalational agents are used in combination, the overall fraction of MAC is approximately the sum of the fractional values of the individual agents. For example, the concurrent administration of 70% nitrous oxide (0.64 MAC) and 0.4% isoflurane (0.36 MAC) achieves an anesthetic effect of approximately 1.0 MAC. MAC for a given anesthetic agent is decreased by the concurrent administration of other CNS depressants, such as opioids, benzodiazepines, barbiturates, and propofol. Finally, there is a decline in the value of MAC as the age of the patient increases.

Gaseous Agents

Nitrous oxide

Nitrous oxide is the most commonly used inhalational anesthetic. It is the only one that is a gas at room temperature and is supplied as a compressed gas in a tank. As shown in Figure 14–5, nitrous oxide is the least soluble inhalational anesthetic and therefore is able to wash in and wash out most rapidly. Its value for MAC is 110% and therefore is not attainable. Most commonly, nitrous oxide is given at concentrations of 50% to 75% in oxygen; an adequate depth of anesthesia is achieved by the concurrent administration of a volatile anesthetic agent, an intravenous agent, or both.

Nitrous oxide is colorless, odorless, and tasteless. It is well tolerated when inhaled by the awake or semiconscious patient. It has minimal effects on organs other than the CNS: it causes little alteration in heart rate, blood pressure, cardiac output, or ventilatory drive. It also causes little muscle relaxation. When nitrous oxide is included in the anesthetic regimen, patients may have a higher risk of postoperative nausea and vomiting. Nitrous oxide is eliminated entirely by exhalation.

Although nitrous oxide is the least soluble anesthetic gas, it is much more soluble in blood than nitrogen. This characteristic may cause problems when nitrous oxide is given to a patient who has gas contained within a closed space (e.g., bowel obstruction, pneumothorax, occluded eustachian tube). Nitrous oxide will diffuse into such a space and either increase its volume (as in the case of bowel distention when an obstruction is present) or increase its pressure (as in the case of increased middle ear pressure when the eustachian tube is occluded). Nitrous oxide is probably best avoided when such pathologic gas collections exist. Nitrous oxide does not trigger malignant hyperthermia.

Volatile Agents

Halothane

Halothane is the prototypical volatile anesthetic. It is termed volatile because it is a liquid at room temperature and is administered by a calibrated vaporizer on the anesthesia machine. Halothane has a value for MAC of 0.75%, and its kinetics are shown in Figure 14–5.

Halothane has a sweet, somewhat pleasant odor and is nonirritating to the respiratory tree. It has excellent bronchodilator properties and may be used to induce anesthesia by inhalation without significant discomfort to the patient. Halothane causes a decrease in ventilatory drive and dose-dependent hypotension, primarily as a result of a decrease in cardiac output. Nodal or junctional cardiac rhythm is common, and halothane increases the sensitivity of the heart to catecholamine-induced ventricular arrhythmias. There is cerebrovascular vasodilation and an increase in intracranial pressure. Halothane produces excellent skeletal muscle relaxation. Splanchnic perfusion is decreased.

The major limitation to the use of halothane is the occurrence of rare, but often fatal, hepatic necrosis. Although the exact mechanism of this effect is unknown, risk factors include obesity and repeated exposure to halothane. Thus, when halothane is used to induce anesthesia by inhalation, it is often replaced by another volatile agent once the patient is adequately anesthetized. All volatile agents, including halothane, may trigger malignant hyperthermia in genetically susceptible persons.

Isoflurane

Isoflurane is the most commonly used volatile anesthetic and its kinetic effects are superior to those of halothane (see Fig. 14–5). Its value for MAC is 1.15%.

Isoflurane has a pungent odor and may cause a burning sensation when inhaled. Like halothane, it decreases ventilatory drive and dilates bronchial smooth muscle. Its cardiovascular effects differ from those of halothane; isoflurane causes hypotension primarily by decreasing systemic vascular resistance, and it has little effect on cardiac output. Although isoflurane often increases the heart rate, arrhythmias are much less common than under halothane anesthesia. Isoflurane causes skeletal muscle relaxation and decreased splanch-

nic perfusion; both of these effects occur to a lesser degree than with halothane.

Enflurane

Enflurane is an isomer of isoflurane and is used less frequently since the introduction of isoflurane. Its value for MAC is 1.68%. Enflurane causes both a decrease in cardiac output as well as peripheral vasodilation, thereby decreasing blood pressure to a greater degree than isoflurane. It causes more profound skeletal muscle relaxation than the other volatile agents.

Desflurane

Desflurane is a newer and the least soluble volatile agent. It therefore has the fastest wash-in and wash-out of the volatile agents. Its value for MAC is 6.0%. Desflurane is also the most irritating of the volatile agents, and coughing and laryngospasm may occur during lighter levels of desflurane anesthesia (such as during induction and emergence). Desflurane has the least effect on cardiac output among the volatile agents, and its hypotensive effect is due to peripheral vasodilation. A rapid increase in the administered desflurane concentration may cause significant hypertension before the onset of hypotension. The concentration of desflurane should be increased slowly.

Sevoflurane

Sevoflurane is the newest volatile anesthetic. It has a value for MAC of 2.0% and a spectrum of cardiovascular effects similar to that of isoflurane. The useful characteristic of sevoflurane is its low solubility (see Fig. 14–5) combined with its pleasant odor and lack of airway irritation; it may be a suitable replacement for halothane when an inhalational induction is indicated. Among newer volatile anesthetics, sevoflurane is unique in that it undergoes significant biotransformation to free fluoride ion. At the concentrations usually achieved, the fluoride ion is not thought to be associated with organ toxicity.

PHARMACOLOGY OF MUSCLE RELAXANTS

Mechanisms of Action

There are two pharmacologic classes of muscle relaxants: depolarizing agents and nondepolarizing agents. Depolarizing agents are agonists at the nicotinic acetylcholine receptor of the neuromuscular junction (NMJ). Administration of a depolarizing muscle relaxant causes an initial intense stimulation of skeletal muscle, manifested as generalized fasciculations, followed by paralysis due to continuing depolarization. Nondepolarizing agents are competitive antagonists of acetylcholine at the NMJ; they prevent acetylcholine, released in response to motor nerve impulses, from binding to its receptor and initiating muscle contraction.

Monitoring of Neuromuscular Blockade

Although alternatives exist, the most common method for quantitating the degree of muscle relaxation is to measure evoked adduction of the thumb initiated by stimulating the ulnar nerve with surface electrodes. The usual stimulus pattern is the train-of-four: four constant-current, square-wave stimuli administered at a rate of 2 Hz.

Ideally, the patient's baseline train-of-four response is determined before the administration of any muscle relaxant (but after the induction of anesthesia, because the stimulus may be uncomfortable). Nondepolarizing agents cause a dose-dependent suppression of twitch manifested as fade; each twitch is weaker than the previous one. Adequate surgical relaxation is often correlated with the disappearance of two or three twitches on the train-of-four. Depolarizing agents cause a diminution in twitch strength without fade.

Indications for Use

Muscle relaxants are used to facilitate endotracheal intubation and to improve surgical conditions by decreasing skeletal muscle tone. Before intubating a patient, the administration of a muscle relaxant results in relaxation of the vocal cords, increasing the ease with which the endotracheal tube may be inserted and decreasing the risk of cord trauma. During surgery, the decrease in skeletal muscle tone may aid in surgical exposure (such as during abdominal surgery), decrease the insufflation pressure needed during laparoscopic procedures, and make joint manipulation easier during orthopedic surgery.

Depolarizing Agents

Succinylcholine

Succinylcholine is the only depolarizing muscle relaxant. A dose of 1 mg/kg results in fasciculations within seconds and excellent intubating conditions in less than 1 minute. Succinylcholine is usually considered the drug of choice when the airway must be quickly secured such as when the patient has a full stomach or has symptomatic gastroesophageal reflux. Succinylcholine may trigger malignant hyperthermia in genetically susceptible persons. Its use in children is controversial because a child may have a genetically determined myopathy that is associated with malignant hyperthermia, but which has not yet become symptomatic (see Chapter 17). Succinylcholine may also be associated with postoperative muscle pain.

A small dose of a nondepolarizing agent (e.g., 0.5 mg of vecuronium) given before succinylcholine prevents the fasciculations caused by succinylcholine. This action may decrease postoperative muscle pain; however, there is controversy regarding this potential benefit. There is a delay in onset (to about 1.5 minutes) of the peak effect of succinylcholine when it is given after a small dose of a nondepolarizing agent.

Succinylcholine is metabolized by pseudocholinesterase, a circulating enzyme. In most people, its duration of action is approximately 5 to 10 minutes. There are a number of inherited abnormalities of pseudocholinesterase that may prolong the duration of succinylcholine.

Short-Acting Nondepolarizing Agents

All short-acting nondepolarizing agents produce similar muscle relaxant effects. After an intubating dose, full relaxation does not usually occur for 2 to 3 minutes.

Vecuronium

Vecuronium produces the fewest adverse effects among the muscle relaxants. It does not cause histamine release or cardiac arrhythmias. The dose given before intubation is approximately 0.08 mg/kg; incremental doses of half the intubating dose are given approximately every 15 to 30 minutes. Vecuronium is metabolized in the liver and is subject to a number of drug interactions. For example, persons taking drugs that induce hepatic enzymes (e.g., phenytoin) metabolize vecuronium more quickly. Vecuronium may have a longer duration in persons with hepatic disease.

Atracurium

Atracurium has a unique mechanism of metabolism: at physiologic pH, the molecule spontaneously hydrolyses. Its pharmacokinetics are therefore unaltered in persons with liver or renal impairment. The dose given before intubation is approximately 0.4 mg/kg; incremental doses of half the intubating dose are given approximately every 15 to 30 minutes. Atracurium may cause histamine release and hypotension; this effect is more likely if the drug is given rapidly.

The commercially available preparation of atracurium contains 10 isomers. Cistracurium is a new agent that is a single isomer of atracurium. This isomer has the highest ratio of NMJ-blocking activity to histamine-releasing activity. Therefore, it causes much less of a hypotensive effect, and its cardiovascular profile is similar to that of vecuronium. It is subject to fewer drug interactions than is vecuronium. The intubating dose of cistracurium is about 0.15 mg/kg.

Mivacurium

Mivacurium is the shortest acting nondepolarizing muscle relaxant. The dose given before intubation is approximately 0.2 mg/kg; maintenance of muscle relaxation is usually by an infusion at a rate of 8 μg/kg/hr. Mivacurium may also cause histamine release, and its duration of action is prolonged in persons with an alteration or deficiency in pseudocholinesterase. Mivacurium use usually does not require reversal (see Reversal of Neuromuscular Blockade).

Rocuronium

Rocuronium is the newest nondepolarizing muscle relaxant. It is slightly faster in onset than other nondepolarizing agents. The dose given before intubation is approximately 0.6 mg/kg; incremental doses of half the intubating dose are given approximately every 15 to 30 minutes.

Reversal of Neuromuscular Blockade

Neuromuscular blockade caused by any of the nondepolarizing agents may be reversed by the administration of a cholinesterase inhibitor such as neostigmine (40 μg/kg) or edrophonium (750 μg/kg). To prevent unwanted parasympathetic effects, such as bradycardia and increased respiratory secretions, the reversal agent is usually given with atropine (16 μg/kg) or glycopyrrolate (8 μg/kg). Inhibition of cholinesterase prolongs and intensifies the neuromuscular blockade produced by succinylcholine.

ADJUNCTS TO GENERAL ANESTHETICS

Sedatives

Diazepam and midazolam are the two most commonly used sedatives in conjunction with general anesthesia. The pharmacology of midazolam is discussed in detail in Chapter 15. Midazolam may be useful as a premedicant given before general anesthesia; it produces sedation, accompanied by decreased anxiety and amnesia. It may decrease the likelihood of recall of events during general anesthesia.

Diazepam is an alternative to midazolam. Despite its longer terminal half-life, the clinical duration of a small number of bolus doses of diazepam is similar to that of midazolam.

Antiemetics

Postoperative nausea and vomiting are the most common adverse effects related to anesthesia and constitute the most common reason for the unanticipated admission of a person scheduled for outpatient surgery. Many classes of drugs have antiemetic activity; any of these agents is more effective if used prophylactically before the induction of general anesthesia. None of these agents is unequivocally more effective than any other; a combination of two or more agents acting via different mechanisms may increase efficacy. These agents are discussed in Chapter 15.

CONDUCT OF GENERAL ANESTHESIA

Stages of General Anesthesia

The classic literature describes four stages of anesthesia: I, analgesia; II, delirium; III, surgical anesthesia; IV, medullary depression.

Stage III is further divided into several planes. Using the medications available in modern times, this nomenclature is somewhat obsolete. For example, when anesthesia is induced with an intravenous agent, the patient passes so rapidly to stage III that the first two stages are not readily observed.

Stage II continues to have important applications during emergence from anesthesia when delirium may occur. In this stage, the patient may appear to be awake but does not follow commands and may make purposeless movements. Airway reflexes are increased, and the larynx is subject to spasm. Thus, stimulation of the airway (e.g., extubation, suctioning) must be avoided during this stage.

Premedication

Most anesthesiologists prefer not to have outpatients take sedating medications before coming to the hospital because their ability to ambulate safely may be impaired. Antiemetics, such as ondansetron or transdermal scopolamine, may be used, if indicated, because they do not produce sedation.

Once the patient has been interviewed and the intravenous catheter inserted, a sedative may be considered for the anxious patient. Midazolam, 1 to 2 mg, or diazepam, 2.5 to 5 mg, may make the patient more comfortable while awaiting surgery; however, there is the possibility that recovery may be prolonged. When an antiemetic is indicated, it should be given before induction.

Induction

A dose of propofol or thiopental adequate to cause sleep and blunt the response to intubation is usually given. An opioid is often given just before, or at the same time, as the induction agent. A muscle relaxant, if needed for intubation, is then given, and the patient is intubated.

Maintenance

An inhalational technique, with nitrous oxide, a volatile agent, or both, may be used. Alternatively, an intravenous technique, consisting of the administration of an opioid and a hypnotic (e.g., sufentanil and propofol), may be used, either by continuous infusion or repeated boluses. A muscle relaxant may also be administered. The doses of the maintenance agents are titrated to minimize autonomic and somatic responses to surgical stimuli, and they are gradually decreased as the end of the procedure nears.

Emergence and Recovery

If residual muscle relaxation is present at the end of the procedure, it is reversed before discontinuing the maintenance agents. The maintenance agents are terminated such that their disappearance (by exhalation, redistribution, or metabolism) is timed to coincide with the end of the procedure. The patient is given

100% oxygen to compensate for likely residual ventilatory depression. If the patient was intubated, the endotracheal tube is removed after the patient emerges from stage II of anesthesia. The patient is then taken to the PACU.

Selected Readings

1. Apfelbaum JL. Muscle relaxants for outpatient surgery: old and new. J Clin Anesth 1992;4(suppl 1):2S.
2. Apfelbaum JL, Grasela TH, Hug CC, et al. The initial clinical experience of 1819 physicians in maintaining anesthesia with propofol: characteristics associated with prolonged time to awakening. Anesth Analg 1993;77(4S):S10.
3. Dershwitz M. Advances in antiemetic therapy. Anesth Clin North Am 1994;12(1):119.
4. Hughes MA, Glass PSA, Jacobs JR. Context-sensitive half-time in multicompartment pharmacokinetic models for intravenous anesthetic drugs. Anesthesiology 1992;76(3):334.
5. Miller RD. Anesthesia. 4th ed. New York: Churchill Livingstone, 1994.
6. Rogers MC, Tinker JH, Covino BG, Longnecker DE. Principles and Practice of Anesthesiology. St Louis: Mosby–Year Book, 1993.
7. Shafer SL, Varvel JR. Pharmacokinetics, pharmacodynamics, and rational opioid selection. Anesthesiology 1991;74(1):53.
8. Victory RA, Pace N, White PF. Propofol: an update. Anesth Clin North Am 1993;11(4):831.
9. Weiskopf RB, Eger EI. Comparing the costs of inhaled anesthetics. Anesthesiology 1993;79(6):1413.
10. White PF. Studies of desflurane in outpatient anesthesia. Anesth Analg 1992;75(4S):S47.

15

Conscious Sedation

Bobbie Jean Sweitzer

Sedation is frequently desirable to minimize the stress and discomfort associated with a surgical or diagnostic procedure. Conscious sedation implies the use of pharmacologic agents either alone or in combination with local or regional anesthesia to provide comfort and safety during both therapeutic and diagnostic procedures. Conscious sedation is defined as a minimally depressed level of consciousness produced by a pharmacologic or nonpharmacologic method that retains the patient's ability to independently and continuously maintain an airway and respond appropriately to physical stimulation and verbal command. The continuum of sedation ranges from minimal sedation such as exists in an awake but relaxed patient to profound sedation resulting in unresponsiveness (Table 15–1).

Primary objectives of conscious sedation include sedation, relief of anxiety, amnesia, and prevention of pain with minimal risk. Supplemental medications also help the patient lie still for relatively long periods on an often uncomfortable operating table in a cold environment. However, to optimize both patient safety and comfort, careful titration of sedative and analgesic drugs, vigilant monitoring of the cardiovascular, respiratory, and neurologic systems, and effective communication with both the patient and surgeon are necessary.

Many patients are resistant to "being awake" for procedures and request to be "knocked out." Often, patients express concern about pain and awareness during their procedures. Anxiety is almost universal in the surgical patient. Most patients prefer to undergo surgery under local anesthesia with sedation compared to receiving local anesthesia alone, and patient satisfaction increases with increasing levels of sedation. The combination of sedation plus analgesia can substitute for general anesthesia for a number of surgical procedures. Because of increasing evidence of the potential benefits of procedures performed under local or regional anesthesia (i.e., decreased cost, reduced hospitalization and long-term recovery, less physiologic derangement), there will be and should be a greater demand for conscious sedation in the future.

PATIENT SELECTION

Most American Society of Anesthesiologists (ASA) class I and II and selected class III and IV patients (Table 15–2) are appropriate candidates for conscious sedation. Even neonates can benefit from this technique. Ambulatory patients, those with significant anxiety or previous unpleasant general anesthetic experiences, and very ill individuals gain maximal benefit from conscious sedation. Even though a procedure may be minor, the anxiety level of outpatients is not. Fear, apprehension, anesthesia, and surgery can cause a variety of potentially harmful cardiovascular and metabolic responses.

The age and physical status of the patient is invaluable in determining sensitivity to medications used for conscious sedation. Other important factors are past experiences with anesthesia, anxiety level, general expectations concerning the procedure, and previous postoperative complications such as nausea and vomiting, excessive pain, or prolonged sedation.

Table 15–1. Definitions

Conscious sedation	A minimally depressed level of consciousness that retains the patient's ability to maintain a patent airway independently and continuously and to respond appropriately to physical stimulation and verbal commands. The drugs, doses, and techniques used are not intended to produce a loss of consciousness.
Deep sedation	A controlled state of depressed consciousness or unconsciousness from which the patient is not easily aroused and is unable to respond purposefully to physical stimulation or verbal command. This may be accompanied by a partial or complete loss of protective reflexes and an inability to maintain a patent airway independently.
General anesthesia	A controlled state of unconsciousness accompanied by a loss of protective reflexes, including loss of the ability to maintain a patent airway independently or to respond purposefully to physical stimulation or verbal command.
Local anesthesia	The introduction of a local anesthetic drug by injection in subcutaneous tissue, in close proximity to a nerve, or applied topically so as to avoid intravascular injection. With sufficient blood levels, all local anesthetics possess both excitatory (seizure) and depressant (loss of consciousness) central nervous system effects and may additionally have profound cardiovascular depressant effects. There may also be interactive effects between local anesthetic drugs and sedative medications.

PROVIDER SELECTION

Conscious sedation can be provided by the operators themselves, which is frequently done in dental, oral surgical, or office-based practices. This entails the added risk of diverting surgeons from their primary focus of performing the procedure. Practitioners who administer drugs for conscious sedation should have the knowledge, skill, and equipment (both for monitoring and resuscitation) to enable them to manage an oversedated patient.

Traditionally, anesthesiologists or certified registered nurse anesthetists (CRNA) have provided care for patients requiring supplemental agents for sedation during surgical procedures. A commonly used term for this is "monitored anesthesia care" (MAC). Even though anesthetists are uniquely trained in conscious sedation techniques, monitoring of physiologic parameters that are often altered with use of pharmacologic agents, and airway management, this expertise and level of functioning may not be necessary or cost effective for many surgical procedures. Many institutions are using (if not training and certifying) registered operating room nurses to administer drugs and monitor patients undergoing operative procedures. Even patients can serve as their own provider of conscious sedation. Patient-controlled analgesic systems, first designed for use in managing postoperative pain, have been modified and adapted for use in the operative setting.

PATIENT PREPARATION

Preoperative preparation of the patient is a valuable but often overlooked aspect of care that has been shown to reduce anxiety, postoperative narcotic needs, and even hospital stay, and to effect a more prompt return to active life and work. Development of a good rapport between the caretakers and the patient is advantageous to the partnership that needs to exist for trust and adequate feedback during the procedure.

Many patients feel anxious and poorly informed before surgery. Preoperative intervention and preparation is most successful when the preoperative fears of the patient are discussed and no new anxieties are introduced. It is important to explore with all patients their personal concerns, which are influenced by the type of procedure, previous experience

Table 15–2. American Society of Anesthesiologists Classification of Physical Status

Category	Description
I	Healthy patient
II	Mild systemic disease—no functional limitation
III	Severe systemic disease—definite functional limitation
IV	Severe systemic disease that is a constant threat to life
V	Moribund patient unlikely to survive 24 hours with or without operation

with surgery, anesthesia, and illnesses, and cultural and societal influences, as well as discussions with family and friends, especially those who have had similar experiences. Specific fears often include fear of the unknown, death, mutilation, loss of control and awareness, nausea, vomiting, and pain. Detailed explanations do not seem to reduce anxiety more than brief explanations. Patients should be given instructions about what and when to eat and what to wear and to bring to the facility. They should be given details about check-in, preparation, and the actual procedure to be performed as well as the recovery and discharge expectations. The more knowledge patients perceive they have (which may not correlate with actual knowledge), the less anxious they are. Therefore, many patients benefit from a factual discussion, written information, video production, or a tour of the facility, as long as it is not too technical.

PHARMACOLOGIC AGENTS FOR CONSCIOUS SEDATION

Preoperative Medications

Premedication reduces fear and anxiety and facilitates venipuncture. Oral medications are generally preferred by patients and offer the additional benefit of administration before a patient's arrival at the operative facility, if appropriate. Intravenous medications must await insertion of an intravenous line but are rapidly effective and reduce anxiety for further preparation such as positioning and injection of local anesthetics. Intramuscular drug administration is usually reserved for patients who are uncooperative (children and mentally or emotionally challenged individuals). Timing of administration is important. The premedicant should be given early enough to be effective.

Amnesia is usually a desirable effect of premedicants, but lack of recall of perioperative events may be disturbing to some patients, particularly those who actually desire to participate and observe their procedure. One of the most effective measures with virtually no undesirable side effects is verbal reassurance and communication. Table 15–3 lists recommended premedications. Many of these drugs are also used intraoperatively for conscious sedation.

Benzodiazepines

Benzodiazepines are the most widely used drugs for preoperative reduction of anxiety and fear. Diazepam has been the most widely prescribed benzodiazepine because it was one of the first available and it is well absorbed orally. Relaxation and drowsiness are evident within 10 to 15 minutes of ingestion. Typically 5 or 10 mg are administered orally 1 to 2 hours before the procedure. Use of larger doses may cause prolonged drowsiness and dizziness. Amnesia is not predictably provided by oral diazepam. Because the metabolite is pharmacologically active, the effects of diazepam may

Table 15–3. Preoperative Medications and Dosages

Medication	Oral	Intravenous	Intranasal
Sedatives			
Midazolam	0.5–0.7 mg/kg	1–3 mg/kg	0.2 mg/kg
Diazepam	0.15–0.3 mg/kg	0.1 mg/kg	
Opioids			
Fentanyl (suckers)	5–15 μg/kg (400 μg max)		
Sufentanil			10–20 μg
Other agents			
Propranolol	10–20 mg		
Clonidine	0.1–0.3 mg		
Antiemetics:			
Metoclopramide	10–20 mg	10–20 mg	
Ondansetron	8–16 mg	4–8 mg	
Droperidol		0.625–2.5 mg	

exceed 30 hours. Repeated doses may result in a cumulative effect. Oral lorazepam provides superior amnesia; however, it too has a long duration of action. Oxazepam is an equally effective anxiolytic and has a much shorter duration of action because of its inactive metabolites.

Midazolam is an excellent preanesthetic medication due to its rapid onset, short duration of action, and anxiolytic and amnesic properties. It is effective when administered intravenously, intramuscularly, orally, rectally, and even intranasally. Midazolam is not available as an oral preparation, but the parenteral preparation can be administered both intranasally and orally. Most commonly, it is administered intravenously, in doses of 1 to 2 mg (see Intraoperative Medications). When administered intranasally, doses of 0.2 mg/kg produce sedation within 10 minutes.

Narcotics

Narcotics administered via novel routes, such as mucosally (oral transmucosal fentanyl suckers), intranasally (sufentanil), or transcutaneously (transdermal fentanyl) have met with some success. These are particularly useful in patients who cannot take medication orally but require medication before an intravenous insertion.

The dose of oral transmucosal fentanyl suckers is based on patient weight with a range of 5 to 15 µg/kg. A dose of 400 µg is recommended for all adults weighing 50 kg or more, to avoid hypoventilation. The suckers are available in 200, 300, and 400 µg strengths. Onset is within 5 to 15 minutes from the start of the lollipop. Maximum reduction in apprehension and peak analgesic effects are noted 20 to 30 minutes from the start of administration. Complete consumption of the lollipop typically takes 10 to 20 minutes. The bioavailability of fentanyl varies depending on the fraction of the dose that is absorbed through the oral mucosa and the portion swallowed. Normally 25% of the total dose is rapidly absorbed from the buccal mucosa and becomes systemically available. The remaining 75% is swallowed and is slowly absorbed from the gastrointestinal tract. Approximately one third of this amount

(25% of the total dose) escapes first pass elimination by the liver and becomes systemically available. Therefore, the bioavailability of transmucosal fentanyl is generally 50%. The latency of onset and duration of action of transdermal fentanyl is prolonged and is only useful if circumstances permit appropriate placement and there is a prolonged opioid requirement.

Sufentanil is an opioid agonist that has a short duration of action and is approximately five to seven times more potent than fentanyl. Sufentanil is an ideal opioid for intranasal administration because of its high potency, which permits use of a smaller volume, shorter duration of action, predictable absorption, and equivalent efficacy with the intravenous route. Sufentanil administered intranasally in a low dose produces effective preoperative sedation. Doses of 10 to 20 µg have a median onset of action of 10 minutes and median duration of action of 40 minutes. Patients appear to be relatively free of common opioid side effects.

Sympatholytic Agents

Beta-adrenergic antagonists have been successfully used to block the sympathetic stimulation that accompanies anxiety. The pounding heart, sweating palms, and butterflies associated with anxiety can be attenuated. Propranolol in doses of 10 to 30 mg orally is commonly used. Central alpha-adrenergic agents such as clonidine are also effective in reducing anxiety when administered preoperatively. Doses of 0.1 to 0.3 mg have an onset within 30 to 60 minutes after intravenous or oral administration with significant sedation, but without respiratory depression. The peak effect is within 2 to 4 hours and the duration of action can be as long as 24 hours with doses of 0.1 to 0.3 mg. The effects of clonidine are additive with sedative and anxiolytic agents administered during the procedure.

Intraoperative Medications

Supplemental intravenous sedative, hypnotic, analgesic, or anxiolytic drugs during local anesthesia or minor diagnostic and therapeutic procedures can improve patient comfort and acceptance of these techniques (Table 15–4).

Benzodiazepines

Traditionally, benzodiazepines have been the most widely used drugs for conscious sedation. These can be administered either alone or combined with sedative-hypnotic agents. Benzodiazepines produce dose-related sedation as well as amnesia and anxiolysis.

Midazolam

Midazolam is a water-soluble benzodiazepine with a rapid onset that produces anxiolysis, sedation, and amnesia. Because of its water solubility, it causes little pain or phlebitis. In relatively low doses (<5 mg), the therapeutic effect is relatively short and the elimination half-life is 2 to 3 hours. The metabolites of midazolam are inactive. Because midazolam does not undergo intrahepatic recirculation, drowsiness does not recur once the patient recovers. However, large doses may result in prolonged drowsiness. Even though midazolam is a potent amnestic agent, retrograde amnesia is not reliably produced. For conscious sedation in the ambulatory setting, midazolam may be titrated in 1-mg doses. It is often given until the patient develops slurred speech and drooping eyelids. The dose response is variable, depending on the patient's overall condition, drug history, and alcohol use.

Soon after its introduction, midazolam was associated with a significant number of incidences of respiratory depression, apnea, cardiac arrests, and deaths. Most of these occurred in elderly individuals undergoing endoscopic procedures, without separate monitoring personnel, outside of the operating room setting, and with little or no monitoring.

Midazolam can be administered by continuous infusion, but careful titration is required to produce the desired level of sedation. The infusion must be terminated soon enough to avoid excessive sedation and prolonged recovery times. A bolus dose or a rapid infusion of a loading dose of 1 to 3 mg is recommended with a maintenance infusion rate of 0.04 to 0.1 mg/kg/hr. Elderly patients require lower loading and maintenance doses.

Diazepam

Diazepam, a benzodiazepine with a long duration of action and active metabolites, has been widely used in the past for conscious sedation. After doses of 0.3 mg/kg, diazepam causes impairment of coordination and reac-

Table 15–4. Intraoperative Medications and Dosages

Medications	Intravenous (Bolus)	Intravenous Infusions	Inhalational
Sedatives			
Midazolam	0.5–1.0 mg	1 μg/kg/min	
Diazepam	2.5–5.0 mg		
Opioids			
Fentanyl	25–50 μg	0.1 μg/kg/min	
Alfentanil	5–10 μg/kg	0.5 μg/kg/min	
Meperidine	12.5–25 mg		
Butorphanol	0.5–1.0 mg		
Sedative-hypnotics			
Propofol	0.5–1.5 mg/kg	25–100 μg/kg/min	
Methohexital	0.5–2.0 mg/kg	0.05–0.15 mg/kg/min	
Ketamine	0.2–0.5 mg/kg	50 μg/kg/min	
Etomidate	10–20 mg	5–8 μg/kg/min	
Droperidol	0.625–2.5 mg		
Inhalational agents			
Nitrous oxide			10%–60%
Enflurane			0.5%
Antagonist agents			
Naloxone	0.04 mg (2 mg max)		
Flumazenil	0.2–0.4 mg		

tive skills (e.g., impaired driving) for up to 10 hours. The addition of opioids to diazepam further prolongs the impairments. Diazepam produces more postoperative sedation and less intraoperative amnesia than midazolam. If diazepam is used, increments of 2.5 mg are appropriate. Again, individual dose response is highly variable, with elderly patients being consistently more sensitive. Because of its pharmacokinetic profile, venoirritation, pain upon injection, and associated phlebitis, diazepam use should be limited to oral premedication.

Narcotics

Fentanyl

Fentanyl is a potent narcotic analgesic, with a peak onset occurring 2 to 4 minutes after intravenous administration. It is the narcotic of choice for outpatient conscious sedation because of its favorable pharmacokinetic profile. Analgesia lasts 30 to 60 minutes after low to moderate doses of less than 5 μg/kg. Incremental amounts of 25 to 50 μg can be titrated to achieve desired sedation and analgesia. Termination of effect is due to redistribution into peripheral tissues with eventual hepatic metabolism. Doses exceeding 10 μg/kg can have a prolonged effect approaching that of morphine. Fentanyl causes sedation and can cause profound respiratory depression that is comparable to that of other opioids. Fentanyl is often administered in combination with a benzodiazepine. This significantly increases respiratory depression compared to use of either an opioid or benzodiazepine alone. Hypoxemia is also more common with this technique. However, in the presence of appropriate monitoring, the combination of a benzodiazepine and opioids causes more profound sedation and improvement in patient cooperation than does benzodiazepine alone.

Alfentanil

Alfentanil is an opioid with 20% the potency of fentanyl and an even shorter duration of action. It has a quicker redistribution half-life and a more rapid elimination half-life than

fentanyl. However, large doses can result in prolonged sedation and respiratory depression. Its pharmacokinetics make it most suitable for infusion techniques. An initial bolus of 5 to 10 μg/kg followed by an infusion of 0.5 μg/kg/min is recommended. The drug must be titrated to the desired effect, and differences in dose requirements must be appreciated. When compared with fentanyl, alfentanil produces more hypotension and rigidity, but it has a shorter duration of respiratory depression.

Agonist-Antagonist Opioids

Nalbuphine and butorphanol have the theoretic advantage of less narcotic side effects such as nausea, vomiting, and respiratory depression. They have analgesic as well as sedative effects. The disadvantage is their relatively long duration of action (3 to 4 hours). Therefore, these are not desirable except for procedures that require significant postoperative pain control.

Other Opioids

Longer acting, classic opioid analgesics such as morphine sulfate and meperidine have been popular in the past. Many practitioners still rely heavily on these agents because of experience and consequent comfort with their use. Morphine sulfate is very sedating. When administered to patients who are not experiencing pain, it can result in significant dysphoria. Its duration of action is long. Meperidine in relatively small doses, not resulting in sedation, causes a pleasant euphoria in most patients. Its duration is intermediate to that of fentanyl and morphine sulfate, but even 75 mg has been shown to cause abnormal tests of coordination and reaction up to 12 hours later. Both morphine sulfate and meperidine cause more nausea and vomiting, dizziness, and a longer duration of respiratory depression than shorter acting opioids. The use of these long-acting narcotic analgesics should be avoided in ambulatory patients except under special circumstances when their excessively long duration of effects is desired.

Sedative-Hypnotic Agents

Propofol

Propofol is a sedative-hypnotic without amnesic or analgesic properties, except when given in doses high enough to induce sleep. Propofol is formulated in a white oil-and-water emulsion. Propofol causes pain on injection, which can be decreased by the addition of lidocaine (50–100 mg) directly to the solution. Lidocaine can be injected previously (10–50 mg) or the propofol can be administered into a larger vein with a rapidly flowing intravenous solution.

Propofol can be administered either as a bolus to achieve a transient loss of consciousness for placement of a local block, for example, or as a continuous infusion. Bolus doses are typically 0.5 to 1.5 mg/kg, and continuous infusion rates of 25 to 50 μg/kg/minute are usually sufficient to produce a sleep-like state in which patients still arouse to verbal stimulation. The dose of propofol should be titrated to desired effect in individual patients. Decreased dosages should be used in elderly patients. Because propofol solution is an excellent medium for bacterial growth, any vials, syringes, or mixtures of propofol should be discarded after 6 hours.

Computer-controlled infusion pumps, designed to achieve a target plasma concentration, have been used successfully. Low-dose infusions of propofol result in predictably rapid recovery with few postoperative side effects. Variable-rate infusions are preferable over intermittent boluses to minimize undesirable cardiorespiratory effects. Because of the pharmacologic profile of propofol, it is an appropriate agent for patient-controlled administration. Typically, patients are awake within 3 to 10 minutes of termination of an infusion, regardless of duration or dosage.

Propofol has been described as euphorogenic, although, when it is administered alone, some patients react dysphorically. Emergence occurs quickly and is associated with a remarkably clear-headed awake state. Recent evidence supports a direct antiemetic effect of propofol, and the incidence of nausea and vomiting after propofol administration is decreased compared with the incidence in patients receiving opioids, inhalational agents, and barbiturates. Doses of propofol adequate to induce sedation have little effect on tidal volume, minute ventilation, end-tidal carbon dioxide ($ETCO_2$) tension, or arterial blood gas values. However, propofol can suppress the ventilatory response to hypoxia.

Propofol causes less postoperative sedation, drowsiness, dizziness, and confusion than midazolam. Midazolam does produce more effective intraoperative amnesia, but it is associated with prolonged amnesia into the recovery period as well as impairment of cognitive function compared with propofol. When amnesia and supplemental analgesia are needed, midazolam and a narcotic such as fentanyl or alfentanil can be added to propofol. When midazolam is given preoperatively or at the beginning of a procedure, it neither delays the rapid recovery seen with propofol alone nor causes additional side effects. This combination takes advantage of the rapid recovery profile of propofol, and the benzodiazepine produces anxiolysis and amnesia intraoperatively.

According to the manufacturer (Zeneca Pharmaceuticals), when propofol is administered for conscious sedation during therapeutic or diagnostic procedures, it should be "administered only by persons trained in the administration of general anesthesia and not involved in the conduct of the surgical or diagnostic procedure. Patients should be continuously monitored and facilities for maintenance of a patent airway, artificial ventilation, and oxygen enrichment and circulatory resuscitation must be immediately available."

Methohexital

Methohexital is an ultra short-acting barbiturate that augments the inhibitory tone of γ-aminobutyric acid (GABA) by occupying receptors adjacent to GABA in the central nervous system. Methohexital produces no analgesia and may actually be hyperalgesic in low doses. Methohexital typically causes a dose-dependent decrease in blood pressure, but heart rate may increase. Methohexital is administered intravenously, either in bolus doses or by continuous infusion techniques for conscious sedation. Typically 30 to 80 mg (0.5–1.0 mg/kg) over 5 to 10 minutes is given, then

0.05 to 0.15 mg/kg/min is administered. Intermittent boluses typically use three times the amount of drug as continuous infusions. Because of its extreme alkalinity, it should not be administered intramuscularly, and methohexital may cause slight discomfort when administered intravenously. Adverse effects can include prolonged sedation and myoclonus.

Etomidate and Ketamine

Etomidate is a unique anesthetic agent, its major advantage being its minimal effects on the cardiovascular system. Typically, it is given in doses of 10 to 20 mg over 5 to 10 minutes, followed by an infusion of 20 to 35 mg/hr or 5 to 8 μg/mm. Etomidate has no analgesic properties. Ketamine is also useful for sedation in some special circumstances. Typical doses are 0.2 to 0.5 mg/kg intravenously as a bolus or 50 μg/kg/min. Ketamine is best combined with a benzodiazepine, such as midazolam, to avoid unpleasant psychomimetic emergence reactions. More cardiovascular stimulation is observed when ketamine is either administered alone or before sedation with a benzodiazepine than when patients are adequately sedated with midazolam before ketamine administration. Its pharmacologic properties are discussed in Chapter 17.

Droperidol

Droperidol is a butyrophenone derivative that produces sedation and a sense of detachment with minimal amnesia. Additionally, it is a potent antiemetic and has been used for many years in various combinations, especially with narcotics, to provide conscious sedation. Typically, 0.625 to 2.5 mg in adults causes minimal sedation and is effective in decreasing the incidence of nausea and vomiting. Droperidol does not have significant respiratory depressant effects. Larger doses may cause prolonged and excessive sedation, hypotension, and extrapyramidal side effects. When given in doses exceeding 5 to 10 mg, some patients can become confused.

Inhalational Agents

Patient-controlled self-administration of nitrous oxide and methoxyflurane has been used to supplement other aspects. With all the anesthetic gases, complete recovery to normal function and discharge criteria are met within 20 to 25 minutes after cessation of administration. Care must be taken to avoid general anesthesia and its potential complications of respiratory and cardiovascular depression, excitement, loss of protective reflexes, and aspiration. For a discussion of nitrous oxide and enflurane, the two most commonly used agents, see Chapter 14.

Antiemetic Agents

Metoclopramide

Metoclopramide is a central and peripheral dopamine antagonist that acts as an antiemetic in the central chemoreceptor trigger zone. It increases motility of the upper gastrointestinal tract and accelerates gastric emptying. The usual dose is 10 to 20 mg intravenously or intramuscularly with onset of action within 1 to 3 minutes or 10 to 15 minutes, respectively, and persists 1 to 2 hours. It is effective when used as prophylaxis or treatment of postoperative nausea. It does not cause sedation but may rarely cause extrapyramidal side effects such as dystonia.

Ondansetron

Ondansetron is a selective serotonin 5-HT$_3$ receptor antagonist and acts both centrally in the chemoreceptor trigger zone and peripherally at vagal nerve terminals. It has no sedative properties. It has an elimination half-life of 4 hours and is metabolized in the liver. Ondansetron can be administered orally or intravenously. The usual dose is 8 to 16 mg orally or 4 to 8 mg intravenously.

Antagonist Agents

Naloxone

Naloxone is a competitive antagonist to narcotics and opioid receptors in the brain and spinal cord. Naloxone is metabolized in the liver and has a clearance half-life of 1 to 4 hours. Naloxone reverses, in a dose-dependent manner, the pharmacologic effects of narcotics. The central nervous system effects are seen within 1 to 2 minutes. The drug is usually administered intravenously but may be given intramuscularly. Recommended dose is 0.04 mg boluses until the desired effect is observed. Maximum dose is usually 2 mg. Naloxone should be titrated carefully as abrupt reversal of opioid effect with onset of pain may be accompanied by dramatic hemodynamic changes (e.g., hypertension, tachycardia).

Flumazenil

Flumazenil is an imidobenzodiazepine and a benzodiazepine antagonist that competitively displaces benzodiazepines at their receptor site. It will not reverse the effects of drugs that bind elsewhere, such as barbiturates, antidepressants, alcohol, or general anesthetics. It has an initial half-life of 7 to 15 minutes and a terminal half-life of 41 to 79 minutes. Flumazenil is indicated for the complete or partial reversal of the sedative effects of benzodiazepines. The recommended dose is 0.2 mg (2.0 mL) intravenously over 30 seconds for partial antagonism and 0.4 mg (4.0 mL) for complete antagonism. The onset of action is within 1 to 2 minutes and peak effects are within 6 to 10 minutes. The duration and degree of reversal are related to plasma concentrations of benzodiazepines as well as the dose of flumazenil administered. Because most benzodiazepines, (except midazolam) have a longer half-life than flumazenil, patients should be monitored for resedation and respiratory depression.

Oxygen

Even though oxygen is not often considered a drug, oxygen is the most valuable adjunctive agent available to the conscious sedation patient. Smith and Crul reported arterial desaturations (SpO_2 75%–88%) in three fourths of patients who were given sedation without the administration of oxygen. The importance of supplemental oxygen during sedation was emphasized by Smith and Crul's abandonment of their prospective evaluation of sedation without supplemental oxygen after only 10 patients had been investigated. It is prudent to admin-

Table 15–5. Additional Equipment

Self-inflating positive pressure oxygen (O_2) delivery system capable of delivering oxygen with an adequate rate, percentage, and duration (at least 60 minutes). This can be accomplished by a bag and mask device (AMBU bag) and oxygen in a standard E cylinder.
Source of suction.
A method and means of notifying additional support personnel such as respiratory therapists and practitioners skilled in airway management, and cardiovascular resuscitation procedures should be identified and clearly posted.
Emergency cart or kit with necessary drugs and equipment for resuscitation and a defibrillator.

ister supplemental oxygen whenever conscious sedation is provided.

CONSCIOUS SEDATION TECHNIQUES

The drugs used to achieve conscious sedation produce dose-dependent central nervous system depression. With the ideal sedation technique, the chosen drug or combination of drugs has sedative, hypnotic, anxiolytic, and amnesic properties. This should be accompanied by a low incidence of perioperative side effects (e.g., hypotension, respiratory depression, hypoxia, nausea, and vomiting) with rapid return to a "clear-headed" state soon after the procedure is terminated.

Intermittent bolus administration of intravenous sedative, hypnotic, and analgesic drugs is the most commonly used technique for conscious sedation. Continuous variable-rate infusion of intravenous anesthetics is associated with less respiratory depression and more rapid recovery. Continuous variable-rate infusions also provide a more stable level of analgesia, fewer side effects, and decreased total dose when compared with the intermittent bolus technique. A level of sedation is achieved by the infusion of a loading dose over a period of 5 to 15 minutes and then maintained by an infusion rate that can be varied to achieve a steady state of patient comfort. The initial dose, with either the intermittent bolus technique or variable-rate infusion method, is based on clinical judgment. The expected length of the procedure, the experience of the surgeon, and the patient's body weight, level of anxiety, general medical condition, and history of narcotic, alcohol, or other drug use should be considered.

One of the most popular techniques involves combined use of benzodiazepines and opioid analgesics. Careful titration is necessary to minimize adverse effects, especially the potential for life-threatening respiratory depression, ablation of protective reflexes, and cardiac depression. Alternatively, inhalational agents can be administered at subanesthetic concentrations to provide conscious sedation. Advantages of inhalational analgesia-sedation are ease of administration, constant anesthetic effect, and rapid reversibility. A disadvantage is the potential contamination of the operating room and exposure of health care workers to the agents.

MONITORING

The most important monitor of conscious sedation is the physician or nurse responsible for the care of the patient. Whenever drugs for conscious sedation are administered, a trained individual should monitor the patient. Vigilance and close verbal and tactile contact with the patient will likely result in recognition of a problem and remedial action sooner than other methods of monitoring. Monitoring involves an ongoing assessment of the desired and undesired aspects of all drugs, patient position, effects of the surgical procedure itself, and the comfort and emotional well-being of the patient. There are limitations to human performance, and human error is one of the most common causes of adverse outcomes.

The choice of monitoring equipment is based on the judgment and experience of the practitioner as well as on the support services available. Many monitoring devices have practical limitations regarding accuracy (e.g., capnography), interference from the electrocautery unit (e.g., pulse oximetry, electrocardiogram), and frequent false alarms due to patient interference. There is also the increasingly important issue of cost benefit. Because there are limitations to all monitoring methods and devices, it is important to use multiple methods as cross-checks to ensure that the monitored data accurately reflect the patient's

physiologic state. Furthermore, additional emergency equipment must be immediately available should complications develop (see Table 15–5).

Respiratory System Monitoring

Hypoxia is a common occurrence during conscious sedation, particularly when combinations of sedatives and opioids are used. Monitoring begins with simple, clinical observation of the respiratory rate, pattern, and chest wall movement. The observer must be watchful for signs of partial or complete airway obstruction, hypoventilation, cyanosis, and apnea. The respiratory rate should be timed by either direct observation or auscultation and should be documented. Palpation of air movement at the mouth or nose while observing cyclical condensation of expired moisture on the inner surface of a face mask is another method to be used. Cyanosis, a decrease in oxygen saturation (SaO_2) shown by pulse oximetry, and changes in vital signs are usually late manifestations of inadequate ventilation.

Auscultation

A precordial, laryngeal, or pretracheal stethoscope is a simple, low-cost, low-maintenance device used to monitor ventilation. A heavy, open-sided receiver connected to a monaural earpiece is the most convenient device. An additional benefit of this technique is that phonation, stridor, or other sounds of impending airway obstruction can be detected early.

The precordial stethoscope is also used to measure heart rate and regularity as well. A stethoscope should be considered the minimum monitoring equipment because it is used to assess heart rate, respiratory rate, and adequacy of tidal volume.

Pulse Oximetry

Pulse oximetry is extremely valuable in conscious-sedation patient monitoring and is rapidly becoming the standard of practice whenever sedative drugs are administered. Pulse oximetry is easy to use, sensitive, reliable, accu-

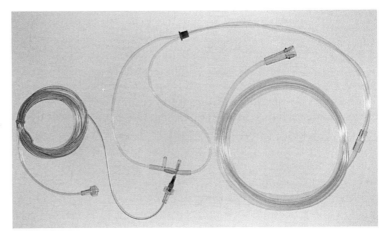

Figure 15–1. Oxygen tubing and nasal cannula for monitoring exhaled P_{CO_2}.

rate, and noninvasive. It provides an early warning of desaturation before the development of clinical signs of hypoxemia, especially cyanosis. Inaccuracies with pulse oximetry occur with (1) profound desaturation; (2) interference from nail polishes, exogenous dyes (e.g., methylene blue), or ambient light; (3) excessive patient movement; (4) use of electrocautery; and (5) presence of abnormal hemoglobins (e.g., carboxyhemoglobin and methemoglobin) or compromised tissue perfusion (e.g., hypotension or vasoconstriction secondary to hypothermia).

Carbon Dioxide Monitoring

Expired carbon dioxide sampling can be obtained by using a device consisting of a nasal cannula or a face mask, a plastic intravenous catheter, and carbon dioxide (CO_2) sampling tubing (Figs. 15–1 and 15–2). A clear capnograph tracing can be achieved in most patients with an acceptable correlation between $ETCO_2$ and arterial P_{CO_2} readings as well as a qualitative estimate of tidal volume and a reliable measure of respiratory rate. Depending on fresh gas flows, the correlation of this sampling readout and $ETCO_2$ and arterial CO_2 varies.

Cardiovascular System Monitoring

Monitoring of the cardiovascular system provides an assessment of patient comfort and of the effectiveness of administered drugs, as well as of the adverse effects from either the drugs used in the procedure itself or those administered for sedation. Cardiovascular stimulation with an increase in heart rate or blood pres-

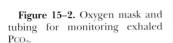

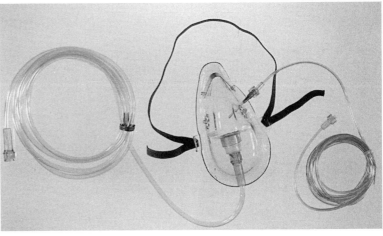

Figure 15–2. Oxygen mask and tubing for monitoring exhaled P_{CO_2}.

sure or the development of arrhythmias results from patient anxiety or pain, general discomfort (e.g., from positioning), drugs (e.g., ketamine, epinephrine), or sympathetic stimulation (e.g., from tourniquet). Cardiovascular depression may be caused by direct myocardial depression (e.g., due to ischemia, beta-blockers, propofol, inhalational agents), peripheral vasodilation (e.g., due to local anesthetics, antihypertensive agents, morphine, inhalational agents, hypovolemia secondary to either inadequate fluid replacement or excessive blood loss), or indirect myocardial depression including bradycardia (e.g., due to vagal stimulation, beta-blockers, fentanyl, alfentanil) and arrhythmias (e.g., due to hypoxia, epinephrine, inhalational agents).

Observation

A readily available monitor is observation of skin, mucous membranes, nailbed color, integrity of pulse, pulse rate, and skin temperature.

Blood Pressure Monitoring

Blood pressure may be determined by manual estimation with a sphygmomanometer oscillotonometric device (most common) or automated ultrasonic device (Doppler). These are indirect methods. Rarely is direct measurement of the blood pressure, requiring an invasive intra-arterial catheter placement, necessary for conscious sedation procedures. Blood pressure alone may be a poor indicator of cardiac output and perfusion in certain patients.

Pulse Oximetry

Pulse oximetry displays a pulse rate that may be more accurate than the electrocardiogram in providing information regarding electrical beats resulting in actual perfusion. If the patient has an arrhythmia that results in electrical activity without adequate mechanical contraction, the pulse oximeter is a more accurate heart rate monitor than the electrocardiogram. Use of a pulse oximeter may be extremely valuable in a patient with a pacemaker to confirm a pulse in association with each electrical impulse. Pulse oximetry typically fails

to generate a signal with marked hypotension or vasoconstriction (secondary to vasopressors or hypothermia) (see Chapter 19).

Electrocardiography

The electrocardiogram provides valuable information about cardiac rhythm, rate, and ischemia. The ASA recommends mandatory monitoring of the electrocardiogram during conscious sedation. Use of standard limb leads and the monitor in "monitor mode" is sufficient for evaluating rate and disturbances in conduction (e.g., bradyarrhythmias, tachyarrhythmias, heart block). Lead II is best for evaluating p waves. A precordial lead V_5 (to detect anterior wall ischemia) and a monitor in the "diagnostic mode" capture 70% to 75% of ischemic episodes. Monitoring lead II detects an additional 10% to 15% of ischemic events. Right ventricular ischemia is more difficult to detect but is best done with a modified precordial lead such as V_5R. By establishing a preanesthetic baseline with the particular pattern of configuration of electrocardiographic leads on an individual patient, any change in the tracing can be compared.

Temperature Monitoring

The most common physiologic deviation from normal during conscious sedation is hypothermia. Heat loss is enhanced by the cold operating rooms and extensive surface exposure, especially during prepping, which is augmented by the evaporation of cleaning solutions from the patient's skin. During conscious sedation cases in which major body cavities are not exposed, the largest decrease in body temperature generally occurs before the time of the skin incision. Reduced heat production is secondary to limited patient activity and drug-induced interference with muscle tone and shivering.

Temperature monitoring in an awake surgical patient has limitations because continuous tympanic, nasopharyngeal, esophageal, and rectal probes are uncomfortable. Monitoring axillary temperature or tympanic membrane temperature intermittently with newer devices is the most practical. The main focus of temperature monitoring is to prevent hypothermia by keeping the room temperature elevated before the patient is draped, covering the patient before heat is lost, and warming intravenous fluids when replacement needs exceed 1 L/h. When shivering occurs, increased oxygen consumption may cause perioperative ischemic events and patient discomfort.

Central Nervous System Monitoring

Evaluation of the central nervous system is essential in evaluating the efficacy of conscious sedation as well as any adverse effects. There is no technologic monitor that ensures that the desired level of sedation, anxiolysis, analgesia, and comfort is reached. Excessive central nervous system depression (i.e., failure to respond to verbal or tactile stimulation) can be caused by overdosage, drug interaction, hypercarbia, hypoxia (respiratory depression), or a primary central nervous system event, which is rare. Many pharmacologic agents have long half-lives, have active metabolites, or accumulate with repeated doses or continuous infusion techniques.

Stimulation of the central nervous system can be a result of drugs (e.g., ketamine, low-dose propofol used alone), local anesthetic toxicity, hypoxia, pain, discomfort, and fear or disorientation resulting in agitation and confusion. A history of prior alcohol or recreational drug use and organic conditions such as dementia predispose certain patients to these adverse occurrences.

DOCUMENTATION

A standard document that is part of the medical record is useful for medicolegal reasons, quality assurance, and future procedures involving any one particular patient. It should document a brief history and results of physical examination, emphasizing the cardiorespiratory system. A family history of adverse events during anesthesia and surgical procedures should be sought. The last food intake time should be documented. The rationale and consent for sedation should be documented, and risk assessment by the ASA physi-

cal status category should be recorded (see Table 15–2).

During the procedure, vital signs (including heart rate, blood pressure, respiratory rate, and patient responsiveness) should be recorded, preferably every 5 minutes. Likewise, oxygen saturation and medication administered (dose, route, time) should be documented.

After the procedure, it is important to record the time of discharge, the patient's condition, and the discharge plan (name of responsible person, patient location). A copy of written patient instructions, including potential unanticipated post-sedation effects and limitations on activities, should remain in the record. A 24-hour emergency contact telephone number must be provided to all patients.

MORBIDITY AND MORTALITY

Complications and deaths have been reported with conscious sedation techniques. Serious complications include idiosyncratic drug reactions, anaphylaxis, respiratory depression, hypoxia, aspiration of gastric contents, malignant hyperthermia, airway obstruction, bronchospasm, hypertension, myocardial infarction, and cardiac dysrhythmias. Intravenous sedation appears to contribute to adverse outcomes in closed claim analysis of factors contributing to unexpected cardiac arrests. Complications occur most often in less experienced hands.

Institutions that have very few complications during conscious sedation attribute this to (1) proper patient selection, (2) proper patient preparation (physical and emotional), (3) careful titration of drugs to produce desired effects, (4) adequate local analgesia, (5) intraoperative monitoring, (6) administration of oxygen, and (7) maintenance of verbal contact with the patient. Continued evaluation of quality control issues, patient safety procedures, and risk recognition as well as efforts to reduce human error are critical to a successful conscious sedation practice.

SUMMARY

Conscious sedation has become a widespread practice in many institutions and is particularly beneficial for the ambulatory surgical population. The explosive growth in numbers of outpatient surgical procedures, the development of minimally invasive surgical techniques, the larger numbers of more seriously ill, aging individuals being treated as outpatients, the development of newer, safer drugs that cause less physiologic perturbations, and advanced noninvasive monitoring techniques have all contributed to the increased opportunities for conscious sedation techniques.

Successful conscious sedation depends on developing the necessary rapport with the patient, careful preoperative evaluation and preparation, careful titration of anesthetic drugs in accordance with the surgical stimulation and response, verbal contact throughout the procedure, and continuous patient monitoring, with pulse oximetry rapidly becoming the standard of care. Optimal patient care results from the knowledge, vigilance, and experience of the conscious sedation provider.

Selected Readings

1. American Society of Anesthesiologists. Standards for Basic Intraoperative Monitoring, ASA House of Delegates, adopted October 6, 1986, amended October 18, 1989.
2. Holzman RS, Cullen DJ, Eichhorn JH, et al. Guidelines for sedation by non-anesthesiologists during diagnostic and therapeutic procedures. J Clin Anesth 1994;6:265–276.
3. Jamison RN, Parris WCV, Maxson WS. Psychological factors influencing recovery from outpatient surgery. Behav Res Ther 1987;25:31–37.
4. Kallar SK. Conscious sedation in ambulatory surgery. Anesth Rev 1990;27:45–52.
5. Smith DC, Crul JF. Oxygen desaturation following sedation for regional analgesia. Br J Anaesth 1989;62:206–209.
6. Smith I, White PF, Nathanson M, et al. Propofol, an update on its clinical use. Anesthesiology 1994;81:1005–1010.
7. Wetchler BV (ed). Anesthesia for Ambulatory Surgery. Philadelphia: JB Lippincott, 1991.
8. White PF. Outpatient Anesthesia. New York: Churchill Livingstone, 1990.
9. White PF. Pharmacologic and clinical aspects of preoperative medications. Anesth Analg 1986;65:963–974.

Chapter 16

Local and Regional Anesthesia

William F. Eckhardt III

Regional anesthesia has a number of applications in ambulatory surgery. Potential advantages include improved postoperative analgesia, shorter recovery time, faster discharge time, diminished nausea and vomiting, reduced risk of aspiration, diminished postoperative nursing service demands, and decreased risk of unanticipated hospital admission. The usual reasons for unanticipated hospital admission after general anesthesia include severe nausea, vomiting, and a generalized hangover feeling. With few exceptions, these are eliminated when regional anesthesia is performed. Patient selection is also important. Patients who are difficult to communicate with because of language barrier or neurologic deficit may be inappropriate for regional anesthesia, as are patients who do not want to tolerate the mild discomfort associated with placement of a regional block.

On the other hand, potential disadvantages with regional anesthesia include (1) the anesthesiologist must be skilled in the technique, (2) surgeons must support this alternative and discuss this with their patients, (3) the surgical procedure must be amenable to this form of anesthesia, (4) there is an additional time requirement necessary for the induction of surgical anesthesia and a system must be in place to accommodate this, (5) complications from both sedatives and local anesthetics may still occur, and (6) even when properly performed, regional anesthetics may not provide completely satisfactory surgical anesthesia.

INFRASTRUCTURE

To successfully perform regional anesthesia for ambulatory surgery patients, several re-

quirements must be satisfied: the patient must have received nothing by mouth (NPO) for a specified period of time (6 hr for liquids in patients at risk for aspiration and altered motility and 3 hr for other patients), a complete airway evaluation must be done, there must be a complete preoperative history and physical examination with review of the patient's pharmacopea, a block induction room or operating room with complete resuscitation equipment must be available, and all of the necessary equipment for performance of the block must be available.

Each patient must follow the NPO guidelines established for the ambulatory surgical center. Regional anesthesia should never be considered an option for those patients who have recently had something to eat or drink for two reasons: (1) virtually every patient who receives a regional anesthetic will require some form of intravenous sedation and (2) occasionally these patients will require general anesthesia, either because the block is not fully adequate or because the surgical procedure outlasts the duration or effectiveness of the block.

For similar reasons, it is imperative that a complete preoperative workup be performed on each patient to detect those patients in whom regional anesthesia is relatively or completely contraindicated. Examples include patients taking warfarin, for whom peridural anesthesia would entail risks of epidural hematoma, or patients with intracerebral mass lesions for whom spinal anesthesia may cause an alteration in cerebrospinal fluid (CSF) dynamics and risk of cerebral herniation.

Evaluation of the airway is an important

151

Table 16–1. Local Anesthetics and Their Properties

	Lipid Solubility	Percentage of Protein Binding	pKa	Potency	Duration	Onset	Maximum Dose (mg/kg) (with epinephrine)	
Aminoesters								
Procaine	1	5	8.9	1	Short	Slow	1000 mg	(14)
2-Chloroprocaine	1	—	9.1	2	Short	Fast	1000 mg	(14)
Tetracaine	80	85	8.6	16	Long	Slow	200 mg	(2)
Aminoamides								
Prilocaine	1.5	55	7.7	3	Moderate	Fast	500 mg	(7)
Lidocaine	4	65	7.9	4	Moderate	Fast	500 mg	(7)
Etidocaine	140	95	7.7	16	Long	Fast	400 mg	(6)
Mepivacaine	1	75	7.6	2	Moderate	Fast	550 mg	(7)
Bupivacaine	30	95	8.1	16	Long	Moderate	225 mg	(3)

part of every preoperative review. Patients with dentures or partial dental plates should always have these removed before a regional anesthetic is begun because it is possible that oversedation, high spinal blockade, or vascular injection of local anesthetic could cause airway compromise. Resuscitation equipment must always be readily available wherever regional anesthetics are performed. At a minimum, this includes suction equipment, laryngoscopes, endotracheal tubes, intravenous access equipment, Ambu bags and masks, an oxygen source, and medications for cerebral and cardiac resuscitation.

Many institutions solve the problem of preparation time for regional anesthesia by designating a block induction room or area within the postanesthesia care unit (PACU) as the location where all regional anesthetics are performed so that the patient's block is fully functional by the start time of surgery. The induction of most regional anesthetic blocks (except spinal and intravenous regional anesthesia) takes more time than does the induction of general anesthesia. Some institutions have different teams of anesthesiologists performing

regional anesthetic blocks; others place a catheter for continuous blockade for those cases of uncertain duration (e.g., brachial plexus catheters). Still others have ancillary or nursing personnel available to start intravenous access, position the patient, and perform skin antisepsis while the anesthesiologist gives report in the PACU on the previous patient. This enables regional anesthetic blocks to be efficiently placed while the operating room (OR) is prepared for the next operation.

LOCAL ANESTHETIC PHARMACOLOGY AND CHOICE OF DRUGS

There are two main classes of local anesthetics: esters (procaine, 2-chloroprocaine, or tetracaine) and amides (lidocaine, prilocaine, etidocaine, mepivacaine, or bupivacaine). The aminoesters are degraded by pseudocholinesterase and the aminoamides are degraded by the liver; their physical properties are described in Table 16–1. Each of these medications has certain applications in local infiltra-

Table 16–2. Local Anesthetics and Their Applications

Medication	Infiltration	Spinal	Epidural	Nerve Block
Procaine (Novocain)	Yes	Yes	No	Yes
2-Chloroprocaine (Nesacaine)	No	No	Yes	Yes
Tetracaine (Pontocaine)	No	Yes	No	No
Lidocaine (Xylocaine)	Yes	Yes	Yes	Yes
Prilocaine (Citanest)	Yes	No	Yes	Yes
Mepivacaine (Carbocaine)	Yes	No	Yes	Yes
Bupivacaine (Marcaine, Sensorcaine)	Yes	Yes	Yes	Yes
Etidocaine (Duranest)	Yes	No	Yes	Yes

Table 16–3. Effect of Epinephrine 1:200,000 on the Onset, Duration, and Maximum Dose of Local Anesthetic

Epidural Medication	Without Epinephrine				With Epinephrine			
	Adult Volume (mL)	Onset (min)	Duration (min)	Maximal Dose (mg)	Adult Volume (mL)	Onset (min)	Duration (min)	Maximal Dose (mg)
Chloroprocaine 2%–3%	15–25	5–15	20–45	800	15–30	5–15	30–90	1000
Lidocaine 1%–2%	15–30	5–15	45–75	300	15–30	10–20	60–180	500
Mepivacaine 1%–2%	15–30	5–15	45–75	400	15–30	10–20	60–180	550
Bupivacaine 0.25%–0.5%	15–25	15–30	90–180	175	15–25	10–30	120–240	225
Major nerve blocks								
Chloroprocaine 2%–3%	25–40	10–20	30–50	800	30–60	10–20	60–120	1000
Lidocaine 1%–2%	20–30	10–20	60–180	300	30–50	10–20	120–240	500
Bupivacaine 0.25%–0.5%	20–30	15–30	180–360	175	20–40	15–30	180–360	225
Mepivacaine 1%–2%	20–30	10–20	60–180	300	30–50	10–20	120–300	500

tion, epidural, spinal, or discrete nerve blocks (Table 16–2).

In addition, each local anesthetic has a recommended maximum dose that may prevent toxicity. The addition of a vasoconstrictor to a local anesthetic often increases the duration of anesthesia and analgesia and often limits toxicity and allows the use of a larger mass (volume × concentration) of local anesthetic (Table 16–3).

There are several pharmacologic alterations that can be performed to improve the physicochemical properties of nerve blockade. Vasoconstrictors added to local anesthetics prolong the duration of anesthesia by limiting absorption and metabolism. They also reduce peak blood levels and aid in the detection of an unintentional intravascular injection when used as part of a test dose. Adding epinephrine to a solution of plain local anesthetic creates a solution with higher pH and may speed the onset of conduction blockade when compared with using a commercially prepared solution of local anesthetic mixed with epinephrine 1:200,000, which has a more acidic pH. To prepare such a solution, 0.1 mL of epinephrine 1:1000 (100 μg) is added to 20 mL of local anesthetic to make a final concen-

tration of 1:200,000 epinephrine (5μg/mL). Phenylephrine is generally used only for spinal anesthesia. When adding vasoconstrictors to local anesthetics for spinal anesthesia, 0.2 to 0.5 mL of epinephrine 1:1000 (200–500 μg) or 0.25 to 0.5 mL of phenylephrine 1% (2.5 to 5 mg) is added.

Altering the pH of local anesthetics by making them more basic (closer to the pKa) speeds the onset by forcing more of the local anesthetic into the non-ionized base form, which penetrates the cell membrane faster. Just before injection of the local anesthetic, commercially prepared sodium bicarbonate 8.4% (1 mEq/mL) is added to the local anesthetic. If the dose recommendations are exceeded, the salt form will precipitate from solution. Table 16–4 lists recommended guidelines.

Some investigators advocate the combination of two local anesthetic agents into a mixture to create a solution with "ideal anesthetic properties," such as an agent with rapid onset (chloroprocaine) combined with one of long duration (bupivacaine). Most studies suggest that the aggregate result is a dilute solution (e.g., 20 mL of 3% 2-chloroprocaine and 20 mL of 0.5% bupivacaine becomes 40 mL of

Table 16–4. Altering Local Anesthetic pH With Bicarbonate

Local Anesthetic	Dose of Sodium Bicarbonate*	pH
Lidocaine	1 mL per 10 mL local anesthetic	7.2
Bupivacaine	0.1 mL per 10 mL local anesthetic	6.4

*Assumes initial concentration of NaHCO₃ is 8.4% (1 mEq/mL).

1.5% chloroprocaine with bupivacaine 0.25%) with few advantages and the potential for additive local anesthetic toxicity.

The risk of systemic local anesthetic toxicity can be minimized by an understanding of its mechanism. Peak blood levels of local anesthetics are determined by four factors: (1) the total dose (mg) of local anesthetic injected, (2) the site of injection, (3) the physicochemical properties of the drug, and (4) the addition of a vasoconstrictor. The higher the total dose of local anesthetic administered, the higher are the resultant peak blood levels. This follows nearly a linear relationship, and peak plasma concentration is reached approximately 20 minutes after injection via simple venous absorption. Different regional anesthetic techniques have variable vascular absorption, blood flow, and protein binding rates, which influence peak blood levels of local anesthetics (Table 16–5).

Regional anesthetic complications such as tourniquet failure during an intravenous regional anesthetic or intra-arterial injection into the vertebral artery during interscalene or cervical plexus blockade rapidly increases peak plasma levels, causing symptoms such as lightheadedness, visual disturbance, muscle twitching, and loss of consciousness in the former example, and grand mal seizure and coma in the latter.

Physicochemical properties such as lipid solubility and the degree of protein binding also influence peak plasma levels. Poorly lipid-soluble drugs such as mepivacaine have higher plasma concentrations than a lipid-soluble drug such as bupivacaine. With high concentration and mass of local anesthetic, the percentage of protein-binding decreases due to saturation of binding sites. When this occurs, peak plasma levels increase.

SEDATION

Intravenous sedation is an important component of both regional anesthesia and monitored anesthesia care. The desired level of sedation should be discussed with the patient, and patients should be reassured that supplemental medications will be available to keep them comfortable during the procedure. Only a minority of patients request no premedication so that they can watch their knee arthroscopy on a video monitor. Most patients prefer some type of premedication with additional sedation during the placement of a "painful" regional block. Despite skin infiltration with local anesthesia, most regional anesthetic blocks are accompanied by some element of discomfort, which, if minimized, improves the overall patient experience. Before performing the block, most patients benefit from receiving an anxiolytic such as midazolam (10–20 µg/kg) and a narcotic such as fentanyl (1–2µg/kg). During the actual procedure, additional sedation may be helpful and may include incremental doses of midazolam (0.5–1 mg), fentanyl (25 µg), or propofol (10–20 mg by bolus) or as an infusion (25 to 150 µg/kg/min). The pharmacology of these agents is reviewed in Chapter 15.

WHY REGIONAL ANESTHESIA? OUTCOME STUDIES

The argument for or against regional anesthetics for ambulatory surgery will be difficult to settle, because arguments can be made from both camps. For an anesthesiologist, a stable, well-executed epidural anesthetic is likely a better option than a general anesthetic for a middle-aged male smoker with heart disease. Despite the variety of short-acting agents such as propofol, midazolam, sevoflurane and desflurane, such patients may react in unpredictable ways to laryngoscopy and intubation or to placement of a laryngeal mask airway. On the other hand, from the surgical perspective, because every regional anesthetic takes more

Table 16–5. Regional Anesthetics and Peak Blood Levels of Local Anesthetics

Regional Anesthetic	Peak Blood Level of Local Anesthetic
Intercostal block	Highest
Paracervical block	
Caudal	
Epidural	
Intratracheal	
Brachial plexus	
Femoral/sciatic	Lowest

time from patient preparation to induction of surgical anesthesia, an extra 10 to 20 minutes per case may translate into an additional 1 to 2 hours of extra 'turnover time' by the end of a busy orthopedic surgical day. Therefore, examining outcome studies may provide a nonbiased perspective on this question. Three studies have looked at this.

Jones and coworkers studied the observation that elderly patients experience delayed recovery after surgery. They studied two groups of elderly patients—one having spinal anesthesia and the other a general anesthetic for knee or hip arthroplasty. They concluded that no anesthetic technique was superior with respect to morbidity and mortality and that the overall results of cognitive function testing revealed no long-term effect on mental function nor any clear benefit to either technique.

The other two studies examined the incidence of unanticipated hospital admission and major cardiopulmonary and cerebral morbidity following ambulatory surgery. Gold and colleagues studied 9616 ambulatory surgical patients, 1% of whom required unanticipated hospital admission. Of the 19 most common reasons for admission, the top six were a direct complication of general anesthesia, including pain, intractable vomiting, postoperative somnolence, aspiration pneumonia, bronchospasm, and airway obstruction, or were associated with these. After multivariate analysis, only four preoperative or intraoperative conditions were predictive for those patients requiring unanticipated admission: (1) the use of general anesthesia, (2) the occurrence of postoperative emesis, (3) laparoscopic or intra-abdominal surgery, and (4) surgical duration of more than 1 hour.

Warner and associates studied 30-day morbidity and mortality following 45,090 ambulatory surgical procedures. Thirty-three patients (0.07%) experienced major morbidity and four patients died (0.00004%) within 30 days of surgery. Of the morbid events, 71% occurred in patients who had received general anesthesia, 16% in those who received regional anesthesia, and 13% in those who had monitored anesthesia care (MAC). The surprising finding was the safety record of ambulatory surgery, particularly because 25% of these patients were classified as American Society of Anesthesiologists (ASA) physical status III patients.

REGIONAL ANESTHETIC BLOCKS AND THEIR APPLICATIONS—THE SURGICAL PERSPECTIVE. WHY SHOULD MY PATIENT HAVE A REGIONAL BLOCK?

Many different surgical procedures are performed in the ambulatory setting, and, for many of them, a regional technique may be an option either for the primary anesthetic or to provide secondary analgesia (in combination with a general anesthetic). Particularly with the introduction of 23-hour recovery room stays, regional anesthetic techniques may provide excellent analgesia and hasten discharge.

The subcutaneous and intramuscular infiltration of any surgical incision with local anesthetic improves the degree of analgesia experienced by the patient and should be a routine part of surgical practice. Even the simple instillation or washing of a surgical wound with local anesthetic may provide postoperative analgesia. Casey reported equivalent postoperative analgesia between two groups of pediatric patients having either local anesthetic wound instillation or ilioinguinal–iliohypogastric nerve blockade following inguinal herniorrhaphy. Wound instillation with 0.25 mL/kg of bupivacaine 0.25% for 2 minutes before closure of the muscle and skin layers provided equivalent analgesia to nerve blockade. Wound instillation has also been reported to improve the analgesia, reduce the opioid requirement, and decrease the respiratory complications following cholecystectomy.

Surgeons often assume the first line in the communication link with the patient regarding anesthetic options. The following discussion describes anesthetic options for all of the common ambulatory surgical procedures as divided into specialties.

General Surgical Procedures

Laparoscopy

Although general anesthesia is most commonly used for laparoscopy, it does necessitate some form of airway intervention such as endotracheal intubation or use of a laryngeal mask airway. For short duration (<1 hour) diagnostic laparoscopy, both *spinal and epidural anesthesia* are viable options, but a relatively high level of blockade (to T4) is required. With these high levels, patients may develop sympathetic nervous system blockade and secondary hypotension requiring use of a vasopressor. In addition, patients may complain of dyspnea from the abdominal distention of pneumoperitoneum or from blockade of sensory afferent fibers from the upper abdomen and chest wall. This can be treated with simple reassurance. Use of epidural narcotic (fentanyl, 50–100 μg, or sufentanil, 30 μg) or intrathecal narcotic (fentanyl, 10–25 μg, sufentanil 10–30 μg, or Duramorph, 0.25 mg) may improve the quality of the regional anesthetic and provide postoperative analgesia.

Cholecystectomy

Although regional anesthesia such as *combined celiac plexus and bilateral intercostal nerve blockade* have been used for open cholecystectomy, most of these procedures are performed with general anesthesia. For ambulatory patients, cholecystectomy is performed laparoscopically, and patients are discharged home after recovery stays of 4 to 23 hours. For a select group of these patients, *spinal, or more commonly, epidural anesthesia* may be an option. These patients must be motivated and often have a fear of "losing control," a history of a previous bad experience with or morbid fear of general anesthesia, or a history of malignant hyperthermia. Under deep epidural anesthesia with sedation, these patients may experience some crampy abdominal discomfort or shoulder pain.

Inguinal Herniorrhaphy

Regional anesthesia is an excellent option for herniorrhaphy because it avoids many of the deleterious aspects of emergence from general anesthesia and extubation (such as straining and coughing). Either *spinal or epidural anesthesia* is a possibility, although the postoperative recovery may be slightly prolonged with spinal anesthesia, and the risk of postdural puncture headache (PDPH) may be slightly higher. Spinal anesthesia differs from epidural anesthesia in several ways: (1) local anesthetic is injected directly into the CSF surrounding the nerve roots so onset of anesthesia is rapid (within minutes), (2) the ultimate extent of anesthesia may be difficult to predict, (3) patients may be at higher risk of PDPH, (4) hemodynamic changes occur more suddenly than with epidural anesthesia, and (5) autonomic blockade may be more profound. Another option would be *ilioinguinal–iliohypogastric neve blockade* with inguinal field infiltration. This block is a complete anesthetic, requires a brief PACU recovery period, and provides analgesia to allow the patient to return home feeling comfortable.

Perianal Surgery

Hemorrhoidectomy, rectal fissures and strictures, and perirectal abscesses are performed in either the lithotomy or prone jacknife position. For surgeons who prefer their patients in the prone position, an alternative to general anesthesia is desirable, because general anesthesia adds an element of complexity and risk regarding airway protection and positioning to avoid neural trauma. Two anesthetic options include *spinal and caudal anesthesia. Spinal anesthesia* has a quick onset and can be adapted to the surgical position desired. For example, in the lithotomy position, a hyperbaric spinal anesthesia may be placed while the patient sits on the OR table. Hyperbaric refers to the density of local anesthetic relative to that of CSF. Thus, hyperbaric solutions are prepared by mixing local anesthetic with 10% dextrose; these are "heavier" than CSF. Isobaric solutions are prepared by mixing local anesthetic with aspirated CSF; these solutions do not spread very far because they are the same density as CSF. Hypobaric solutions are prepared by mixing local anesthetic powder or solution with sterile water to create a solution that is "lighter" than CSF. In this case, the hyperbaric solution would sink and pool toward lower lumbar and sacral roots while the patient was in the sitting position, effectively creating perianal anesthesia with little cephalad spread.

For surgery in the prone jacknife position, a spinal needle can be placed in the position of surgery (patient prone, table flexed in slight Trendelenburg position). When a hypobaric spinal anesthetic is injected, it tends to "float upward" to the highest body position (in this case the buttocks), causing perirectal anesthesia. The only problem with placing spinal needles with the patient in the prone jacknife position is that it is difficult to flex and open the normal lumbar lordotic curve. For this reason, I prefer to place spinal needles via a lateral paramedian approach rather than midline for the prone jacknife position.

The addition of intrathecal narcotics (e.g., fentanyl, 10–25 μg, sufentanil, 10–30 μg, or Duramorph 0.25 mg) improves the quality and duration of spinal analgesia.

Caudal anesthesia is another possibility. In adults, the spinal cord extends to L1 or L2 and the dural sac extends to S2. A needle inserted via the sacral hiatus provides a very low epidural block. In young adults, the volume of local anesthetic injected (usually 15–25 mL) will fill the epidural space as well as the proximal nerve root sleeves. Thus, one does not usually get extensive cephalad spread of local anesthetic, and the risk of sympathetic nervous system blockade is low. On the other hand, in elderly patients, more extensive cephalad spread can occur, leading to sympathetic nervous system blockade. This is thought to occur because of connective tissue changes in elderly persons that limit lateral spread into the epidural space along the nerve roots. This can be avoided by decreasing the volume of local anesthetic, which is injected (using 8–15 mL), and by injecting smaller dose increments with longer time intervals between injections. Caudal anesthesia is less popular than spinal anesthesia because of its slower onset time (taking 12–20 minutes to set up for surgical anesthesia).

Intravenous Access Procedures

A variety of different central venous lines may be inserted to facilitate hemodialysis or to provide long-term venous access for chronic antibiotic administration or chemotherapy. Techniques vary in complexity from percutaneous insertion of Permacaths using Seldinger technique to surgical cutdowns and creation of subcutaneous tunnels for Hickman catheters, Portacaths, and Groshong catheters. Regional anesthetic options can include *simple skin infiltration* with intravenous sedation, placement of *superficial and deep cervical plexus blocks* (which provide a cape-like zone of anesthesia from the lateral neck, shoulder, and chest infraclavicularly to an area above the nipples), *intercostal nerve blockade, and thoracic epidural blockade.* The superficial cervical plexus block is risk free and easy to perform, whereas the deep cervical plexus block requires injection of local anesthetic at the transverse processes of C2, C3, and C4. Thus, the deep cervical plexus block may cause phrenic nerve blockade and carries a potential risk of intravascular injection (into the vertebral artery causing grand mal seizure) and central nervous system depression (via subdural root sleeve injection).

Simple Mastectomy and Lumpectomy

There are three regional anesthetic possibilities for breast surgery: *circummammary and retromammary field block, intercostal nerve blockade, and thoracic epidural anesthesia.* With concomitant sedation, they are all excellent regional anesthetic options. Thoracic epidural anesthesia may be the simplest option because it involves a single-needle insertion to permit the injection of local anesthetic or insertion of a catheter to permit injection of the same.

Intercostal nerve blockade of the third through sixth intercostal nerves requires four separate injections in the mid or posterior axillary line and carries the theoretical risk of pneumothorax.

Circummammary and retromammary field block requires the injection of 50 mL of dilute local anesthetic (e.g., lidocaine 1–2% with epinephrine 1:200,000) into the space between the breast and the pectoral muscles. It provides excellent anesthesia and hemostasis but involves minor discomfort during performance of the block. When using any of these regional blocks, it is important to provide space around the conscious patient's face to prevent causing a suffocating claustrophobic sensation once the drapes are applied. I often use an ether screen and oxygen insufflation with 6–10 L/min.

Pediatric Surgical Procedures

Regional anesthetics are commonly used in pediatric anesthesia, although they are most often applied as part of a combined technique with general anesthesia. Simple wound infiltration with local anesthesia can provide analgesia after surgery on any part of the body, although specific nerve blocks are most commonly used. Regional anesthesia can be used for upper or lower extremity, urologic, and lower abdominal surgery. These blocks may include blockade of the ilioinguinal, iliohypogastric, genitofemoral, and penile nerves; caudal or epidural anesthesia; and brachial or lumbosacral plexus blockade.

Circumcision

This procedure may be performed at any patient age and is usually done under anesthesia for all patients other than newborns. Three regional anesthetic options exist: *simple penile ring block, penile nerve block, and caudal anesthesia.* Concomitant general anesthesia is given (usually by inhalation induction with nitrous oxide-halothane or sevoflurane) and the block is applied after insertion of an intravenous catheter.

The penile ring block is simple and reliable. It involves the subcutaneous injection of local anesthetic around the base of the shaft of the penis. Any local anesthetic may be used, but bupivacaine 0.25% to 0.375% (1 cc for neonates, 2 cc for children, and 4 cc for adults) is most popular because of its long duration. Whichever local anesthetic is selected, it must not contain epinephrine because this could cause skin vasoconstriction and sloughing.

The penile nerve block is performed using a syringe with a 26 or 27-gauge needle. Two injections of local anesthetic (0.4 mL per dose for neonates, 1 mL per dose for children, and 2 mL per dose for adults) without epinephrine are made at the 10 o'clock and 2 o'clock positions on the base of the penis. The needles are aimed posteromedially and inserted 3 to 5 mm beneath the skin until entering Buck's fascia. After negative aspiration is obtained, the local anesthetic is injected. This block carries a risk of hematoma and intravascular injection.

Caudal anesthesia is usually performed in children younger than 6 years old. The patient is turned into the lateral decubitus position, standard landmarks are identified (the paired posterior superior iliac spines, the paired sacral cornua, and the tip of the coccyx), and the skin prepared with a topical antiseptic. There are several anatomic differences between the caudal space of children and adults—the subarachnoid space extends to S2–3 or S3–4, rather than S1–2 as it does in adults; thus the distance from the sacral hiatus to the subarachnoid space is only 2.5 cm in children. This increases the potential risk of subarachnoid puncture with subsequent spinal anesthesia. A 22-gauge 1.5- or 2.5-inch Quincke spinal needle or 16-, 18-, or 20-gauge intravenous catheter is advanced through the skin at the sacral hiatus at a 60° angle until the tip "pops" through the sacrococcygeal ligament and contacts the ventral surface of the sacrum. The needle is withdrawn slightly, the tip of the needle is directed more cranially, and the needle is advanced. After aspiration to confirm the absence of blood or CSF, bupivacaine 0.125% to 0.25% with or without epinephrine 1:200,000 is injected. Fentanyl, 1 μg/kg, may be added to the mixture to prolong postoperative analgesia. Local anesthetic test doses may be unreliable in pediatric patients due to the physiologic tachycardia that is common in young patients, although an intravascular injection of epinephrine may still cause a brief hypertensive response. Accepted caudal anesthetic dosing regimens are summarized in Table 16–6. The duration of caudal analgesia with bupivacaine averages 4 to 6 hours, with greater degrees of motor blockade accompanying the use of more concentrated local anesthetics. Young children may be discharged before complete resolution of motor and sensory blockade with instructions to protect the affected extremities. Urinary retention is rarely encountered in pediatric patients, but these children should be monitored and the surgeon or anesthesiologist notified if there has been a failure to void after 8 to 10 hours. Other complications include vomiting with an incidence of 11% to 70%, although this may be related to the concomitant nitrous oxide-halothane anesthetic commonly used in these published studies.

Table 16–6. Caudal Analgesia Regimens for Pediatric Anesthesia

Study	N	Surgery	Ages	Local Anesthetic	Dose	Duration	Complications
Bramwell (1982)	181	Circ Hernia Orch	1–12 yr	Bupivacaine 0.25%	0.5 mL/kg 1 mL/kg 1.25 mL/kg	1.5–4 hr	Vomiting, 18%
Markham (1986)	52	Hernia Orch	1–12 yr	Bupivacaine 0.5%	1 mL/yr + 2 mL	>6 hr	Vomiting, 11% Urine retention, 46% Unable to walk, 54%
Cross (1987)	41	Hernia Orch	1–13 yr	Bupivacaine 0.2%–0.25%	1–1.25 mL/kg	3–6 hr	Vomiting, 70% Pain-free at 6 hr, 50%
Hannallah (1987)	44	Orch	1–12 yr	Bupivacaine 0.25%	2.5 mL/yr		Vomiting, 45%

Circ = circumcision, Hernia = herniorrhaphy, Orch = orchidopexy.

Inguinal Herniorrhaphy

There are several regional anesthetic options for inguinal herniorrhaphy: *spinal, caudal, epidural, and ilioinguinal–iliohypogastric nerve block*, but only the latter two are commonly used. Caudal anesthesia has been previously described.

The *ilioinguinal–iliohypogastric nerve block* may be useful for inguinal herniorrhaphy, orchiectomy, and orchidopexy. These nerves provide sensation to the anterior lower abdominal wall. They can be blocked at the anterior superior iliac spine (ASIS) where they emerge from the internal oblique muscle and travel inferomedially between the internal and external oblique muscles. The iliohypogastric nerve provides sensory innervation to the skin over the lower part of the rectus abdominis muscle. The ilioinguinal nerve enters the spermatic cord and supplies the anterior one third of the scrotum, the root of the penis, and the upper and medial part of the groin. A needle can be inserted 1 cm medial to the ASIS and local anesthetic injected inferomedially and inferolaterally through the external oblique muscles. Typical dosing regimens are 0.5 to 2 mg/kg of bupivacaine 0.25%. Analgesia should persist for 4 to 12 hours. In adults, these blocks can be combined with blockade of the genitofemoral nerve and infiltration of the skin along the line of the incision to permit hernia surgery without the need for general anesthesia. As with caudal anesthesia in pediatric patients, the concomitant general anesthetic probably influences the complication rate. The incidence of vomiting varies from 11% to 66%, and transient femoral nerve blockade has been reported in 2% to 28% of cases.

Scrotal procedures such as orchiectomy, orchidopexy, and testicular torsion may be performed using *caudal anesthesia* or *ilioinguinal–iliohypogastric nerve blockade* with inguinal field block as the best regional options. These have been previously described.

Ventral or Umbilical Herniorrhaphy

Ventral or umbilical herniorrhaphy can be performed with *caudal anesthesia* for postoperative analgesia.

Extremity Surgery

Although spinal and epidural anesthesia can be performed in pediatric patients, most children still require concomitant general anesthesia, thus negating some of their advantages. The most common options for postoperative analgesia of the extremity include general anesthesia with *blockade of the brachial plexus or lumbar plexus, or combined femoral and sciatic nerve blocks*, depending on the site of surgery. Each of these techniques is best guided by use of a nerve stimulator. Advantages include prolonged postoperative analgesia, with the degree of motor blockade depending on the concentration of the local anesthetic.

For pediatric dosing of brachial plexus blocks, most authors recommend 0.5 mL/kg without exceeding the upper guidelines on a milligram per kilogram basis.

Lumbar plexus 3-in-1 blockade or fascia iliaca

block is useful for closed reduction of femur fractures, surface operations on the thigh (i.e., for wounds, skin grafts, abscesses), and orthopedic procedures. A 3-in-1 block is a technique in which a single injection of local anesthetic provides combined blockade of the femoral, lateral femoral cutaneous, and obturator nerves. To place a 3-in-1 block, the inguinal ligament is identified from the ASIS to the pubic tubercle. The junction of the femoral artery is marked with this line. A point is selected that is 0.5 to 1 cm below the inguinal ligament and lateral to the femoral artery. A 2.5 to 3.5-inch, 22-gauge needle is inserted in a cephalad direction with the needle angled 30° to the skin until a quadriceps contraction or femoral nerve paresthesia is elicited. Firm but gentle pressure is applied to the leg below the needle entry, and local anesthetic is injected according to the following regimen: 0.7 mL/kg for children weighing less than 20 kg, 15 mL for children weighing 20 to 30 kg, 20 mL for children weighing 30 to 40 kg, 25 mL for children weighing 40 to 50 kg, and 27.5 mL for children weighing more than 50 kg. Pressure on the leg during injection may force the local anesthetic more proximally toward the nerve roots. Many authors report that this is rarely a 3-in-1 block, but rather a 2-in-1 block, often missing the obturator or lateral femoral cutaneous nerve.

The *fascia iliaca block* is similar. After drawing a line from the ASIS to the pubic tubercle and dividing it into thirds, a point is marked that is 0.5 cm caudal to the spot where the lateral third joins the middle third. A 3.5-inch, 22-gauge needle attached to an air- or saline-filled syringe is advanced perpendicularly to the skin with gentle pressure on the plunger. A give and loss of resistance is felt as the needle traverses the fascia lata and a second give and loss of resistance is felt as the fascia iliaca is pierced. After negative aspiration and test dose, dosing of local anesthetic proceeds as described for 3-in-1 blocks with firm pressure maintained to the leg below the needle entry site.

For *femoral and sciatic nerve blocks*, pediatric dosing recommendations are 0.2 mL/kg for femoral nerve blocks and 0.3 mL/kg for sciatic nerve blocks using bupivacaine 0.5%.

Gynecologic Surgery

There are only two commonly used regional anesthetic techniques for ambulatory gynecologic surgery—*spinal and epidural anesthesia.* Common ambulatory gynecologic procedures include dilatation and curettage, dilatation and evacuation, cervical cone biopsy, laparoscopy, anterior and posterior repairs, and vaginal hysterectomy, the latter two sometimes done with patients having 23-hour PACU stays. For spinal anesthesia, the challenge is in performing the block with minimal risk of PDPH and delayed recovery. The use of small-gauge pencil-point needles such as 24 to 27-gauge Sprotte or Whitacre needles has reduced the risk of PDPH to less than 1% (Table 16–7). In addition, the use of spinal lidocaine in concentrations from 0.5% to 5% with the addition of intrathecal fentanyl can provide surgical anesthesia of up to 90 minutes duration with excellent postoperative analgesia and minimal recovery problems such as bladder dysfunction. Epidural anesthesia is well suited to procedures of uncertain duration if a catheter is inserted to allow top-off doses, and it has a lower incidence of PDPH. Compared with spinal anesthesia, however, it has a higher incidence of backache and requires a longer onset time to reach surgical anesthesia.

Orthopedic and Plastic Surgery

A variety of orthopedic procedures are performed in the ambulatory setting, and regional anesthesia is appropriate for many of them.

Hand Surgery

Hand surgery can be performed under *brachial plexus or intravenous regional anesthesia.* The deciding factor relates to the anticipated duration of the surgery and whether a surgeon will require the use of an occluding tourniquet or will need to examine nerve or muscle function immediately after the completion of surgery.

There is no block more appropriate for outpatient surgery than the *intravenous regional.* It is simple, has a rapid onset, and is short acting

Table 16–7. Spinal Anesthesia and Incidence of Postdural Puncture Headache

Study	N	Type of Needle	Gauge	PDPH (%)	Success (%)	Epidural Blood Patch (%)*	Patient Age (yr)
Dittman (1994)	2378	Quincke	29	1.2	98.3	0	10–101 (mean 33)
Liew (1994)	30			0	100	NA	
	15	Pencil point	26				
	15	Cutting	29				
Brattebo (1993)	133	Quincke	27	4	96	20	15–45
Hurley (1992)	4108	Quincke	26	5.2	NA	NA	NA
			27	2.5			
		Whitacre	25	1.1			
		Epidural	17	1.3			
Kang (1992)	730	Quincke		5.5	NA	36%	18–86
			26	9.6		39%	
			27	1.5		20%	
Ross (1992)	132	Sprotte	24	1.5	NA	0	NA
Quaynor (1990)	106	Quincke	26	7.5	100	0	18–70
Sarma (1990)	160	NA		9.4	NA	13	18–87
			25	18.2			
			26	4.8			
Thornberry (1988)	80	NA	25	40	NA	9.4	19–39
			26				

*Percentage of patients with PDPH who received epidural blood patch.
PDPH = postdural puncture headache.

and reliable, but it offers little in the way of postoperative analgesia. After exsanguination of the limb, an occluding tourniquet is inflated on the upper arm and local anesthetic is injected into a vein in the hand or wrist. The veins become distended with a dilute solution of local anesthetic, which diffuses out to block the small nerves and nerve endings. Anesthesia begins immediately, and surgery may follow. Once the local anesthetic is injected, the tourniquet must stay inflated for at least 20 minutes to minimize the risk of systemic local anesthetic toxicity. If the tourniquet must be deflated before 45 minutes has passed, a two-stage deflation may be used, wherein the cuff is deflated for 5 to 10 seconds, then reinflated for 1 minute, before final release of the tourniquet. This technique allows a slower wash-out of local anesthetic and lower peak blood levels.

Brachial plexus anesthesia is an excellent choice for hand surgery because it provides postoperative analgesia, although the prolonged sensory and motor blockade may necessitate that these patients be discharged with their arm in a padded sling until recovery of neurologic function. There are three approaches to the plexus—interscalene, supraclavicular, and axillary—depending on the desired level of upper extremity blockade. A nerve stimulator or paresthesia technique may be used to localize the nerves. The *axillary approach* is used for procedures on the hand, wrist, and lower arm. At this level, it blocks the individual nerves. The *supraclavicular approach* provides anesthesia for the entire plexus (at the level of the nerve trunks) and is useful for surgery on the hand, wrist, and elbow. There is a risk of pneumothorax with this technique. The *interscalene approach* is useful for upper arm and shoulder surgery because it blocks both the cervical and brachial plexus at the nerve root level. The ulnar nerve is often spared with this technique, and it carries a risk of phrenic nerve blockade and diaphragmatic dysfunction.

Motor function and adequacy of brachial plexus blockade can be tested by checking the following functions:

- Flexion at the elbow—musculocutaneous nerve
- Thumb opposition—median nerve
- Finger abduction—ulnar nerve
- Wrist and elbow extension—radial nerve

The axillary approach is the one block most commonly used for hand surgery, although the supraclavicular approach may also be appropriate. The musculocutaneous and median nerves lie superior to the axillary artery and the ulnar and radial nerves lie inferior to it. Upon localization of the brachial plexus using a nerve stimulator or presence of a paresthesia, 40 mL of local anesthetic is injected in divided doses after negative aspiration is obtained.

Alternatively, the needle may be advanced until it punctures the axillary artery and, while aspirating on the syringe, it is advanced posteriorly until it passes through the posterior wall. Twenty milliliters of local anesthetic is injected posterior to the artery, and the needle is withdrawn, again with constant aspiration until it is anterior to the artery. An additional 20 mL of local anesthetic is injected there as well. The axillary artery transfixation technique may be relatively contraindicated in patients with severe atherosclerotic vascular disease.

The musculocutaneous nerve provides sensation to the forearm and is often missed with the axillary approach. This can be blocked by injecting 5 to 10 mL of local anesthetic into the body of the coracobrachialis muscle, superior to the axillary artery and lateral to the border of the pectoralis muscle. If a tourniquet is to be used, the intercostobrachialis nerve should also be blocked by injecting 5–10 mL of local anesthetic subcutaneously in a circumferential ring around the arm in a line parallel to the axillary skin crease.

For the supraclavicular approach, the midpoint of the clavicle is identified and a 1.5 inch, 23-gauge needle is advanced caudally in the supraclavicular fossa toward the first rib. A paresthesia technique or nerve stimulator may be used. If the rib is contacted, the needle should be "walked off" posteriorly or laterally. Any medial direction of the needle risks apical lung puncture and pneumothorax. Twenty-five to 40 mL of local anesthetic is injected once the needle is in the proper location. If a tourniquet is to be used, blockade of the intercostobrachial nerve may be required. For patchy blocks, the individual nerves—radial, median, and ulnar—can be blocked individually at the elbow or at the wrist to complete the anesthetic.

Foot Surgery

There are five regional anesthetic options available for foot surgery: *spinal, epidural, com-* *bined femoral and sciatic, ankle blockade, and intravenous regional.* Spinal and epidural have been previously described.

Combined femoral and sciatic nerve blockade are useful for operations on the lower extremity. The femoral artery pulse and inguinal ligament are identified. The femoral nerve lies lateral to the femoral artery and may be localized by using a nerve stimulator or seeking a paresthesia and infiltrating 15 to 20 mL of local anesthetic lateral to the arterial pulsation. The femoral nerve may also be blocked at the knee (the saphenous nerve) for operations on the foot, ankle, and lower leg. The medial tibial condyle and gastrocnemius muscle are identified and 10 mL of local anesthetic is infiltrated subcutaneously and to the bone to provide anesthesia over the medial aspect of the foot and lower extremity.

There are two common approaches to *sciatic nerve blockade* at the hip—the classic posterior approach and lithotomy variations.

For the classic posterior approach, the patient is placed in the Sims' position (lateral decubitus with the leg to be blocked uppermost and flexed at the hip and knee) and the greater trochanter of the femur and posterosuperior iliac spine (PSIS) are identified. A straight line is drawn to connect them and, at the midpoint, a perpendicular line is dropped 4 cm. This point overlies the sciatic nerve as it emerges from the sciatic foramen. A 3.5 inch, 22-gauge needle is inserted perpendicular to the skin and is connected to a nerve stimulator set to 2.5 mA. The needle is advanced until it strikes bone, where it is then redirected, or until a motor contraction is noted in the sciatic distribution (e.g., foot dorsiflexion or plantar flexion, contraction of the hamstring or gastrocnemius muscle, paresthesia in the leg or foot). Forty milliliters of local anesthetic is then injected.

For the lithotomy approach, the patient is placed supine and the leg to be blocked is flexed at the hip and placed in stirrups or held by an assistant. The greater trochanter and ischial tuberosity are identified and a line is drawn between these two points. At the midpoint along this line, a 3.5-inch, 22-gauge needle attached to a nerve stimulator is inserted perpendicular to the skin and the needle advanced until a motor contraction is noted in the sciatic distribution. Thirty to 40 mL of local anesthetic is injected in divided doses after a negative test dose is obtained.

The sciatic nerve can also be blocked at the knee for operations on the foot and lower leg. The patient is placed in the prone position and the knee is flexed to 30° to define the borders of the popliteal fossa. The following landmarks are identified: the knee crease inferiorly, the biceps femoris laterally, and the semimembranosus and semitendinosus tendons medially. A vertical line is drawn inferiorly along the femur until it bisects the knee crease. A 2.5-inch, 22-gauge needle is inserted at a point 6 cm above the knee crease and 1 cm lateral to the midline. A nerve stimulator is used to localize the nerve. Twenty to 30 mL of local anesthetic is injected in divided doses.

The *ankle block* is useful for foot or toe surgery. The five nerves supplying the foot are terminal branches of the two main nerves innervating the leg—the femoral and sciatic nerves. They are easily blocked at the ankle and do not require identification with a paresthesia or use of a nerve stimulator. The deep peroneal nerve is located lateral to the dorsalis pedis artery and between the extensor hallucis longus tendon (identified by extension of the great toe) and the anterior tibialis tendon (identified by dorsiflexion of the foot). A 1.5-inch, 22-gauge needle is inserted between the tendons until contacting bone. The needle is withdrawn slightly, and 5 to 10 mL of local anesthetic is injected.

The superficial peroneal nerve is blocked by injecting a subcutaneous wheal of local anesthetic from the skin insertion point for the deep peroneal nerve block lateral to the lateral malleolus (5 mL is usually sufficient). The saphenous nerve is blocked in similar fashion by extending the subcutaneous wheal medially toward the medial malleolus with 5 mL of local anesthetic. The sural nerve is blocked by inserting the needle midway between the lateral malleolus and the Achilles tendon until contacting bone. The needle is withdrawn slightly and 5 mL of local anesthetic is injected in a fan pattern. The posterior tibial nerve is located posterior to the posterior tibial artery pulse and behind the medial malleolus. Five to 10 mL of local anesthetic is injected in a fan-shaped pattern, and some patients may report a paresthesia to the sole of their foot.

Intravenous regional anesthesia of the lower extremity may be used for operations on the toes, foot, ankle, and lower leg. The technique is similar to that for intravenous regional blocks of the upper extremity; however, systemic local anesthetic toxicity is a greater risk for this block due to the larger volume (50–100 mL) of local anesthetic injected and the conical shape of the thigh, which may hinder tourniquet occlusion. As with intravenous regional blocks of the upper extremity, this block is time limited to surgery of less than 90 minutes to prevent ischemia and tourniquet pain.

Arthroscopy

Arthroscopy is commonly performed on the knee, ankle, elbow, and shoulder and is amenable to many forms of regional anesthesia. For knee arthroscopy, *spinal, epidural, and lumbar plexus anesthesia* are all appropriate and have been described. For ankle arthroscopy, *spinal, epidural, intravenous regional, and femoral and sciatic nerve blocks* are all options. For elbow arthroscopy, *brachial plexus blockade* using the interscalene or supraclavicular approach is a potential option.

For shoulder arthroscopy, the *interscalene approach to the brachial plexus* is the best choice. The ipsilateral sternocleidomastoid muscle is identified, as are the anterior and middle scalene muscles. The groove between the anterior and middle scalene muscles is marked at a point where it overlies the transverse process of C6 (Chaissagnac's tubercle at the level of the cricoid cartilage). A paresthesia technique or nerve stimulator may be used. After careful aspiration to detect intravascular or subdural root sleeve placement, a 1-mL test dose is injected, followed by the remainder of 30 to 40 mL in divided doses. Potential complications for this block include pneumothorax, cervical epidural or central nervous system anesthesia, recurrent laryngeal nerve blockade, grand mal seizure from vertebral artery injection, and phrenic nerve blockade.

Urologic Surgery

Many urologic procedures are performed in the ambulatory setting, including cystoscopy, ureteral stent placement, circumcision, inguinal herniorrhaphy, and scrotal procedures such as orchiectomy and orchidopexy. As previously discussed, *spinal and epidural anesthesia* may be appropriate options. When performing regional anesthesia for cystoscopy, a T10 level is desired. When cystoscopy is combined with a ureteral procedure such as stent placement or retrograde injection, a higher level of anesthesia to T4 is desired. Other options for urologic surgery include *penile ring blocks, penile nerve blocks, caudal anesthesia, and ilioinguinal–iliohypogastric nerve blockade.*

Ophthalmologic Surgery

Cataract extractions and lens implantations are frequently performed in the ambulatory setting. Two regional anesthetics are appropriate for this type of surgery: *the retrobulbar and peribulbar blocks.* The retrobulbar block requires facial nerve blockade to provide periorbital sensory block and motor blockade of the eyelid, while the retrobulbar block anesthetizes the sensory and motor nerves of the posterior orbit. There are a number of potential complications with this block. Among them are hematoma, systemic local anesthetic toxicity, globe perforation, retrobulbar hemorrhage, bradydysrhythmias, optic nerve trauma, and central nervous system anesthesia from subdural spread. For these reasons, the peribulbar block was developed; it involves the injection of local anesthetic outside the muscular cone of the extraocular muscles, from which it diffuses much more slowly than the retrobulbar block, thus having a slower onset of surgical anesthesia. Peribulbar block complications include intravascular injection, globe perforation, and bradydysrhythmias. These blocks are not useful for extraocular muscle repair.

PATIENT FOLLOW-UP AND QUALITY ASSURANCE

The standard of anesthetic care necessitates that a postoperative visit be made for every patient recovering from an anesthetic. With the increasing popularity of ambulatory sur-

gery, this becomes difficult. Thus, a follow-up telephone call should be made to every patient on the day after surgery to inquire about specific anesthetic issues such as nausea, vomiting, adequacy of analgesia, duration of a peripheral nerve block, and dental or lip injury. If the patient is not home, simply leaving a telephone message with a telephone number where someone may be reached gives the patient the peace of mind that someone is available. Every patient who has a subsequent unanticipated hospital admission should be seen.

Upon discharge from the ambulatory surgery center, each patient should receive a card containing telephone contact numbers for both the surgeon and the anesthesiologist. In addition, some centers have a problem sheet that may be sent home with the patient describing any unanticipated or perioperative problem that occurred, particularly those that might impact on future surgical care. Examples might include details about a suspected adverse drug reaction or intraoperative problem such as difficult intravenous access, difficult intubation, cardiac dysrhythmia, bronchospasm, or laryngospasm.

Finally, quality assurance data should be compiled and discussed at departmental conferences to better understand infrequent but expensive problems such as inadequate analgesia, delayed recovery room discharge, persistent nausea and vomiting, urinary retention, PDPH, and subsequent unanticipated hospital admission, because some of these may necessitate that a change be made in the anesthetic technique or medications that are used for therapy, and others may be due to a system-based problem.

Selected Readings

1. Arthur DS, McNichol LR. Local anaesthetic techniques in paediatric surgery. Br J Anaesth 1986; 58:760–778.
2. Davis WJ, Lennon RL, Wedel DJ. Brachial plexus anesthesia for outpatient surgical procedures on an upper extremity. Mayo Clin Proc 1991;66:470–473.
3. Dittmann M, Schaeffer HG, Renkel F, et al. Spinal anaesthesia with 29 guage Quincke point needles and post dural puncture headache in 2,378 patients. Acta Anaesthesiol Scand 1994;38:691–693.
4. Gold BS, Kitz DS, Lecky JH, et al. Unanticipated admission to the hospital following ambulatory surgery. JAMA 1989;262(21):3008–3010.
5. Jones MJT, Piggott SE, Vaughan RS, et al. Cognitive

and functional competence after anaesthesia in patients aged over 60: controlled trial of general and regional anaesthesia for elective hip or knee replacement. BMJ 1990;300:1683–1687.

6. Mulroy MF. Regional Anesthesia: An Illustrated Procedural Guide. Boston: Little, Brown, 1989.

7. Mulroy MF. Regional anesthetic techniques in: White PF, ed. Anesthesia for Ambulatory Surgery. International Anesthesiology Clinics. Vol. 32(3). Boston: Little, Brown, 1994.

8. Raj PP. Clinical Practice of Regional Anesthesia. New York: Churchill Livingstone, 1991.

9. Scott DB. Techniques of Regional Anaesthesia. Norwalk, CT: Appleton & Lange/Mediglobe, 1989.

10. Selzer JL. Is regional anesthesia preferable to general anesthesia for outpatient surgical procedures on an upper extremity? (Editorial). Mayo Clin Proc 1991;66:544–547.

11. Warner MA, Shields SE, Chute CG. Major morbidity and mortality within 1 month of ambulatory surgery and anesthesia. JAMA 1993;270(12):1437–1441.

12. Casey WF, Rice LJ, Hannallah RS, et al. A comparison between bupivacaine instillation versus ilioinguinal/iliohypogastric nerve block for postoperative analgesia in children. Anesthesiology 1990;72:637–639.

13. Thornberry EA, Thomas TA. Posture and postspinal headache. Br J Anaesth 1988;60:195–197.

14. Bösenberg AT. Lower limb nerve blocks in children using unsheathed needles and a nerve stimulator. Anaesthesia 1995;50:206–210.

17

Managing the Pediatric Outpatient

Terrance A. Yemen

More than 55% of pediatric surgeries at the University of Virginia Medical Center are performed on outpatients. For the past 5 to 10 years, numerous changes have occurred in this medical field. Ambulatory surgery has become increasingly complex, the patient's medical conditions are increasingly severe, and age limits suitable for outpatient anesthesia have evolved to include even the neonate. This chapter reviews the changes that have occurred over the past 10 years in pediatric anesthesia and provides an update regarding the preoperative selection, preparation, intraoperative management, and postoperative care of the pediatric outpatient.

SELECTION OF PEDIATRIC PATIENTS

Basic Considerations

In general, the purpose of ambulatory care is to decrease the costs of anesthesia and surgery and to increase patient convenience and satisfaction while maintaining the same standard of care and outcome afforded to inpatients. This goal cannot be obtained without carefully selecting suitable children for pediatric outpatient surgery. The decision to schedule a child for outpatient surgery should encompass three fundamental premises: (1) the medical condition of a child should not require extensive evaluation or preoperative admission, (2) the surgery planned should not worsen the medical condition of the child, and (3) the care provided should not result in a prolonged or complicated postoperative stay.

These premises are closely interrelated and cannot be separated, but, as a whole, they allow appropriate selections to be made. For example, a child with severe cystic fibrosis is a suitable candidate for ambulatory surgery if the nature of the surgery does not significantly alter the child's condition or require extensive postoperative management. If such a child is scheduled for a myringotomy or an inguinal hernia repair, ambulatory surgery may be appropriate despite the severe medical condition of the patient. Neither surgery has significant impact on the medical condition of this child, and postoperative care should be uncomplicated.

On the other hand, healthy children scheduled for extensive surgical procedures are often unsuitable outpatients because these operations have significant physiologic consequences. An example of the aforementioned is a healthy child scheduled for a femoral osteotomy. Although the surgical procedure can be accomplished in an outpatient setting, these children have considerable postoperative pain that cannot be managed by oral medications alone. These cases are best treated in an inpatient setting where other pain modalities are available. The selection of patients must, therefore, consider the whole picture and not just the type of surgery or the medical condition of the child.

Although the duration of anesthesia and surgery has often been considered a factor in the decision to perform outpatient surgery, the length of anesthesia is a poor indicator. The length of surgery and anesthesia has only minimal impact on the ability of the patient to be ready for discharge by the day's end.

Improved anesthetic delivery techniques and anesthetic agents allow anesthesia to be delivered over several hours without an accumulation of anesthetic effect. There is no evidence to support beliefs that children anesthetized for 1 hour have a better outcome than those anesthetized for 2 or 3 hours. For example, a child may be scheduled for bilateral otoplasties. This surgery often lasts more than 2 hours, but the surgery has little impact on the medical condition of the child, and the postoperative pain is easily managed with oral medications. The type of surgery and the medical condition of the patient are more important than the time it takes to perform the surgery. If a child's surgery is scheduled to last for 2 or 3 hours, it should be scheduled as one of the first cases in the morning. This allows adequate time after the surgery is completed for the child to recover and to make appropriate adjustments. By the time the ambulatory unit is ready to close, these children have been safely discharged home.

Preoperative Investigations

Patients scheduled for pediatric ambulatory surgery should not require an extensive preoperative clinical workup. The need for a comprehensive preoperative evaluation on the day of surgery results in considerable delays in the operative schedule. The reasons for the delays are logistical. Substantial coordination is required to ensure that children with complex or multiple illnesses have the appropriate examinations completed. This information, along with any necessary laboratory values, must then be received and interpreted before an appropriate decision can be made regarding the patient's suitability for outpatient surgery. Occasionally, further investigations are warranted. The failure to notify the anesthesiologist about clinically important anomalies in the preoperative workup commonly leads to cancelation of surgery just before the scheduled time of the surgery. The end result is confusion in the operating room schedule.

In the 1990s, freestanding ambulatory surgical units have become popular. Most freestanding clinics lack the necessary laboratory facilities to provide chemical or hematologic assays beyond a simple spun hematocrit or blood glucose level. In most cases, laboratory specimens must be sent to another institution and analyzed. The resultant values must then be transferred back to the freestanding unit before a decision to proceed with surgery can be made. This often produces significant delays and confusion. Therefore, those children who require laboratory investigations beyond measuring glucose or hemoglobin level should have this work done at the time the surgery is originally contemplated. These values are then available to an anesthesiologist before the day of surgery and appropriate decisions can be made regarding the patient's suitability for ambulatory surgery. Such a system avoids unnecessary cancelations on the day of surgery. Physicians should also consider that children who require extensive and complicated preoperative laboratory tests often require the same tests intraoperatively or postoperatively.

In contrast to the aforementioned problems, some children with significant medical conditions (for example, chronic renal failure) may be appropriately scheduled for ambulatory surgery. Hemoglobin and serum electrolyte values can be measured before surgery. If these values are acceptable, the child may undergo a minor surgical procedure on the following day.

All ambulatory surgical centers should be capable of measuring hemoglobin levels. There is always the possibility of blood loss, and all ambulatory units, freestanding or otherwise, must be able to assess blood loss. This is particularly true for institutions scheduling tonsillectomies, functional endoscopic sinus surgery, and orthopedic surgery involving osteotomies. Such children may suffer either intraoperative or postoperative blood loss requiring an assessment of anemia.

It is also essential that ambulatory centers be able to monitor glucose values in children who are diabetic or in young infants in whom the risk of hypoglycemia must be considered, especially after a prolonged fast. Glucose levels are easily monitored using a variety of glucometers available commercially.

The need for a routine preoperative laboratory workup in healthy pediatric patients has caused considerable debate over the past 10 years. In the 1980s, most centers required that children have, as a minimum, a hemoglobin level and a urinalysis. However, by the end of the decade, many investigators questioned the validity and necessity of such testing and studies investigating this issue were conducted.

Two such studies were done in large pediatric centers and demonstrated concurring results. In both studies, healthy children scheduled for outpatient surgery had hemoglobin levels measured. All the children studied received care that was independent from the preoperative knowledge of the value. Children who were anemic had hemoglobin levels so marginally below the normal age-related values that they had no effect on either the anesthetic or surgical care. The investigators concluded that preoperative hemoglobin measurements in otherwise healthy children did nothing to alter their outcome after surgery. They recommended that routine hemoglobin measurements should not be required for healthy children but should be required when preoperative knowledge of the extent of the anemia would change the care of the patient.

At the University of Virginia, the aforementioned recommendations have been followed over the past 5 years and routine laboratory investigation is not ordered for otherwise healthy children. In children with preexisting medical conditions, the attending surgeon orders the laboratory investigations that are appropriate for the safe conduct of anesthesia and surgery before the day of surgery. If surgeons are unsure which values the anesthesiologist needs for the planned surgery, they should communicate their concerns to the anesthesiologist in advance so that a consensus can be reached as to which investigations are appropriate. The elimination of routine laboratory workup in healthy children has not affected the outcome of care. This policy has achieved a true cost saving and reduced some suffering endured by children during venopuncture for unnecessary tests.

Preexisting Medical Conditions

Although there have been many changes in the past decade regarding the appropriate selection of pediatric outpatients, three preexisting medical conditions that affect the anes-

thesiologist in particular are discussed in this chapter. Children with such conditions are (1) the ex-premature infant, (2) the child with a cold, and (3) the child with a history of malignant hyperthermia.

The year 1982 marked the first publication of literature identifying premature infants as more prone to complications after minor surgery than are full-term infants. In particular, premature infants were noted to have life-threatening apnea while recovering from general anesthesia. This finding was supported by subsequent studies and, over the ensuing years, investigations were conducted to answer a number of question: Why do these children have apnea after anesthesia? What is the risk of apnea after anesthesia? How can this complication be prevented? Further studies demonstrated that, in addition to premature infants, ex-premature infants are also at risk of apnea after general anesthesia, necessitating a general consensus regarding the gestational ages at which infants are at risk of postoperative apnea. None was reached, but, by the end of the 1980s, many institutions accepted that premature infants up to 60 weeks' gestational age were at risk of life-threatening apnea after general anesthesia.

In addition to the studies involving premature and ex-premature infants, a variety of case reports appeared, illustrating that full-term infants younger than 44 weeks' postconceptual age at the time of surgery can also have life-threatening apnea after general anesthesia. These reports strengthened the resolve to more clearly define the risk of apnea in infants after general anesthesia.

At the Hospital for Sick Children in Toronto, a study was conducted to define the risk of apnea after general anesthesia in premature and ex-premature infants. In this large, well-conducted prospective study, it was shown that the risk of apnea after general anesthesia in infants is approximately 5% in children younger than 44 weeks' gestation. In this same study, there were no children with apnea who were older than 44 weeks' gestation. Most recently, the data from all previously published papers submitted by several pediatric institutions were combined and analyzed to provide a more accurate analysis as to which infants are truly at risk of postoperative apnea. The results of this most recent paper suggest that the risk of postoperative apnea is increased significantly in children who are premature and decreases substantially in those greater than 44 weeks' gestation. The exact gestational age at which infants are not at risk of postoperative apnea can still not be accurately defined; it can only be predicted that the probability of postoperative apnea appears to be 1%, or less, for healthy ex-premature infants greater than 50 weeks' gestational age at the time of surgery.

The exact nature and cause of this apnea after anesthesia is also an enigma. Most experts think that there is an immaturity in the regulatory centers of respiration. However, gestational age is not the sole risk factor. The general health of the child and the anesthetic technique must also be considered.

Investigators have studied the influence of anesthetic agents and techniques on the risk of postoperative apnea. Controlled, prospective studies have demonstrated that the choice of general anesthetic agents has only moderate influence over the incidence of apnea, with apnea occurring following the use of all sedative and anesthetic drugs. However, several studies have demonstrated that infants who receive spinal anesthesia, unsupplemented by intravenous sedative agents, do not have apnea postoperatively.

Studies have also been conducted to look at the correlation of anemia and postoperative life-threatening apnea. The findings have been equivocal, with some studies showing a direct correlation and others showing no correlation. Much debate still exists as to why life-threatening apnea should occur after general anesthesia and, until regulatory mechanisms of respiration in premature infants are fully understood, complete understanding of the problem is unlikely.

At the University of Virginia Medical Center, an outpatient policy regarding premature, ex-premature, and full-term infants has been implemented based on the preceding information. Currently, only full-term infants who are 4 weeks old and 44 weeks' postconceptual age at the time of their ambulatory surgery are accepted. In regard to ex-premature infants, only infants who are at least 46 weeks' gestational age at the time of surgery are accepted.

Additionally, they must not be receiving treatment for or monitoring of apnea at home. Some centers take a more conservative viewpoint, requiring ex-premature infants to be at least 60 weeks' gestational age at the time of surgery and off all monitoring and therapy for apnea. This position is ultraconservative and not supported by any of the studies conducted in the past decade.

The child with a cold presents perplexing problems for the anesthesiologist, pediatrician, and surgeon. The process of deciding whether a child with a cold is suitable for anesthesia often involves more emotion than scientific fact.

Studies involving children with respiratory tract infections having general anesthesia are scattered throughout the medical literature. None of the studies conducted in the past 10 years was well controlled. In all investigations, preselection of patients was made before study enrollment, with those children who had obvious signs of a lower respiratory tract infection being excluded from the study. As such, a bias was introduced into these studies before they even began. Even so, these same studies have demonstrated general agreement in their findings: children with upper respiratory tract infections are more prone to minor complications and intraoperative respiratory events than are children without such an infection. Hypoxic events resulting from laryngospasm or bronchospasm were found to be more common in children with upper respiratory tract infections. These complications were observed in both operating and recovery rooms. Life-threatening hypoxic events resulting from upper respiratory tract infections did not result in an increased incidence of unplanned hospital admissions. Studies examining the outcome of children with significant lower respiratory tract infections are not available. The management of these children remains questionable.

A straightforward approach to the child with a cold is to first distinguish allergic and vasomotor rhinitis from infective respiratory disorders. Second, upper respiratory infections are distinguished from lower respiratory tract infections by determining the child's baseline, whether there is nasal discharge, whether the child is febrile or there is other evidence of systemic infection, whether there is a productive, croupy cough, and whether rhonchi are audible. In general, surgery is only canceled when the child has a productive cough, croup, rhonchi, or a fever greater than 38.5°C.

Parents of children with colds should be included in the decision-making process as to whether to proceed with the surgery or to reschedule. Parents of a child with an upper respiratory tract infection should be comfortable in proceeding with the surgery after receiving a full explanation of the risks involved and the possible outcome. If the parents are unhappy with the prospect of any increased risk of anesthesia and surgery, then they may reschedule the procedure. This gives the parents an opportunity to participate in their child's care, particularly when there are difficulties in presenting the child for surgery. Some parents travel several hours to arrive at an ambulatory surgical center. Many parents take time off from work. Many children have chronic ear infections and constantly have one infection after another, enduring a runny nose most of the time. These children's procedures are often canceled, only to be rescheduled a few weeks later when the child has yet another runny nose and cough. Therefore, the decision to proceed with the anesthesia and surgery is a balance of the past history of the child, the child's current condition, and the opinion of the parents at the time of surgery. This allows safe and rational care for children with a cold without unnecessarily canceling those children who probably do not benefit from rescheduling.

Malignant hyperthermia is a rare but lethal disorder that appears uniquely related to anesthesia. This hypermetabolic disorder occurs in less than 1:10,000 applications of anesthetics, more commonly in children than adults. It is characterized by a hypermetabolic state involving all tissues but most notably striated muscle. Clinically, metabolic hyperthermia can manifest in a variety of manners but the classic presentation is rapidly progressive muscle rigidity, mottled skin, cardiac dysrhythmias, hyperthermia, hyperkalemia, and myoglobinuria, all of which lead to death unless recognized and treated quickly.

In the past, children with a personal or familial history of malignant hyperthermia were seen only as inpatients; however, these patients may be suitable for outpatient surgery. The volatile anesthetics and succinylcholine are the only proven provocative agents of malignant hyperthermia in humans, so it may be possible for a "malignant hyperthermia safe" anesthetic to be given in the outpatient setting. Recent investigational studies have been conducted to investigate this possibility.

In a large study of patients at risk of malignant hyperthermia in Canada, children of all ages were given such safe anesthetics and monitored for evidence of malignant hyperthermia. None of the children were given dantrolene prophylaxis. Episodes or events related to the development of malignant hyperthermia intraoperatively or postoperatively did not occur. The data in this study support the conviction of many anesthesiologists: that is, given appropriate anesthetic drugs, malignant hyperthermia patients can be safely anesthetized. Malignant hyperthermia did not occur postoperatively after these uneventful anesthetics, which is important because the objective is to send the children home shortly after recovering from their anesthetic. Concern that these children might require monitoring for malignant hyperthermia postoperatively appears unfounded, although the size of related studies makes broad and sweeping conclusions unrealistic.

At the University of Virginia ambulatory center, outpatient anesthesia is provided for patients at risk of malignant hyperthermia. This is based on the University of Virginia experience and that of others, combined with published studies addressing this issue. Dantrolene and the necessary equipment to monitor and treat a malignant hyperthermia episode is available at all times. If the children have an uneventful stay in the operating and recovery rooms, they are sent home. The parents of these children are given specific instructions to call or come back to the hospital if any of the described signs of malignant hyperthermia appear the next day.

PREOPERATIVE PREPARATION

Orders to give children nothing by mouth (NPO) have been wildly debated in the past and remain a source of heated discussion in surgical centers. Over the past few years, a general consensus has been reached (at least in the anesthesia literature) that fasting times should be adjusted according to the age of the child. There is no demonstrated advantage in keeping newborns to children 2 years of age NPO for more than 2 to 3 hours or in keeping children older than 2 years of age NPO for more than 4 to 6 hours. Extending NPO times past these limits results in greater discomfort to the child, annoyance to the parents, and an increase in the incidence of hypoglycemia, headache, and dehydration. Dehydration results in difficult intravenous access and an increased incidence of hypotension upon induction of anesthesia.

At the University of Virginia, parents are encouraged to use the following NPO guidelines: offer infants and toddlers clear fluids 2 to 3 hours before their scheduled surgery time, even if the child must be awakened; maintain an NPO period of 4 hours in children older than 2 years of age (breast milk is not considered a clear fluid; it contains considerable fat, activating the digestive process and resulting in increased gastric acid); and do not feed children after midnight, regardless of what time the surgery is scheduled.

These moderated NPO guidelines work well as long as the time of surgery does not change extensively. If children are scheduled for surgery in the midafternoon and are subsequently rescheduled for noon, they will not have been NPO for the appropriate amount of time. Children should be scheduled as the first cases in the morning. Infants should be scheduled first and the older children afterward. This arrangement still allows some flexibility in the schedule later in the day.

In addition to the physiologic challenge that pediatric patients present for anesthesia, they are also psychologically challenging. Although children represent a wide spectrum of psychological development, basically they can be divided into three psychological categories: (1) the dependent years between infancy and 2 years of age, (2) the so-called "golden years" between 2 and 5 years of age, and (3) the period of reasoning from age 5 years through adolescence. Each of these developmental stages carries its own unique psychological needs. Surgical centers providing care for pediatric patients need to be able to provide for the needs of each stage of development.

To make a child calm and cooperative requires: (1) adequate preoperative psychological preparation for the parents and the child, (2) empathetic and understanding preoperative nursing, (3) the appropriate use of preoperative medications when necessary, and (4) the skills of an anesthesiologist comfortable with children.

Many ambulatory centers allow both the parents and children to visit the center and become oriented to its routine before the day of surgery. This is particularly useful for children between the ages of 4 and 12 years. However, many toddlers and a few older children simply cannot be "talked through" the preoperative preparation and induction. A preoperative medication is appropriate in this situation.

The ideal premedication for outpatient pediatric anesthesia would be simple to administer and would take effect in just a few minutes. It would cause minimal cardiac and respiratory depression. It would not require special monitoring or nursing care. It would not cause nausea or delay discharge. The ideal premedicant has not been discovered, but improvements in existing medications have been made.

Substantial improvements have been made with oral premedication in particular. Oral midazolam is both effective and safe in healthy children. A dose of 0.5 mg/kg has an onset of action in approximately 20 minutes and is effective for approximately 30 to 45 minutes. Midazolam itself is unpalatable and, as such, it is traditionally administered combined with a sweet liquid such as cherry acetaminophen syrup or a sweetened soda drink. Oral midazolam does not provoke nausea and is a mild respiratory depressant when given without narcotics. There have been no case reports of apnea or hypoxia when oral midazolam is the sole sedative. Children demonstrate marked anxiolysis and mild sedation. When the drug is used appropriately, children are able to cooperate with either an intravenous or mask induction and they demonstrate little or no distress.

Ketamine can also be used as a preanesthetic medication. It is given orally in a dose of 6 mg/kg. It is effective in 10 to 20 minutes and has an effective duration of approximately 30 to 45 minutes. It appears to produce a state of apparent calm but does not have the anxiolytic effect of midazolam. Amnesia commonly occurs. The effect of oral ketamine is less aesthetic from a parental point of view (due to its dissociate properties as described in Chapter 14) compared with oral midazolam, but it is more palatable and therefore easier to administer.

Intravenous preparations of both synthetic and naturally occurring narcotics can be given as oral premedication. However, they have the disadvantage of producing chest wall rigidity, respiratory depression, nausea, and vomiting, and often delay discharge even after short, minor procedures.

Because preoperative medications such as midazolam and ketamine do not delay discharge, they should be considered in any child who is particularly frightened or difficult to manage. Preoperative medications should not be withheld form children simply because they are ambulatory patients. They should receive the same attention to alleviating their anxiety and fear as if they were inpatients.

In addition to using preoperative teaching and premedication for children, the presence of parents can facilitate inductions. The presence of a parent can be used with rectal, intravenous, or inhalational inductions. Either an induction room or operating suite can be used. At the University of Virginia, most pediatric inductions with parents present take place in an induction room, thus bypassing the need for parents to change into operating room attire. This results in a decrease in parental and child anxiety. The use of an induction room also allows the operating room nurses to prepare the operating room while anesthesia is induced. Parental presence at induction is particularly useful if the parents are motivated, well prepared, and do not transmit their anxiety and fears to their child.

ANESTHETIC MANAGEMENT

There are several methods of anesthetic induction for infants and children. Intravenous, intramuscular, inhalational, and rectal induc-

tions have all been used successfully in pediatric outpatients. The choice of technique and selection of induction agents has more to do with the personal experiences and preferences of the parents, child, and anesthesiologist than does outcome. In general, the more techniques practiced, the better the care.

Rectal induction of anesthesia with 30 mg/kg methohexital is a particularly useful technique for children younger than 3 years of age. It is easy to administer and can be given in the preoperative holding area. Children generally fall asleep in 5 to 7 minutes. Rectal methohexitol fails to induce anesthesia in approximately 5% of patients. Even if the child is not asleep, most children are sufficiently sedated to allow a quiet transfer to the operating room. Apnea has been associated with rectal methohexital, but not in healthy children. Even so, an anesthesiologist should be in attendance after administration because it is an induction technique and not a premedication. The disadvantage of this technique is the 5 to 7 minutes that it requires to be effective and that the anesthesiologist must remain in attendance during this time. There are few studies regarding the impact of this technique on discharge times. Serum methohexital levels consistent with anesthesia are measurable in many children 1 to 2 hours after administration. Rectal methohexital is an appropriate induction agent for children scheduled for procedures lasting 1 hour or longer and does not appear to delay discharge in such cases. However, procedures such as myringotomy and ear tube placement often last only 5 to 10 minutes. Rectal methohexital is probably not the ideal choice for such cases.

Induction of anesthesia by intramuscular injection is reserved generally for those children who are completely uncooperative or when other techniques are either not desired or inappropriate. Ketamine, given as a 3 mg/kg intramuscular injection, is effective in 2 to 3 minutes and produces a light state of anesthesia. Children can then be readily separated from their parents. Subsequently, either an inhalational or intravenous anesthetic can be used for the duration of the surgery. Spontaneous respiration is maintained with ketamine and there is little cardiac depression. A dose of 3 mg/kg does not significantly affect discharge times for operations lasting greater than 1 hour.

Intravenous inductions have the advantage of being rapid, reliable, and safe. They also have the disadvantage of needing intravenous access in place before induction. Obtaining intravenous access is difficult in certain pediatric populations. Needle phobia is a regional issue, varying from community to community. Needles are well tolerated and accepted by some communities, loathed by others. The use of Emla cream, a eutectic mixture of local anesthetics, helps to improve the acceptance of intravenous induction in children. Emla cream is applied to the back of the hands, covering those veins desired for intravenous access, and an occlusive dressing is applied. In 1 to 2 hours, profound analgesia occurs in the treated areas and an intravenous line can then be inserted without pain. There are three problems: (1) the patient must be available 1 to 2 hours before surgery so that the cream can be applied in time to be effective, (2) Emla produces some venoconstriction, occasionally hindering venopuncture, and (3) the individual inserting the intravenous needle must still convince the child that the skin is anesthetized and the needle will not hurt. Educating the patient about the use of Emla cream before the day of surgery eliminates many of these problems.

Propofol has recently become particularly popular for both induction and maintenance of anesthesia in children with an intravenous line in place. It is rapid in onset and has a very short effective half-life, making it ideal for outpatient anesthesia. Unlike many intravenous anesthetics, it is easily administered for the maintenance of anesthesia as well as for the induction of anesthesia, because accumulation of effect is minimal. Propofol appears to have its own antiemetic effect, lasting approximately 2 to 4 hours. Intravenous propofol injection does produce localized venous discomfort. By adding Xylocaine to the propofol before injection, the discomfort is largely negated.

Pentothal remains the gold standard regarding the intravenous induction of children and remains popular. It produces little or no discomfort on injection. However, it is antianalgesic and has no antiemetic effect. Compared with propofol, discharge times for very short procedures may be slightly longer but are inconsequential clinically.

Induction of anesthesia with inhalational agents is a well-established practice. Induction with halothane by mask, in particular, is generally well tolerated. Inhalational inductions are ideal in children with needle phobia or in children with poor veins. Upon completing the induction, an intravenous line can be inserted and the anesthesia care continued. The disadvantage of inhalational induction is that the anesthesiologist is preoccupied with the airway while the induction takes place. If laryngospasm or other complications occur during the induction, the anesthesiologist may be dependent on other operating room personnel to provide the intravenous access and administer any medications as necessary. None the less, many pediatric anesthesiologists are highly skilled in conducting inhalational induction and their patients do very well.

Isoflurane and desflurane are highly pungent inhalational agents, making them unsuitable for mask induction in children and adults. They commonly provoke laryngospasm and bronchospasm and are best regarded as maintenance agents. The advantage of these two drugs is that they are both relatively insoluble agents. Once the vaporizer is turned off, their anesthetic effect quickly dissipates. Emergence from anesthesia using desflurane is extremely rapid.

Sevoflurane is the most recent inhalational agent to be approved for use in the United States. Like desflurane, it is relatively insoluble and therefore produces a rapid onset of anesthesia and a short emergence. Unlike isoflurane and desflurane, sevoflurane is sweet smelling and nonirritating to the airway. It is well tolerated by children, even those with colds, for anesthetic induction and has become my anesthetic induction agent of choice for children.

The decision to control the airway or have the child breathe spontaneously depends on the needs of the surgeon, the medical condition of the patient, and the preference of the anesthesiologist. Many outpatient procedures are highly suited to spontaneous ventilation by either a face or laryngeal mask.

The laryngeal mask airway (LMA) is easy to

insert and provides a stable airway. It has the advantage of liberating the hands of the anesthesiologist to perform other tasks and is less tiring. The airway can be secured at lower levels of anesthesia compared to that required for endotracheal intubation. The incidence of a sore throat with an LMA is comparable to that of an oral airway or endotracheal tube. The LMA is particularly useful in cases that are readily amenable to spontaneous ventilation, but the surgery (such as an excision of a cyst around the face of a child) requires that the anesthesiologist's hands and face mask be out of the way. The LMA has been used for controlled ventilation in some centers, but this is not currently recommended and the LMA should be reserved for patients breathing spontaneously. The LMA does not protect the airway against pulmonary aspiration. The LMA is particularly useful when anesthetizing a child with a cold. Because the LMA is placed above the vocal cords, the laryngospasm and bronchospasm associated with colds and endotracheal intubation is avoided.

An endotracheal tube should be inserted when the airway must be protected against aspiration or when controlled ventilation is necessary. In the past, concerns were expressed that the endotracheal intubation of children would result in postextubation croup, thereby preventing or delaying discharge of the children home. This has not been supported by either experience or current research. The incidence of postextubation croup is extremely low when an air leak around the endotracheal tube at an inflation pressure less than 30 mm Hg can be demonstrated. At the University of Virginia postextubation croup occurs in less than 0.5% of intubated children.

Currently, all sizes of cuffed and uncuffed endotracheal tubes are available for children. Most children do not require a cuffed endotracheal tube. However, they are useful in children whose preexisting pulmonary conditions negatively affect pulmonary compliance or in those rare circumstances when aspiration of blood might occur during the surgery. Children with cystic fibrosis represent the former, and functional endoscopic sinus surgery is an example of the latter.

The drugs and techniques selected for anesthetic maintenance are predicated on the principles of providing good operating conditions for the surgeon while allowing a short recovery, free from pain and nausea, for the child. Anesthetic approaches that combine the use of general anesthesia with local anesthetic techniques are highly popular and readily applicable to pediatric outpatients. Ideally, most anesthesiologists providing care for children should try to become proficient with common regional anesthetic techniques including penile blocks, ilioinguinal blocks, and caudal blocks. The use of these blocks has been shown to be both safe and efficacious. They are readily learned and easy to perform with experience. Contrary to the concerns of many, these techniques are not time consuming. Regional techniques often shorten operating room time by allowing for a very rapid, pain-free emergence.

The addition of a local anesthetic technique to the general anesthetic reduces intraoperative anesthetic requirements and reduces or eliminates the need for postoperative narcotics. Postoperative pain and narcotic use are the two most important factors causally related to nausea, vomiting, and delayed discharge from the recovery room. If, by using local anesthetic techniques, postoperative pain and subsequent use of narcotics can be eliminated, the care of children is both improved and shortened.

When local anesthetic conduction blocks are not possible, it is helpful for the surgeon to infiltrate the wound edges before closure. Surgeons should be aware of the appropriate doses of amide anesthetics. For subcutaneous infiltration of bupivacaine, the total dose should be restricted to 1 mL/kg when using 0.25% bupivacaine and 0.5 mL/kg when using 0.5% bupivacaine. These formulas give the maximum safe dose of bupivacaine as 3 mg/kg. Epinephrine may be added to these preparations but does not change the maximum safe dose significantly. If Xylocaine is used for infiltration, doses should be restricted to 7 to 8 mg/kg. The benefit of bupivacaine infiltration lasts much longer than most physicians think and can provide 8 or more hours of pain relief.

A number of new nonnarcotic analgesics have become available over the past few years. Most notable among these drugs is ketorolac.

Ketorolac is a nonsteroidal anti-inflammatory agent. Although this drug is not approved for use in children by the Food and Drug Administration (FDA), many pediatric centers have obtained good results with its use. Traditional dosing is 0.5 to 1.0 mg/kg given as a single intravenous or intramuscular injection. It should not be used in children with a history of aspirin sensitivity and nasal polyps, because it may provoke severe bronchospasm. It should also be avoided in children with renal insufficiency. Ketorolac has been quoted to be the equivalent to 0.09 mg/kg of morphine, but personal experience has not found it to be as effective as this implies. Ketorolac is nonsedating and does not delay discharge. It is not known to produce nausea and vomiting. It is a useful adjunct in patients with some residual discomfort that does not warrant further doses of narcotics. This medication seems to be ideally suited for outpatient surgery.

Other nonsteroidal anti-inflammatory pain medications can be used to provide analgesia intraoperatively and postoperatively. Rectal acetaminophen or indomethacin are commonly used, with the suppository being inserted after anesthesia is induced. Combined with local infiltration, these drugs are effective for the prevention and reduction of pain in the immediate postoperative period. The effective rectal dose of acetaminophen is uncertain, with recent studies suggesting that doses of 25 to 30 mg/kg are necessary to obtain therapeutic levels. Bleeding secondary to the use of nonsteroidal anti-inflammatory drugs such as ketorolac or aspirin remains to be defined. Recent studies have shown that bleeding was increased in children when they were given ketorolac for post-tonsillectomy pain. Further studies are needed to define the risk of bleeding for other operations.

Muscle relaxants are commonly used in pediatric anesthesia. In the past, the most commonly used muscle relaxant was succinylcholine. Recently, however, there has been considerable controversy over its routine use in pediatric patients. Succinylcholine is a rapid-onset, short-acting muscle relaxant ideally suited to provide endotracheal intubating conditions. It is a depolarizing muscle relaxant and the onset of action is heralded by fasciculations resulting from the depolarization of motor endplates. In some circumstances, the motor endplates are not discrete. If the motor endplates are not discrete, the use of succinylcholine may result in a massive depolarization of the entire muscle membrane and ensuing life-threatening hyperkalemia. This has occurred in children with burns, demyelinating injuries, upper and lower motor neuron deficits, and a variety of myotonias.

Most recently, the FDA reviewed the elective use of succinylcholine in children, particularly male infants. This review was prompted by case reports in which several male children experienced hyperkalemic cardiac arrests after receiving succinylcholine. Most of the children were subsequently discovered to have Duchenne's muscular dystrophy. Although this event would appear to be uncommon, occurring in approximately 1 in 1,000,000 patients, it did result in drug vial labeling changes and revised indications for the use of succinylcholine. Presently, the drug is not recommended for routine use in children, male or female. Succinylcholine is reserved for situations in which rapid intubation of the trachea is necessary or for the emergent treatment of laryngospasm.

Nondepolarizing muscle relaxants, particularly suitable to day care surgery, are available. These include mivacurium, atracurium, vecuronium, and rocuronium. These drugs have a relatively rapid onset of 2 to 3 minutes. The duration of relaxation is approximately 10 to 20 minutes in the case of mivacurium and 45 to 60 minutes for atracurium and rocuronium. Vecuronium is the longest acting of these muscle relaxants with a duration of approximately 1 hour. Intermediate-acting muscle relaxants add flexibility to anesthetic management, allowing the anesthesiologist to use a nondepolarizing muscle relaxant in cases lasting less than 1 hour. This was not possible with curare or pancuronium (see Chapter 14).

Most pediatric day surgery cases are short in duration, but allowances should be made for heat loss. Most heat loss occurs by convection and conduction. A warm room and table surface, combined with overhead heating lamps, sharply reduces heat loss, particularly during the induction of infants. Additionally, efforts to conserve heat, by the use of in-line humidification and warming mattresses, are appropriate in prolonged cases.

Routine anesthesia monitoring guidelines for pediatric patients have been set forth by the American Society of Anesthesiologists. These guidelines recommend that there be continuous monitoring of cardiorespiratory parameters and that temperature monitoring also be available. This includes use of an electrocardiogram (ECG), noninvasive blood pressure, pulse oximetry, and a precordial stethoscope. If the patients are intubated or have an LMA inserted, continuous CO_2 waveforms and values should be monitored. Patients requiring intra-arterial or central venous monitoring are rarely, if ever, suitable for outpatient surgery.

POSTOPERATIVE CARE

Care of children in the recovery room is often overlooked by physicians and left to the discretion of recovery room nurses, but the successful management of problems that occur during emergence from anesthesia is essential to maintain a productive outpatient center. Recovery from anesthesia and surgery and discharge home is the rate-limiting step for most outpatient centers. Failure to deal with common recovery room complications in a timely manner can result in a backlog of patients in the surgical suites while they await a recovery room bed and in prolonged recovery room hours at the end of the day.

The recovery room is also the source of last impressions given to the child and family. It is a time of great transition for both children and parents. Children are often frightened and disorientated upon emergence. They commonly feel unwell and may be uncomfortable or in pain. Children often do not understand these sensations and require a great deal of comfort and support to cope with these new and unpleasant experiences. Parents commonly have mixed emotions during their child's recovery phase. The concern parents have for their child is often mixed with feelings of guilt and intimidation. The degree of comfort parents have in accepting responsibility for the care of their own child shortly after surgery varies significantly among individuals. Subsequently, recovery room personnel must

be capable of dealing with the many social issues that arise.

Ideally, the care provided in the recovery room merely represents the last step in a continuum of sound care that started with the appropriate selection of suitable patients and was followed by the use of anesthetic techniques appropriate for outpatient anesthesia. However, even the best centers have problems, and a number of common problems can be anticipated. Most unplanned overnight hospital admissions are the result of one of five situations: (1) inappropriate selection of surgical procedure or screening of patients, (2) bleeding, (3) intractable nausea and vomiting, (4) pain, and (5) respiratory complications secondary to airway management.

The pressures of cost savings in medicine, combined with social pressures from referring physicians and parents, not infrequently results in the inappropriate selection of pediatric patients. Such patients commonly require extensive medical resources and personnel in the recovery room and thereby distract from the care that is expected and needed by others. For example, the need for mechanical ventilation in the recovery room is disruptive and destroys the efficiency of the entire ambulatory surgical center. Many recovery room personnel are untrained or uncomfortable with such equipment, necessitating that care be personally provided by an anesthesiologist or respiratory therapist, distracting that person from the care of others. It only takes one such case to disrupt an entire day. This is particularly true when working in a busy freestanding outpatient surgical center. These centers are rarely equipped to handle patients requiring such care and must transport them to a nearby inpatient facility. Such transfers are labor intensive and not in the patient's best interest. Finally, cost savings are realized only when complications are minimal. Good ambulatory surgical centers have an admission rate of less than 1%. To be competitive with these results, careful patient selection is required.

Whereas bleeding from the surgical wound is not uncommon, particularly with oral or nasal surgery, it rarely requires hospital admission. Bleeding most commonly occurs with tonsillectomies and functional endoscopic surgery. Although surgical technique remains the most important factor in reducing postoperative bleeding, the use of drugs that inhibit platelet function, given either preoperatively or intraoperatively, can increase the incidence of bleeding. Recently several studies have examined the incidence of postoperative bleeding when either intravenous ketorolac or rectal ibuprofen were used as analgesics after tonsillectomies. The findings were consistent with a demonstrated increase in post-tonsillectomy bleeding with the use of either drug.

The management of postoperative bleeding centers on maintaining adequate hydration and early notification of the surgeon. Few patients should ever require transfusion. Complications arising from postoperative bleeding are almost invariably related to the failure to appreciate the extent of blood loss or the subsequent failure to maintain adequate intravenous hydration. Estimating blood loss can be difficult, especially after oral surgery. Children usually swallow the drainage and it is not until they vomit copious amounts of blood that the actual extent of the bleeding is appreciated. Those patients who bleed to the point that a transfusion is considered should be taken back to the operating room to achieve adequate hemostasis. Children needing either a second visit to the operating room for hemostasis or transfusion of red cells should be admitted overnight. Children at risk of delayed postoperative bleeding (e.g., outpatients undergoing tonsillectomies) should be discharged home only if the parents live close to a facility capable of managing such a problem.

Postoperative nausea or vomiting is the most common postoperative complication requiring admission to hospital. The incidence of nausea is related not only to the choice of anesthetic but also to the type of surgery. Strabismus repair, tonsillectomy, and the creation of a pneumoperitoneum are all associated with a high incidence of nausea and vomiting. The most common pediatric outpatient surgical procedures, myringotomy and inguinal hernia repair, are infrequently associated with nausea.

The choice of anesthetic agents can also affect the incidence of nausea and vomiting. The use of narcotics can cause or exacerbate nausea; therefore, whenever possible, local anesthetic techniques that treat postoperative pain are preferable. The incidence of nausea is comparable with all narcotics, synthetic or naturally occurring. Withholding narcotics solely to avoid nausea and vomiting, however, is not always appropriate. Children who are experiencing pain often have nausea or vomiting. In such cases, treating the pain may reduce the incidence of nausea.

A number of antiemetics have been demonstrated to be effective in reducing the postsurgical incidence of nausea and vomiting in children. The major tranquilizers and sedatives such as promethazine and droperidol are effective antiemetics but they produce significant sedation and prolong recovery and discharge times. Metoclopramide, a dopamine antagonist, is an equally effective antiemetic that produces minimal sedation. Additionally, serotonin antagonists such as odansetron are highly effective antiemetics and produce insignificant sedation. The high cost of the serotonin antagonist drugs has limited their routine use. For reasons that are not well elucidated, children are more prone to agitation and other parkinsonian side effects associated with antiemetics. When administering antiemetics to children, it is advisable to use the lowest effective dose, avoid repeated dosing, and carefully observe for side effects before their discharge.

In the 1980s, it was routine for many surgical centers to require that children demonstrate the ability to drink and retain oral liquids before being discharged. But several papers have been published in the past 4 years demonstrating that this practice increases the incidence of nausea and vomiting, delays discharge, and is not predictive of the child's ability to retain fluids at home. Children who are at significant risk of nausea should be well hydrated before discharge, thereby avoiding the urgency for oral intake on the day of surgery. Many children become nauseated during the car ride home. Having a full stomach upon discharge only worsens the situation.

The best treatment for postoperative pain is an intraoperative appreciation of the painful nature of the surgery and its preemptive treatment in the operating room. Withholding pain treatment until the patient is in the recovery room results in an unpleasant and painful anesthetic emergence. Because pain control is easier to maintain than to obtain, children who awaken in pain require substantially more medication than would have been necessary had the pain been treated intraoperatively. The end result is that these children must be sedated almost to the point of unconsciousness to achieve adequate pain control, and discharge is delayed. Once again, the use of intraoperative local anesthetic techniques can dramatically reduce the incidence of pain and subsequent use of sedative narcotics, allowing shorter discharge times.

Although respiratory complications are not the most common cause of pediatric morbidity in the outpatient recovery room, they are the most serious. Most respiratory complications involve (1) upper airway obstruction, including laryngospasm, (2) croup, and (3) postobstructive pulmonary edema.

Upper airway obstruction is either the result of soft-tissue collapse in the oropharynx or hypopharynx or of laryngospasm. Both can occur with any procedure but airway obstruction is most commonly associated with tonsillectomies and oral surgery. In both, treatment must be immediate, because both are life threatening. The failure to treat these problems quickly and effectively remains a significant cause of anesthetic morbidity and mortality. Initial treatment consists of giving oxygen using a face mask and, while maintaining a tight seal around the patient's nose and mouth, applying continuous positive pressure. In the case of severe hypoxia or cardiac compromise, the use of a muscle relaxant and immediate reintubation is appropriate. The differentiation between soft-tissue obstruction and laryngospasm can be difficult, and both may occur at the same time. Although airway obstruction can occur in awake patients, it most often occurs during early emergence from anesthesia or with excessive sedation. The incidence of both can be avoided by the careful timing of extubation and the elimination of oral secretions that irritate the airway.

Croup has become a relatively uncommon recovery room problem, occurring in only 0.5% of intubated patients. The most common cause of croup in the recovery room is postextubation croup, and it appears directly related to the use of excessively large endotracheal tubes. For uncuffed endotracheal tubes, an audible leak should be demonstrable at a peak inspiratory pressure of 25 to 30 mm Hg. Children between the ages of 1 and 4 years are at greatest risk of croup, as are children with Down's syndrome. Upper respiratory tract infections do not appear to increase the incidence of postextubation croup. Initial treatment of croup involves cold humidified oxygen via a croup tent (ideally) or by face mask. For most children, the croup resolves with application of these simple measures. For children who are in distress or hypoxic despite initial therapy, 0.5 mL of 2.25% racemic epinephrine diluted in 5 mL of saline can be nebulized and taken orally over 5 minutes. Dexamethasone 0.3 mg/kg may also be used but will not be effective for several hours and is more appropriately given intraoperatively as a prophylaxis to prevent croup. Children with croup who do require treatment with racemic epinephrine should not be discharged home until the effects of the therapy have dissipated. In this manner, the physician can avoid having discharged a child home only to have the condition rebound necessitating a subsequent visit to the emergency room for further therapy. If more than one dose of racemic epinephrine is necessary, the child should be admitted.

Postobstructive pulmonary edema is a relatively uncommon respiratory complication, which, for unknown reasons, has been seen with increasing frequency over the past 5 years. This entity is most common in infants who have laryngospasm complicated by significant hypoxia. The exact mechanism of postobstructive pulmonary edema is both multifactoral and incompletely understood. Certainly, an obstructed airway and hypoxia are two important factors. The onset of the pulmonary edema is rapid and often fulminant. Hemodynamic instability is uncommon. Treatment involves supportive oxygen therapy including continuous positive airway pressure and intubation if necessary. Diuretic therapy is of no value and the pulmonary edema resolves over several hours. Hospital admission is almost always required overnight. The morbidity and mortality rate from postobstructive pulmonary edema is exceedingly low and the outcome is almost always favorable as long as the airway is managed appropriately in the acute phase. Recent reports have implicated the use of vasoactive drugs in producing pulmonary edema after nasal surgery. This complication clinically appears similar to postobstructive pulmonary edema but the mechanism of injury is probably different, although the therapy is the same.

Discharge criteria vary among institutions. Many centers use a standardized point system based on an ongoing assessment of cardiorespiratory and neurologic parameters. When children reach a critical point total, they are discharged. The advantage of such scoring systems is that they remove individual judgments and biases in the discharge decision-making process, particularly when physicians do not see the patients before the discharge. However, that is also the downfall of such systems. When each patient is seen before discharge and each case is handled on an individual basis, then there is a personal touch to patient care and there is immediate feedback regarding successes and failures. It also provides an opportunity to be sure that no child is discharged before the parents are ready to assume responsibility for that child's care, and last minute assurances can be given to the family (see Chapter 9).

All parents should be given a telephone number at which a care provider affiliated with the ambulatory center can be reached 24 hours a day. All parents should be called the following morning as a follow-up to any problems that may have occurred since discharge. Such a system provides important feedback on how the children have done over the past 18 to 24 hours, which is vital to the quality assurance of any ambulatory surgical center.

Selected Readings

1. Alderson PJ, Lerman J. Oral premedication for pediatric ambulatory anesthesia: a comparison of midazolam and ketamine. Can J Anaesth 1994;41(3):221–226.
2. Cohen MM, Cameron CB. Should you cancel the operation when a child has an upper respiratory tract infection? Anesth Analg 1991;72(3):282–288.
3. Cote CJ, Zaslavsky A, Downes JJ, et al. Postoperative apnea in former preterm infants after inguinal herniorrhaphy. A combined analysis. Anesthesiology 1995;82(4):809–822.
4. Efrat R, Kadari A, Katz S. The laryngeal mask airway in pediatric anesthesia: experience with 120 patients undergoing elective groin surgery. J Pediatr Surg 1994;29(2):206–208.
5. Hackman T, Steward DJ, Sheps SB. Anemia in pediatric day-surgery patients: prevalence and detection. Anesthesiology 1991;75(1):27–31.
6. Littleford JA. Patel LR, Bose D, et al. Masseter muscle spasm in children: implications of continuing the triggering anesthetic. Anesth Analg 1991;72(2):151–160.
7. Martin TM, Nicolson SC, Bargas MS. Propofol anesthesia reduces emesis and airway obstruction in pediatric outpatients. Anesth Analg 1993;77(2):297–304.
8. O'Flynn RP, Shutack JG, Rosenberg H, Fletcher JE. Masseter muscle rigidity and malignant hyperthermia susceptibility in pediatric patients. An update on management and diagnosis. Anesthesiology 1994;80(6):1228–1233.
9. Piertopaoli JA Jr, Keller MA, Smail DF, Abajian JC. Regional anesthesia in pediatric surgery: complications and postoperative comfort level in 174 children. J Pediatr Surg 1993;28(4):560–564.
10. Patel RI, Hannallah RS. Preoperative screening for pediatric ambulatory surgery: evaluation of a telephone questionnaire method. Anesth Analg 1992;75(2):258–261.
11. Schreiner MS, Nicolson SC, Martin T, Whitney L. Should children drink before discharge from day surgery? Anesthesiology 1992;76(4):528–533.
12. Steward DJ. Screening tests before surgery in children. Can J Anaesth 1991;38(6):693–695.
13. Ummenhofer W, Frei FJ, Urwyler A, et al. Effects of ondansetron in the prevention of postoperative nausea and vomiting in children. Anesthesiology 1994;81(4):804–810.
14. Veyckemans F, Van Obbergh LJ, Gouverneur JM. Lessons from 1100 pediatric caudal blocks in a teaching hospital. Regional Anesthesia 1992;17(3):119–125.
15. Weir PM, Munro HM, Reynolds PI, Lewis IH, Wilton NC. Propofol infusion and the incidence of emesis in pediatric outpatient strabismus surgery. Anesth Analg 1993;76(4):760–764.
16. Welborn LG, Greenspun JS. Anesthesia and apnea. Perioperative considerations in the former preterm infant. Pediatr Clin North Am 1994;41(1):181–198.
17. Weldon BC, Watcha MF, White PF. Oral midazolam in children: effect of time and adjunctive therapy. Anesth Analg 1992;75(1):51–55.
18. Yentis SM, Levine MF, Hartley EJ. Should all children with suspected or confirmed malignant hyperthermia susceptibility be admitted after surgery? A 10-year review. Anesth Analg 1992;75(3):345–350.

18

Special Considerations for Laparoscopic Surgery

Stephen D. Small

As laparoscopic surgery has evolved since the turn of the century, it has presented anesthesiologists with both basic science and clinical issues to resolve. First, as related to biopsy and diagnosis, laparoscopic procedures became much more frequent with the advent of minimally invasive therapy for gynecologic disorders in the late 1960s. The next phase of development began with the introduction of laparoscopic cholecystectomy 20 years later. Its rapid eclipse of open cholecystectomy as the procedure of choice for most patients with symptomatic cholelithiasis is a testament to the current focus on quick postoperative recovery, patient satisfaction, and containment of health care costs. Although this chapter is concerned with ambulatory anesthesia and surgery, videoscopic surgery for intrathoracic conditions as well as numerous intra-abdominal conditions is also gaining fast acceptance. Progress in this area can be described as a tradeoff between the postoperative benefits and the new intraoperative risks and physiologic trespass. Although they are relatively rare, complications still can be catastrophic.

Several factors have driven a new wave of clinical experimentation in this field. First, the surgical stimuli and patient positioning requirements for laparoscopic cholecystectomy and Nissen fundoplication differ substantially from anesthetic considerations for pelvic surgery. These operations may also expose patients to the consequences of prolonged pneumoperitoneum. Second, there has been a change in the epidemiologic makeup of pa-

tients who undergo this new array of laparoscopic procedures. The spectrum has been broadened from primary focus on young, healthy females to include older patients of both sexes with higher incidences of atherosclerosis, diabetes, pulmonary insufficiency, and other pathologic conditions. Third, the movement toward increasing outpatient care and reducing costs has prompted greater numbers of older, sicker patients subjected to short periods of intense physiologic and social stress to be included in the patient envelope. Finally, the ready availability and safety of both noninvasive and invasive monitoring techniques have led to their application in this group of patients.

Within the context of recent investigations and experience with new laparoscopic procedures, this chapter focuses on considerations unique to the patient who undergoes ambulatory laparoscopic surgery.

ISSUES UNIQUE TO LAPAROSCOPIC SURGERY

Physiology

Cardiovascular Factors

Numerous factors affect the hemodynamic variables that are routinely monitored during laparoscopic surgery. These include patient comorbidities, the effects of regional and general anesthesia, surgical stimuli, patient positioning, positive pressure ventilation, pneumoperitoneum, and absorption of insufflated gas from the abdomen. Other important variables such as transmural right atrial pressure and cardiac output are also affected but not measured routinely because of tradeoffs such as increased risk, expense, and uncertain benefit.

The patient who undergoes ambulatory laparoscopic surgery is most likely to be completely free of comorbidities or to carry a diagnosis of one or two stable chronic diseases. More patients are being scheduled with severe systemic disease that limits activity but is not incapacitating (ASA III). The need for invasive monitoring or special postoperative care usually steers patients away from ambulatory pathways. However, it is not unusual for ambulatory surgery patients to have a history of prior myocardial infarction, hypertensive cardiomyopathy, or congestive heart failure that is well-controlled on medical management.

Arrhythmias

Patients taking beta-blockers can present challenges to anesthetic management when their heart rates slow because of narcotic administration, vagal stimuli from peritoneal stretching, or traction on viscera. Similar drug interactions likely to occur in this setting may result from administration of propofol or agents to reverse neuromuscular blockade. Vasoactive drugs used to control blood pressure during light anesthesia may also induce bradycardia because of beta-blockade or direct effects on the sinoatrial node or atrioventricular nodal pathways. Rescue from significant bradycardias, slow junctional rhythms, or even (uncommonly) asystole may be necessary. Usual small doses of ephedrine or atropine may not suffice, and although phenylephrine elevates blood pressure, it may induce reflex bradycardia. It may be necessary to use small doses of vasoactive drugs with beta-agonist and chronotropic properties and for the surgeon to relieve the patient's intra-abdominal pressure (IAP) and level the operating table if the patient is in steep head-up position. Moving the patient to the Trendelenburg position is controversial (see Hemodynamics).

When an acceptable heart rate is regained, deepening of anesthesia has been reported to prevent further recurrences of bradycardia

due to vagal stimulation. Reports of arrhythmias occurring during laparoscopic surgery date from the era of routine halothane administration and include cases of spontaneous ventilation. Even though a more recent review suggests that arrhythmias are more likely to occur early in the insufflation period, there is no substantiating evidence. Until more data concerning patients with cardiovascular and pulmonary disease undergoing laparoscopic surgery are available, it remains prudent to be vigilant during the initiation of insufflation, when decreases in cardiac output and increases in afterload have been shown to be most marked.

Hemodynamic Factors

Numerous factors affect hemodynamic variables during laparoscopic surgery. They include patient positioning, intrinsic cardiopulmonary factors peculiar to the patient, intravascular volume, insufflation of the abdomen with carbon dioxide, absorption of carbon dioxide and stimulation of the sympathetic nervous system, general anesthesia and anesthetic agents chosen, positive pressure ventilation, and surgical stimuli.

Early reports from the era of active study of pelvic laparoscopy in the Trendelenburg position essentially agreed on the finding of hypertension, tachycardia, and increased end-tidal carbon dioxide ($ETCO_2$) with intra-abdominal insufflation of carbon dioxide. However, there was controversy surrounding the measurement of cardiac output. Some patients ventilated spontaneously, others were mechanically ventilated, and IAP varied.

Not until IAP reached 40 mm Hg did hypotension ensue in healthy patients. Current practice uses a variable flow insufflator that keeps IAP at 12 to 15 mm Hg in most cases. The effects of increased IAP were thought to be secondary to both forced pooling of blood in the lower extremities and squeezing of volume into the central circulation. Increased IAP increases thoracic pressures, rendering exact interpretation of central compartment hemodynamics difficult. Mechanical and humoral factors increase systemic vascular resistance (SVR) because the increase in resistance outlasts the pneumoperitoneum. Intra-abdominal organ blood flow decreases dramatically with insufflation as well. There are no outcome data on the significance of this change.

In the following discussion, the newest physiologic investigations in this field are briefly critically discussed and summarized.

In a report by Wittgen and colleagues in 1991, one of the earliest of the recent reports to study the hemodynamic effects of laparoscopic cholecystectomy, 20 healthy and 10 ASA II and III patients were included. In this preliminary but oft-quoted paper, routine monitoring was used and the only invasive test was the sampling for arterial blood gases. Cardiac output was not measured, but it was hypothesized to increase because of the increase in mean arterial pressure and heart rate with insufflation of the abdomen with carbon dioxide. Hypercarbia was judged to be responsible for these changes because it increased peripheral vascular resistance and inotropy. This hypothesis has not been verified in more recent studies using Swan-Ganz (SG) catheters and transesophageal echocardiographic (TEE) assessment. The sentinel finding reported in the Wittgen study was the increase in arterial carbon dioxide underestimated by $ETCO_2$ in the sicker group of patients. In one patient, intra-abdominal insufflation was stopped and the abdomen opened to complete the procedure because there was uncontrollable hypercarbic acidosis. However, no mention was made of the possibility of subcutaneous or mediastinal emphysema or of trochar misplacement. In addition, the minute ventilation in the acidotic patient was not significantly increased before conversion to an open procedure. Another criticism of the study is that preoperative pulmonary and cardiovascular data necessary to accurately classify the patients were not available. Although this is one of the few studies to report hemodynamic data in sicker patients undergoing a laparoscopic procedure, few if any generalizations can be made.

In 1993, Cunningham and Brull studied 13 healthy patients undergoing laparoscopic cholecystectomy with TEE. Left ventricular function was maintained throughout insufflation and changes in patient positioning. Systolic, diastolic, mean arterial (MAP), and peak airway pressures all increased significantly. Left ventricular end-systolic area dropped minimally with insufflation and subsequently increased to normal. End-systolic wall stress increased by 25%. Changes in left ventricular end-diastolic area were less marked, except when the patient was put in the reverse Trendelenburg position, when there was a 20% decrease. Although $ETCO_2$ increased 10% by the conclusion of the study, minute ventilation was held constant, reducing generalization of findings to clinical practice. In summary, in a small group of healthy patients, ejection fraction was maintained despite small changes in loading conditions.

In 1992, McLaughlin and associates conducted another study that used TEE in a similar setting. It confirmed the typical heart rate and blood pressure findings of previous work. However, decreases in stroke volume (27%) and cardiac index (24%) occurred 30 minutes after insufflation and positioning. Whereas central venous pressure increased 60%, the effects of positive pressure ventilation and increased IAP were not taken into account. Urine output did not decrease, despite the observation previously made regarding significant decreases in renal blood flow with insufflation. McLaughlin and associates cautioned that patients with cardiac disease may be at increased risk for previously unrecognized problems with the procedure.

Finally, in 1993, Joris studied 15 nonobese patients without cardiorespiratory disease during laparoscopic cholecystectomy and used SG catheters to characterize changes in hemodynamic variables. In addition, mean thoracic pressure was measured by an esophageal balloon. The most marked finding was a 50% decrease in cardiac index (CI) 5 minutes after insufflation. This was thought to be caused by head-up tilt, increased IAP, and the effects of anesthesia. However, CI improved significantly during surgery to preinsufflation values without a clear explanation. $ETCO_2$ was controlled by changing minute ventilation, and $PaCO_2$ was not significantly altered in these healthy patients. With IAP maintained at 14 mm Hg, intrathoracic pressures increased approximately 9 mm Hg. Only a 10° head-up tilt was used; this was associated with a small but significant decrease in right atrial pressure and pulmonary capillary wedge pressure (Table 18–1).

Table 18–1. Hemodynamic Changes During Laparoscopic Cholecystectomy

	After Induction	Head-up	Pneumoperitoneum			After Surgery
			5 min	15 min	30 min	
Mean arterial pressure	↓	↓↓	↑↑	↑	↓	↑
Heart rate	↑	↓	↑	↑	↔	↓
Right atrial pressure	↔	↓↓	↑↑	↔	↔	↓
Pulmonary capillary wedge pressure	↔	↓	↑↑	↔	↓	↓
Cardiac index	↓↓	↓	↓	↑	↔	↑
Systemic vascular resistance	↑	↑	↑↑↑	↓	↔	↓
Peripheral vascular resistance	↑	↓	↑↑↑	↓	↓	↓

Modified from Joris JL, Noiret D, Legrand et al. Hemodynamic changes during laparoscopic cholecystectomy. Anesth Analg 1993;76:1067–1071.

The authors observed that MAP remained the same before induction and after initial insufflation, when there was the greatest decrease in CI. They concluded that an increase in SVR was responsible and suggested that both mechanical and humoral factors were involved because, at the end of the procedure, correction took several minutes after IAP was released. Right atrial pressure minus the extracardiac pressure measured via esophageal balloon did not change much, reducing the significance of changes in venous return on CI.

In summary, several new studies have characterized in a few healthy patients mostly minor physiologic perturbations during laparoscopic cholecystectomy in the head-up tilt position. A transient well-tolerated decrease in CI of as much as 50% may be seen. Caution must be used in generalizing these results to sicker patients in the absence of prospective data. Postoperative benefits may exceed the risks of controlled hemodynamic changes. Indeed, anecdotal reports of experienced clinicians suggest that this may be the case despite prolonged insufflation times in patients with complex conditions.

Pulmonary Factors

Multiple variables affect respiratory mechanics and gas exchange during laparoscopic procedures. These include increased IAP, decreased diaphragmatic excursion, absorption of carbon dioxide, patient tilt, positive pressure ventilation, decreased cardiac output, reduced incisional pain, and patient factors such as body weight and cardiorespiratory disease. Information concerning pelvic laparoscopic procedures in the head-down position has been well reviewed, but there are numerous contradictions traceable to experimental and anesthetic techniques. This discussion focuses mainly on reviewing general issues and recent studies.

Increased IAP limits diaphragmatic movement and induces atelectasis and shunt that may be partially offset by head-up tilt and the administration of positive end-expiratory pressure (PEEP). Functional residual capacity (FRC), total lung volume, and lung compliance are also reduced. This is further exacerbated in obese patients, who are highly represented in the population of patients with cholecystitis. Head-down tilt compounds atelectasis and is also a risk factor for the creation of a functional right main-stem intubation as the abdominal viscera displace the lungs cephalad. The unsuspected presence of the endotracheal tube at the carina may cause a mistaken diagnosis of light surgical anesthesia.

Carbon dioxide is favored as the insufflating gas because of its high solubility; hence, the risk of frequency and severity of gas embolism is reduced. In addition, it is not combustible. The absorption of carbon dioxide has been studied in pelvic laparoscopy under local anesthesia, general anesthesia with spontaneous ventilation, and in laparoscopic cholecystectomy with mechanical ventilation. Respiratory rate, not tidal volume, is increased to regulate carbon dioxide in the presence of high IAP in awake patients. With anesthetic depression, spontaneous ventilation is inadequate to meet the increased carbon dioxide load and IAP. When the patient undergoes mechanical ventilation in the head-up position with increased

IAP, initial research has suggested that increasing minute ventilation by 12% to 16% is sufficient to maintain carbon dioxide homeostasis, but that $ETCO_2$ may not accurately reflect $Paco_2$ if large volumes of carbon dioxide are insufflated and $ETCO_2$ is greater than 41. Although an exacerbation of this situation has not been verified in a large number of patients with significant cardiorespiratory disease during laparoscopic procedures, experienced clinicians already hold $ETCO_2$ suspect in this population in routine nonlaparoscopic surgery (Table 18–2).

Absorption of carbon dioxide may actually be limited by high IAP that is caused by compression of peritoneal small vessels; the reduction in organ flow has already been alluded to. Marked increases in $ETCO_2$ may be seen if carbon dioxide escapes the high IAP environment of the peritoneal cavity and is more rapidly absorbed from subcutaneous tissues or pleural surfaces. However, in a recent study by Lister and colleagues, carbon dioxide absorption was not found to be linearly related to IAP pressure. In this pig study, the initial increase in carbon dioxide production (VCO_2) was hypothesized to be caused by increased peritoneal surface area being exposed during insufflation. After an IAP of 10 mm Hg was achieved, VCO_2 did not increase much. However, $Paco_2$ continued to increase as IAP was driven from 10 to 25 mm Hg. This was accounted for by increasing areas of wasted ventilation, or physiologic dead space. Suspiciously, however, cardiac output was not decreased and hemodynamic parameters did not change significantly over the range of IAPs achieved. This may have been caused by the large and continuous fluid loading of the animals.

Several factors may act in concert to shift more of the lung to a West's zone 1, or area of increased ventilation:perfusion, and result in an increase in dead space. Decreased cardiac output caused by anesthesia, increased IAP, and increased SVR may occur as discussed. Increased intrathoracic pressure may accomplish the same result. Finally, if minute ventilation is not adjusted, the smaller tidal volumes accompanying higher peak inspiratory pressures may cause a reduction in alveolar ventilation in addition to the prior increase in dead space.

Several investigators have recently studied the putative benefits of laparoscopic surgery on postoperative respiratory mechanics. Abdominal incisions—especially upper abdominal incisions—are associated with postprocedure lung volume loss. This includes forced vital capacity (FVC), FRC, and tidal volume. In addition, forced expiratory flow (FEF) measurements are reduced, not only because of obstruction but also because of this loss of lung volume. The relief of pain with regional postoperative anesthetic practices does not totally restore these volumes to normal in patients with upper abdominal incisions, implicating diaphragm dysfunction and other incompletely understood factors.

Immediately postoperatively, Frazee and associates were able to show in healthy patients that laparoscopic cholecystectomy was associated with a 25% improvement in FVC, FEF (25%–75%), and forced expiratory volume in 1 second (FEV_1) over open cholecystectomy. This was not, however, linked to any change in outcome or reduction in complications. A more in-depth and expanded study by Putensen-Himmer and colleagues of the same question found large differences in FVC favoring the laparoscopic group that persisted to 3 days postoperatively. Changes in FRC, while not as marked, showed the identical trend. FEV_1 decreased markedly in the open cholecystectomy group in the first 6 hours after surgery, remained low for 24 hours, and

Table 18–2. Changes in Pulmonary Mechanics and Gas Exchange

↑	Intra-abdominal pressure
↓	Diaphragmatic excursion
+	Pressure ventilation
	↓
↓	Functional residual capacity
↓	Total lung capacity
↓	Compliance
↑	Transthoracic pressure
↑	Intrathoracic pressure
↓	Cardiac output
	↓
↑	Atelectasis
↑	Shunt
↑	Alveolar/end-tidal gradient
	↓

Add positive end-expiratory pressure
Increase FIO_2
Increase minute ventilation
Measure arterial blood gas when necessary

then increased to lag behind the laparoscopic group by 10% at 3 days. Although oxygenation was statistically better in the laparoscopic group, it was not clinically significant. There was no difference in $PaCO_2$ or pH. Whereas the pain scores of the two groups were the same, the open group had significantly higher analgesic requirements. Again, no outcomes or complication rates were studied.

A sophisticated study of diaphragmatic and abdominal muscle activity after laparoscopic cholecystectomy revealed no changes in FRC and residual volume. There were, however, decreases of 20% when maneuvers requiring maximal inspiratory effort were performed. Diaphragm function was deemed to be intact during quiet breathing postoperatively, but it was impaired if stressed by maximal breathing. Improvement over historic control studies of open procedures was documented, and the authors attributed the results to less abdominal wall trauma with the laparoscopic approach.

To summarize, laparoscopic surgery is associated with numerous trespasses on the patient's gas exchange and respiratory mechanics, some of which are unique to the procedure. Attention to maintaining and increasing minute ventilation, being suspicious of falsely low $ETCO_2$ values in certain settings, using PEEP judiciously, checking endotracheal tube position, and considering extraperitoneal movement of large volumes of carbon dioxide in the hypercarbic patient all mark proficient performance.

Metabolic Factors

A number of recent papers have addressed the stress response associated with laparoscopic surgery. These are of special interest to the anesthesiologist, because one of the prime functions of the administration of anesthesia is to control somatic and autonomic responses to surgical trauma. The selection of patients for ambulatory procedures precludes the conduct of major surgical operations, but it is of interest to briefly review how the stresses of ambulatory laparoscopic surgery compare with open procedures.

Jakeways and associates found that laparoscopic surgery stimulates a significant stress response. Changes in cortisol levels have been found to be no different between laparoscopic and open procedures, whereas changes in glucose and C-reactive protein were significantly less in the laparoscopic group. This supports the finding that regional anesthesia for upper abdominal surgery attenuates hyperglycemia and catecholamine release but does not alter the cortisol response, perhaps because there is incomplete inhibition of visceral afferents. The equivalent decline in albumin and plasma proteins in both laparoscopic and open procedures indicates that microvascular permeability accompanies both equally. However, interleukin-6 (IL-6) has been shown to correlate with the magnitude of the surgical insult, and laparoscopic procedures are clearly associated with smaller elevations in this major cytokine.

Jakeways and associates also looked at postoperative fatigue and muscle weakness and suggested that the greater acute stress response in the open procedures group was responsible for the later recovery of those patients. Another study by Rademaker and coworkers confirmed that patterns of cortisol secretion and glucose homeostasis in laparoscopic surgery mirrored those seen in open cholecystectomy, and their conclusion was that the rapid recovery seen with laparoscopic procedures was not due to a reduced endocrine stress response. Thoracic anesthesia in one of the study groups provided pain relief but did not improve lung function or stress marker levels.

Because the intraoperative anesthetic requirements for open and closed procedures are similar, the ability to provide acceptable ambulatory care for these patients has been facilitated by the introduction of numerous potent, short-acting, predictable anesthetic agents. Even though the IL-6 stress response is significantly lower in laparoscopic cholecystectomy, other factors must also be responsible for the quick recovery that these patients experience. These probably include, as discussed previously, less abdominal wall trauma and improved respiratory mechanics. Pain is discussed in later paragraphs.

Positioning

There are some specific patient positioning concerns in laparoscopic surgery. Padding of bony prominences and prevention of stretching of neurovascular plexuses is standard. However, the often steep head-up and head-down tilts required by surgeons necessitate that special care be given by the anesthesiologist. The patient's arms may become dislodged, hyperextended, or adducted, with unsuspected pressure being put on radial or ulnar nerves or with the brachial or cervical plexuses being stretched. Shoulder braces must be positioned opposite the coracoid process to avoid plexus injury also.

The head-down position (Trendelenburg position) has been studied in a variety of clinical situations. There are essentially no consistent, well-documented, predictable hemodynamic changes that can be ascribed to the assumption of this position. Clinical variables include intravascular volume, comorbidities, degree of tilt, position of lower extremities, surgical considerations (e.g., packing or increased IAP), and level of modification of baroreceptor function. The changes that have been observed in healthy volunteers are neither statistically nor clinically significant. Although some surgeons request an initial head-down position for inserting trochars into the abdominal cavity, hemodynamic variables during this maneuver were not reported in the recent studies discussed. The placing of any patient in a head-down position should be a cue to the anesthesiologist to recheck the position of the endotracheal tube.

The head-up position has not received much attention; however, Joris and colleagues documented significant decreases in right atrial pressure, pulmonary capillary wedge pressure, and CI after the patient was put in a 10° head-up position before carbon dioxide insufflation.

Potential Complications

Gas Embolism

The introduction of carbon dioxide or air into the vascular system is both rare and catastrophic. Although carbon dioxide is soluble, it can cause an air lock in the right heart if enough gas is rapidly entrained. Injury to a vessel, thus exposing it to high IAP, or the

inappropriate placement of the carbon dioxide injector into an organ or vessel may be the inciting cause. Early recognition is key to rectifying the problem; however, the classic signs of gas embolism are rarely all present. Shock, tachycardia, cyanosis, arrhythmias, a millwheel murmur, and, in large emboli, electrocardiographic evidence of right heart block or strain may occur. The $ETCO_2$ may increase briefly before it declines as a result of excretion of carbon dioxide that has been absorbed into the blood. Patients with any reason to have high right-sided pressures may be more susceptible to transfer of embolized gas across a patent foramen ovale. Treatment includes administering 100% oxygen, increasing ventilation to increase carbon dioxide excretion, placing the patient into left lateral decubitus and head-down position to allow the gas to rise away from the pulmonary circulation, and, possibly, inserting a multiple-orifice central venous catheter to aspirate gas.

Air embolism may occur as a rare complication of the use of the air-cooled Nd:YAG laser. A jet of air may be directed into an organ, viscus, or vessel, causing signs similar to those discussed for carbon dioxide embolism. Because of its low solubility in blood, an air embolism requires much less air to cause cardiac arrest than does a carbon dioxide embolism. In addition, less hypotension may be seen immediately with an air embolus, because a carbon dioxide embolism can cause a rapid decline in resistance. Treatment is identical.

Absorption of Irrigating Fluid

Patients undergoing hysteroscopic surgery may be at risk for a type of transurethral resection of prostate (TURP) syndrome because of the rapid and continued absorption of large amounts of relatively hypotonic fluid into the vascular system. In addition, patients merely receiving large volumes of irrigating fluid through the laparoscope may be at risk if no one is monitoring the output from the abdomen. The symptoms and signs of volume overload, pulmonary edema, and hyponatremia should alert the clinician to this possibility. In patients under general anesthesia, recognition may be difficult. Ethanol labeling of the irrigating fluid coupled to a breath ethanol analysis device has been proposed. Treatment includes fluid restriction postoperatively, and, for more critical cases, Lasix with hypertonic saline administration.

Escape of Carbon Dioxide From the Abdomen to Other Body Cavities or Subcutaneous Tissue

Gas may escape from the abdomen to a variety of locations—one or both pleural spaces, the pericardium or mediastinum, or the subcutaneous tissue. Clinical signs may vary from shock and respiratory failure resulting from a tension pneumothorax to delayed recognition of facial and neck swelling with crepitation. Treatment depends on the clinical acuity of the problem and when it is recognized. If carbon dioxide accumulates in the pleural space, nitrous oxide should be turned off, 100% oxygen administered, PEEP applied, and the surgeon notified. In the case of carbon dioxide accumulation, chest tube placement may be deferred until the patient is reassessed after IAP is normalized because spontaneous resolution may be expected. Some clinicians have adopted conservative management of patients with signs of significant head and neck emphysema, delaying extubation and elevating the head of the bed after surgery.

Laparoscopic fundoplication for symptomatic hiatal hernia has been gaining acceptance recently. There are minimal data concerning the management of these cases. In one recent case report describing 13 patients, it was observed that no patients experienced shock or ventilatory difficulties. Despite the long duration of the procedures, there were no serious complications. Mediastinal emphysema, pneumopericardium, and subcutaneous emphysema resolved within 4 hours after the operation. With more experience, skilled manipulation of the gastroesophageal junction, and mobilization of the esophagus, such complications should become less frequent, although gas may still enter the thoracic cavity through congenital diaphragmatic hernias.

Fluid may also migrate from the abdomen, by vigorous irrigation, a misplaced trocar, or the presence of a large volume of ascites during a laparoscopic procedure, causing a tension hydrothorax.

Pulmonary Aspiration of Stomach Contents

There are no data to suggest that patients undergoing ambulatory laparoscopic procedures are at a higher risk for gastric aspiration than other ambulatory patients. A cohort with cholecystitis may have a higher number of patients who are obese or suffering from reflux. Patients who undergo laparoscopic fundoplication are treated as if they had full stomachs. Controversy exists regarding the risk of aspiration in the merely anxious patient. There is some evidence that the gastroesophageal barrier to reflux is maintained during increased IAP and Trendelenburg positioning, and the upper esophageal protective sphincter should be unaffected.

Surgical Complications

Surgical complications pertinent to the anesthesiologist include misplacement of the insufflating trochar (causing carbon dioxide embolism or tracking of carbon dioxide to other body cavities); laceration of a hollow viscus or solid organ (e.g., liver, spleen); injury from the trocar insertion before insertion of the laparoscope, causing bleeding abdominal wall vessels, avulsion of adhesions, and omental disruptions; and bile peritonitis and bleeding from liver biopsy. One case report documented urinary bladder perforation that was detected by the collection bag filling with carbon dioxide. Although large vessel injuries are rare, they can occur, as can unsuspected, enlarging retroperitoneal blood collections. Distortion by video cameras and working in a darkened room can impair cue perception. Vigilance and a good working relationship with the surgeon are necessary to satisfactorily diagnose and manage these problems.

Carbon Monoxide Production

A recent report by Beebe and colleagues pointed out that pyrolysis of tissue in a hypoxic environment can produce carbon monoxide (CO). Although extremely high levels of CO were found in insufflation gas after the use of cautery, patients did not have notable carboxy-hemoglobin levels. Numerous hypotheses for these results were suggested, including there being a low uptake from peritoneal capillaries, there being a low diffusion coefficient for CO in the lung, and the possible inhibition of CO uptake by hemoglobin in peritoneal capillaries because of the 100% carbon dioxide environment. The authors suggested the use of routine scavenging of laparoscopic exsufflation gases when cautery is performed.

PATIENT SELECTION

There are few absolute contraindications to ambulatory laparoscopic surgery. The presence of congestive heart failure or severe angina dictates the avoidance of induction of high systemic vascular resistance and a decrease in CI. Patients with high intracranial pressure might tolerate the possible hypercarbia and high intrathoracic pressures poorly. The insufflation of gas into the abdomen would also be dangerous for someone with a peritoneal shunt to the atrium or cerebral ventricles in place. Finally, the hypovolemic patient would first need to be volume resuscitated. Most of these patients would not qualify for ambulatory care. Surgical considerations may more likely dictate the decision to use an open procedure. Whereas some physicians cautiously approach the patient with cardiorespiratory disease, others think that the postoperative benefits far outweigh controlled hemodynamic perturbations.

THE PERIOPERATIVE PERIOD

Preoperative

Medications for the ambulatory patient undergoing laparoscopic surgery need no special mention. Routine prophylaxis for gastric aspiration is not standard practice for all patients. Controversy exists surrounding premedication with nonsteroidal agents to reduce opioid requirements postoperatively. A single 18- or 20-gauge cannula is satisfactory in most instances for intravenous access. Placement in a large

vein in the nondominant antecubital fossa obviates the concerns associated with propofol-induced pain and phlebitis. Standard monitoring devices are used. If a patient requires central venous access for invasive monitoring and intra-arterial pressure monitoring, that patient should not be considered eligible for ambulatory care, although standards may change. Doppler devices are not considered routine to monitor for presence of carbon dioxide or air embolism.

The choice of anesthetic technique is usually limited to general anesthesia for upper abdominal procedures. In an ambulatory setting, the use of combined epidural–general anesthesia offers limited benefit. Laparoscopic pelvic surgery may be accomplished under local, regional, or general anesthesia. Advantages of general anesthesia include securing of the airway in a patient with increased IAP, control of ventilation in the setting of an increased carbon dioxide load, provision of adequate analgesia and good operating conditions if much discomfort is to be expected from visceral traction, and avoidance of expected sedation with concomitant pneumoperitoneum. Advantages of local and regional anesthesia include avoidance of narcotics and other agents linked to causing emesis, avoidance of large doses of hypnotic drugs, and having an awake patient to monitor. If a relatively long ambulatory procedure is contemplated later in the day, however, urinary retention caused by some types of regional block may limit timely discharge. The use of the laryngeal mask airway for laparoscopic procedures is controversial, because it does not protect against aspiration and may not seal adequately at the peak inspiratory pressures required if the patient is not spontaneously ventilating.

Intraoperative

Propofol is usually recommended for induction of anesthesia because of its antiemetic properties, even when infusion is not contemplated. In addition, its other qualities of providing euphoria, reducing incidence of increased airway reflexes, and allowing early ambulation have made it the first choice of ambulatory anesthetists. If regional anesthesia is not contemplated, muscle relaxation for the patient is necessary. Choice of relaxant and techniques for maintenance of anesthesia are identical to those for other ambulatory anesthetic procedures. In patients who may require intraoperative cholangiograms, the use of narcotics that may cause spasm of the sphincter of Oddi is controversial; anesthetists should work closely with surgeons on their philosophies of this issue as well. In addition, when spasm occurs, it may be reversed by naloxone or glucagon. The choice of vasoactive drugs or inhalation agents to lower SVR might lean to ones with vasodilating properties. Many anesthetists provide emesis prophylaxis to laparoscopic patients, because there is a high rate of nausea and vomiting in this population. This prophylaxis may consist of a small dose of droperidol, Reglan, or odansetron; passage of an orogastric tube to empty the stomach of air and fluid; or the avoidance of nitrous oxide and inhalation agents and the use of propofol infusion. Combination therapy with antiemetic agents with different sites of action may be most efficacious. Emergence from general anesthesia may be accompanied by emesis; therefore, the patient's airway reflexes must be fully recovered before extubation.

Postoperative

Postoperative pain control and treatment of nausea and vomiting do not differ from other regimens used in the ambulatory population. Goals are early oral intake, voiding, and ambulation, as well as pain control and control of nausea. Occasionally, shoulder pain after exsufflation of gas can be troublesome.

SUMMARY

The provision of anesthesia for the patient undergoing laparoscopic day surgery entails the taking on of new perioperative risks for postoperative benefits, especially in the case of older patients with more complex problems who undergo stimulating upper abdominal manipulation. As more prospective, controlled outcome data are generated for these patients, it may become possible to use sophisticated invasive intraoperative monitoring and still consider the patient eligible for same-day discharge.

Selected Readings

1. Beebe D, Swica H, Carlson N, et al. High levels of carbon monoxide are produced by electrocautery of tissue during laparoscopic cholecystectomy. Anesth Analg 1993;77:338.
2. Couture J, Chartrand D, Gagner M, et al. Diaphragmatic and abdominal muscle activity after endoscopic cholecystectomy. Anesth Analg 1994;78:733.
3. Cunningham AJ, Brull S. Laparoscopic cholecystectomy: anesthetic implications. Anesth Analg 1993;76:1120.
4. Cunningham AJ, Turner J, Rosenbaum S, et al. Transesophageal echocardiographic assessment of haemodynamic function during laparoscopic cholecystectomy. Br J Anaesth 1993;70:621.
5. Frazee RC, Roberts JW, Okeson GC, et al. Open versus laparoscopic cholecystectomy—a comparison of postoperative pulmonary function. Ann Surg 1991;213:651.
6. Jakeways MSR, Mitchell V, Hashim IA, et al. Metabolic and inflammatory responses after open or laparoscopic cholecystectomy. Br J Surg 1994;81:127.
7. Joris J. Anesthetic management of laparoscopy. In: Miller R, ed. Anesthesia. Vol II. 4th ed. New York, Churchill Livingstone, 1993:2011.
8. Joris J, Noirot D, Legrand M, et al. Hemodynamic changes during laparoscopic cholecystectomy. Anesth Analg 1993;76:1067.
9. Lister D, Rudston-Brown B, Warriner C, et al. Carbon dioxide absorption is not linearly related to intraperitoneal carbon dioxide insufflation pressure in pigs. Anesthesiology 1994;80:129.
10. McLaughlin JG, Bonnell BW, Scheeres DE, et al. The adverse hemodynamic effects related to laparoscopic cholecystectomy. Anesthesiology 1992;77:A70.
11. Overdijk L, Rademaker B, Ringers J, et al. Laparoscopic fundoplication: a new technique with new complications? J Clin Anesth 1994;6:321.
12. Putensen-Himmer G, Putensen C, Lammer H, et al. Comparison of postoperative respiratory function after laparoscopy or open laparotomy for cholecystectomy. Anesthesiology 1992;77:675.
13. Rademaker B, Ringers J, Odoom J, et al. Pulmonary function and stress response after laparoscopic cholecystectomy: comparison with subcostal incision and influence of thoracic epidural analgesia. Anesth Analg 1992;75:381.
14. Wahba RWM. Ventilatory requirements during laparoscopic cholecystectomy. Can J Anaesth 1993;40:206.
15. Wilcox S, Vandam LD. Alas, poor Trendelenburg and his position! A critique of its uses and effectiveness. Anesth Analg 1988;67:574.
16. Wittgen C, Andrus C, Fitzgerald S, et al. Analysis of the hemodynamic and ventilatory effects of laparoscopic cholecystectomy. Arch Surg 1991;126:997.

19

Evaluation and Monitoring of the Patient

PART I
Preoperative Evaluation of Outpatients

William T. Ross, Jr. • James Thomas Cox

Few aspects of ambulatory surgery are more important than the preoperative evaluation. Not only is preoperative evaluation relevant to surgical and anesthetic outcome but also the patients' perceptions of the success of surgery are influenced through preoperative assessment. Patients may arrive on the day of surgery with anxiety related to anticipated operative pain, fear of untoward complications, and concern about anesthetic side effects. The goals of the preoperative evaluation go beyond merely classifying a patient's physical status. Preoperative visits, whether in the surgeon's office, in a structured preoperative setting, or upon arrival on the day of surgery, provide surgeons and anesthesiologists opportunities to obtain informed consents, to allay patient concerns regarding surgery and anesthesia, to ascertain the patient's current medical condition, and to gather indicated historical and laboratory data. Preoperative evaluation is essential if the patient is to undergo a safe, uneventful outpatient surgical procedure. This chapter outlines important aspects of the preoperative evaluation for anesthesia, including patient assessment, the appropriate use of preoperative screening tests, and preoperative patient education.

PATIENT ASSESSMENT

Schemes for preoperative assessment programs vary from a limited history and physical examination on the morning of surgery to a more formal evaluation by either an anesthesiologist or nurse practitioner before the day of surgery. Each ambulatory surgical center should institute a standardized preoperative evaluation protocol based on its particular needs to ensure an effective and efficient preoperative assessment. At the Virginia Ambulatory Surgery Center (VASC), patients complete a Health Assessment Questionnaire in the surgeon's office or clinic at the time the decision for surgery is made. Patients provide information on current drug therapy, allergies, medical history, and previous surgical procedures, and they give a systems review. This is not a substitute for a skillful history and physical examination, but rather a means to facilitate patient data accumulation.

Oral Intake Status

Traditionally, patients have been instructed to take nothing by mouth after midnight before the day of surgery. From a clinical standpoint, this is a simple, effective way to ensure adequate fasting before elective surgery. Over the past several years, as the understanding of gastrointestinal physiology has improved, this practice has undergone modification in many centers. Our practice is to have adult patients take no solid food after midnight before the day of surgery. Clear liquids are allowed up to 3 hours before surgery, thus permitting patients their morning tea or coffee. The addition of cream to the coffee is not encouraged, but studies by Roger Maltby indicate that the amount of particulate matter from cream is inconsequential and should not preclude or delay surgery if taken more than 3 hours before anesthesia. In fact, several ounces of water 30 minutes to 3 hours before surgery may promote gastric emptying and increases gastric pH. Prudence suggests that patients with known delays in gastric emptying (e.g., patients with hiatal hernia, gastroesophageal reflux, diabetes with gastroparesis, central nervous system [CNS] disease) should have a minimum preoperative fast of 8 hours and not take clear liquids during this time.

Personal Support

Regardless of the operative procedure or the type of anesthesia, the patient should not drive home. A designated driver (usually a friend or family member) should be identified by the surgical facility staff during the preoperative interview.

Physical Status

Patient assessment begins with the history and physical examination, which provides the anesthesiologist with information to determine the patient's physical status using the American Society of Anesthesiologists (ASA) classification. The ASA physical status designations are given in Chapter 9 as part of preoperative assessment criteria.

Historically, only patients with ASA classifications of 1 or 2 were considered appropriate candidates for ambulatory surgery. With the accrued knowledge of expanding and evolving ambulatory surgery practices, patients with more significant systemic disease (i.e., ASA 3 and 4) may undergo surgery in the ambulatory setting. For these patients, the objective is to determine whether the patient's disease process is stable and under adequate control.

Commonly Encountered Disease States

This section discusses several frequently encountered disease processes that may influence the risks and outcomes of ambulatory anesthesia and surgery. Important elements of the preoperative history, physical examination, and additional anesthetic concerns unique to these diseases are reviewed.

Diabetic Patient

The spectrum of diabetes ranges from well-controlled, diet-treated non–insulin-dependent diabetes mellitus to poorly controlled insulin-dependent diabetes mellitus. The history (including past medical records) and physical examination should identify sequelae of long-standing diabetes such as ischemic heart disease, cerebrovascular disease, peripheral neuropathy, or renal dysfunction. The most common cause of morbidity associated with diabetes is ischemic heart disease. Chest pain may not manifest as a symptom of myocardial ischemia in patients with long-standing diabetes; but, instead, they may have shortness of breath as their anginal equivalent.

Instructions given to diabetic patients regarding the use of medications the morning of surgery must be clear and concise. The patient taking oral hypoglycemics should be instructed to forgo the morning dose on the day of surgery. Oral hypoglycemics can produce hypoglycemia for many hours after the dose is given (e.g., up to 36 hours in the case of chlorpropamide). It is important to determine the blood sugar concentration of all diabetic patients upon their arrival for surgery; this can be conveniently accomplished when the intravenous line is established by testing a single drop of blood with a glucose meter. We suggest that the insulin-dependent diabetic patient be instructed to bring insulin on the morning of surgery. One half the normal morning insulin dose may then be given upon the patient's arrival at the ambulatory surgical center where intravenous dextrose can be provided if necessary. This may be especially important for patients traveling long distances for surgery or for those who have difficulty controlling their blood sugar. Ideally, diabetic patients should be scheduled for surgery early in the day to minimize prolonged fasting and interruptions to their regular medication and feeding schedules.

Cardiac Patient

With increasing acceptance of ambulatory surgery, the anesthesiologist and surgeon are challenged frequently by patients with significant coexisting cardiovascular disease. Patients with a history of cardiovascular disease may be considered candidates for ambulatory surgery. The challenge is to determine which patient is likely to experience perioperative myocardial ischemia. Coronary artery disease frequently coexists in patients with poorly controlled hypertension, diabetes mellitus, left ventricular hypertrophy, or a history of digoxin use; these patients have a substantial risk of experiencing perioperative myocardial ischemia. All information about a patient, including medical evaluations, objective data such as stress test results, echocardiogram reports, and results of cardiac catheterization, must be considered. Also important in the evaluation of such patients is an accurate assessment of their cardiovascular performance based on exercise tolerance. Typically, patients who are able to climb one flight of stairs without angina or dyspnea have adequate cardiorespiratory reserve to withstand the physiologic demands of anesthesia for many outpatient surgical procedures; those who cannot require additional evaluation.

Patients with a history of myocardial infarction present many difficulties to the evaluating physician. The history and physical examination should identify those patients with postinfarction symptoms of chest pain, arrhythmias, or congestive heart failure. Such findings may suggest the existence of "myocardium at risk," poorly preserved left ventricular function, or the potential for sudden death. All of these findings deserve further medical evaluation before elective surgery. The rate of perioperative reinfarction may be as high as 37%, when anesthesia and surgery follow the original infarction within 3 months. As indicated in Table 19–1 this incidence appears to stabilize at 5% to 6% once 6 months have elapsed.

It has been suggested that the anticipated physiologic impact of the surgical procedure should guide the preoperative selection of ambulatory surgery patients following myocardial infarction. A conservative viewpoint is to delay elective and outpatient surgical procedures for patients who have sustained a myocardial infarction until at least 6 months after the infarction.

In summary, patients with cardiovascular disease should be carefully evaluated before outpatient surgery. The anesthesiologist should be consulted early regarding patients with complex cardiac or medical histories. Patients determined to have well-managed, stable conditions without a myocardial infarction in the prior 6 months may be expected to tolerate outpatient surgery with little expectation of adverse perioperative events.

Patient With Pulmonary Disease

In patients with pulmonary disease (i.e., chronic obstructive pulmonary disease [COPD], asthma), the history and physical examination should disclose elements of conditions that are reversible. Both the incidence and severity of postoperative pulmonary complications are decreased with preoperative treatment of COPD. For example, a productive cough and symptoms consistent with infection should be treated with antibiotics. The use of β-agonists can enhance airflow when bronchospasm is observed preoperatively. Regular use

Table 19–1. Incidence of Perioperative Myocardial Reinfarction

Time Elapsed Since Prior Myocardial Infarction (mo)	Tarhan, et al. (%)	Steen, et al. (%)	Rao, et al. (%)	Shah, et al. (%)
0–3	37	27	5.7	4.3
4–6	16	11	2.3	0
>6	5	6		5.7

of inhaled steroids can markedly improve airway function, help control airway inflammation, and, often, help in preparing patients for surgery.

Additional medications encountered when evaluating pulmonary patients include anticholinergics, cromolyn, and theophylline. Anticholinergic agents such as ipratropium bromide or glycopyrrolate bromide can enhance bronchodilation by blocking muscarinic receptors in airway smooth muscle. The occurrence of peak bronchodilator effect at 15 to 30 minutes therefore makes them useful for preoperative administration. Cromolyn, although more commonly used in children for its anti-inflammatory effect, can be of added value in adults. The mechanism of action of cromolyn is undetermined, but is believed to include the inhibition of inflammatory chemical mediator release. Because cromolyn is of little benefit in treating bronchospasm once it has occurred, it should be part of the long-term management of asthma. Theophylline, once considered first-line treatment for asthma, is currently a secondary adjunct. Upon obtaining a history of theophylline use, it is helpful to obtain serum levels of the drug. Its potential side effects include cardiac dysrhythmias (potentiated by halothane inhalational anesthesia) and CNS stimulation. Systemic steroids may also be used in the management of asthma or severe COPD; however, the effects on wound healing and immunosuppression must be weighed against the beneficial effects on the airways. It is not logical to taper or discontinue effective, even aggressive, treatment of severe pulmonary disease (including asthma) with systemic steroids and other long-term agents in the immediate preoperative period. In addition, patients who have received steroid therapy in the previous 6 months may require supplemental "stress dose" steroids at the time of surgery.

Alternatives to general anesthesia in patients with severe COPD include regional block or local anesthesia with monitored sedation when surgery is superficial or when it involves the extremities. Preoperative instruction in incentive spirometry, breathing exercises, and aggressive perioperative pulmonary toilet are all parts of the care of patients with COPD.

Perhaps the most important advice a physician can give to surgical candidates with smoking-related COPD is to quit smoking well before surgery. Not only does the patient make a positive lifestyle change, but also the incidence of postoperative complications is decreased with cessation of cigarette smoking. Although reduced pulmonary complications of statistical significance are only demonstrated when smoking has been stopped for more than 8 weeks, the reduction of carbon monoxide (which has a half-life of 4 hours) and the decrease in airway reactivity attributed to smoking suggest that any abstinence from smoking is beneficial.

Geriatric Patient

Elderly persons are becoming a greater proportion of the population in the United States. Because of this demographic shift, it is expected that ambulatory surgery centers will be caring for increasing numbers of elderly patients. Although age alone should not be a criterion for restricting ambulatory surgery, a reasonable assessment of the patient's functional status (or "physiologic age") should be sought. In general, aged patients can be characterized as having decreased margins of reserve in organ function and consequently a decreased capacity for adaptation to the changes associated with anesthesia and surgery. Among other things, this may be reflected in prolonged elimination times of medications. Elderly patients often take multiple medications and the possibility of drug interactions must be appreciated by physicians assessing these patients.

In addition to assessment of drug therapy, a general assessment of the patient's nutritional status should be obtained. Elderly patients are prone to malnourishment, which can interfere with their ability to respond to surgical stress. In addition, the changes in body habitus that occur with aging require greater perioperative vigilance in preventing hypothermia. Dorsal kyphosis, which limits thoracic wall motion, may present as restrictive lung disease. Cardiovascular reserve is difficult to assess in inactive elderly patients. In addition, there is a decreased responsiveness of the aged cardiovascular system to stress. Finally, elderly patients often have multiple concurrent diseases that may need further evaluation and treatment.

Obese Patient

Obesity is the most common nutritional disorder in the United States. The definition of obesity is not uniform. Different medical organizations have attempted to define obesity objectively as a way to relate it to various morbidities. Insurance companies typically define obesity as body weight 20% above ideal weight and morbid obesity as twice ideal body weight. The body mass index (BMI) is useful in classifying patients based on weight and height and is calculated as:

$$BMI = \frac{Weight\ (kilograms)}{Height\ (meters)^2}$$

A normal BMI is 20 to 25. Outcome studies by Pasulka suggest that moderately overweight patients with a BMI of 26 to 29 have only minimally increased morbidity rates following inpatient surgery. However, those patients with a BMI of more than 30 demonstrate increased perioperative mortality, especially an increased incidence of postoperative infection.

Adverse changes associated with obesity affect metabolic function, cardiovascular performance, respiratory function, and hemostasis. Pulmonary function changes are manifested by a restrictive lung disease pattern and, in some patients, pulmonary hypertension. The pickwickian syndrome is a complicated form of obesity characterized by episodic somnolence and hypercapnia. These patients have respiratory acidosis, arterial hypoxemia, polycythemia, and pulmonary hypertension and may have associated right ventricular failure. Such patients (i.e., those with the full-blown syndrome) should be admitted for postoperative observation of their respiratory status. Generally, they will not be suitable for outpatient surgery if general anesthesia is required.

In addition to a greater incidence of postoperative wound infection, obese patients present significant risk for deep vein thrombosis (DVT) and subsequent pulmonary embolism. This is especially true for those with pulmonary hypertension. DVT prophylaxis should be strongly considered even though ambulatory surgical procedures are typically shorter in duration and are amenable to early postoperative ambulation.

Obese patients also present technical challenges during the conduct of anesthesia. Intravenous cannulation, blood pressure determination, and airway management are all more difficult. The airway of the obese patient is particularly prone to passive obstruction, thus appropriate precautions must be exercised during induction and following extubation. Provision of supplemental oxygen is the cornerstone of the management of obese patients.

In summary, the changes in body habitus associated with obesity are likely to increase morbidity and mortality in this patient population. No studies define what degree of obesity renders a patient unsuitable for outpatient surgery. Patients are not excluded from ambulatory surgery based solely on body weight. However, the physiologic impact of obesity on other organ systems and the anticipated physiologic stresses of anesthesia and surgery should be carefully evaluated when considering obese patients for ambulatory surgery.

Patient With Gastroesophageal Reflux Disease

No contraindications exist to general anesthesia in patients with gastroesophageal reflux disease (GERD). It is important, however, to identify those patients with GERD to select an appropriate anesthetic induction technique. Typically, a rapid sequence induction while maintaining cricoid pressure is often used in patients with a good airway who are judged to be easy to intubate. A rapid sequence induction reduces the risk of passive reflux and subsequent aspiration of gastric contents. At most institutions, premedication with H_2 antagonists or metoclopramide is not routine.

Physical Examination of the Airway

The physical examination of the upper airway is of utmost importance during the anesthetic preoperative evaluation. The anesthesiologist must ascertain whether difficulty with either ventilation by mask or with tracheal intubation is expected. Clues to a difficult laryngoscopy include a short, muscular neck, a receding mandible (this may be hidden in bearded men), protruding front upper incisors, and poor mandibular mobility. One simple maneuver used to evaluate patients for possible difficulty in laryngeal visualization is to have patients open their mouth and protrude the tongue. Mallampati has correlated the difficulty in laryngeal visualization with the examiner's ability to visualize the faucial pillars, soft palate, and uvula. Typically, when all three pharyngeal structures are visualized, laryngoscopic visualization of the glottic aperture is performed easily. When the examiner can visualize only the soft palate because the base of the tongue obstructs view of both the uvula and faucial pillars, then direct laryngoscopy more often provides inadequate glottic visualization.

The ability to align the laryngeal, pharyngeal, and oral axes should be assessed by evaluating cervical spine mobility and temporomandibular joint mobility. Documentation of loose, chipped, or missing teeth and the presence of dental prostheses (i.e., caps, permanent bridge) is important so that the postoperative discovery of dental abnormalities is not mistakenly attributed to damage occurring with laryngoscopy and tracheal intubation.

When laryngoscopy is anticipated to be difficult, the anesthesiologist may choose to proceed with an awake intubation (e.g., in patients unable to widely open their mouth following radical head and neck surgery and subsequent radiation therapy). The goals of an awake intubation are to maintain spontaneous respiration and laryngeal reflexes, thereby maintaining ventilation and airway protection. Intravenous, topical, or regional anesthesia is provided. Tracheal intubation may be facilitated by either blind nasal, fiberoptic, transillumination, or direct laryngoscopic assistance while the patient is awake.

PREOPERATIVE SCREENING TESTS

Historically, the preoperative medical assessment was based on a thorough patient interview and physical examination. However, with the advent of readily accessible laboratory testing, physicians began across-the-board preoperative laboratory screening as a routine. Recent outcome studies demonstrate little evidence to support extensive baseline preoperative laboratory studies to either change or predict outcome in healthy patients. Cost–benefit analyses provided by these studies suggest that preoperative laboratory tests are overused and contribute to increased medical care costs out of proportion to any benefit realized. The need to provide cost-efficient medical care combined with the realization that patient outcome is not influenced by screening test results has resulted in redefined standards for minimum preoperative screening studies. Current recommendations regarding the chest radiograph, electrocardiogram (ECG), and selected laboratory tests are discussed in this section.

Chest Radiograph. Several investigators have attempted to define the utility of a baseline preoperative chest radiograph (CXR). Sommerville retrospectively studied 797 patient records, of which 6% of preoperatively ordered CXRs identified clinically significant abnormalities. Older patients were more likely than younger patients to have these positive findings. Whereas 17% of patients older than 60 years old had important CXR findings, only 2% of patients younger than 60 years had abnormal radiographic findings. Other investigators report a similarly low incidence of radiographic abnormalities in otherwise healthy patients. In 1993, Archer and colleagues published results of a meta-analysis of the value of routine preoperative chest radiographs concluding that omitting the routine preoperative chest radiograph is justifiable in the absence of specific medical indications. The 12 studies in the analysis support the selective use of preoperative chest radiography.

Despite these studies, which indicate clinical evaluation of the patient alone should guide the decision to order a preoperative chest radiograph, a consensus group of representatives from several university hospitals currently suggests routine chest radiographs for patients aged 60 years and older.

Electrocardiogram. The ECG is used to identify and characterize electrical abnormalities of the cardiac cycle in patients with diseases such as hypertension, atherosclerotic peripheral vascular disease, diabetes mellitus, certain malignancies, collagen vascular disease, and electrolyte abnormalities. In patients with a history of heart disease, the ECG is useful in detecting previous transmural myocardial infarction or ongoing ischemia. However, the ECG is of limited value in uncovering occult ischemic heart disease. Based on the reasonable premise that older patients are more likely than younger patients to benefit from preoperative ECG screening, age has been proposed as a criterion for ordering a preoperative ECG. The guidelines for the American College of Physicians and the majority opinion of recently surveyed university hospitals both recommend that patients at increased risk for occult heart disease, men older than 40 years of age, and postmenopausal women (i.e., 50 years and older) all undergo screening preoperative ECGs.

Blood Counts. The complete blood count (CBC) is useful in identifying significant anemia in patients with poor nutrition and chronic disease. In addition, there are several subsets of patients that have a high prevalence of anemia in which a preoperative CBC is warranted. These patients include those who are institutionalized, elderly, pregnant with inadequate prenatal care, and recent immigrants from Third World countries, especially those with apparent malnutrition.

The recommendations for preoperative CBC screening vary among medical specialty organizations. The state of Maine has instituted practice parameters on an experimental basis that provide liability protection for those physicians who comply with certain designated practice standards. Maine's guidelines are the most inclusive and recommend a preoperative hematocrit for women aged 15 and older as well as men aged 50 and older. The Mayo Clinic requires a CBC for any patient 60 years and older and those needing a concurrent type and screen or crossmatch. We currently recommend that specific clinical indications rather than age should determine the need for a preoperative CBC.

Prothrombin Time, Partial Thromboplastin Time, and Bleeding Time. The utility of preoperative coagulation studies as screening tests to detect unsuspected bleeding disorders has never been validated. Currently, the American College of Physicians does not recommend such routine preoperative screening for patients without clinical evidence of a coagulopathy. Clinical indications include a personal or family history of a bleeding disorder; prolonged nosebleeds; excessive bleeding or bruising following injuries, dental extraction, or previous surgical procedures; possible liver disease; malnutrition; and malabsorption.

Bleeding time study is not routinely recommended. For patients requiring elective operations, aspirin should be discontinued 5 to 7 days before surgery. This is based on the fact that a single aspirin tablet inhibits thromboxane B_2 production for at least 5 days following ingestion. Studies indicate that preoperative aspirin ingestion prolongs bleeding time and increases operative blood loss depending on the nature of the surgical procedure. Many surgeons provide patients with a list of aspirin-containing medications to avoid during the week preceding surgery.

Serum Chemistry Analysis. Several medical organizations, including the state of Maine's, have specific indications for laboratory evaluation of serum creatinine and blood urea nitrogen in patients older than 60 years of age. We think specific clinical indications should determine the need for these tests, regardless of age.

Concurrent Medication Therapy and Coexisting Disease States. The indication for ordering many laboratory tests and preoperative screening studies stems from concurrent medication usage or coexisting disease. Specific drug therapies and selected disease states with suggested preoperative screening tests are listed in Table 19–2.

CONCLUSION

Thorough preoperative patient education facilitates an uneventful ambulatory surgical experience. Patients receiving complete, clear, and concise preoperative instruction are more prepared for surgery and usually present fewer problems involving unexpected delays. Important elements of preoperative patient education include instruction on status of oral

Table 19–2. Recommended Preoperative Screening Tests for Selected Medical Situations

Medical Condition	Preoperative Screening Tests
Cardiovascular disease	BUN, creatinine, CXR, ECG, Hgb
Pulmonary disease	CXR, ECG, possible ABG
Renal disease	Electrolytes, BUN, creatinine, Hgb, platelet count
Hepatic disease	PT, PTT, SGOT, alkaline phosphatase, platelet count
Diabetes	Electrolytes, platelet count, glucose, ECG, BUN, creatinine
Hypertension	ECG, BUN, creatinine, electrolytes with diuretic usage
Seizure disorder	Serum anticonvulsant level
Possible pregnancy	β-hCG
Steroid use	Blood glucose, platelet count
Use of Prior Test Results	
CXR	A chest radiograph showing normal results that was performed within 1 year of surgery can be used if there has been no intervening clinical event.
ECG	An ECG showing normal results that was performed within 6 months of surgery can be used if there has been no intervening clinical event.
Blood Tests	Tests performed within 6 weeks of surgery that show normal results can be used if there has been no intervening clinical event.

BUN = blood urea nitrogen; CXR = chest radiograph; ECG = electrocardiogram; Hgb = hemogloblin; ABG = arterial blood gas; PT = prothrombin time; PTT = partial thromboplastin time; SGOT = serum glutamic-oxaloacetic transaminase; β-hCG = β-human chorionic gonadotropin.

From University Hospital Consortium Technology Advancement Center. Technology Assessment: Routine Preoperative Diagnostic Evaluations. Oak Brook, IL, 1994.

intake and identification of a "responsible person" to provide postoperative assistance.

With increasing reliance on ambulatory surgery, physicians will be challenged to provide safe and effective care to patients with significant medical conditions. The key to continued successful outpatient surgery will rest on appropriate patient selection and thorough preoperative evaluation. A skillful history and physical examination provide a basis for preoperative anesthesia evaluation of surgical patients. Replacement of routine across-the-board screening tests with specific, clinically indicated preoperative tests provides cost-effective health care. With the focus on the patient interview, high-quality anesthesia and surgical care will be provided in the rapidly evolving medical environment.

Selected Readings

1. Archer C, Adrian RL, McGregor M. Value of routine preoperative chest X-rays: a meta-analysis. Can J Anaesth 1993;40(11):1022–1027.
2. Hollenberg M, Mangano DT, Browner WS, et al. Predictors of postoperative myocardial ischemia in patients undergoing noncardiac surgery. JAMA 1992; 268:205–209.
3. Mallampati SR, Gatt SP, Gugino LD, et al. A clinical sign to predict difficult tracheal intubation: a prospective study. Can Anaesth Soc J 1985;32:429–434.
4. Narr BJ, Hansen TR, Warner MA. Preoperative laboratory screening in healthy Mayo patients: cost-effective elimination of tests and unchanged outcomes. Mayo Clin Proc 1991;66:155–159.
5. Pasulka PS, Bistrian BR, Benotti PN, et al. The risks of surgery in obese patients. Ann Intern Med 1986;104:540.
6. Rao TLK, Jacobs EH, El-Etr AA. Reinfarction following anesthesia in patients with myocardial infarction. Anesthesiology 1983;59:499–505.
7. Shah KB, Kleinman BS, Sami H, et al. Reevaluation of perioperative myocardial infarction in patients with prior myocardial infarction undergoing noncardiac operations. Anesth Analg 1991;71:231–235.
8. Sommerville TE, Murray WB. Information yield from routine preoperative chest radiography and electrocardiography. S Afr Med J 1992;81(4):190–196.
9. State of Maine S.P. 495-L.D. 1333 Medical Liability Demonstration Project. Anesthesiology Specialty Practice Parameters and Risk Management Protocols. Department of Professional and Financial Regulation, Board of Registration in Medicine, 1991.
10. Steen PA, Tinker JH, Tarhan S. Myocardial reinfarction after anesthesia and surgery. JAMA 1978; 239:2566–2570.
11. Stoelting RK, Dierdorf SF, eds. Anesthesia and Co-Existing Disease. 3d ed. New York: Churchill-Livingstone, 1993.
12. Tarhan S, Moffitt EA, Taylor WF, et al. Myocardial infarction after general anesthesia. JAMA 1972; 220:1451–1454.
13. University Hospital Consortium Technology Advancement Center. Technology Assessment: Routine Preoperative Diagnostic Evaluations. Oak Brook, 1994.
14. Warner MA, Divertie MB, Tinker JH. Preoperative cessation of smoking and pulmonary complications in coronary artery bypass graft patients. Anesthesiology 1984;60:380–383.
15. Wetchler BV, ed. Anesthesia for Ambulatory Surgery. 2d ed. Philadelphia: JB Lippincott, 1991.

PART II
Postoperative Monitoring and Evaluation

Kenneth Haspel

The ambulatory surgical center, whether freestanding or affiliated with an inpatient facility, must have a postanesthesia care unit (PACU), a specialized unit devoted to monitoring, evaluating, and giving treatment to patients as they recover from the effects of anesthesia and surgery. Patient safety is paramount; comfort, convenience, and cost are additional issues that must be considered as the individual makes the transition from the operating room to discharge. This is especially true as more complete procedures are being performed on outpatients. Patients with more severe underlying disease processes [American Society of Anesthesiologists (ASA) class III and IV] are undergoing outpatient surgery, and previously held restrictions on ambulatory surgery for the very young and old are falling by the wayside. These trends will continue, necessitating appropriate preoperative assessment, intraoperative management, and vigilant postoperative care in a specialized environment to ensure that these changes in practice patterns are safe for the patient.

DESIGN AND STAFFING OF THE POSTANESTHESIA CARE UNIT

Specific requirements for the design of a PACU have been published and should be consulted. Two key elements of design are to provide an appropriate amount of space for recovery room beds with an acceptable ratio of recovery beds to operating rooms. This ratio depends on the number of operating theaters and immediacy of patient needs. Generally, the ratio is between 1:1.25 and 1:1.6, operating rooms to recovery bays. There should be a recovery lounge where patients can be closely observed by nursing personnel for a period of time after leaving their bed before discharge

home. The patient can take fluid by mouth or void in this setting, important factors to assess in determining readiness for discharge. Discharge from the recovery room bed to home is neither convenient nor acceptable in most cases. Space must be allocated for a pharmacy and a basic laboratory if the PACU is not adjacent to an inpatient facility. There is usually a provision for plain film radiologic studies. Planning must include an appropriate number of electrical outlets with a rating sufficient to handle the load of modern medical technologic equipment.

Each PACU bed must have a wall source of oxygen and oxygen delivery system. Measuring pulse oximetry has become the standard of care in the postoperative setting and there should be monitoring for each patient. There should be a continuous electrocardiogram (ECG), preferably with the provision for multiple lead display. Additionally, many modern monitors can provide ST segment and arrhythmia analysis. A monitor for the display of invasive pressure measurements should be available. The blood pressure must be checked regularly (automatic cuffs are widely used). In the PACU, there should be a nerve stimulator and there must be provision to monitor body temperature. A fully stocked "code cart" and a defibrillator are essential.

The key to a well-run PACU is to have a high-quality nursing staff. To provide safe, competent care, nurses should have an appropriate patient load (no more than 1:3 in the outpatient setting, with a lower ratio if they are caring for "higher acuity" patients). A dedicated physician designated as medical backup for the PACU (almost always an anesthesiologist) should be immediately available as should adequate ancillary medical staff (i.e., respiratory therapists and laboratory and radiology technicians).

ADMISSION

All patients undergoing surgical procedures, regardless of the type of anesthesia, should be evaluated before discharge home from the PACU. Occasionally, a young healthy patient will have a superficial procedure under a field block and will require minimal assessment before discharge, but most patients warrant a formal admission to the PACU.

Patients receiving sedation, regional or general anesthetic should be transported to the PACU by the anesthetist involved with the case as well as a member of the surgical team. On arrival, the anesthetist should provide a complete summary of the patient's past history, especially any active medical problems. A list of medications, their doses and when they were last taken, when the patient last took anything by mouth (NPO status), allergies—especially to medications and the type of reaction that ensued (e.g., rash, anaphylaxis)—and past anesthetic history should be conveyed. The anesthetist should detail the type of procedure and anesthetic technique and elaborate specifically on any airway difficulties if they have occurred. A summary of intravenous fluids given and estimated blood loss should be provided with any relevant preoperative or intraoperative laboratory values.

The anesthetist details any specific concerns or problems intraoperatively (e.g., bronchospasm, hypotension, arrhythmia) and relays to the PACU personnel a report on the anticipated recovery course. There should be documentation of when the last pain medication was given and the doses required. Before the anesthetist leaves, the PACU should be informed of the location of the anesthesia and surgical teams involved with the care of the patient in case problems arise. Supplemental oxygen should be provided to all appropriate patients before their arrival at the PACU.

Vital signs are recorded, including heart rate, blood pressure, and respiratory rate. Patients should have continuous ECG monitoring, pulse oximetry, and temperature monitoring. Vital signs should be recorded at regular intervals, usually every 5 minutes for the first 15 minutes and then every 15 minutes unless clinical circumstances warrant more frequent appraisal. A more specific assessment should be done if there is any reason to anticipate difficulty in the recovery room (i.e., "sleepy" patients, or patients typed ASA III or IV), with continued vigilance to the status of the patient being the key to a safe recovery. If a regional block was performed, an assessment of sensory and motor function is essential. The affected limbs must be protected from accidental injury, and positioning with particular reference to pressure points is needed.

AIRWAY ASSESSMENT

Frequent assessment of the airway is needed because it is common that the stimulation provided by moving a patient from the operating room to the PACU is sufficient to maintain an airway; however, as the stimulation subsides, the patient may become resedated and hypoventilate or the airway may become obstructed. It is unlikely that the ambulatory patient will be brought to the PACU intubated, but this does occasionally occur. Careful observation of the patient provides much information (Table 19–3). A good oximeter reading should not be used as sole evidence of an adequate airway. Supplemental oxygen is routinely prescribed for postoperative patients; thus, significant hypoventilation can be seen with an acceptable oxygen saturation. The patient should be observed, with focus on the respiratory rate and pattern. There should be good chest movement with respiration, implying an adequate tidal volume is being generated. There should not be discordant chest movement (rocking) and accessory muscle use, and there should be no evidence of upper airway obstruction (e.g., snoring, "tugging"). If there is evidence of upper airway obstruction, simple maneuvers such as extension of the neck or a jaw thrust often resolve the obstruction, but the necessity of these inter-

Table 19–3. Airway Assessment

Patient stimulation may be sufficient to maintain an airway.
  Lack of stimulation may lead to resedation or
    hypoventilation and obstruction.
Pulse oximetry is not a monitor of ventilation.
Respiratory rate and pattern are extremely important.
Jaw thrust frequently relieves obstruction.
Cause of obstruction should be determined.

ventions identifies this patient as one who will require close observation. If simple interventions do not resolve an obstructed airway, providing a lubricated nasal or oral airway may suffice. The physician must be satisfied that the airway is secured; if not, the physician must remain with the patient.

It is important to determine whether the cause for airway obstruction is anatomic, due to residual drug effect, a combination of the two, or perhaps an indicator of a more ominous situation (e.g., stroke). The most common cause is residual sedation from intraoperative medication; thus, it may be desirable to carefully titrate a specific narcotic antagonist (e.g., naloxone, 40 μg boluses) or a benzodiazepine receptor antagonist (e.g., flumazenil, 0.2 mg boluses) to effect. The patient must be observed closely to confirm improvement. The half-life of the antagonist may be shorter than that of the drug that it antagonizes, so resedation must be observed. Overzealous use of these antagonists may precipitate the arousal of an agitated patient in a great deal of pain. Naloxone may precipitate myocardial ischemia or narcotic withdrawal in predisposed patients. Therefore, it must be used carefully and cautiously (see Chapter 15).

ASSESSMENT OF CIRCULATION

Adequacy of circulation and end-organ perfusion can usually be confirmed by observation. A patient who is awake and alert, who has good color and warm extremities, and who makes urine is perfusing adequately. This patient is not frequently seen on admission to the PACU. Observing that the patient appears to have a good mental status implies adequate perfusion of the brain, but anesthetic drugs frequently cloud the sensorium even with perfectly adequate perfusion. Blood pressure should be obtained on arrival in the PACU, with the expectation that values will be within 20% of preoperative values. In the initial assessment, hypotension is generally of more concern than hypertension, but either extreme is unacceptable and often requires treatment. In addition to the blood pressure, the heart rate and rhythm must be observed. A

three-lead ECG should be applied to allow continuous monitoring of rate and rhythm.

TEMPERATURE

Patients returning from the operating room are frequently cold. The frequency of temperature monitoring is dictated by the initial measurement and the condition of the patient, but often measurements at admission and discharge suffice. Hypothermia is a more common problem than hyperthermia. Heat loss is an especially critical issue with pediatric patients. Most heat lost from the patient in the operating room occurs by radiation (approximately 60%). Conduction and convection do not contribute greatly to intraoperative heat loss, but evaporative heat loss (via the skin and lungs) accounts for approximately 25% of the heat lost by patients. Some additional factors intraoperatively that contribute to hypothermia include the relatively cool temperature of most operating rooms, the use of nonwarmed intravenous or irrigation fluids, and the changes in heat production due to decreased body metabolism while the patient is under anesthesia. The best strategy regarding hypothermia is prevention. Given the large heat loss from radiation, heating the operating room is the best prevention for heat loss, especially until the patient is covered with surgical drapes.

NEUROLOGIC ISSUES

When regional anesthetic technique is used, an initial assessment of the level of the block is made with an attempt to differentiate the degree of sensory and motor blockade. A motor block generally recedes before a sensory block, which resolves before autonomic function or proprioception returns to normal. This is attributable to the type of local anesthesia used. It is therefore possible that the affected limbs may have return of motor function without sensory function. The patient could move the limb but not have sensation, increasing the likelihood of damage to the affected extremity. There may be pressure points that could impair perfusion to the limb or result in unacceptable traction on the neurovascular bundle. The limb must be safely protected and positioned until there is a return of sensory function.

MONITORS

The most effective "monitor" is an attentive, experienced health care provider (nurse or physician). Increasingly, highly technical equipment is relied on to provide clinical information. Several monitoring devices have proven to be invaluable and the current standard of care dictates their routine use.

Pulse Oximeter

Oximetry has found widespread application in the health care environment. It is a relatively cheap, noninvasive, reliable technique that is easy to use, is well tolerated by patients, and provides real-time evaluation of important clinical information. The pulse oximeter uses two light-emitting diodes (LEDs) at 660 nM and 940 nM with a detector to determine arterial oxygen saturation. Different forms of hemoglobin absorb light at different wavelengths. At 660 nM, deoxyhemoglobin absorbs approximately 10 times as much light as oxyhemoglobin. At 940 nM, the other wavelength of light used in the oximeter probe, oxyhemoglobin absorbs more light than deoxyhemoglobin. The second principle upon which pulse oximetry is based is that absorbance of light at these wavelengths has a pulsatile (AC) component due to the arterial pulsations in the vascular bed between the light source and the detector (i.e., the finger) and a nonpulsatile (DC) component. Baseline absorbance (DC) represents absorbance of the tissue bed including venous and capillary blood. The pulse oximeter measures the AC and DC absorbance at 660 nM and 940 nM and then compares the respective ratios to calculate an R value. The R value thus determined can be compared with a previously determined calibration curve, and saturation is calculated.

Technical factors that may introduce error to this measurement come from the assumption that the light emitted is monochromatic.

The light is never truly monochromatic but is centered around the desired wavelength. The actual central wavelength shifts, thus introducing error due to the nonpulsating component (the venous component); thus, conditions with significant vasoconstriction or vasodilation that affect this component impair the accurate measurement of the oxygen saturation. Conditions associated with a decreased pulse amplitude (i.e., poor perfusion) make the instrument more sensitive to the influence of electronic (i.e., cautery) or physiologic (i.e., muscle artifact) noise.

A pulse oximeter measures pulse amplitude based on the assumption that the only forms of hemoglobin contributing to light absorption are oxyhemoglobin and deoxyhemoglobin. The presence of carboxyhemoglobin introduces an error of approximately 1% for every 10% of carboxyhemoglobin; thus, a patient could have serious carbon monoxide poisoning in the setting of a normal oximeter reading. Methemoglobulinemia gives an oximeter reading of 85%. The presence of significant anemia or sickle cell disease affects the measured oxygen saturation to a small degree.

Blood Pressure

Blood pressure is a fundamental physiologic measurement; yet, there is controversy as to how it should be measured. A variety of noninvasive methods have been developed, with the auscultation of Korotkoff sounds being the most common. The systolic blood pressure is taken as the reading at which the first muffled sounds are heard as the cuff is slowly deflated. This has been shown to correlate with directly measured systolic pressure (within 10 mm Hg) 84% of the time. The correlation with a directly measured diastolic blood pressure is not nearly as good, occurring 56% of the time (within 10 mm Hg). It is difficult to know whether diastolic pressure should be taken at the point of the muffling of sound, which is usually 3 to 4 mm Hg above measured diastolic, or at the disappearance of sound, which is approximately 7 mm Hg below directly measured diastolic blood pressure.

A crucial assumption is made that the cuff

size chosen is correct when one refers to these measurements. The cuff width should be approximately 40% of the circumference of the limb or 65% of the length of the limb. A cuff that is too small yields an artificially elevated reading as does an appropriately sized cuff that is loosely applied. Conversely, too large a cuff gives an artificially low reading.

Automatic blood pressure cuffs have become common. A piezoelectric crystal is used with a microprocessor to detect the motion of the vessel wall as an occluding pressure is applied and then slowly released. The point where the vessel wall begins to move as blood flows through it is taken as the systolic pressure, with the point of maximal vessel wall oscillation generally viewed as the mean arterial pressure. The diastolic pressure is a calculated number based on these measured values. This method relies on the detection of small movements. Therefore, motion artifact can be troublesome with this method. Prolonged cuff inflation times can be uncomfortable to an awake patient and may occlude an intravenous line in the arm.

Direct measurement of the blood pressure with an intra-arterial catheter is rarely used for ambulatory surgery.

Electrocardiography

In the PACU setting, a bipolar three-lead system to view the standard limb leads (with an additional precordial lead if the index of suspicion for ischemia is high) is standard. Continuous display of a single lead should be routine.

COMMON POSTOPERATIVE PROBLEMS

Hypoxemia and Hypoventilation

A small decrease in arterial oxygen saturation in the early postoperative period is common. Oxygen saturation below 90% occurs 30% of the time. A more significant decrease (<85%) is observed up to 12% of the time. Both of these occur in healthy patients (ASA I and II) and are not associated with any nega-

tive sequelae. Although there are no studies to confirm the need for supplemental oxygen, it seems prudent to supply oxygen nonetheless. Desaturation is especially common in certain patient populations such as in obese patients or those with a history of asthma; thus, a recommendation can be made that supplemental oxygen should be given to all patients after general anesthesia and in most cases should be done with intravenous sedation or regional anesthesia with sedation. Patients with a history of coronary artery disease are especially vulnerable to desaturation. These patients constitute a class of individuals who should always receive supplemental oxygen. Use of supplemental oxygen should be waived only if it is specifically directed by the anesthesiologist.

The most common cause of hypoventilation and hypoxemia is depression of the respiratory drive due to the residual effects of anesthetic agents. Respiration is stimulated by the decrease in the pH of the cerebrospinal fluid (CSF) due to the rapid diffusion of carbon dioxide into the CSF.

Anesthetic medications, including inhalational agents, benzodiazepines (in conjunction with other medications), and, in particular, narcotics, shift the carbon dioxide response curve of the respiratory center. Hypoventilation is thus commonly observed even with minimal levels of medication. Additionally, the carotid body is responsive to the arterial PaO_2 and increases afferent neural input to the respiratory center, stimulating the drive to breathe if the PaO_2 is less than 60. Very low concentrations of inhalational agents completely blunt this response. The effects of these depressant agents is additive. Even with new, potent, short-acting medications, once noxious stimulation is removed, a degree of resedation is almost uniform. This must be anticipated, monitored, and, if needed, treated in the PACU.

In addition to pharmacologically induced respiratory depression, intraoperative changes in lung mechanics contribute to hypoxemia. Within minutes of the induction of general anesthesia, there is a decrease in functional residual capacity (FRC) due to a decrease in the normal elastic recoil of the chest wall. Microatelectasis then develops, further decreasing compliance and altering the ventilation perfusion ratio of lung units. A critical factor that may contribute to increased airway resistance is upper airway obstruction due to the position of the tongue or laryngospasm. Obstruction at the level of medium-sized airways, seen as bronchospasm, may be precipitated by any number of causes. Occasionally, hypoxemia or hypercarbia is observed because of a hypermetabolic state such as sepsis or shivering (where $\dot{V}_{O_2}$ max increases 300%–500%), but these diagnoses should be obvious (Table 19–4).

After general anesthesia, an important potential cause of hypoventilation is residual muscle weakness due to neuromuscular blocking drugs used intraoperatively. This is seen when the wrong muscle relaxant was chosen (there is probably no place for long-acting agents such as pancuronium in the outpatient setting), an insufficient amount of time has elapsed since reversal agents were given (reversal may take 30 minutes if only a single twitch was seen on train-of-four stimulation), or a low dose of reversal agent was given. Return of function should be assessed with a nerve stimulator intraoperatively; however, use of a nerve stimulator in the PACU can be very painful and judicious use is suggested. There are clinical guidelines to judge reversal of blockade. The patient can be asked to squeeze the examiner's hand or cough, a very subjective gauge of strength. The best clinical predictor of adequate muscle strength is a sustained head lift for more than 5 seconds. A measured vital capacity should be at least 10 to 12 mL/kg and if measured, the negative inspiratory force should be more than 25 mm Hg. All clinical indicators should confirm adequate muscle strength in order to protect the airway and permit gas exchange. The clinician must

Table 19–4. Hypoxemia and Hypoventilation

Pulse oximetry is not a monitor of ventilation.
Most common cause is due to residual anesthetics and narcotics.
Normal stimulators of ventilation are blunted easily and quickly by many drugs.
Changes in lung mechanics secondary to general anesthesia include decreased functional residual capacity, atelectasis, and upper airway obstruction.
Hypermetabolism can lead to decreased PaO_2.
Residual muscle relaxation may contribute to both.

be aware of factors that make residual blockade more likely. The metabolism or clearance of these drugs may be slowed by renal or hepatic disease, hypothermia (which prolongs the action of relaxants), electrolyte disturbances (e.g., acute hypokalemia, hypermagnesemia, hypocalcemia), acid-base status (respiratory acidosis makes antagonism more difficult), and other drugs (e.g, aminoglycoside antibiotics potentiate nondepolarizing muscle relaxants; local anesthetics augment neuromuscular blockade). Some patients (e.g., those with myasthenia gravis, muscular dystrophy, Eaton-Lambert syndrome) are extremely sensitive to the effects of muscle relaxants.

Hypotension

Hypotension is best defined in clinical terms as a blood pressure less than 80% of the patient's "normal" pressure or a low blood pressure with evidence of inadequate end organ perfusion. The clinician should not focus on a particular number but more on the overall clinical picture. A young healthy patient can almost certainly tolerate a blood pressure considerably less than 80% of the preoperative value, whereas an elderly patient with vascular disease may not tolerate a decrease in blood pressure of this magnitude. In the PACU, hypotension is almost always attributable to either relative hypovolemia or to the effect of administered drugs. There are other less common but important causes for hypotension such as heart failure (due to ischemia, arrhythmia, valve incompetence), impaired venous return (e.g., tension pneumothorax after central line placement in the operating room, supine positioning of the pregnant patient), a drug reaction, or pulmonary embolus (e.g., clot, air, fat). These cases, although less common, must be ruled out quickly.

Hypotension due to hypovolemia is not always accompanied by signs of sympathetic activation (e.g., tachycardia, cool extremities). Numerous perioperative factors may contribute to hypovolemia in this setting including a preoperative fast, bowel prep, or intraoperative blood or fluid loss (e.g., ascites). Inadequately replaced fluid loss or third space losses secondary to tissue manipulation and dissection contribute greatly to hypovolemia.

Hypotension is commonly caused by drugs given in the perioperative period. Induction agents often cause decreased vascular resistance, direct myocardial depression, or decreased sympathetic outflow, and similar effects are seen with inhalational agents. Depending on the dosages and the length of the surgical procedure, the effects of these drugs may persist into the postoperative period. Furthermore, narcotics and benzodiazepines may cause peripheral vasodilation. The hypotensive effects of these classes of drugs are synergistic. Other drugs administered perioperatively (e.g., droperidol, Dilantin, vancomycin) may also contribute to hypotension.

If the degree of hypotension warrants treatment, it should be directed at the underlying cause. In most cases, a small, rapidly infused fluid bolus with crystalloid clarifies the diagnosis and is therapeutic. Pharmacologic support of the blood pressure must address the underlying cause of the hypotension. In most cases, if hypotension persists despite adequate blood volume repletion, a relative low-tone state exists and an alpha-agonist (i.e., phenylephrine titrated to effect) is appropriate therapy. Treatment of other causes of hypotension must address the cause (e.g., ischemia treated with nitrates with or without beta-blockers), not just the symptom—the low blood pressure (Table 19–5).

Hypertension

Elevated blood pressure is also commonly seen in the PACU. It is usually a transient phenomenon, but, left untreated, it may be prolonged and have detrimental effects (e.g., increased bleeding, congestive heart failure, myocardial ischemia in the susceptible patient). It is vitally important not to overlook other potentially dangerous causes of hypertension such as hypoxemia, hypercarbia, or elevated intracranial pressure. These are diagnoses that would warrant immediate treatment directed at the underlying cause. After ruling out the common and potentially life-threatening causes of an elevated blood pressure, less common explanations such as bladder distention or shivering should be entertained.

Pain and anxiety or arousal on emergence from anesthesia are the most common causes of postoperative hypertension. The diagnosis is easily made and treated, usually with calm reassurance and a small dose of short-acting narcotic (e.g., fentanyl, 25–100 μg intravenously) or benzodiazepine (e.g., midazolam, 0.5–2.0 mg intravenously) titrated to effect. Because NPO is a standard instruction perioperatively, many patients do not take their regularly prescribed antihypertensive medication. Rebound hypertension, especially if the patient is on a beta-blocker or clonidine, can be seen as a result. Restarting the appropriate class of drug is usually all that is needed.

Treatment of postoperative hypertension is directed at the underlying cause. In the PACU, commonly used drugs for blood pressure control include nifedipine S/L, 10 to 20 mg; labetalol, 5 to 40 mg intravenously; propranolol, 0.5 to 5 mg intravenously; and furosemide, 5 to 40 mg intravenously. If rapid, readily titratable blood pressure control is needed, a nitroglycerin (20–200 μg/min) or nitroprusside (5–200 μg/min) infusion can be started, although, if this is deemed necessary, an intra-arterial line for blood pressure monitoring should be introduced and serious consideration for overnight admission to the hospital must be made (Table 19–6).

Myocardial Ischemia

Many patients undergoing outpatient surgery have significant coronary artery disease. In some of these patients, perioperative ischemia may develop, which must be quickly recognized and treated. A high index of suspicion with continuous monitoring of a precordial lead, usually V_5, goes a long way to achieving

Table 19–5. Hypotension

Definition: Greater than 20% decrease from patient's normal blood pressure or decreased blood pressure with evidence of inadequate organ perfusion
Causes
    Hypovolemia—most common cause
    Drug induced
    Cardiogenic (ischemia, arrhythmia)
    Impaired venous return

Table 19–6. Common Causes of Postoperative Hypertension

Life threatening causes
Hypoxemia
Hypercapnia
Elevated intracranial pressure
Less life threatening causes
Bladder distention
Shivering
Pain
Anxiety and arousal
Failure to take prescribed medications

these goals. The clinician must not rely solely on symptoms to diagnose myocardial ischemia in the postoperative setting. "Silent" ischemia is common, particularly when the residual effects of anesthetic agents or narcotics may cloud the sensorium of the patient. In addition, it may be difficult for the patient to distinguish ischemic discomfort from that due to the surgical procedure. In patients with a history of coronary artery disease, a postoperative 12-lead ECG should be considered. The threshold for performing such a test should be low. This recommendation must be tempered with the fact that "minor" ECG changes (especially T wave changes) are common and are frequently not due to ischemia but may be due to factors such as electrolyte disturbances, low temperature, or lead positioning (bandages sometimes cover usual lead locations). If ischemia is suspected, it should be treated by controlling hemodynamics and instituting specific anti-ischemic therapies. A patient thought to have had perioperative ischemia should not be discharged home without formal assessment.

Hypothermia

A mild degree of hypothermia is common in the early postoperative period after general anesthesia. Anesthetic agents depress the threshold for triggering thermoregulatory vasoconstriction, usually to 33°C to 35°C, but, once activated, the intensity is unaltered. There may be benefits to mild hypothermia, such as lengthening the "safe" length of ischemia before tissue damage secondary to reduced oxygen requirements for cellular function at a lower temperature. The disadvan-

tages, however, are typically of more clinical relevance. These include a large increase in oxygen requirements (up to 500% increase) and a large increase in minute ventilation and cardiac output seen if the patient shivers, as well as the increased pain and suture line stress that accompanies shivering. Other detrimental features of hypothermia include an unpredictable lengthening of the duration of drug action due to reduced metabolism and clearance. Platelet dysfunction with hypothermia is well described, putting the patient at increased risk of bleeding complications. Pharmacologic treatment for shivering includes Demerol, 25 to 50 mg intravenously, or clonidine, 75 to 150 μg intravenously (not presently available in the U.S.).

The maintenance of normothermia should be a priority. Most (90%) heat is lost via the skin surface to the environment. The amount lost is proportional to the gradient between the body temperature and the ambient temperature; thus, warming the room is a practical measure. The skin surface should be kept completely covered except to provide surgical exposure. Active rewarming is only marginally successful, especially when interventions such as infrared lights or water mattresses are used. Forced air heaters have become widely available and can elevate core temperature by approximately 1.5°C per hour.

Mental Status Changes

Patients are rarely brought to the PACU "completely themselves" because of the changes that have occurred intraoperatively, including the administration of medications, a change in temperature or metabolic status, or the development of a significant problem perioperatively. The patient may be severely obtunded or agitated.

If obtunded, the first priority of the medical staff must be attention to the "ABCs," or airway, breathing, circulation, with establishment of a secure airway and adequate ventilation. The specific treatment depends on the underlying cause of the decreased level of consciousness, but the importance of these basic tenets of resuscitation are paramount. The residual effect of anesthetic medication is the most common explanation for an obtunded patient, and the anesthesia record should be consulted with particular reference to the doses and time of most recent administration of narcotics, benzodiazepines, or other sedating medications, such as droperidol. If needed, a specific antagonist medication can be administered, although most commonly the patient must simply be observed postoperatively for a longer than routine length of time. A patient with residual neuromuscular paralysis usually appears weak rather than obtunded, but the presence of multiple medications may make this distinction difficult.

A nonpharmacologic cause of a decreased level of consciousness includes moderate to severe hypothermia, which can directly depress consciousness and prolong the action of some drugs. A variety of metabolic disturbances can explain obtundation including hypoglycemia, hyperglycemia, hypo-osmolality, electrolyte disturbances, and hypercarbia. A primary neurologic cause of a decreased level of consciousness should be considered if other causes have been ruled out. Increased intracranial pressure from any cause can manifest in this manner as it may in the patient with an intracranial hemorrhage or a thromboembolic event.

Agitated patients are often disruptive and can be a challenge to deal with in the PACU. In most cases, a straightforward cause such as pain or anxiety is obvious and easily treated. Hypoxemia as a cause of agitation must not be ignored. Diagnosis is facilitated with the use of pulse oximetry and should be seen infrequently if supplemental oxygen use in the PACU is routine.

Some patients have a true emergence delirium characterized by disorientation, agitation, restlessness, and moaning. This syndrome is more commonly seen in children and young adults. The common causes of delirium must be ruled out with a systematic assessment. Hypoxemia or significant hypotension with impaired cerebral perfusion should be immediately identified and treated. Easily treated causes of agitation include a distended bladder or the removal of restraints, which, in some people, worsens a situation more than helps. Metabolic derangements that may cause agitation include electrolyte abnormalities such as

hyponatremia seen with transurethral prostatic resection.

Agitation postoperatively is commonly due to medications such as phenothiazines, tricyclic antidepressants, benzodiazepines, and anticholinergic medication. A "central anticholinergic syndrome" has been described and is attributed to the central nervous system effects of anticholinergic medications, although other classes of drugs have also been implicated. Agitation and disorientation are common features. It occurs most commonly in the elderly patient and can often be treated successfully with pyridostigmine, 1 to 2 mg intravenously. Severe agitation due to other medications can often be dealt with by using a calm reassuring voice, especially by a family member, and giving frequent verbal reassurance. Pharmacologic treatment may be needed, with haloperidol being the drug of choice. This medication has a very high therapeutic ratio and can be titrated to effect. A starting dose is 0.5 to 1.0 mg intravenously with the dose doubled every 20 minutes until the desired sedation is achieved. Peak effect is after approximately 30 minutes, so it is important to give the drug adequate time to work before administering additional drug. The clinician should be aware of the potential extrapyramidal side effects occasionally seen when this drug is used (Table 19–7).

NAUSEA AND VOMITING

Postoperative nausea and vomiting is a significant problem. When intractable, it may result in admission to an inpatient facility, increased patient discomfort, and an increased

Table 19–7. Common Causes of Mental Status Changes

Hypoxia
Hypercarbia
Residual anesthetic agents (most common cause)
Metabolic disturbances
    Hyperglycemia
    Hypoglycemia
    Hypo-osmolality
    Hyponatremia
    Hepatic encephalopathy
Primary neurologic event
Bladder distention

risk of aspiration. It is important for the anesthetist to identify patients at high risk of nausea and vomiting preoperatively so that treatment is anticipated and initiated early. Subgroups of patients known to be at increased risk include those with a previous history of postoperative nausea and vomiting and a history of motion sickness. Younger patients, obese patients, and women are most likely to experience postoperative nausea and vomiting. In this group of patients, regional rather than general anesthesia should be considered when feasible. The type of surgical procedure also affects risk of nausea and vomiting. Strabismus surgery, middle ear surgery, orchiopexy, herniorraphy, and laparoscopic procedures are associated with higher than average risk of postoperative nausea and vomiting. In the high-risk patient, preoperative and intraoperative management should include antiemetics and adequate hydration. Care should be taken to move the patient slowly. An orogastric tube to empty the stomach is a practice of questionable utility.

Adequate analgesia, even if this requires narcotics, significantly reduces nausea and vomiting. In susceptible patients, consideration should be given to use of nonnarcotic analgesics. Ultimately, however, pain relief is the top priority. In addition to adequate pain relief, antiemetics should be liberally used. All phenothiazines and butyrophenones are antiemetics. The two most commonly used are droperidol, (0.625–1.25 mg intravenously) and prochlorperazine, 10 mg. Scopolamine patches have not been widely used in this setting. The newest class of drugs used that have proven to be very effective are the serotonergic drugs, with the most commonly used being ondansetron. Other techniques such as hypnosis or acupuncture may have utility in selected circumstances. Despite all efforts, intractable nausea and vomiting require admission approximately 2% of the time.

PAIN

Intravenous access is generally available in all but the most trivial procedures, and this route should be initially used to quickly control postoperative pain. Fentanyl, a potent analgesic with rapid onset, is commonly used (0.5–2.0 μg/kg as a starting dose) with titration to effect. Morphine (2.5–5.0 mg intravenously) can also be used, but its peak effect occurs 15 minutes after administration, and a drug with a more rapid onset of action is more appropriate for the patient in severe pain. A critical issue in the use of intravenous narcotics is the careful titration of small doses of medication at the bedside to obtain adequate analgesia without dangerous respiratory depression or a decreased level of consciousness.

In some settings, intravenous access is not reliable or the intravenous line has been discontinued in anticipation of discharge. If analgesia is needed, intramuscular medication (codeine, 1.0–1.5 mg/kg; morphine 0.05–0.1 mg/kg; or meperidine, 0.5–0.75 mg/kg) can be used. The oral route is an acceptable route of administration of medication if the patient can tolerate it. There are many potent oral analgesics (e.g., oxycodone preparations, meperidine), and most patients are discharged with a prescription for a drug of this class.

There is increasing recognition of the role that inflammation plays in pain. This has resulted in greater use of anti-inflammatory medications (e.g., nonsteroidal anti-inflammatory drugs such as acetaminophen, ketorolac) perioperatively, in addition to traditionally prescribed narcotic analgesics. These medications can be used as a primary treatment or in conjunction with narcotics, limiting the untoward and unwanted side effects.

Regional anesthesia is used in the outpatient setting and the residual effects of a dense block required for surgical anesthesia intraoperatively often result in continued perioperative analgesia that may be adequate for up to 24 hours, depending on the specific local anesthetic chosen by the anesthetist and the type of regional block used. The use of local blocks to supplement a general anesthetic has also become commonplace, especially in pediatrics, and usually results in very good postoperative pain relief.

SUMMARY

The economic and psychologic benefits of having patients undergo an outpatient surgical procedure with a rapid return to their normal surroundings are well accepted. The transition from the operating room to the PACU to discharge is a journey the outpatient must take under the watchful eye of the PACU staff. Successful transition is dependent on frequent assessment of the patient with attention paid to the potential problems commonly encountered in this setting with appropriate treatment initiated in a timely fashion.

Selected Readings

1. Breit SN, O'Rourke MF. Comparison of direct and indirect arterial pressure measurements in hospitalized patients. Aust N Z Med 1974;4:485.
2. Cromwell EB, Ketchum JS. The treatment of scopolamine induced delirium with physostigmine. Clin Pharmacol Ther 1967;8:409.
3. Cuss FM, Colaco CB, Bersh JB. Cardiac arrest after reversal of effects of opiates with naloxone. BMJ 1984;288:363.
4. Hudson RBS. Pattern of work in the recovery room. J Soc Med 1979;72:273.
5. Knill RL, Gelb AW. Ventilatory responses to hypoxemia and hypercapnia during naloxone sedation and anesthesia in man. Anesthesiology 1978;49:244.
6. Patel RI, Nannallah RS, Murphy LS, et al. Pediatric outpatient anesthesia. A review of post anesthetic complications in 8995 cases. Anesthesiology 1986;65:A435.
7. Sessler DI. Temperature regulation and anesthesia. ASA Refresher Course. 1993;153:1.
8. Tanaka G. Hypertensive reaction to naloxone. JAMA 1974;228:25.
9. Tremper KK, Berker SJ. Pulse oximetry. Anesthesiology 1989;70:98.
10. Tyler IL et al. Continuous monitoring of arterial oxygen saturation with pulse oximetry during transfer to the recovery room. Anesth Analg 1985;64:1108.
11. Willock MM, Willock GM. Design of the recovery room. In: Israel JS, Dekornfelt TJ, eds. Recovery Room Care. Chicago. Year Book Publishers, 1987.

Section

6

Procedures and Techniques for Ambulatory Surgery

BASIC GENERAL SURGERY

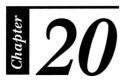

Head and Neck

Ranès C. Chakravorty

Recently, the percentage of surgical procedures done on a hospital inpatient basis has diminished significantly, primarily because many surgical procedures do not need hospital admission and because third-party payers give reimbursement incentives for ambulatory procedures. For the surgeon, however, safety of the patient is the primary concern.

The head and neck area comprises the skin and soft tissues of the head and neck, the upper portions of the respiratory and digestive tracts, and their glandular (exocrine and endocrine) derivatives. The eyes and the intracranial contents are generally excluded, as are problems of the vascular tree. Surgical problems here fall under the care of various groups of specialists such as general surgeons, otorhinolaryngologists, and plastic surgeons. This discussion focuses on the scope of ambulatory surgery as performed by the general surgeon.

PROCEDURE AND PATIENT SELECTION

As with all ambulatory surgery, the suitability of a head and neck procedure to be performed on an ambulatory basis depends on the nature of the problem, the condition of the patient, and the ability of the patient to be safely followed postoperatively. The procedure should be reasonably short. The thoracic cavity should not be entered. Prolonged or significant postoperative pain or complications should not be anticipated, nor should significant drainage. The patient should not have

other significant systemic diseases that preclude safe performance of the procedure.

The patient should be aware of the procedure planned, agree to its performance as an outpatient, and understand the postoperative protocol and what to do in case of unexpected problems. The distance of travel to and from home should not be excessive, and there should be effective medical help available close to the patient's home.

PREOPERATIVE WORKUP

Head and Neck Examination

The skin of the head and neck should be diligently searched for lesions, especially for suspected melanomas. Common areas that may be omitted by the physician are the hair-bearing scalp and the back of the ears.

The oral cavity should be inspected with good, clear, shadowless light. I use the gloved fingers of both hands to systematically inspect and palpate the intraoral structures. The floor of the mouth is best viewed by moving the tongue border medially. Masses in the submaxillary triangles should be examined bidigitally.

The lateral and anterior neck areas are examined with the patient's head bent slightly forward (to relax the investing layer of the deep cervical fascia). Visual inspection is done both from the front and the lateral sites. Palpation of the neck for abnormal masses is done from the front. Thyroid nodules are best felt with the examiner standing behind the patient and feeling the central area of the neck with the finger tips. The midline structures are pushed to one side and the contralateral thyroid lobes palpated against the hard larynx and trachea. The patient is asked to swallow. Motion of a mass with swallowing is characteristic of a thyroid nodule. A substernal goiter may be visible and palpable only when the patient swallows.

Fiberoptic endoscopes have made detailed clinic examination of the nasal cavity, nasopharynx, oropharynx, piriform sinuses, hypopharynx, and larynx easy. A short burst of Xylocaine spray in each nostril is all the anesthesia that is required. The endoscope is lubricated with clear, water-soluble lidocaine jelly. The patient is given a glass of water to sip with a drinking straw. This helps wash down phlegm that obscures the lens of the endoscope. The base of the tongue, piriform sinuses, hypopharynx, and larynx are carefully examined. Mobility of the vocal cords is checked.

Figure 20–1 shows some of the common site-specific lesions in the neck area.

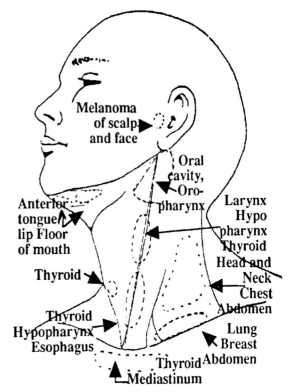

Figure 20–1. Common etiologic sites of lesions resulting in cervical adenopathy.

Preoperative Tests

Ambulatory head and neck surgical procedures can be divided into the following three major groups:

1. Those that can be done with local infiltration anesthesia or local nerve block (such as excision of small skin lesions)
2. Those that need to be done under fairly heavy sedation requiring the presence in the room of an anesthetist (monitored anesthesia care), such as endoscopies and superficial excisions requiring complicated plastic repairs
3. Procedures done under general anesthesia, such as complicated plastic repairs and parotidectomies

No particular preoperative laboratory investigation is needed for patients having surgery under local anesthesia unless the patient has a history of liver disease or coagulopathy. For suspected coagulopathy, however, the usual tests of prothrombin time and partial thromboplastin time do not necessarily identify potential bleeding problems. A thorough history of unusual bleeding is more important than the tests alone. A bleeding time or other more specific testing may be indicated by the history.

Preoperative laboratory testing for patients undergoing surgery under monitored anesthesia care or general anesthesia customarily includes a complete blood count, measurement of selected blood chemical constituents, a chest film (if none has been obtained within a year), and, in patients older than 45 years or with a history of heart disease, an electrocardiogram. The need and value of such "routine" tests is currently under scrutiny because they are expensive and may have little clinical yield.

ANESTHETIC TECHNIQUES

Local Anesthesia

Infiltration of local anesthesia is generally performed by the surgeon. Infiltration anesthesia produces quick local numbing following intradermal or subcutaneous administration, although the duration of anesthesia varies based on the agent used. The total amount of anesthetic used should be monitored to prevent toxic effects. When large areas are to be anesthetized, the anesthetic must be diluted and given slowly. The properties of the usual anesthetics given at my institution are listed in Table 20–1.

Because of its acidic nature, injections of lidocaine can be quite painful. This pain is ameliorated by the addition of 1 mL of 8.4% sodium bicarbonate for each 10 mL of lidocaine solution, and 0.1 mL of 8.4% sodium bicarbonate for each 10 mL of bupivacaine.

Nerve Blocks

Mental Nerve Block

The mental nerve emerges from the mental foramen of the mandible at about the level of the canine tooth on a vertical line joining the notch for the exit of the supraorbital nerve on the ridge of the eyebrow and the pupil of the forward-looking eye (Fig. 20–2). The foramen is palpated, a fine needle is inserted through anesthetized skin to the foramen, and 2 to 4 mL of the anesthetic is injected. Bilateral infiltration is wise because there is some overlapping of the supply, especially near the midline. This anesthetizes the lower lip and chin. Occasionally, some added anesthetic may be needed in the alveobuccal sulcus.

Supraorbital Nerve Block

The supraorbital notch is palpated. A fine needle is inserted immediately superior to the notch through the anesthetized skin (Fig. 20–

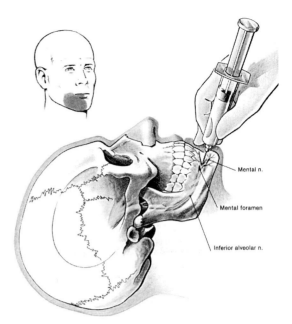

Figure 20–2. Placement of mental nerve block. The area around the mental foramen, which lies directly under the canine tooth, is infiltrated to produce anesthesia of the lower lip and ipsilateral chin (see shaded area). (From Katz J. Regional Anesthesia. 2d ed. Norwalk, CT: Appleton & Lange, 1994:29.)

3A). Two to 4 mL of anesthetic solution is injected. An additional 2 to 4 mL injected medially also anesthetizes the supratrochlear nerve. This block anesthetizes the skin of the upper eyelid and the medial part of the forehead.

Infraorbital Nerve Block

The infraorbital foramen of the maxilla lies on the vertical line connecting the supraorbital notch and the mental foramen. The infraorbital notch is palpated and a fine needle is introduced approximately 1 cm inferior to it and advanced laterally and cephalad toward the notch (see Fig. 20–3B). Three to 4 mL of anesthetic solution is injected in the neighborhood of the foramen. The cheek and the upper lip are numbed by this block. It is advisable to block both sides because of overlapping nerve supply near the midline.

Superior Laryngeal Nerve Block

The patient lies on his or her back with the neck extended. The hyoid bone is displaced

Table 20–1. Drugs Used for Local Anesthesia

	Lidocaine	Bupivacaine
Concentration (%)	0.5–1.0	0.25–0.5
Max dose (mg)		
Plain solution	300	175
With epinephrine	500	225
Duration (min)		
Plain solution	30–60	120–240
With epinephrine	30–90	180–420

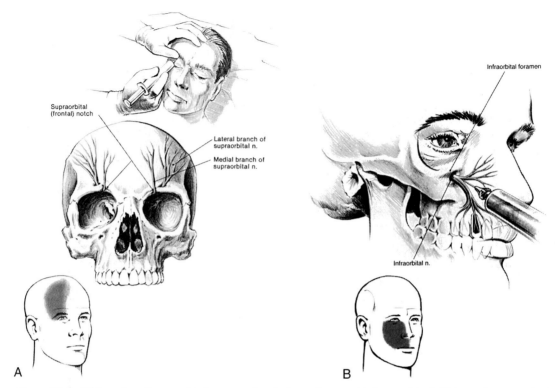

Figure 20–3. (A) Location of supraorbital nerve and technique of supraorbital nerve block. This produces anesthesia of the ipsilateral upper eyelid, eyebrow, and forehead. (B) Infraorbital foramen and technique of infraorbital nerve block. Anesthesia of the ipsilateral medial cheek, lower eyelid, and upper lip results. (From Katz J. Regional Anesthesia. 2d ed. Norwalk, CT: Appleton & Lange, 1994:9, 15.)

laterally, and a 25-gauge needle is inserted below the greater cornu. It is advanced 2 to 3 mm through the thyrohyoid membrane (the membrane can generally be felt as it is traversed). Then, 2 to 3 mL of anesthetic solution is placed superficial and deep to the membrane. The procedure is repeated on the opposite side to anesthetize the interior of the larynx and the epiglottis.

Transtracheal Block

With the patient lying supine, 3 to 5 mL of lidocaine is injected into the trachea through a plastic cannula (mounted on a needle) introduced through the cricothyroid membrane. The position should be verified by aspiration of air. The patient coughs, distributing the solution and anesthetizing the infraglottic larynx and trachea.

Intraoral Blocks

Much of the minor oral surgery of the tongue, cheek, and alveolar margins can be done by blocking the mandibular and lingual nerves. Dentists may be asked to put in these blocks because of their frequent use of these techniques.

BIOPSIES

In evaluating lesions of the head and neck, a definitive diagnosis is essential for determining the best treatment method. The entire lesion might be removed by an excisional biopsy. On occasion, if the lesion is large or fixed to vital structures, an incisional biopsy to obtain an adequate sample of the suspicious tissue is done. In such cases, the superficial tissues should be closed in layers to decrease the chances of fungation of an underlying cancer. For this same reason, the nature of a swelling in the neck must be determined before attempted incisional drainage.

The placement of the incision in an open biopsy must be planned so that it can be excised at the time of later definitive surgery.

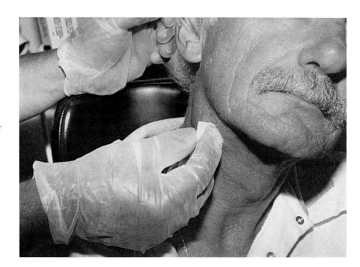

Figure 20–4. Needle aspiration biopsy of a suspicious neck mass. The overlying skin is prepared with an antiseptic solution.

Small lesions can be excised using a Martin punch. Punches are also useful for sampling larger lesions.

Tissue sampling can also be done from deep-seated structures with a fine needle or with a special cutting needle with a thicker bore (trocar) that allows a cored sample to be removed. The former technique, known as *fine-needle aspiration biopsy*, is quick, inexpensive, and safe. The sample obtained shows the cells only—a good pathologist can generally decide the nature of the tissue from the cytologic smear. Fine-needle aspiration of lesions can provide an accurate histologic diagnosis in as many as 96% of head and neck lesions. Samples obtained with a special cutting needle with an obturator give the pathologist a specimen for histologic examination that might be preferable to cytologic study; however, the technique is more expensive and potentially more hazardous.

I use fine-needle aspiration extensively as an outpatient procedure using inexpensive, readily available material. The equipment needed is shown in Figures 20–4 through 20–9. The technique is as follows: Informed consent is obtained. The patient usually sits for the procedure. The skin and subcutis over the mass is prepared with a 10-second scrub with 70% isopropyl alcohol (see Fig. 20–4) and anesthetized with 0.5% lidocaine with epinephrine and sodium bicarbonate using a 25-gauge needle bent at an angle with the bevel pointing downward (see Fig. 20–5). Slow injection minimizes pain. When a cutting needle is to be used, the skin is nicked with the

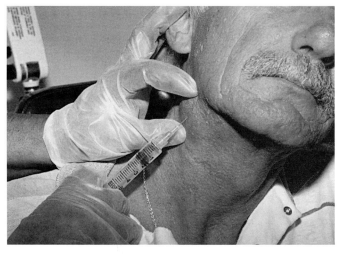

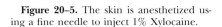
Figure 20–5. The skin is anesthetized using a fine needle to inject 1% Xylocaine.

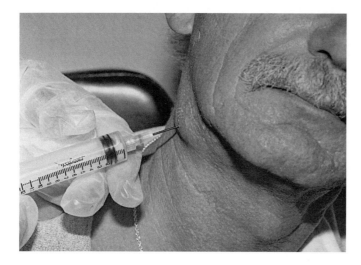

Figure 20–6. A 16-gauge needle is inserted into the mass, aspirating a sample of tissue into the needle.

tip of a number 15 scalpel blade. A 16- to 20-gauge needle attached to a fresh syringe, with the plunger slightly pulled out, is used to transfix the suspect mass (see Fig. 20–6). Suction is applied by pulling out the plunger farther, and the needle is withdrawn and advanced in the mass a number of times in different directions while maintaining suction. The suction is released and the needle withdrawn.

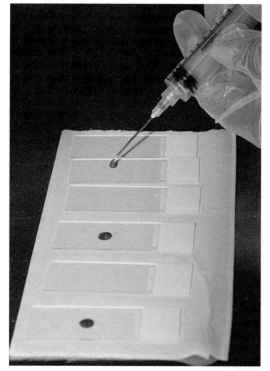

Figure 20–7. The aspirated material is placed on slides.

The material obtained is expressed on slides (see Fig. 20–7), smears are made (see Fig. 20–8), and the slides are immediately placed in the fixative preferred by the pathologist (see Fig. 20–9). The use of a needle with an obturator makes obtaining the specimen easier but is seldom needed. The smears should not be allowed to dry because this interferes with interpretation.

Firm pressure is placed on the needle entrance site for 1 to 2 minutes to achieve hemostasis. A light dressing may be applied, although it is generally not needed. On occasion, needle biopsy may be done under ultrasound guidance.

Needle aspiration biopsy has been particularly useful in lesions of the thyroid gland, in lesions of the salivary glands, and in lymph nodal swellings. The diagnostic yield and accuracy of fine-needle aspiration depends on the expertise of the surgeon and the pathologist.

Biopsy specimens from intraoral structures—nasopharynx, oropharynx, and hypopharynx—are best obtained with the use of punch biopsy instruments. These are easily used and obtain an adequate tissue specimen from surface lesions in most cases. Frozen section on biopsies is seldom indicated when cytologic study is adequate.

Pitfalls

Biopsy results from cancers of the base of the tongue, the piriform sinus area, and the

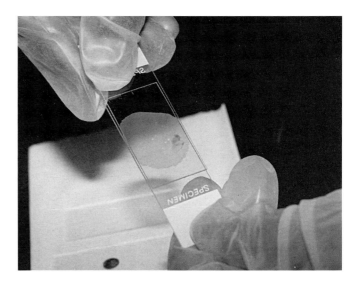

Figure 20–8. Smears are made.

supraglottic larynx are occasionally falsely negative. If there is a strong clinical suspicion, the patient should undergo rebiopsy. Under such circumstances, a frozen section examination is justified. Proper biopsy can be difficult in large necrotic tumors and also following radiation therapy. Biopsy specimens from the larynx and nasopharynx should be carefully observed for persistent bleeding. Applying pressure with a cotton pad soaked in 1/100,000 adrenaline

solution helps stop persistent bleeding in these areas.

SKIN LESIONS OF THE HEAD AND NECK

The skin of the head and neck area comprises approximately 9% of the total body surface. All the lesions seen in the skin and soft tissues on the rest of the body are also seen here, although some are more common. Exposure to sunlight and the elements makes the skin of the head and neck particularly susceptible to certain types of benign, premalignant, and malignant lesions. Although many of these can be treated on an outpatient basis, extensive and complicated lesions need specialized attention and general anesthesia.

INFECTIOUS LESIONS

Furuncles

Furuncles are generally caused by *Staphylococcus aureus*. A particularly recalcitrant form is sometimes seen in men when the hair of the beard coils in on itself. The condition is most commonly seen in blacks. Apart from treatment with the usual antibiotics and local measures such as compresses and drainage, patients must keep their faces meticulously clean,

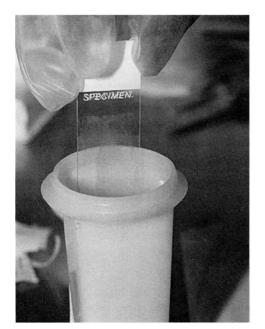

Figure 20–9. The smears are immediately dipped in the preservative solution.

including regularly scrubbing themselves with a cloth.

BENIGN DEGENERATIVE LESIONS

Seborrheic Keratoses

Seborrheic keratoses are generally seen in elderly patients. The lesions are found in the skin all over the body, including the head and neck area and the trunk. Characteristically, they are brownish in color and somewhat greasy to feel. Some can grow in thickness to be raised above skin level. They are benign and rarely undergo malignant transformation. They can be ignored.

Actinic Keratoses

Actinic keratoses may be seen at all ages in adults, although numbers increase with age. The areas vary from slightly reddened irregular spots less than 1 cm in any dimension to whitish irregular areas that are flaky. These are considered premalignant. Some early basal cell cancers cannot be visually distinguished from actinic keratoses. Therefore, persistent areas should be excised, frozen, or treated with 5-fluorouracil cream.

Cutaneous Papillomas

Cutaneous papillomas are small excrescences from the skin, generally with an irregular surface. They may be treated with podophyllum resin or tincture, frozen, or excised superficially. Many of them are of viral origin and tend to recur.

Skin Tags (Acrochordon)

Skin tags are soft protrusions of the skin. The surface is smooth, in contrast to papillomas. They may be frozen or excised if needed.

Cutaneous Horn

Cutaneous horns are long, fairly hard, and often curved protrusions arising from the skin that grow very slowly. They should be excised if they cause inconvenience.

Keratoacanthoma

Keratoacanthoma is a benign lesion that mimics a squamous cancer in its appearance (Fig. 20–10). However, it grows rapidly for a period of a month or so and then involutes equally rapidly. The lesion resolves spontaneously in 6 to 8 weeks.

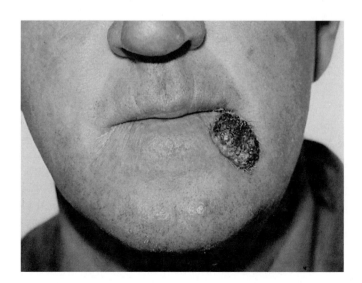

Figure 20–10. Keratoacanthoma. The lesion appeared 2 weeks earlier.

Table 20–2. Classification of Skin Cancers

Nonmelanoma skin cancers	
Dermal	Basal cell cancers
	Squamous cell cancers
Appendages	Hidradenocarcinoma
	Sebaceous gland carcinoma
Neuroendocrine	Merkel cell cancers
Melanoma	Lentigo maligna
	Superficial spreading (thin)
	Nodular (thick)

MALIGNANT NEOPLASMS OF THE SKIN

Skin malignancies are particularly common on the face. Their clinical aggressiveness (local invasion, distant metastases, threat to life) vary enormously. Currently, they are divided into two broad groups: melanomas and nonmelanoma skin cancers (Table 20–2).

Sunburn increases the incidence of both melanomas and nonmelanoma skin cancers. Significant sunburn in childhood is particularly dangerous. Pigmentation is protective, hence skin cancers are seen more commonly in lightly pigmented persons, especially persons with very pale skin, gray or light-blue eyes, and red hair. The incidence of skin cancer has increased rapidly among people who frequently indulge in sunbathing and suntanning. Patients with skin cancer must be counseled about exposure to sunlight, direct or reflected (as from snow or water), and the use of sunscreens. Even nonmelanoma skin cancer patients should have regular follow-up for the appearance of new lesions. Even though most new basal and squamous cell skin cancers in patients who received previous treatment occur within a year, quite a few also develop later. A friend or family member should therefore be instructed in regular and systematic review of the entire skin (including that of the scalp) for new or suspicious lesions. Immune deficiency (as in acquired immunodeficiency syndrome) or immune suppression (as in transplant patients) increases the rate of appearance of skin cancers and may increase the aggressiveness of the lesions. Patients with albinism and xeroderma pigmentosum are particularly susceptible to development of multiple skin cancers.

Basal Cell Skin Cancer

The classic appearance of a basal cell carcinoma is that of a small pearly outgrowth on the skin (Fig. 20–11). As the lesion enlarges, the central portion may necrose to give rise to a typical "rodent" ulcer with somewhat serpiginous margins. Sometimes, a local pigmentary reaction in the adjacent skin can make these pigmented basal cell cancers difficult to differentiate from melanomas.

Basal cell cancers are generally slow growing and metastasize very rarely. However, if the cancer involves the mucosa of the nose or conjunctiva, it spreads extensively and rapidly, and the margins are difficult to judge clinically. Occasionally, basal cell cancer can be quite aggressive locally. I have seen two instances of a basal cell cancer invading the underlying parotid gland after crossing the parotid–masseteric fascia (Fig. 20–12). In both instances, wide excision with in-continuity superficial parotidectomy has controlled the disease.

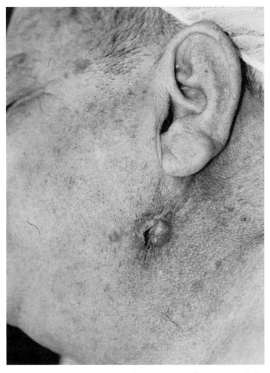

Figure 20–11. Long-standing basal cell cancer of the face that recurred after excision many years earlier.

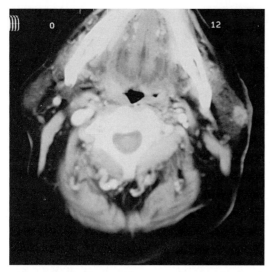

Figure 20–12. Computed tomography scan showing focus of basal cell cancer in the left parotid gland continuous with a lesion in the skin.

Squamous Cell Cancers

Squamous cell cancer is generally ulceroproliferative. The lesions seldom have the pearly appearance of basal cell cancers. They are more likely to infiltrate and metastasize to neighboring lymph nodes. Patients should be examined for possible lymph nodal metastases at initial examination and on follow-up visits. Lesions arising on the vermilion border or the lip mucosa are almost always squamous cell cancers.

Melanoma

Melanomas are an increasing clinical problem in North America. The persistent desire of light-skinned persons to darken themselves has fostered sunbathing and suntanning in salons. The result has been an alarming increase in the incidence of all skin cancers, including melanomas (see Chapter 36).

In contrast to the nonmelanoma skin cancers, melanomas are prone to metastasize and therefore significantly threaten the patient's life. Melanomas spread both by the lymphatic and the arteriovenous pathways and are known to metastasize to sites where other cancers rarely appear. Thus, melanomas can be seen in the gastrointestinal tract, spleen, cardiac muscle, pericardium, and the eye.

The common diagnostic features of melanomas include the following:

- Variegated black pigmentation
- Rapid growth
- Pruritus
- Bleeding
- Satellite nodules

There might also be local or regional lymphadenopathy or evidence of distant spread.

Head and neck area melanomas usually are of three clinical varieties, each with a fairly characteristic natural history. These types are lentigo maligna, superficial spreading, and nodular.

Lentigo maligna melanoma is also known as the *superficial melanotic freckle of Hutchinson. Lentigo malignas* arise on the skin of elderly people. They are generally irregular in their outline and have a variegated pigmentary appearance. They are considered to be in situ melanomas. After a prolonged period, their benign nature changes and they become full-fledged invasive melanomas.

All melanomas have two components of development. One is radial or horizontal and the other vertical. When the radial or horizontal growth propensity is most marked, the lesion is called a *superficial spreading melanoma.* These lesions spread laterally and tend not to invade in depth. Consequently, they have a low tendency to metastasize.

Preferential growth in the vertical dimension produces a *nodular* melanoma. Because of invasion of deeper structures, the possibility of distant metastases is higher in this group and consequently the disease-free survival time is lower.

In patients in whom the clinical findings suggest melanoma, a full-thickness biopsy should be done—either excisional or incisional. The depth of the lesion must be measured critically, both in millimeters and histologically to the level of invasion by melanoma cells. This is the single most crucial factor determining the natural history of a given lesion.

Treatment of melanomas of the head and neck requires excision with adequate margins to prevent local recurrence. However, excessive skin removal makes acceptable cosmetic appearance and reconstruction more difficult. A recent National Institutes of Health consensus conference suggested a 0.5-cm. margin for in situ melanomas (lentigo maligna), a 1-cm margin of excision for superficial melanomas (less than 1 cm in diameter), and a 2-cm margin for nodular lesions of 2- to 4-mm depth. Wide excisions generally require closure with rotated flaps or with skin grafts. The type of closure does not seem to affect the result. Surgery is best done under general anesthesia, although same-day discharge is often possible for smaller lesions.

The need for a prophylactic lymphadenectomy is still controversial. Elective node dissection is probably not indicated for patients with stage I disease. In patients with palpable cervical nodes, a superficial parotidectomy should be done at the time of the neck dissection because the intraparotid nodes are frequently involved in head and neck melanoma metastases. This is probably beyond the scope of ambulatory surgery.

GENERAL PRINCIPLES OF TREATMENT OF SKIN CANCERS

Items to consider in the treatment of skin cancer are the following:

1. Establishment of histologic nature via excisional or incisional biopsy
2. Potential for local recurrence
3. Potential for metastases, sites of metastases, and choice of treatment methods for metastases
4. Cosmetic results

The importance of cosmetic results varies with the lesion being treated. Although a good scar is important, the degree to which a good scar is a priority depends on many factors. Closure of a facial defect with a local flap generally gives a better cosmetic result than a rotated flap closure or a skin graft. However, closure with a flap is more complicated, time-consuming, and expensive. Closure with a skin graft may be acceptable to older persons or to those with sun-damaged skin, even though the ultimate result is somewhat inferior to repair with a flap. Theoretically, a rotated flap may

hide recurrence in the excision bed for some time. That is true of skin graft replacement also.

TREATMENT METHODS FOR SKIN CANCERS OF THE HEAD AND NECK

Nonsurgical Methods

One nonsurgical method to treat skin cancers of the head and neck is radiation therapy, which may be used as primary treatment for lesions of the lip, where its efficacy is equal to surgical excision.

Photodynamic therapy is being used in certain settings to treat skin cancer, but, again, this is not the primary mode used for most lesions, particularly those with any malignant potential. Another nonsurgical treatment used primarily for premalignant lesions, such as actinic keratoses, is the application of fluorouracil ointment or cream to the lesion.

Cryosurgery

Cryosurgery, also known as "freezing," is an effective method for many superficial skin lesions. Liquid nitrogen is the agent commonly used. The liquid nitrogen is kept contained in an insulated tank from which it can be released either as a spray or as a local contact coolant. Applicators of diverse sizes allow differing size areas to be cooled.

The area cooled is generally slightly larger than the lesion itself. For small areas, local anesthesia is often not needed. The appropriate size of the cooling head is determined, a light coating of water-soluble jelly is applied on the head, and it is pressed in contact with the lesion. As the liquid nitrogen is circulated through the cooling head, the jelly freezes and is seen as a white rim around the cooling head. The head adheres to the skin and is gently lifted off the deeper tissues to prevent unnecessary freezing of the deeper structures. The frozen tissue becomes white and gradually expands. Freezing is maintained from 30 to 45 seconds depending on the thinness of the skin and the size of the lesion. At the end of the procedure, the skin is allowed to thaw and the applicator is removed when it is no longer adherent.

As the tissue thaws, some patients complain of burning pain that might require analgesics for a short while. A blister and then a black eschar develop, which falls off by itself after a few days. The area may be kept exposed and dry. On occasion, there is some depigmentation of the frozen area.

Small and superficial lesions of actinic keratoses and basal cell and squamous cancers can be treated with cryosurgery. Lentigo maligna and melanomas should not be frozen. Skin tags can have their bases frozen, following which they fall off. Cutaneous horns are better excised.

Freeze–thaw cycles using subcutaneous temperature probes have also been advocated. In this technique, the probe is inserted to a point approximately 1 mm deep to the center of the lesion. The temperature at the probe tip is brought down to $-25°C$, maintained at that level for 1 minute, then allowed to gradually thaw.

Surgical Excision

Many small skin lesions are eminently suitable for excision as an ambulatory procedure.

Little patient preparation is required. The patient is allowed to have a light breakfast and take regular medications (if any) at the usual time. The patient may be given a small dose of an antianxiety agent 30 minutes before surgery if needed. In general, a relative or attendant should be available to drive the patient to and from the hospital. Excisions are done under full surgical precautions with appropriate preparation of the skin, use of local infiltration anesthesia, and sterile conditions.

Most superficial lesions are seen in older people and the laxity of the skin permits excision with primary closure. The affected skin and the surrounding area are prepared with Betadine solution and draped. The extent of excision around the area is marked with a skin pencil. Whenever possible, excision should follow skin lines to minimize scarring. Details of the technique of determining appropriate incision alignment with skin lines are given

in Chapter 34. On occasion, a small lesion fragments during excision so that examination of the edges is unsatisfactory. That is why preoperative indication of the margin of excision is important.

The area is infiltrated with 1% lidocaine with 1/10,000 epinephrine and sodium bicarbonate solution. For superficial lesions, the anesthetic solution is injected just deep to the dermoepidermal junction. This raises up the lesion and makes adequate excision in depth easy. If mobilization of the edges of the excision is needed for tension-free closure, further injections in the same plane facilitate appropriate dissection.

The margin of excision in melanomas has been examined critically to prevent local recurrence. However, the margin of clearance has not been looked at critically in basal cell or squamous cell cancers of the skin of the face. A 5-mm margin is adequate in my experience. In recurrent lesions or when the edges seem to be diffuse, frozen sections of the lateral and deep margins should be examined to ensure complete excision. The excised specimen is put on a piece of Telfa or similar material and a diagram made of the orientation of the specimen. This enables the pathologist to identify the orientation of a margin that might be involved with neoplasm. In primary excisions, this step can generally be safely avoided to cut down on time and expenses.

Hemostasis is obtained with the electrocautery set at the lowest effective setting for coagulation. Deeper tissues are approximated with interrupted sutures of polyglactin if needed. The edges of the excision are approximated with fine nonabsorbable sutures, and a light dressing is applied. The patient is returned to the discharge unit after the written postoperative instructions are explained. Depending on the degree of tension on the closure, the sutures are removed between the fourth and seventh day postoperatively. By this time, the histologic results should be available and discussed with the patient.

If the microscopic examination shows a margin to be involved, I inform the patient of this circumstance. In the case of basal cell cancer, I examine the patient at 3-month intervals if the excision is judged to have adequate margins. Less than 10% of such lesions have recurred locally following this wait and watch policy. When the margins may be involved in a squamous cell cancer, the scar may be reexcised. In most instances, the scar is found to have no residual tumor; however, because squamous cell cancers are known to metastasize and basal cell cancers seldom do, it is safer to be more aggressive with squamous cell cancers.

Local Flaps

Satisfactory tension-free closure often requires the use of local flaps. Some useful techniques are shown in Figures 20–13 and 20–14. Only those flaps that can be safely used by the general surgeon in an ambulatory setting are shown. More complicated resections should be undertaken by a plastic surgeon and might require overnight admission.

Small lesions of the forehead are usually best excised with a transverse elliptical excision parallel to skin creases and primary closure. Larger lesions may be closed using double rotation flaps.

Lesions of the ear are best treated with wedge excision and closure.

Lesions of the nose are particularly difficult with respect to cosmetic considerations. Closure of the defect after excision of small lesions on the nose may be done using a trans-

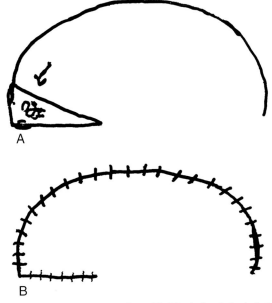

Figure 20–14. Rotation flap. (**A**) The lesion is included in the triangle of tissue to be excised. (**B**) Rotation of the pedicle of skin forward allows coverage.

position flap (see Fig. 20–13). Large lesions and distal lesions near the tip of the nose can be covered with an axial frontonasal flap. Lesions near the ala are best closed with a nasolabial transposition flap.

Lesions removed from the cheek can be covered using either a rhomboid flap (see Fig. 20–13) or a rotation flap (see Fig. 20–14).

An alternative to using flaps in most of the areas described is the use of fibrin-glued full-thickness skin grafts for coverage of the excised lesion. Skin grafts may be another alternative when cosmetic considerations are less important.

Lesions of the Lips

The skin immediately adjacent to the mucosa of the lower lip and the lower lip mucosa itself are often the site of basal cell or, more commonly, squamous cell cancers. Lesions extending to one third of the lip can be removed by excision and primary closure. Bilateral mental nerve block gives excellent anesthesia. Occasionally, some anesthetic must be placed in the lower alveolabial sulcus. The excision should be done in the form of a shield, other-

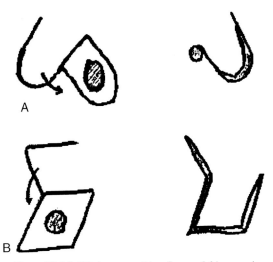

Figure 20–13. (**A**) A transposition flap useful in covering excised areas of the nose. (**B**) A rhomboid flap, useful for covering excised areas of the cheek.

wise there is an unsightly depression on the lip margin. The vermilion border should be accurately brought together. Fine polyglactin sutures can be used to bring together the deeper tissues and the orbicularis oris muscle. The mucosal apposition is done with the same material, and the skin is sutured with fine monofilament nylon.

Lesions on the upper lip are much less common than on the lower lip and can be similarly excised (when small) with bilateral infraorbital nerve block. Larger upper lip lesions may require a cheek advancement flap.

Both the lower and (less commonly) the upper lip mucosa can show leukoplakia or multiple small areas of superficial cancers. This can be treated by a "lip shave." Bilateral mental (or infraorbital) nerve blocks are placed. The entire mucosa is then carefully removed from the underlying muscle layers. The oral mucosa is dissected back as a flap for a short distance and then sutured to the skin with multiple closely placed fine nylon sutures. The cosmetic results are surprisingly good.

Excision and Skin Grafting

On occasion, a defect is best closed with a skin graft. Full-thickness skin grafts provide a more pliable coverage than split-thickness grafts. The former generally gives better cosmetic results and is less likely to break down from trauma.

After the lesion is excised, an impression of the defect is made on a piece of Telfa. The impression is transferred to a previously prepared locally anesthetized donor site. Even though the retroauricular region serves as a satisfactory donor site for small grafts, I prefer to take the graft from the supraclavicular or infraclavicular skin. A full-thickness graft is obtained, including some of the subcutaneous fat. This makes subsequent closure of the donor defect easier.

The graft is "defatted" by putting it on a finger deep side up and using curved iris scissors to remove the subcutaneous fat until the white dermis is evenly seen. After defatting, the graft is applied to the defect (which should have perfect hemostasis) and anchored securely in place. Generally, this is done with

multiple fine sutures that are tied over a bulky "bolster" dressing. The same effect can be quickly and easily obtained by using fibrin "glue" prepared from the patient's blood.

Fibrin glue is prepared from fibrinogen precipitated from approximately 10 mL of the patient's blood by a solution of ammonium sulfate. The precipitate is suspended in a solution of calcium chloride. This mixture is applied to the defect simultaneously with a solution of (commercially available) thrombin and epsilon-aminocaproic acid. The fibrinogen solution can also be prepared from cryoprecipitate obtained from the blood bank. I prefer to use autologous fibrinogen because transmission of disease is prevented and a nonreplaceable resource is not wasted. The fibrin glue can be produced in the laboratory with readily available equipment within 15 minutes.

The mixture of the two solutions produces a visible gel almost instantaneously. The donor graft is pressed down on the defect for 15 to 20 seconds, which fixes it satisfactorily. It is protected with an appropriate appliance or by multiple Steri-Strips applied over covering pieces of Adaptic and Telfa that are slightly larger than the graft.

The patient is advised to avoid disturbing the graft, especially while sleeping. The dressings are changed carefully on the fifth or sixth postoperative day. Although the graft is well adherent by then, some care is still advisable. The graft may then be kept exposed, although I prefer to apply a light water-soluble jelly over it. The protective covering used previously is discarded unless the patient is very restless while sleeping.

Fibrin "glue" grafting has been uniformly successful and is eminently suitable for small defects anywhere on the face (such as on the tip of the nose or on the ear) where suturing a skin graft is technically unwieldy. Full-thickness grafts have been successfully glued to the underlying mucosa after excising a basal cell cancer on the nasal ala together with the cartilage under it. Similarly, full-thickness skin grafts have been successfully placed on the exposed skin of the medial side of the helix after excision of a basal cell cancer and underlying helical cartilage from the lateral side. The lax skin of the cheek makes flap closure easy and cosmetically satisfying. Full-thickness grafts are therefore seldom used in that area. Either flaps or a graft can be used on the forehead.

In areas where the skin is adherent to the underlying firm or hard tissues (e.g., forehead, nose, ear) a defect can be left to heal by epithelialization from the margins. Although this takes some time, the cosmetic results are often quite satisfactory.

Over a period of more than 5 years and 300 cases, graft "take" and the cosmetic results have been quite satisfactory. The color match is generally good, although some pigmentary changes can be seen in a small number of patients. When applied on defects in thick skin (e.g., the tip of the nose in some obese persons), the graft sometimes gives a depressed scar. When cosmesis is not a paramount consideration, the use of "glued" full-thickness skin grafts is a fast and effective alternative to skin flaps and even sutured-in grafts (Fig. 20–15).

Chemosurgery by Moh's technique is a time-consuming method of destruction of thin layers of the tumor, reexamination of margins by immediate microscopy, and further reexcision if needed. Although it is useful in extensive lesions or invasive lesions, the method is highly specialized and time-consuming. Eminently suited to ambulatory surgery, the method is limited to special units with appropriately trained personnel.

SOFT-TISSUE LESIONS

Soft-tissue tumors arising in the rest of the body can also arise in the soft tissues of the head and neck area. These include masses such as epidermal inclusion cysts, sebaceous cysts, pilar cysts, and benign neoplasms (e.g., lipomas and fibromas). They are treated as elsewhere by simple excision (see Chapter 35).

Special soft-tissue masses in this region include the dermoid cysts and the branchial cleft cysts. Both groups are developmental in origin. The dermoid cysts usually arise along the lines of fusion of the embryonic protrusions forming the infant's face. They are most commonly seen at the outer edge of the eyebrows, although they can arise anywhere along the eye and along the fusion line of the nose and the cheek. They are eminently suitable for removal on an ambulatory basis.

Branchial cleft cysts are seen in the upper part of the neck laterally. Even though they are of developmental origin, they are often not recognized until youth or early adulthood (Fig. 20–16). Cystic in feel, they can be removed by same-day surgery also. As with dermoid cysts, incisions should be made in the crease lines of the face or the neck.

Thyroglossal duct cysts arise from the remnants of the thyroglossal duct. The duct originates in the foramen cecum of the tongue, passes down in the midline through the substance of the tongue, between the upper and lower developmental blocks of the hyoid bone, and ends at the top of the pyramidal lobe of the thyroid gland on the front of the trachea. Generally, these slow-growing cysts present during youth or middle age. The classic subcutaneous position below the hyoid and above the thyroid cartilage can be seen in Figure 20–17. They are removed by a transverse

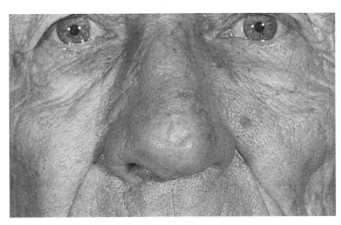

Figure 20–15. Fibrin-glued full-thickness skin graft on the tip of the nose, 6 months after surgery.

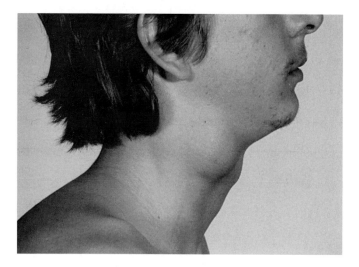

Figure 20–16. Appearance of a branchial cleft cyst.

incision—if possible, in a skin crease. The mass is easy to remove. The probability of a recurrence is diminished by excising the central portion of the hyoid bone (this does not cause any noticeable morbidity). If hemostasis

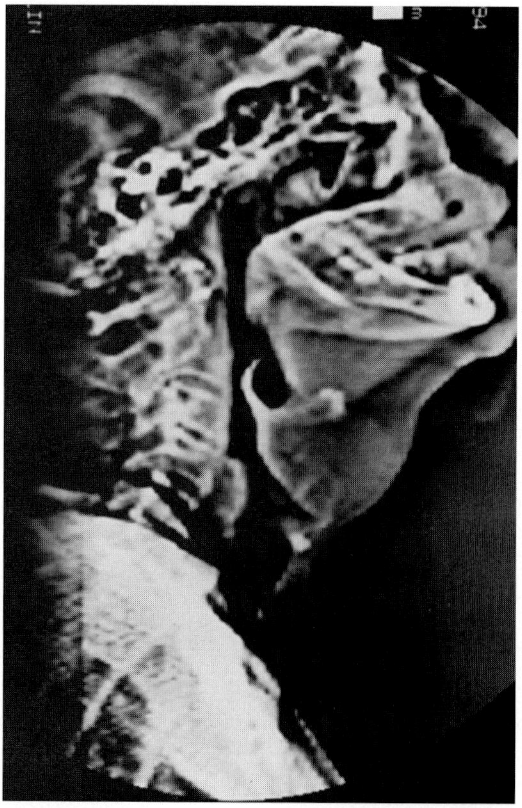

Figure 20–17. A lateral soft-tissue radiograph of the submental region showing the classic position of a thyroglossal duct cyst.

is achieved, the patient can be discharged after a short period of observation.

INTRAORAL LESIONS

Some small intraoral lesions can be safely removed by same-day surgery. Very small lesions can be excised under local anesthesia. However, most patients benefit from deep sedation and monitored anesthesia care. For lesions situated in the posterior oropharynx, general anesthesia may be advisable to gain adequate access and ensure satisfactory oxygenation.

Local infiltration gives satisfactory numbing but puts some tension on the closure of the mucosal edges. A nerve block using Xylocaine with epinephrine solution is useful in many instances.

Lesions that can be satisfactorily removed without admitting the patient include fibromas and small areas of leukoplakia on the buccal mucosa, small benign lesions of the tongue (e.g., papillomas and pyogenic granulomas), small benign lesions of the soft palate and uvula, and lesions on the jaw mucosa. Malignant neoplasms need wider excision and reconstruction and often must be done under general anesthesia. Small areas of leukoplakia may be treated with cryosurgery.

SALIVARY GLAND LESIONS

Salivary glandular tissue is found in two large aggregations in the parotid and submandibular glands bilaterally and diffusely distributed in the oral mucosa. Infection of these glands has become rare as a result of improved dental and oral hygiene. The only common nonneoplastic lesion of the salivary glands is a salivary duct stone in Wharton's (submandibular gland) ducts. The typical history is of mild discomfort on salivation and occasional swelling underneath the jaw when eating. If infected, a submandibular sialoadenitis is quite painful and may go on to cause respiratory distress.

Submandibular duct stones may or may not be palpable under the oral mucosa on bidigital palpation of the floor of the mouth. When palpable, the stones can be removed by a small incision made in the sublingual mucosa over the stone. The incision is not closed. If the stones cannot be located or if they are in the substance of the gland, the gland is removed by an incision in the skin of the submandibular triangle. Special care is needed to identify and preserve the ramus marginalis mandibuli branch of the facial nerve in reflecting the upper skin flap. Damage to the nerve causes permanent weakness of the lower lip on that side and the patient might drool.

The space left after removing the gland may or may not have to be drained. The patient may be discharged home after recovery from anesthesia. The drain should be removed in 24 to 48 hours.

Neoplasms of the salivary glands are uncommon. They arise most often in the parotid glands and are classically situated in the space between the back edge of the mandible and the mastoid process. Neoplasms arising in the tail of the gland can be mistaken for lymph nodes. Even though the glands can be imaged by radioactive nuclear scan, more information is gained by a computed tomography (CT) scan with intravenous contrast. The location, extent, and even the nature of the tumor can be seen and any suspect neck nodes visualized.

Aspiration biopsy of a parotid mass is easy and is generally diagnostic. Parotid neoplasms are more commonly benign than malignant. Because all parotid neoplasms are best treated by surgery, some surgeons do not think that a preoperative diagnosis is necessary.

The parotid gland is removed through an incision as shown in Figure 20–18. The incision

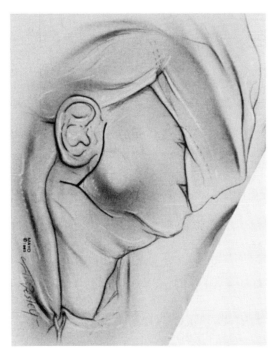

Figure 20–18. An incision that may be used to perform parotidectomy. The incision is often straight up and down starting in the vertical crease in front of the tragus and traveling down the neck with a slight anterior curve to follow an appropriate crease line. The author actually prefers to make a Y extension (behind the ear) rather than the T type extension pictured. (From Beahrs OH, Kiernan PD, Hubert JP Jr., eds. An Atlas of the Surgical Techniques of Oliver H. Beahrs. Philadelphia: WB Saunders, 1985:51.)

is deepened down through the skin to the level of the deep (parotidomasseteric) fascia. The sternomastoid muscle is identified and the posterior edge of the gland dissected forward from the anterior border of the muscle. The great auricular nerve usually crosses the field and must be transected. Occasionally, the nerve divides into an anterior and a posterior branch, and only the former has to be divided.

Dissection along the anterior border of the muscle is deepened until the styloid process can be palpated at the depth of the wound. The facial nerve is identified here by careful blunt dissection done on a transverse plane, parallel to the course of the nerve. Once the nerve is identified, it is traced forward along its individual branches through the substance of the gland until the branches emerge out of the anterior border of the gland. Removal of the portion of the gland superficial to the nerve is generally adequate because most neoplasms arise in the superficial "lobe." For a total parotidectomy, the deep portion of the gland can be dissected out from underneath the nerve branches. Apart from preservation of the branches of the facial nerve, the auriculotemporal nerve coursing along with the superficial temporal artery should also be spared. Injury to this structure may produce the annoying (Frey's) gustatory syndrome postoperatively.

A drain is used after a total parotidectomy and often after a superficial lobe resection. Depending on the extent of resection, the dead space left, the amount of drainage, and the patient's convenience and condition, the patient may or may not be discharged home after appropriate postanesthetic recovery.

THYROID LESIONS

Thyroid gland disorders fall in the domain of the surgeon only when there is a diffuse or localized swelling of the gland. Thyroid nodules are common, although only a small fraction are malignant. Various diagnostic tests are used to establish the nature of a thyroid mass. These include measurement of serum thyroid hormone levels, radioactive iodine uptake and imaging studies of the gland, and CT scans and ultrasound examination of the gland and surrounding tissues. Any of these may be useful in a given patient to decide on optimal treatment. However, the most cost-effective and important diagnostic procedure is a needle biopsy of the thyroid mass. A large-bore cutting needle can be used to obtain a core sample. Alternatively, fine-needle aspiration is probably safer and equally informative. This is often the appropriate first diagnostic test in the evaluation of a thyroid mass.

In a fine-needle aspiration, the suspect nodule is identified, the skin and overlying subcutaneous tissues are infiltrated with a local anesthetic after skin preparation with alcohol, and a fine needle is inserted into the mass. Suction is applied to the piston, and the needle is withdrawn almost to the skin and reinserted with suction. The patient should be asked not to move and, if possible, not to breathe during the needle aspiration. It is important to insert the needle into the mass in separate passes so

that the needle does not cut the mass. The aspiration pressure on the syringe is stopped before the needle is withdrawn from the skin. Firm pressure should then be applied over the area for 2 to 3 minutes and the patient should be observed to be sure there is no sign of continued bleeding.

The diagnostic yield from needle aspiration of the thyroid is satisfactorily high. Malignant or cytologically indeterminate nodules as well as cysts that recur within a year after aspiration should be resected, especially when occurring in children, males, or postmenopausal women. I do not aspirate nodules of toxic adenoma or diffuse toxic goiter.

After a partial or total thyroidectomy, the operative field may be drained. Significant, even life-threatening, respiratory distress follows rapidly expanding fluid collections in this space. The drain acts more to indicate persistent oozing after thyroidectomy rather than as a safety valve for the pressure caused by the collected blood. Therefore, in my practice, I generally admit thyroidectomized patients after operation for observation until the drain is removed in 24 to 48 hours. Drainage after thyroidectomy is not universal, however, and many surgeons do not routinely drain such wounds.

In recent years, outpatient thyroidectomy has been reported to be safe in selected patients. This is particularly true if only a lobectomy or subtotal resection is performed and parathyroid function is not likely to be compromised. Patients who live within a short distance of the hospital are discharged home after several hours of observation. They should be alert to signs of hypocalcemia, especially if there is any question of operative dissection in the area of the parathyroid glands.

ENDOSCOPY

Carcinomas of the upper aerodigestive tracts are often multifocal. Therefore, the upper respiratory and digestive tracts should be thoroughly examined before definitive treatment of a cancer. With the fiberoptic flexible laryngoscope, the nasal cavities, nasopharynx, oropharynx, hypopharynx, and larynx can be examined reasonably well in the outpatient clinic. For a more thorough examination and to biopsy suspect areas, endoscopy is done in the endoscopy suite after appropriate preparation.

Deep sedation and monitored anesthesia care is adequate for most patients. The oral mucosa is numbed with topical application of a surface anesthetic. Bilateral superior laryngeal nerve block and a transtracheal block adequately anesthetizes the interior of the larynx.

The base of the tongue, the hypopharynx, and the interior of the larynx are best examined with a rigid laryngoscope; the tracheobronchial tree and the esophagus are generally examined with flexible endoscopes. Appropriate biopsy samples are obtained. Further details on upper endoscopy are given in Chapter 42 and on bronchoscopy in Chapter 43.

METASTATIC CERVICAL NODES WITH AN UNKNOWN PRIMARY

Quite a few patients present to the head and neck clinic with an enlarged neck node as their first and only symptom. If the involved nodes are in the supraclavicular area, the thoracic and abdominal organs, especially the lungs, pancreas, and stomach, are suspect as the site of the primary lesions. Aspiration biopsy of isolated cervical nodes shows squamous carcinoma in most cases, implicating the upper respiratory tract and the lungs as the site of the primary lesion. Adenocarcinomatous metastases may be from the abdominal organs, the breast, the salivary glands, or the thyroid.

Ninety percent to 95% of patients have the primary site identified on careful head and neck examination, including office endoscopy. In the remaining 5% to 10%, the primary site cannot be identified despite thorough examination at the time of initial diagnosis. If careful examination does not reveal the primary site, a radical neck dissection followed by external beam radiation therapy to the neck is in order. In one third of these patients, the primary lesion ultimately reveals itself. Approximately one third of these patients survive free of disease for 5 years, and, in them, the site may never be identified.

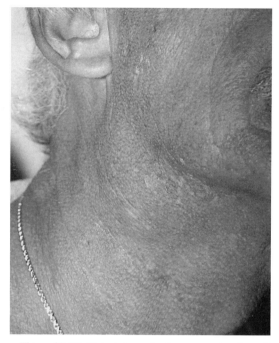

Figure 20–19. Metastatic nodes from a previously undiagnosed base of the tongue cancer.

Common sites of occult primary malignancies of the head and neck are the nasopharynx, the piriform sinus, and the base of the tongue (Figs. 20–19 and 20–20). If the primary site of cancer cannot be identified in the pa-

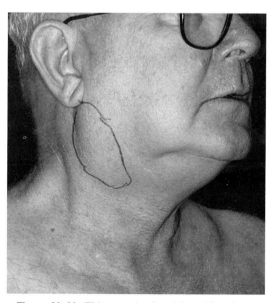

Figure 20–20. This mass in the right midjugular area resulted from a primary site of cancer in the right piriform sinus.

tient with isolated cervical adenopathy, a careful endoscopy and blind biopsies should be performed from these sites.

Adenopathy of the medial supraclavicular nodes (scalene nodes) can pose a diagnostic problem. A fine-needle aspiration is helpful in this situation. The biopsy may show inflammation, lymphoma, or cancer. Metastases to the scalene nodes from carcinomas of the thoracic cavity, breasts, or the head and neck area showed no predilection for spread to the ipsilateral or contralateral side in one study. Abdominal primaries, however, metastasized almost uniformly to the left side.

MISCELLANEOUS DIAGNOSTIC BIOPSIES

The surgeon is occasionally asked to perform diagnostic tests for internist colleagues. Four such procedures are lip mucosal biopsy, temporal artery biopsy, lymph node biopsy, and scalene node biopsy.

Lip Mucosal Biopsy

Lip mucosal biopsy is of use in the diagnosis of generalized amyloidosis. The mucosa of the lower lip on its inner side is anesthetized with a local anesthetic. An elliptic segment of the lip mucosa, together with the underlying submucosal glands, is sharply excised. The edges of the excised segment are brought together with simple sutures of 4-0 polyglactin, placed deep enough to achieve hemostasis.

Temporal Artery Biopsy

Temporal artery biopsy is used in the diagnosis of temporal arteritis. The superficial temporal artery comes up vertically through the parotid gland and in front of the ear. At a variable distance above the zygoma, it divides into an anterior and a posterior branch. The branches can always be felt and sometimes seen. The anterior branch is generally biopsied. The branches should be palpated on both sides to determine whether there are any nodularities. If not, a 3- to 4-cm segment is isolated after infiltrating and incising through the overlying skin. The artery is suture ligated behind and in front of the specimen excised. Trauma to the specimen should be minimized. Bilateral biopsies increase the yield significantly.

Lymph Node Biopsy

In many cases, a fine-needle aspiration biopsy gives the diagnosis in lymph node biopsy. If a node does have to be removed, this is done after appropriate skin preparation through a transverse incision over the node. Details of lymph node biopsy are given in Chapter 21. Cervical lymph node biopsies carry certain specific risks. In the anterior cervical triangle, the surgeon must be careful to avoid injuries to the structures of the carotid sheath: the carotid artery, internal jugular vein, and vagus nerve. In the submandibular area, the mandibular branch of the facial nerve must be preserved (see Salivary Gland Lesions). In the posterior triangle, injury to the accessory nerve should be avoided because this leads to disabling trapezius palsy and weakness of the shoulder.

Scalene Node Biopsy

With the introduction of mediastinoscopy, scalene node biopsies have become infrequent. The technique of scalene node biopsy and its attendant risks are detailed in Chapter 21.

Selected Readings

1. Bearcroft PW, Berman LH, Grant J. The use of ultrasound guided cutting needle biopsy in the neck. Clin Radiol 1995;50(10):690–695.
2. Cervin JR, Silverman JF, Loggie BW, Geisinger KR. Virchow's node revisited. Analysis with clinicopathologic correlation of 152 fine-needle aspiration biopsies of supraclavicular lymph nodes. Arch Pathol Lab Med 1995;119(8):727–730.
3. Chakravorty RC. Head and neck cancer. In: Kahn SB, Love RR, Sherman C, Chakravorty RC, eds. Concepts in Cancer Medicine. New York: Grune & Stratton, 1985:577–596.

4. Chakravorty RC, Sosnowski K. Autologous fibrin glue in full-thickness skin grafting. Ann Plast Surg 1989;23:488–491.

5. Diagnosis and treatment of early melanoma. NIH Consensus Development Conference. January 27–29, 1992. Consensus Statement 1992;10(1):1–25.

6. Hruza GJ. Moh's micrographic surgery. Otolaryngol Clin North Am 1990;23(5):845–864.

7. Lo Gerfo P, Gates R, Gazetas P. Outpatient and short-stay thyroid surgery. Head Neck 1991;13:97–101.

8. Martin HE, Ellis EB. Aspiration biopsy. Surg Gynecol Obstet 1934;59:578–589.

9. Martin HE, Ellis EB. Biopsy by needle puncture and aspiration. Ann Surg 1930;92:169–181.

10. Shaha AR, Webber CA, Marti JR. Fine needle aspiration in the diagnosis of cervical adenopathy. Am J Surg 1986;152:420–423.

11. Sharma AK. Advantages of short-stay parotidectomy (letter). Am J Surg 1994;167(4):459–460.

12. Sinclair RD, Dawber RP. Cryosurgery of malignant and premalignant diseases of the skin: a simple approach. Austr J Dermatol 1995;36(3):133–142.

13. Steckler RM. Outpatient thyroidectomy: a feasibility study. Am J Surg 1986;152(10):417–419.

14. Wang CY, Brodland DG, Su WP. Skin cancers associated with acquired immunodeficiency syndrome. Mayo Clin Proc 1995;70(8):766–772.

15. Woeber KA. Cost effective evaluation of the patient with a thyroid nodule. Surg Clin North Am 1995;75(3):357–363.

21

Lymph Node Biopsy

Herbert C. Hoover, Jr.

The general and oncologic surgeon often participates in the evaluation and diagnosis of patients with lymphadenopathy. This chapter discusses when a lymph node biopsy is indicated, the general approaches to lymph nodes in different anatomic sites, and the problems that can occur along the way.

INDICATIONS FOR LYMPH NODE BIOPSY

Not all palpable lymph nodes require an immediate diagnosis. In both children and adults, some palpable lymph nodes are seen normally. This is especially so for cervical nodes (0.5–1 cm) in children and inguinal nodes (0.5–2 cm) in adults. These are typically referred to as "shotty" nodes and are almost invariably palpable in thin individuals in whom there is scant subcutaneous fat to obscure the nodes. Otherwise, most palpably enlarged lymph nodes at all ages are present in association with various benign and malignant pathologic conditions. The challenge is to determine those conditions that warrant the inconvenience and expense of lymph node biopsy. Generally, diffuse lymphadenopathies associated with systemic symptoms suggestive of a viral syndrome in otherwise healthy individuals are of less concern than regionally localized lymphadenopathy. Patients with diffuse adenopathy should generally be followed up closely at 4 to 6 weeks to determine whether spontaneous resolution will occur. A workup for systemic disease in these patients should generally be directed by the primary care physician.

Persistent lymphadenopathies, especially when localized to a single anatomic site, prompt the bulk of the referrals and require a thorough and thoughtful evaluation. These patients range from those with a single node to those with multiple matted nodes. Adenopathies in certain anatomic sites are more frequently associated with certain diseases, a fact that weighs heavily in the differential diagnosis. Table 21–1 gives a correlation between the different anatomic sites and the cause of the lymphadenopathy.

It is often difficult to decide when to biopsy an enlarged lymph node, especially in a child. Inflammatory enlargement usually resolves within 4 to 6 weeks and a biopsy is not indicated. Discrete, hard, enlarged nodes should be biopsied as soon as possible. There is a large zone of uncertainty in between these two straightforward situations. Mature clinical judgment is necessary to decide when a biopsy is indicated. The usual situation is that of lymphadenopathy in one or more nodes in a single node-bearing area where an acute localized infectious process has been effectively ruled out. Delay beyond a few weeks of observation is not indicated if the enlarged nodes are not clearly regressing.

GENERAL PRINCIPLES OF LYMPH NODE BIOPSIES

Lymph nodes, especially those in the deep cervical and axillary areas, are often much deeper than anticipated from the physical examination, which reveals nodes "just beneath

Table 21–1. Correlation Between Location and Cause in Lymphadenopathy

Location	Cause
Occipital	Scalp infections, insect bites, ringworm, rarely lymphoma or metastatic tumor
Posterior auricular	Rubella
Anterior auricular	Eyelid and conjunctiva infections, keratoconjunctivitis
Posterior cervical	Toxoplasmosis
Posterior cervical and submental	Scalp and dental infections, tuberculosis
Anterior cervical	Tuberculosis, Hodgkin's lymphoma, oral and pharyngeal infections
Supraclavicular	Metastases from thoracic or abdominal carcinoma
Axillary	Upper extremity infections, cat scratch disease, brucellosis, sporotrichosis, non-Hodgkin's lymphoma
Epitrochlear	
Unilateral	Infection in hands
Bilateral	Viral diseases in children, sarcoidosis, tularemia
Inguinal	
Unilateral	Lymphogranuloma venereum, syphilis
Bilateral	Gonococcal, herpetic venereal infections, mycoplasma, urethritis
Progressive enlargement (without infection)	Metastatic carcinoma, lymphoma
Pulmonary hilar	
Unilateral	Metastatic lung carcinoma
Bilateral	Sarcoidosis, tuberculosis, histoplasmosis, coccidioidomycosis
Mediastinal, asymmetrical	Hodgkin's lymphoma
Intraabdominal and retroperitoneal	Lymphoma, metastatic carcinoma, tuberculosis in mesenteric nodes
Regional involvement in systemic infections	Infectious mononucleosis, viral hepatitis, cytomegalovirus disease, rubella, influenza
Generalized lymphadenopathies	Sarcoidosis, hyperthyroidism, autoimmune hemolytic anemia, lymphoma

From Ioachim HL. The lymph node biopsy. In: Ioachim HL, ed. Lymph Node Biopsy. Philadelphia: JB Lippincott, 1982.

the skin." The surgeon must prepare the patient that the procedure will require their cooperation. These procedures can be technically challenging when nodes are deep, large, and fixed to surrounding structures. They should not be assigned to an inexperienced junior resident without senior assistance.

Except in children, who almost always require general anesthesia, biopsies in the cervical, supraclavicular, scalene, axillary, and inguinal areas can be performed under local anesthesia in an ambulatory setting, unless physical or neuromuscular disorders prevent adequate stability or positioning of the patient on the operating room table. Xylocaine (1%) with epinephrine with 1 mL of sodium bicarbonate in 20 mL of Xylocaine is the usual local anesthesia.

Incisions should routinely be oriented in a transverse or slightly oblique direction as dictated by the skin lines. In a head and neck primary tumor that would potentially prompt a radical neck dissection, the incision should be oriented, when possible, in such a way that it could be excised as part of the neck dissection. Because all lymph nodes are located adjacent to blood vessels, meticulous dissec-

tion and hemostasis is critical. Cutaneous nerves and any significant blood vessels or other structures can usually be dissected away from the nodes and spared. There is usually one major vascular pedicle to the node that should be clamped and tied before it is cut, lest it retract into the deep recesses of the incision where control can be difficult or impossible.

If there is only one enlarged node, that node should be removed entirely with an intact capsule, if technically possible. When there are multiple enlarged nodes, the most firm, large node and one or two adjacent enlarged but smaller nodes should be removed. Pathologic nodes can be surrounded by nodes that are enlarged by histologically normal hyperplastic changes. Large nodes may be almost entirely necrotic and be unsatisfactory for histologic analysis but can provide important bacteriologic data. Occasionally, for the complete and definitive diagnosis of lymphoma, a second biopsy is necessary at a later date. Inflammatory changes in the nodes adjacent to the original biopsy site often make the nodes unsuitable for analysis, so a distant site should be chosen when possible.

All incisions are closed with absorbable sutures to the subcutaneous tissue or the superficial fascia with a subcuticular skin closure with absorbable suture reinforced with Steri-Strips. Cervical and inguinal sites are usually not drained, whereas axillary sites that were extensively dissected usually are drained with a small closed suction drain that is removed in 2 or 3 days in the usual patient. Occasionally, drainage is prolonged and the drain should not be removed until there is minimal drainage. Pressure dressings are not necessary if proper hemostasis is achieved.

All lymph node excisions should be sent fresh for pathologic study in a saline-moistened container in no contact with a dry sponge, which can distort the architecture of a small node. A pathologist familiar with the special processing necessary for making a definitive diagnosis must be the person to handle the fresh material. Often, touch preps, special cultures, electron microscopy, flow cytometry, and other tests that require fresh tissue are necessary. The pathologist should be notified in advance if special studies are desired. A thorough clinical history should be recorded on the pathology requisition, with a personal phone call made to the pathologist if special handling is requested.

LYMPH NODE BIOPSY IN SPECIFIC SITES

Cervical Lymph Node Biopsy

Not all cervical masses are lymph nodes. The differential diagnosis includes sebaceous cysts that may not have an obvious punctum, lipomas and other benign soft-tissue masses, malignant soft-tissue masses, and branchial cleft and thyroglossal duct cysts. All of these nonnodal masses should be excised to clarify their histologic makeup, except in the unusual situation when their size or extension prohibits excision under local anesthesia.

No cervical lymph node biopsy should be performed before the patient has undergone a thorough physical and endoscopic examination of the oropharyngeal and nasopharyngeal areas in those clinical situations when the lymphadenopathy could represent the metastatic spread of squamous cell carcinoma of the head or neck. In such cases, diagnosis and biopsy of the primary tumor are essential steps in treatment and preclude the need for diagnostic lymph node biopsy.

Although considered "minor surgery," cervical lymph node biopsies can be associated with significant complications unless utmost care and skill are used while working within a very small space containing a large number of important or even vital structures. Complications include hemorrhage, vocal cord paralysis, lymphatic or chylous (left neck) fistulas, pneumothorax, hemothorax, cervical esophageal fistulas, air embolism, cardiac arrhythmias or arrest, stroke, hypoglossal or facial nerve branch damage (especially ramus mandibularis), salivary fistula, and infection.

Cervical lymph node areas include the anterior and posterior triangles, and the supraclavicular and scalene node areas.

The technique of anterior cervical lymph node biopsy follows:

1. The patient's neck is slightly hyperextended and the head turned away from the side of interest.

2. A transverse incision is made directly over the node and deepened through the platysma muscle.

3. Enlarged anterior jugular nodes may be immediately palpable. If so, one or two should be excised with minimal dissection, with the dissection staying just outside the capsule of the node and the surgeon taking care not to injure surrounding structures such as the jugular vein or vagus nerve.

4. Deep jugular nodes require careful dissection and retraction of the jugular vein, vagus nerve, and carotid artery for proper exposure. Low in the left neck the surgeon must avoid injury to the thoracic duct or perform a careful repair or ligation when injury is unavoidable.

5. The platysma is closed with a running 3-0 or 4-0 absorbable suture with skin closure made by a running 4-0 absorbable subcuticular suture reinforced with Steri-Strips and a light dressing.

6. Patients are instructed to keep the wound dry for 1 to 2 days. After that, normal bathing can resume, with the Steri-Strips remaining in place until they fall off.

Scalene Lymph Node Biopsy

Scalene nodes drain primarily the mediastinum and intrathoracic cavities. These nodes are embedded in a fat pad located on the surface of the fascia of the scalenus anticus muscle, at the angle of confluence of the subclavian and internal jugular veins, beneath the superficial layer of the deep cervical fascia. These nodes should be distinguished from those in the subcutaneous fat superficially, the supraclavicular nodes. The distinction is important in that only the scalene nodes normally drain the mediastinum. Scalene node biopsies are performed much less frequently since the use of mediastinoscopy became widespread, but they are still occasionally indicated. Palpable scalene nodes are positive in 85% to 90% of patients with carcinoma of the lung, so scalene biopsy is preferred over the more dangerous and invasive mediastinoscopy in those patients. For patients with lung cancer and nonpalpable nodes, mediastinoscopy is thought to have a higher yield, which justifies its use despite its higher morbidity and expense. Scalene node biopsy can be a very effective method of confirming the diagnosis of sarcoidosis, even with nonpalpable nodes.

The procedure must be performed skillfully to prevent serious complications such as pneumothorax, hemorrhage from the subclavian or jugular veins, air embolism, infection, lymph or chyle fistulas, vocal cord paralysis, paralysis of the hemidiaphragm, and even death from mediastinitis.

The technique of scalene node biopsy follows:

1. The patient's neck is hyperextended and the head rotated to the opposite side.

2. A 4- to 5-cm incision is made 2 cm above and parallel to the clavicle, medially over the midportion of the sternocleidomastoid muscle (Fig. 21–1). It is carried through the platysma muscle.

3. The two bellies of the sternocleidomastoid muscle are spread to enter the prescalene space.

4. Readily palpable nodes can be easily removed without a formal dissection.

5. If the biopsy is being performed as a staging procedure in which there are no palpably enlarged nodes, the deep cervical fascia should be incised to expose the prescalene fat pad. It is bounded medially by the jugular vein, laterally by the omohyoid muscle, and inferiorly by the subclavian vein. Medial retraction of the jugular vein enhances the exposure (Fig. 21–2).

6. The fatty tissue filling the prescalene triangle is totally removed down to the anterior scalene muscle fascia, with the surgeon taking care not to injure the phrenic nerve, which lies on top of the muscle (Fig. 21–3).

7. By having the patient cough or perform a Valsalva maneuver at the end of the dissection, bleeders and lymphatic leaks can be easily identified and ligated. With careful technique, drainage is not routinely necessary.

8. Closure is accomplished as discussed for cervical node biopsy.

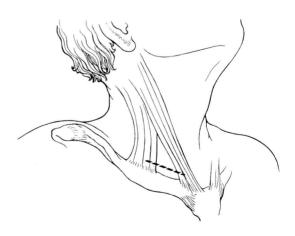

Figure 21–1. Incision for scalene lymph node biopsy. (From Preston FW. General surgery. In: Kassity KJ, McKittrick JE, Preston FW, eds. Manual of Ambulatory Surgery. New York: Springer-Verlag, 1982.)

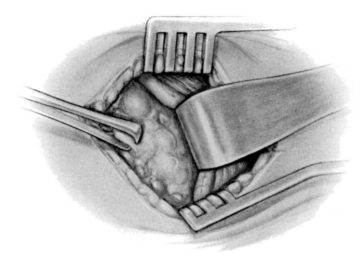

Figure 21–2. The lymph nodes are above and behind the clavicle and lateral to the internal jugular vein. (From Preston FW. General surgery. In: Kassity KJ, McKittrick JE, Preston FW, eds. Manual of Ambulatory Surgery. New York: Springer-Verlag, 1982.)

Supraclavicular Lymph Node Biopsy

Biopsy of the supraclavicular lymph nodes is a much simpler procedure because of their superficial location. None of the potentially serious complications associated with scalene node biopsy should occur. The technique is identical to that of scalene node biopsy except that the dissection is limited to the superficial tissues.

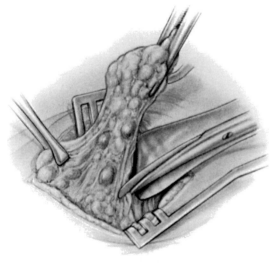

Figure 21–3. Removal of scalene lymph nodes and lymph-node-bearing connective tissue (From Preston FW. General surgery. In: Kassity KJ, McKittrick JE, Preston FW, eds. Manual of Ambulatory Surgery. New York: Springer-Verlag, 1982.)

Axillary Lymph Node Biopsy

Enlarged axillary nodes may be the most difficult of all regional nodal groups to expose because they are often obscured by axillary fat or are difficult to distinguish from the normal axillary fat pad. They are commonly enlarged secondary to minor cuts or scrapes on the hands or arms. They also can herald the first sign of lymphoma, breast cancer, or other malignancy and, therefore, require careful evaluation.

Pitfalls in the biopsy of axillary adenopathy, especially for the inexperienced surgeon, relate to their difficult exposure in some patients. Without proper positioning of the patient, high axillary nodes can be several inches deep in some patients. Optimal exposure is critical to success in adequate excision and avoidance of complications commonly seen such as brachial nerve damage, hemorrhage, lymph fistula, and infection.

The technique of axillary lymph node excision follows:

1. With the patient supine, the upper extremity is flexed 90° at the shoulder and adducted 30°; the forearm is pronated fully and flexed 100° at the elbow. The forearm is suspended in a small towel secured to an overhead anesthesia screen if needed. This position serves to displace the pectoralis major muscle medially and superiorly (Fig. 21–4). This maneuver shifts the lateral border of the

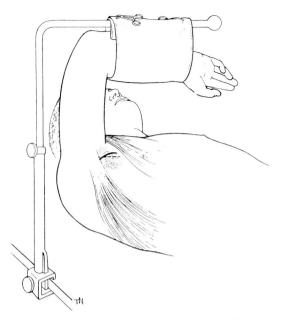

Figure 21–4. Method of securing arm in position described. Solid line indicates usual orientation of incision. Broken line is an alternate choice. Note that incisions are limited to hair-bearing (stippled) area. (From Parker GA, Chretien PB. Axillary lymph node biopsy. Arch Surg 1977;112:1124.)

pectoralis major muscle medial to the apex of the axilla and positions the apical axillary lymph nodes immediately deep to the hair-bearing area of the axillary skin.

2. A 2- to 5-cm transverse incision is made in the hair-bearing area of the axilla, depending on the anticipated depth of the dissection. The depth is minimized with this positioning.

3. The desired lymph node is grasped with a Babcock or similar clamp and the soft-tissue attachments are clamped, divided, and ligated. It is important that lymphatics not be left open and that hemostasis be meticulous.

4. If the dissection is deep it is not unreasonable to leave a small closed suction drain brought out through the wound edge or preferably through a separate incision. A bulky dressing is unnecessary.

5. Closure is routine, as discussed.

Inguinal Lymph Node Biopsy

Masses in the inguinal area present a more extensive differential diagnosis than the other

lymph node basins discussed in this chapter. This list includes lymphadenopathy from a variety of inflammatory and venereal diseases, metastatic carcinoma from anorectal or genital organs, melanomas of the lower extremity, abdominal wall, or perineal area, lymphoma or nonlymphoid masses such as dermoid or other benign cysts, lipomas, soft-tissue sarcomas, inguinal and femoral hernias, undescended testicle, hydrocele of the cord, lipoma of the cord, and femoral aneurysms. Lymphadenopathy can usually be determined preoperatively with a reasonable degree of certainty but there is always the possibility of a different diagnosis.

Inguinal nodes are either superficial or deep. Those in the superficial group are adjacent to the saphenous vein and its tributaries and are the usual nodes subjected to biopsy. Inguinal lymph node biopsy is associated with few complications except that wound infection is more common than in other sites. Nerve trauma or hemorrhage is possible if care is not exercised during deep node excisions.

The technique of inguinal lymph node biopsy follows:

1. The incision is made in a transverse or oblique manner directly over the node.

2. Dissection through the subcutaneous fat should easily reveal the enlarged nodes, which are grasped and totally excised. Multiple branches of the saphenous or femoral vein and branches of the femoral artery may require ligation.

3. Drainage is rarely used. A small pressure dressing may help prevent seroma formation in this area, which is subject to the motion of ambulation.

4. Closure is routine.

SPECIAL CONSIDERATIONS

HIV-Infected Patients

Surgeons are increasingly being asked to participate in the diagnostic workup of human immunodeficiency virus (HIV)–infected patients. Numerous studies reveal that lymph node biopsy can significantly alter therapy in HIV-infected patients. Surgeons will be increasingly involved with these patients, who are likely to be seen more frequently in the future.

There is nothing special about the technical aspects of lymph node biopsy in these patients except for the usual precautions against contamination of the surgeon and the operating room, transport, and pathology laboratory staff. It is critical that all personnel be informed that HIV-infected material is being handled. Fine-needle aspiration may be diagnostic if performed skillfully and when adequate preparation and interpretation are available.

Lymph Node Mapping (Sentinel Node Biopsy)

Several recent studies suggest that identifying the sentinel node that drains a melanoma accurately reflects the likelihood of involved regional lymph nodes. If the sentinel node is negative, studies suggest that there is no benefit to performing a prophylactic node dissection with its associated morbidity. Vital dyes or radioisotopes injected into the primary melanoma site drain first to the sentinel node, which can be localized by visual methods or nuclear detectors and excised under local anesthesia on an outpatient basis. Only patients with positive sentinel nodes undergo node dissection with this approach. The question of which patients with melanoma potentially ben-

efit from prophylactic node dissection is still unresolved, so the ongoing studies of sentinel node biopsy could make this issue irrelevant. It will require several years of additional follow-up to determine the efficacy of this innovative approach. Similar studies are underway in patients with invasive breast cancer.

Selected Readings

Alex JC, Krag DN. Gamma-probe guided localization of lymph nodes. Surg Oncol 1993;2:137–143.

Giuliano AE, Kirgan DM, Guenther JM, et al. Lymphatic mapping and sentinel lymphadenectomy for breast cancer. Ann Surg 1994;220(3):391–401.

Ioachim HL. The lymph node biopsy. In: Ioachim HL, ed. Lymph Node Biopsy. Philadelphia: JB Lippincott, 1982:14–31.

Lee YM. Tumors. In: Hill GJ, Wickland E, ed. Outpatient Surgery. 3rd ed. Philadelphia: WB Saunders, 1988:99–105.

Morton DL, Wen D, Wong JH, et al. Technical details of intraoperative lymphatic mapping for early stage melanoma. Arch Surg 1992;127(4):392–399.

Palumbo LT, Sharpe WS. Scalene node biopsy correlation with other diagnostic procedures in 550 cases. Arch Surg 1969;98(1):90–93.

Parker GA, Chretien PB. Axillary lymph node biopsy. Arch Surg 1977;112:1124.

Pierce EH, Gray HK, Dockerty MB. Surgical significance of isolated axillary adenopathy. Ann Surg 1957;1:104–107.

Preston FW. General surgery. In: Kassity KJ, McKittrick JE, Preston FW eds. Manual of Ambulatory Surgery. New York: Springer-Verlag, 1982:72–78.

Wong R, Rappaport W, Gorman S, et al. Value of lymph node biopsy in the treatment of patients with the human immunodeficiency virus. Am J Surg 1991; 162(12):590–593.

22

Management of Breast Abnormalities

Marcia Moore • *Charles Harris*

This chapter reviews an efficient surgical approach to the management of breast masses, with practical approaches for avoiding common clinical pitfalls.

Even as recently as two decades ago, diagnostic breast biopsies were commonly performed only for palpable masses. With the widespread use of screening mammography, there has been a dramatic increase in the number of biopsies being performed for mammographically detected nonpalpable abnormalities. For example, from 1988 to 1994, the number of biopsies performed at the University of Virginia Health Sciences Center doubled for mammographically detected abnormalities. Slightly more than 1% of the 10,000 patients undergoing screening mammograms yearly had a lesion classified as sufficiently suspicious to warrant biopsy. With more biopsies being performed for nonpalpable lesions, there has been a concomitant increase in the number of early stage cancers detected, and a slow, steady trend toward increased survival that one would expect to see as a corollary. The number of in situ cancers being diagnosed and treated has increased significantly as well.

The approach to palpable and nonpalpable abnormalities is discussed separately because the surgical techniques for excision of palpable and nonpalpable lesions are quite distinct.

PALPABLE ABNORMALITIES

Not infrequently a patient comes to the surgeon's office having noticed a palpable ab-

normality on breast self-examination. On examining this patient, the surgeon may not be able to confirm a suspicious finding. Often the patient feels a prominent area of breast tissue, which is physiologic. When the lesion is not thought to be pathologic, it is my practice to offer the patient reassurance and to schedule her for a repeat breast examination after her next menstrual cycle or in 1 month's time. If on the second examination the patient is still concerned about the area, it is prudent to obtain a tissue diagnosis of the area, despite a lack of clinical suspicion. Sometimes an incidental in situ lesion is found. More importantly, obtaining a tissue diagnosis of the area offers reassurance to the patient as well as legal protection for the surgeon. If cancer develops in the area of prior suspicion, it is important for the area to have been investigated when the patient brought it to the surgeon's attention.

In investigation of an area of the breast to confirm that there is benign ductal tissue present, a fine-needle aspiration (FNA) done as an office procedure is appropriate. This office procedure is also cost effective for confirming that a highly suspicious lesion is a carcinoma. On review of a recent series of FNAs performed at the University of Virginia for palpable lesions considered by the surgeon to be highly suspicious for carcinoma, FNA revealed 73% to be carcinomas. An unsatisfactory needle biopsy of any suspicious lesion— that is, one having insufficient material for analysis or one showing benign ductal epithelium that does not explain the presence of a palpable mass—should *always* dictate an open biopsy procedure.

Information on core biopsies is insufficient to assess clearly the extent to which this technique may replace the FNA procedure for the office diagnosis of palpable masses. Nevertheless, initial studies suggest that core biopsy may have higher utility, especially when FNA is not commonly performed and skilled cytopathologists may not be available for evaluation of the material. A recently published prospective series showed that nine of nine cancers were diagnosed by core biopsy and that 26 of the 29 core biopsies were diagnostic. A review of a 20-institution trial in which core biopsies were performed on 6152 lesions showed that the false-negative rate for diagnosing cancer was only 1.2% and that none of 1268 fibroadenomas diagnosed by means of core biopsy proved to be malignant on surgical excision.

One advantage of the core biopsy over FNA is that the pathologist has a larger fragment of tissue to analyze. Moreover, the diagnostic limitations of FNA do not exist in core biopsy. Because a larger, 16-gauge needle is used, the architecture of the lesion is preserved so that a carcinoma in situ can frequently be distinguished from an invasive carcinoma. Estrogen and progesterone receptor information can be obtained on core needle specimens. Although rare, the complications of hematoma and infection have also been reported after core needle biopsy in 0.2% of the 3765 cases for which follow-up information was available.

BREAST CYSTS

Cystic changes are the most common pathologic condition of the breasts. Cystic disease of the breast is often seen in middle-aged women, and it is essential to distinguish dominant cystic masses of the breast from malignancies. If a single fluctuant mass is present, suggesting a solitary macrocyst of the breast, aspiration is recommended for initial assessment. This is adequate therapy if (1) the mass completely disappears with aspiration, (2) there is no blood in the aspirated fluid, and (3) the mass is not palpable when the breast is reexamined 1 month after aspiration. Before the aspiration

is performed, a *mammogram* should be obtained to ascertain that there are no additional areas of concern in either breast. Finally, ultrasound is a useful adjunct to determine whether the palpable mass is indeed a simple cyst.

Bloody fluid return, with or without a residual mass, should be submitted for cytologic examination because 19% of these lesions are malignant. If the fluid is clear, the probability of finding any malignant cells within it is so small that cytologic examination is not cost effective.

Approximately 20% of aspirated cysts recur. If the cyst does recur, it is my practice to excise it. Reaspiration with cytologic examination is an acceptable alternative practiced by others. However, it is especially important to counsel all patients who have had recurrent cysts never to ignore the appearance of a new mass in the breast. Whether cystic disease predisposes the patient to a malignancy of the breast is very much debated. However, it is certainly a tragedy when the existence of previous breast cysts interferes with early diagnosis of a malignancy.

FIBROADENOMAS

Fibroadenomas of the breast are the most frequently seen solid breast masses in women younger than age 25 years. These tumors rarely occur before menarche and their frequency rapidly decreases after menopause. They may be diagnosed with a needle or core aspiration in the clinician's office. However, because it is not unusual for fibroadenomas to become massive in size, it is reasonable to offer the woman the option of having them excised to prevent them from becoming difficult to approach surgically.

TECHNIQUES OF BIOPSY

Good technique is important to maximize diagnostic accuracy when performing breast biopsies. It is advantageous to have a reasonably high volume of biopsy samples to achieve optimal results. The watchword is caution: if a question arises as to the adequacy of tissue obtained, a second biopsy of the area in ques-

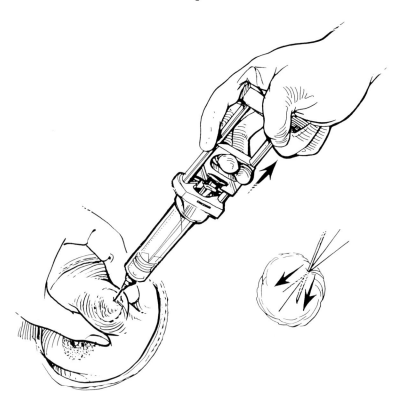

Figure 22–1. Technique of fine-needle aspiration. The surgeon localizes the lesion between the index finger and thumb of the nondominant hand. The fine needle, mounted in a biopsy trigger guide, is passed into the skin and negative pressure is exerted on the syringe as the needle is passed several times through the lesion. Negative pressure is then released and the needle withdrawn. The cellular material within the needle is then prepared and analyzed.

tion must be undertaken. At times, this may require using an alternative method of biopsy.

TECHNIQUES OF FINE-NEEDLE ASPIRATION

The sensitivity for FNAs has been reported to range from 68% to 93%. Specificity has ranged from 88% to 100%, with insufficient sampling rates ranging from 0% to 38%. These wide ranges suggest the importance of careful technique. The best results are reported when an experienced surgeon and cytopathologist work together.

For both FNA and core biopsy, the needle tract should be angled in such a way as to be encompassed by subsequent definitive surgery. In an evaluation of 2000 core biopsies performed recently, the seeding of tumor cells was noted along the core biopsy tract in three cases. Although this is a low rate of seeding, it is a preventable complication when the needle tract is excised by subsequent definitive surgery.

FNA is carried out with a 19- or 21-gauge needle attached to a syringe, which is mounted

in a guide (Fig. 22–1). Several passes are made into the mass, without the needle being withdrawn from the breast tissue. Negative pressure is maintained on the syringe with one hand and the mass is stabilized between the thumb and index finger of the other hand. The material aspirated is placed on a microscopic slide and fixed in 95% ethanol immediately before being sent for pathologic examination. Satisfactory specimens from this technique range from 89% to 98%.

Open Surgical Biopsy

Open biopsy is necessary when needle aspiration procedures yield equivocal results. It is also advisable for cysts that recur despite aspiration and for enlarging fibroadenomas. Some patients prefer to have a dominant mass in the breast excised rather than have a needle biopsy performed. When the patient wants removal of the mass to relieve symptoms of tenderness or if she finds it troubling to feel the mass while doing breast self-examination, a needle biopsy does not resolve the problem and therefore should not be performed. Instead, it is sensible to streamline the approach and go directly to open excision of the mass.

Surgical Approach to Open Biopsy

The open surgical biopsy under local anesthesia is often performed as an office procedure. If the mass is large or deep, it is advisable to proceed with the addition of intravenous sedation in the ambulatory operating room setting.

A patient aged 35 years or older who is undergoing an open surgical biopsy should have a mammogram before the biopsy. This may identify an occult lesion that can be biopsied at the same time and one that may be more important than the original lesion for which the biopsy is planned. It is frustrating to perform an open biopsy only to find a lesion 2 or 3 months later on a planned mammogram, necessitating a second trip to the operating room.

Breast lesions can be adequately excised using rather small incisions by following a few surgical principles. A curvilinear incision over-

lying the lesion is preferred for a lesion located very superiorly or inferiorly in the breast. For a lesion that is central, a circumareolar incision is ideal both oncologically and cosmetically. Because the biopsy incision must be removed at the time of the subsequent definitive surgical procedure for cancer, a biopsy incision should be placed appropriately. At times, it is essential to know whether a patient would elect breast-conserving therapy or a mastectomy to optimally place the biopsy incision. If the patient prefers breast-conserving therapy, a very peripherally located lesion should be removed through a peripheral incision, avoiding a long tunnel that must be excised in a subsequent procedure. Contamination of a long-tunneled tract may eliminate the potential for breast-conserving therapy. If a subsequent mastectomy would be the patient's choice, the biopsy incision should be placed at a central location (Fig. 22–2).

It is important to examine the patient both sitting and supine before prepping and draping the breast. When a patient is lying down, it is often difficult to palpate a lesion that was easy to feel when the patient was sitting. The

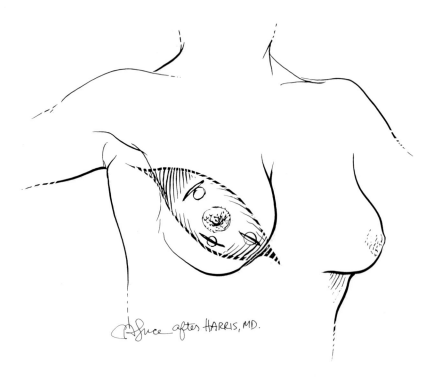

Figure 22–2. Location of open breast biopsy. Whenever mastectomy may serve as definitive treatment of carcinoma, the surgeon must be careful to place the open biopsy incision within the area to be removed with the mastectomy incision.

patient and the surgeon must agree on the location of the lesion to be biopsied before the breast is prepped and draped for the procedure. Betadine prepping solution tends to make the skin somewhat tacky, thereby decreasing the surgeon's tactile sensitivity. Marking the lesion with a non–alcohol-soluble pen before prepping and draping is advisable.

No antibiotic prophylaxis is required for these clean procedures, but careful attention to sterile technique is.

Because hematoma formation is the most common complication of a breast biopsy, it is worthwhile to view the use of lidocaine with epinephrine with some skepticism. The half-life of epinephrine is 15 to 20 minutes, and it is possible that small vessels that are not bleeding at the time of skin closure are in vasospasm secondary to the epinephrine. A hematoma may form from a subsequent reflex vasodilatation after the incision is closed. There are excellent data in animal models suggesting that the risk of infection, presumably secondary to transient ischemia during surgery, is also increased by the addition of epinephrine to lidocaine. Therefore, it is my practice to use lidocaine without epinephrine. Bicarbonate added to the lidocaine just before administration neutralizes the pain of the injection caused by the acidity of the lidocaine.

Absorbable sutures, chromic or Vicryl, are used in the deep tissues because of the poor blood supply of the breast tissue. Because of this limited blood supply, there is a tendency toward infection. Permanent sutures that might serve as a nidus for infection should therefore be avoided. To achieve ideal cosmetic results, the deeper tissues should not be reapproximated. If the biopsy cavity is reapproximated, there is the potential problem of puckering of the skin. Allowing the breast biopsy cavity to fill with seroma ultimately gives the breast a natural contour. One excellent method of skin closure is obtained with a monofilament subcuticular skin suture, which is removed in 4 to 7 days. This suture minimizes inflammatory reaction and avoids the problem of unsightly suture marks on the skin.

A drain should be avoided, if possible, because it negatively affects the cosmetic outcome of the procedure by changing the breast contour. In rare cases, the placement of a drain for 24 hours may be unavoidable. A drain is used in patients who are taking anticoagulants or in those in whom hemostasis is difficult during the operation. The drain tract must also be excised in a subsequent procedure if cancer is diagnosed; therefore, it should be placed centrally in the breast if a mastectomy is contemplated.

A very large lesion that is highly suspected of being carcinoma is best approached by an *incisional* biopsy rather than by undertaking an extensive operation that will be subsequently negated by mastectomy.

Cosmetically, the most difficult lesions are those that are in the upper inner quadrant. It is worthwhile to discuss with the patient preoperatively that this incision will be visible when she wears a low-necked garment. Likewise, patients in whom a large mass is to be excised should be cautioned that they may notice postsurgical changes in the contour of the breast. In rare cases, a patient may be a candidate for breast reconstruction surgery if a very large benign mass or several moderately sized masses must be removed from the same breast.

In a large-breasted patient, seeing into the depths of the incision can be difficult unless an adequate self-retaining retractor is available. A headlight is a useful aid for good visualization as well. After irrigation of the tissues, the skin can be closed with a subcuticular monofilament suture, which is removed 1 week postoperatively when the patient returns to discuss her pathology report. The patient can be given acetaminophen with codeine for postoperative pain, although most patients are comfortable with taking acetaminophen only. I also counsel them to wear a supportive bra continuously for 2 to 3 days after surgery.

All specimens resected from the breast should be sent to the pathologist for evaluation immediately after excision. The specimen should be sent on ice, because there is evidence that hormone receptors deteriorate with periods of warm ischemia. Warm ischemia time exceeding 30 minutes may lead to falsely negative binding assay for estrogen and progesterone receptors. While immunohistochemical staining for hormone receptors can be performed on formalinized fixed tissues, this technique is not always available.

Use of Frozen Sections

The first priority in the evaluation of any breast lesion is to arrive at an accurate diagnosis. The Association of Directors of Anatomic and Surgical Pathology has recently stated that a frozen section is not mandatory on every breast biopsy and is often contraindicated. If the gross lesion is small (less than 1 cm in greatest dimension), a frozen section may not yield a definitive diagnosis and permanent sections from that frozen block may be degraded by freezing artifacts. The conservation of tissue that has never been frozen is a high priority for optimal diagnosis. I therefore explain to any patient who has a small lesion of the breast that a frozen section may not be optimal and that a final pathology report will be available on her postoperative office visit. At that visit, I remove the suture, assess wound healing, and discuss the biopsy results in detail.

Biopsies of some benign lesions (such as epithelial hyperplasia with atypia) carry an increased risk for future development of carcinoma. This necessitates additional discussion with the patient and her family.

A recent review of 100 biopsies of solid breast lesions performed at the University of Virginia showed a total of 22 malignancies. Of these, eight were less than 1 cm in size and only four were more than 2 cm. Two of these palpable malignancies were ductal carcinomas in situ.

Breast Stereotactic Core Needle Biopsies

The most common presentation of breast abnormalities originates from an abnormal mammogram of a nonpalpable lesion. The increased use of high-quality mammograms has resulted in a dramatic shift in surgical practice. Here, communication between the surgeon and radiologist is paramount because there is a substantial variability in radiologists' interpretations of mammograms. Clinical input from the surgeon, including a review of all previous abnormal mammograms, reduces the number of negative biopsies and improves the overall management of patients. In addition, it is strongly recommended that double read-

ings of the mammograms be obtained. The radiologists' perceptual threshold can cause an important abnormality to be overlooked. No matter how experienced the observer, the rate of cancer detection with double reading is reported to be increased by 15%. The evolving capacity to digitize mammograms makes the potential for future double reading more feasible, because images can then be reproduced at distant sites.

Traditionally, the removal of nonpalpable abnormalities has required surgical biopsy with a needle localization wire. There is new evidence that core needle biopsies of these lesions will have a high positive predictive value. Core needle biopsies have been performed for 6 months at our institution with 95% sensitivity in more than 250 biopsies.

As confidence in this technique grows, the applications for its usefulness may extend. It will not, however, completely replace the necessity for performing wire-guided surgical biopsies of occult breast lesions. There will be times when the core biopsy results are inconclusive or when the lesion itself is ill defined and not amenable to approach by core needle techniques. Indeed, as the number of surgical biopsies decreases, it is more important than ever that the surgeon be comfortable with these techniques.

Technique of Needle-Localized Breast Biopsy

Successful needle-localized breast biopsy of occult lesions requires cooperation among the surgeon, radiologist, and pathologist. Here, careful attention to technical considerations yields dividends.

Numerous techniques have been described for performing surgical biopsies of nonpalpable lesions. However, most surgeons have found that the use of a hooked localization wire gives the most satisfactory results. The hooked guide wire is difficult to dislodge during the dissection of the breast. By localizing the lesion quite precisely, it also permits the surgeon to minimize the amount of tissue that must be removed, therefore limiting cosmetic deformity.

Successful removal of the lesion requires

that the needle be placed close to the abnormality. Because the anatomic relationship between the abnormality and the wire shifts when the patient is sitting with her breast compressed in the mammography unit as opposed to when she is lying supine on the operating table, a wire eccentrically placed several centimeters from the lesion does not have the same ultimate relationship to the lesion as that demonstrated on placement mammograms. Placing the wire very close to, or, ideally, through the abnormality, aids in removing the lesion. Placement of the wire within 1 cm of the lesion is considered adequate. In a review of 100 consecutive needle localizations performed at the University of Virginia, 95% of the wires were placed through the lesion or within 1 cm of it. Even though some reports document unsuccessful biopsy rates as high as 22%, it seems clear that, with cooperation between the surgeon and the radiologist, the rate of missed lesions can be in the 1% to 3% range.

The technique is typically performed using local anesthesia and averaging 20 mL of 1% lidocaine (Xylocaine) per biopsy. In rare cases when a large-breasted woman has a very large or deep-seated lesion, general anesthesia may be required. Intravenous sedation with midazolam or fentanyl can be a good supplement to local anesthesia.

Before the breast is prepared and draped, the wire from needle localization should be cut approximately 5 to 10 cm from the skin (Fig. 22–3). If the wire is cut too short, there is a risk of pulling the wire inside the breast during the biopsy.

The surgeon must carefully evaluate the wire localization radiographs and understand the orientation of the hook and wire with respect to the breast abnormality before ap-

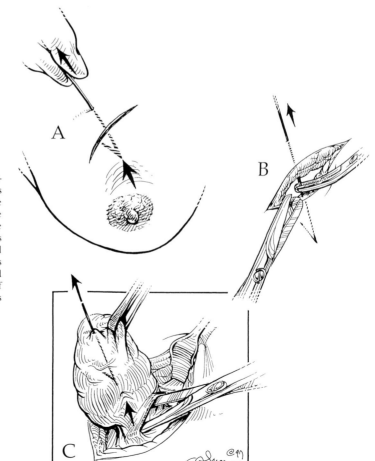

Figure 22–3. Technique of needle localization biopsy. (**A**) A hooked wire is placed under mammographic guidance by the radiologist. The tip of the wire should ideally be within 1 cm of the lesion and the wire should pass through the lesion. (**B**) An elliptical incision of skin containing the wire is made. (**C**) The incision is deepened to include an appropriate cylinder of tissue, which contains the wire at its center.

proaching biopsy. This is an essential prerequisite to an accurate excision and minimizes the necessity for removing a great deal of extra breast tissue. In surgical planning, the surgeon should place the incision directly over the lesion, not over the wire. The surgeon can then minimize the amount of tunneling through the breast tissue. When biopsying a soft-tissue mass, the surgeon must examine the specimen carefully to ensure that the nodule has been removed. The wire itself may have been deflected by a very dense nodule and the target nodule may therefore be missed. Furthermore, the wound should be carefully palpated before closure to detect any additional areas of density that may warrant removal. Intraoperative ultrasound may be used for additional screening.

As the specimen is removed from the biopsy cavity, the wire should be left in place in the specimen. This aids the radiologist in confirming the position of the specimen. In particular, the wire should never be pulled out through the wire tract, because this would potentially contaminate the tract with cancer cells.

If the specimen mammogram indicates that the lesion has not been removed, it is my practice to excise a second specimen after speaking with the radiologist directly. In rare cases, the lesion may be a cyst that was punctured during the procedure, making the specimen mammogram difficult to interpret. When the lesion has not been excised, the specimen may contain landmarks that suggest the direction for proceeding with removal of the second specimen. It is imperative, for this reason, that specimens be oriented. A mnemonic to help in remembering suture placement is to place a *l*ong suture in the *l*ateral position and a *s*hort suture on the *s*uperior pole of the lesion. If the second specimen does not contain a lesion, the surgeon should consider terminating the procedure and having a repeat localization performed at a second sitting.

LUMPECTOMY

Patients with ductal carcinoma in situ or an early-stage invasive carcinoma are often good candidates for local excision of the lesion as an ambulatory procedure. It is ideal for these patients to have a lumpectomy performed at their initial procedure, followed by radiation therapy for control of residual disease within the breast.

When the patient is a candidate for breast-conserving therapy, it is worthwhile to place clips in the biopsy cavity in preparation for subsequent radiation therapy, because this obviates the need for reopening the biopsy cavity for clip placement. The clips allow the radiation therapist to fine-tune the "boost" of radiation given to the biopsy site as part of the treatment for early invasive breast cancer or ductal carcinoma in situ. In our review of 50 early-stage breast cancer patients who were offered this option, 90% of them had an adequate excision to negative margins in their initial biopsy. The common lesions with positive margins are ductal carcinoma in situ lesions, whereas invasive carcinomas are often more clearly demarcated. When a lesion has been identified as highly suspicious for carcinoma in situ, the surgeon may be well advised to aim for wider margins because it is common to underestimate the extent of the lesion.

DUCT EXCISION FOR PERSISTENT NIPPLE DISCHARGE

The patient who presents with spontaneous nipple discharge, whether it is clear, blood-tinged, or bloody, usually has a benign lesion. The most common such lesion is an intraductal papilloma. The possibility of a carcinoma cannot be excluded without duct excision. With a solitary papilloma, the lesion is usually small and is not palpable. Mammographic evidence may show only a dilated duct resulting from the obstruction by the papilloma. Excision of the duct and the tissue surrounding it is the treatment of choice. Other less frequent causes of persistent nipple discharge include duct ectasia, papillomatosis, subareolar infections, and fibroadenoma. In a series of 448 patients with nipple discharge, 140 underwent biopsy and were given the following diagnoses: intraductal papilloma, 43.6%; carcinoma, 29.3%; and cystic disease, 11.4%.

Often the quadrant involved with the nipple discharge and not the duct itself can be identified preoperatively. In such a case, an areolar quadrantectomy is the surgical procedure of choice. A pathologist who understands the clinical situation carefully reviews the specimen and frequently can identify the dilated duct and papilloma.

Microscopically, the intraductal papillomas are seen as a proliferation of ductal epithelium that projects into the dilated duct. Multiple papillomas, in contrast to a solitary papilloma, consist of many grossly visible papillomas that arise from several different ducts. The multiplicity is obvious to the pathologist on tissue review. Because multiple papillomas recur after local excision, it may often be necessary to control the disease by multiple excisions. Although multiple papillomas may occasionally evolve into carcinoma, we treat this symptomatically rather than to perform prophylactic mastectomy.

GYNECOMASTIA—BREAST LESIONS IN THE MALE

Although true gynecomastia is a common clinical finding, distinction between this and the more rare but deadly carcinoma of the breast is crucial. Whereas gynecomastia is rarely associated with fatal disease, breast cancer in men is fatal in 33% of those affected.

Gynecomastia may present as an asymptomatic, incidental finding or as an acute, unilateral or bilateral painful, tender subareolar mass. There are three distinct peak times for gynecomastia to occur in the life of a male. The first is in the neonatal period, when, because of transplacental passage of estrogens, 60% to 90% of all newborns have transient development of palpable breast tissue. The second peak occurs during puberty, beginning at age 10 years and peaking between ages 13 and 14 years, with a subsequent decline in incidence thereafter. The third and last peak is among 50- to 80-year-old men.

Pubertal Gynecomastia

Pubertal gynecomastia develops in an estimated 40% of adolescent males. This condition disappears in 75% of affected boys within 2 years and 90% within 3 years. It appears to be due to increased conversion of adrenal androgens to estrogens in tissue sites such as the breast at a period in life when daytime secretion of testosterone is low. Typically, the glandular tissue is less than 4 cm in diameter and resembles the early stages of female breast budding.

Macrogynecomastia

Macrogynecomastia is described when the breast tissue extends 5 cm or more in diameter and the breasts are dome shaped. Gynecomastia in this subset of patients is unlikely to regress spontaneously and requires treatment that may include surgical excision.

Causes of Gynecomastia

The exclusion of pathologic causes of gynecomastia is important and can be done with a simple history and physical examination. A history of medications taken detects the 10% to 20% of gynecomastia caused by drugs. Calcium channel blockers, digoxin, H_2-antagonists, neuroleptics, ketoconazole, spironolactone, and marijuana are the more common agents implicated. A physical examination reveals the findings associated with cirrhosis and malnutrition (8%), testicular tumors (3%), secondary hypogonadism (2%), hyperthyroidism (1.5%), or renal disease (1%) as possible causes; 25% of gynecomastia cases are idiopathic.

Therapy

Because gynecomastia is so common, an elaborate workup is seldom indicated. After the history and physical examination, serum chemistry evaluations of hepatic, renal, and thyroid function are the only other tests indicated in most cases.

Medical therapy for gynecomastia has included androgen supplementation (dihydrotestosterone, danazol) and antiestrogen agents (clomiphene citrate, tamoxifen, testolactone) with complete responses to therapy ranging from 25% to 80%. The effectiveness of medical therapy is difficult to evaluate because of the high rate of spontaneous regression. If gynecomastia has been present more than 12 months, increased stromal hyalinization and reduction in epithelial proliferation results in inactive fibrotic tissue that is unlikely to respond to medical therapy. It is this patient population that comprises most surgical referrals for this problem.

Surgery is indicated to relieve the anxiety and embarrassment that usually attends pubertal gynecomastia. Although medically benign, the patient's symptoms can be of sufficient magnitude to cause avoidance of participation in athletic activities. If gynecomastia persists in the older man who has stopped taking the implicated drug for more than 1 month, an excisional biopsy is indicated. A small or moderately sized mass can be excised through a circumareolar incision under local anesthesia. A simple mastectomy may be required in the older patient to prevent recurrence. Eccentric breast enlargement on examination raises the concern of carcinoma, even though other benign conditions such as lipomas, dermoid cysts, neurofibromas, lymphangiomas, and hematomas can present similarly. Sterility, schistosomiasis, ionizing radiation therapy, and Klinefelter's syndrome (sex chromosomes XXY) are identified risk factors for male breast cancer, with a 16-fold increased incidence in men with Klinefelter's syndrome. The presence of gynecomastia does not seem to be associated with an increased risk of male breast cancer, although microscopic changes of gynecomastia have been associated with 40% of male breast cancer patients. Findings of a hard, fixed mass with nipple discharge or retraction warrants an aggressive and expedient evaluation for cancer, starting with needle biopsy. The standard surgical approach to male breast cancer remains modified radical mastectomy.

APPROACH TO THE ELDERLY PATIENT

Breast disease, like other conditions requiring surgical procedures, necessitates individualization to treat each patient appropriately. In particular, frail elderly patients with invasive breast cancer who are not candidates for cyto-

toxic chemotherapy may not benefit from an axillary dissection. The disadvantage of the axillary dissection is that it requires a general anesthetic, which an elderly patient in poor health may not tolerate well. If the axilla is clinically negative and the patient is not well enough to undergo cytotoxic chemotherapy, the benefit of staging with an axillary dissection is small enough that it may well be counterbalanced by the risks of the anesthetic. Therefore, a lumpectomy or simple mastectomy performed under local anesthesia may be the single best procedure for patients with multiple medical problems who are poor anesthesia risks.

CONCLUSION

As the biologic factors of breast cancer become better understood and as additional treatment modalities arise, the trend toward less extensive surgical procedures may accelerate, thus allowing for an increasing number of breast procedures to be performed in the ambulatory care setting.

Selected Readings

1. Balch CM, Singletary SE, Bland KI. Clinical decision-making in early breast cancer. Ann Surg 1993; 217:207–225.
2. Carty NJ, Ravichandran D, et al. Randomized comparison of fine needle aspiration cytology and biopsy–cut needle biopsy after unsatisfactory initial cytology of discrete breast lesions. Br J Surg 1994;81:1313–1314.
3. Donegan WL. Evaluation of palpable breast mass. N Engl J Med 1992;327:937–942.
4. Elmore JG, et al. Variability of radiologists' interpretations of mammograms N Engl J Med 1994;331:1493–1499.
5. Frykberg ER, Masood S, Copeland EM 3rd, Bland KI. Ductal carcinoma in situ of the breast. Surg Gynecol Obstet 1993;177:425–440.
6. Graham NL, Bauer TL. Early detection of occult breast cancer: the York experience with 678 needle localization biopsies. Am Surg 1988;54:234–239.
7. Kopans DB. The accuracy of mammographic interpretations. N Engl J Med 1994;331:1521–1522.
8. Perdue P, Page D, et al. Early detection of breast carcinoma: a comparison of palpable and nonpalpable lesions. Surgery 1992;111:656–659.
9. Sullivan DC. Needle core biopsy of mammographic lesions. Am J Radiol 1994;162:601–608.
10. Wilhelm MC, Wanebo HJ. Technique and guidelines for needle localization biopsy of nonpalpable lesions of the breast. Surg Gynecol Obstet 1988;167:439.

Hernias: Traditional Approach

Arthur I. Gilbert • Michael F. Graham

The classic repair of inguinal hernia was established by Edoardo Bassini of Padua and Henry Marcy of Boston in the last half of the 19th Century. Bassini focused on rebuilding tissues to repair a direct hernia. After ligation of the peritoneal sac at the level of the deep inguinal ring, he opened the herniated posterior wall, then reconstructed it in multiple layers. He appreciated the importance of restoring the obliquity between the deep and superficial inguinal rings and did so by closing the external oblique aponeurosis over the cord. Marcy clearly concentrated on indirect hernias caused by incompetency of the internal ring. In 1871, he repaired two indirect hernias by ligating the peritoneal sac, then he recomposed the internal ring using the medial and lateral crura of the transversalis fascia. He showed that restoring the failed mechanism of the deep ring is the essential measure for permanent repair of an indirect hernia. Even though Bassini and Marcy worked independently, the sum of their efforts remains the bedrock of modern inguinal hernia surgery.

Bassini's classic three-layer repair uses the transversalis fascia and the aponeurosis of the transversus abdominis and internal oblique muscles, sewn together with a single layer of interrupted silk sutures to the shelving edge of Poupart's ligament. His repair features solid myofascial reconstruction of the posterior wall while preserving the obliquity of the canal. Results in 262 patients, with better than 90% follow-up, showed a failure rate of 3%. Halsted's repair added a fourth layer by including the external oblique aponeurosis to reconstruct the posterior wall. Direct apposition of the deep and superficial rings sacrifices

the obliquity of the canals, resulting in an unacceptably high rate of recurrent indirect hernias. Both the Bassini and Halsted techniques actually narrow the inguinal canal rather than truly repair the defect.

Halsted, Ferguson, Andrews, and others used much of the work of Marcy and Bassini as the basis for their versions of hernia repair. Before the turn of the century, the pureness of the Bassini repair was compromised by Bull and Coley of New York. They omitted opening the posterior wall; the internal oblique muscle was sutured directly to Poupart's ligament over the spermatic cord. Halsted, as much as any other surgeon, was responsible for the North American modification of Bassini's operation. His alteration is much the same as Bull's version except Halsted placed the cord above the repair.

The Cooper's ligament repair was introduced by Georg Lotheissen in 1898. In a patient whose inguinal ligament was destroyed, he successfully substituted Cooper's ligament. Anson, Morgan, and McVay popularized the Cooper's ligament repair, emphasizing that it was the truest anatomic repair of the canal. By studying numerous cadaver dissections, they determined that the plane of the transversus abdominis aponeurosis is closer to Cooper's ligament than to Poupart's ligament. This repair, with or without relaxing incisions, has been used by many surgeons. The procedure requires transition sutures from Cooper's ligament to the inguinal ligament to avoid compression of the iliofemoral vein. Breakdown of this essential suture line often occurs when the tissues are approximated under tension to Cooper's ligament. For this reason and because of the current availability of excellent prosthetics, many surgeons have abandoned this repair.

Relaxing incisions in the rectus fascia became popular to reduce tension on the sutured posterior wall or between the anterior muscles sutured to Poupart's or Cooper's ligaments. First described by Wolfer and then popularized by Halsted, making relaxing incisions became common in most repairs in adults. In current hernia surgery, suture line tension in pure tissue repairs is avoided by use of prosthetic mesh.

In 1945, E. E. Shouldice opened a hernia surgery clinic in Toronto. In a six-bed facility, he and his first associate, Nicholas Obney, began to do hernia repair using local anesthesia. This innovative approach, coupled with their excellent later results, attracted the interest of surgeons worldwide. The clinic has since grown to a 62-bed hospital devoted exclusively to hernia surgery. The procedure that Shouldice first used was similar to Bassini's operation. In it, the cremasteric fascia is excised and the cord thinned. The posterior wall is opened from the internal ring to the pubic tubercle. A four-layer continuous posterior wall reconstruction is done with two strands of stainless steel wire. Initially, the cremasteric vessels and genital branch of the genitofemoral nerve were preserved. Because early failure rates were high, Shouldice subsequently improved the procedure by dividing the cremasteric bundle including the genital branch of the genitofemoral nerve and the cremasteric vessels. This step facilitated clear exposure of the entire posterior wall and resulted in a significant reduction of failures.

The Shouldice repair for primary and recurrent hernias has stood the test of time. With impressive follow-up in more than 200,000 patients operated on at the Shouldice Hospital, the failure rate is less than 1%. More than any other institution, the Shouldice clinic has been responsible for exposing surgeons to a better quality of hernia surgery. For surgeons who visit there, its success is seen in each surgeon's keen knowledge of groin anatomy and the technique of the detailed dissection performed in each operation. If there is any shortcoming in the Shouldice operation for inguinal hernia, it is the high incidence of femoral hernia that occurs following inguinal hernia repair. There are two contributing factors. The innominate fascia is routinely opened in the thigh to check for a femoral hernia; in the inguinal component of the repair, Poupart's ligament is pulled cephalad enough to encourage the development of a femoral hernia. After many years of reluctance to alter the pure tissue repair, the Shouldice group recently reported that, by using mesh repairs, they have obtained better results in cases of difficult recurrent hernias.

The era of prosthetic repairs began in 1958 with the work of Usher. Initially, use of prosthetics was resisted by surgeons. They feared foreign body reactions, infection, and possible oncogenic consequences related to the materials. In patients with incisional hernias that resulted from extensive tissue loss, polyethylene mesh was successfully used to bridge fascial defects. The technique allowed lasting repairs of large abdominal wall hernias that would have failed if closed under tension by fascial suture techniques. Initially, mesh was used to supplement tissue approximation repairs. Currently, a preferable technique is to accept the defect and to patch it with a mesh graft. Polypropylene (the successor of polyethelene), polytetrafluoroethylene, and Mersilene are permanent prosthetics suitable for hernia repair.

Avoiding tension in the suture line is necessary for success in hernia surgery. When recurrent hernias are subsequently repaired, it is often evident that failure was caused by sutures that tore through tissues. In time, mesh became accepted in groin hernia repair, first in treating recurrences and currently in making primary repairs. Our contribution to "tension-free" repairs for indirect hernia is to show the use of the internal ring as a natural passageway to the preperitoneal space (Fig. 23–1). A polypropylene prosthetic mesh (Prolene mesh) is folded as an umbrella plug. It is inserted through the internal ring into the actualized preperitoneal space where it opens and blocks the internal ring and the medial portion of the posterior wall, thereby instantly repairing the indirect hernia and protecting against any incipient or future direct hernia. This technique has been used for the past 6 years and

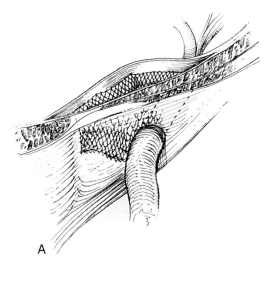

A

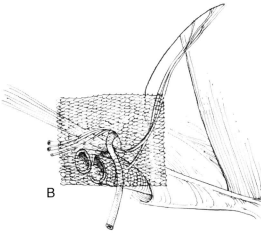

B

Figure 23–1. (A) Anterior view, prosthetic mesh opened in preperitoneal space. **(B)** Posterior view, prosthetic mesh opened in preperitoneal space.

has significantly facilitated the repair of all indirect hernias.

The introduction and trials of the laparoscopic approach to hernia repair have heightened the use and value of mesh for all repairs. Many surgeons who attempted laparoscopic herniorrhaphy, including the majority who have abandoned it, gained useful knowledge as a result of their efforts. They now have clearer understanding of groin and abdominal wall anatomy, and they better appreciate the value and safety of mesh.

Open hernia repair is often done through a posterior approach. The approach was initially described in the late 19th Century. Cheatle reported using it in the 1920s; Henry en-

hanced it in the 1930s. Nyhus and Condon popularized it in later years. When the repair was done with pure tissue, it was effective for indirect hernias but could not be performed satisfactorily for direct hernias. This problem eventually was solved when mesh was used to patch direct defects. Stoppa and Rives developed a procedure designed to wrap the entire pelvic peritoneal bag. This technique obviated the need to patch or suture myofascial defects in the myopectineal orifice. The procedure has proven to be valuable for the surgeon who attempts to repair the most difficult of recurrent hernias. An adaptation of this approach was designed by Wantz, who has successfully used it in unilateral recurrent hernias. A more detailed discussion of prosthetic material repair can be found in Chapter 24.

INDICATIONS FOR OPERATION

Operative repair is indicated for most patients who are seen with groin hernias. All symptomatic hernias should be repaired. It is recommended that all indirect and femoral hernias be repaired regardless of the absence of symptoms. In general, small, asymptomatic direct inguinal hernias can be safely managed without an operation, perhaps by a truss or in some cases simply by expectant, repeated observation. The risk in this approach is that, in preoperative clinical examination, even experienced surgeons are unable to reliably differentiate direct from indirect hernias with impressive accuracy. Because of this uncertainty, it is probable that many asymptomatic direct hernias are repaired that could have safely been observed. The downside of nonoperative treatment is that there is a severe increase in morbidity and a significant incidence of mortality if an emergency operation is required for hernia. When nonoperative recommendations are made, much weight is placed on the patient's history of being completely unaware of the hernia until it was diagnosed by a primary physician.

Once the diagnosis is confirmed, timing of the surgery becomes important. Repair can be done electively in most cases of chronic hernia that is not painful or tender. If the patient complains of pain and the hernia is confirmed, repair should be done promptly. Hernias that are painful and tender or that are seen with acute incarceration should be repaired as emergencies. Patients in whom an acutely painful groin mass suspicious of an incarcerated hernia develops should undergo urgent or emergency surgery. If surgery is delayed for a symptomatic reducible hernia, the patient is advised to use a soft truss to temporarily contain the herniating mass.

Many patients ask to know the risks associated with deferring hernia repair. There are potential dangers in delaying the operation, even one that is clearly elective. In addition to increasing the ever-present chance of strangulation, extended delay encourages enlargement of a hernia and allows for additional fibrosis to develop between the hernia sac and vital elements of the spermatic cord. Both enlargement and fibrosis contribute to an increased incidence of postoperative testicular problems. When a patient has been advised to undergo hernia surgery and declines, the surgeon is well advised to record the patient's refusal.

DIFFERENTIAL DIAGNOSIS

Differentiating a hernia from other groin masses is not too difficult. A hernia is usually obvious when the patient stands or increases intra-abdominal pressure by coughing or straining. Unless it is incarcerated, a hernia usually recedes within the abdominal cavity when the patient is supine. The differential diagnosis of a groin mass that remains unchanged when the patient is supine includes inflamed lymph nodes (lymphogranuloma venereum or cat-scratch fever), an incarcerated femoral hernia, and an inguinal hernia. When the diagnosis is in doubt, it is safer to do a surgical exploration than to risk development of gangrene of a strangulated loop of bowel in an incarcerated hernia.

Occasionally, a patient describes the presence of an acute groin mass related to straining, yet on examination the mass cannot be reproduced. This occurs in the early phase of some acute indirect hernias that still have tight internal rings. In such a case, the patient should return when the mass is evident. In an

otherwise asymptomatic patient, nothing is lost by delaying the operation until the hernia can be clearly identified. Such patients are permitted to continue their normal activities. Repair is advised when the hernia reappears and is confirmed by a reliable source, preferably the surgeon.

Every surgeon sees patients who complain of groin pain but have no palpable hernia. This is a difficult problem to diagnose and even more difficult to treat successfully. Generally, the patient who complains of groin pain without an identifiable hernia is an enigma to the referring physician and the surgeon. Important considerations that are difficult to evaluate in only one or two appointments include the patient's social background, work ethic, pain threshold, and whether ulterior motives exaggerate the complaints. In the patient without a palpable hernia who has never before had surgery, the cause of groin pain usually is of myofascial origin. Hip bursitis, nerve root irritation, and urinary tract inflammation or calculi should be considered. Diverticulitis, inflammatory bowel disease, appendicitis, and retroperitoneal lesions are also part of the differential diagnosis. A reducible hernia that is not tender rarely causes much pain.

PATHOGENESIS

The formation of direct hernias is correlated with numerous factors, including (1) abnormally thinned transversalis fascia, (2) failure of the arching fibers of the internal oblique muscle or aponeurosis to extend low enough to reach the pubic tubercle, resulting in loss of the muscular shutter mechanism that protects the posterior wall, and (3) failure of the aponeurotic fibers of the transversus abdominis muscle to extend far enough laterally on Cooper's ligament, leaving only the fascia of the transversus abdominis muscle to be fused with the transversalis fascia.

Indirect hernias form as the result of a persistent patent processus vaginalis with an abnormally widened internal ring. In an infant, hernias occur when the internal ring is incompletely formed or has not closed sufficiently to withhold the abdominal contents when the infant increases intra-abdominal pressure. Indirect hernias that form in adult patients usually are due to a congenital peritoneal sac and the degenerative breakdown of the musculature of the internal ring. Some indirect hernias develop outside the internal spermatic fascia of the spermatic cord; these often have bladder as the protruding component.

CLASSIFICATION

We have classified inguinal hernias into five types, each of which is repaired with measures specifically directed at correcting the defect unique to the type. Types 1, 2, and 3 are indirect. Types 4 and 5 are direct (Fig. 23–2). The three factors that must be evaluated to determine the hernia type are (1) the presence or absence of a peritoneal sac, (2) the size of the internal ring, and (3) the integrity of the posterior wall. Use of this anatomic and functional classification facilitates the exact typing of the hernia and suggests the best repairs to use for each type.

PREOPERATIVE PREPARATION

Some centers have categorically denied elective surgery to overweight patients. At the Hernia Institute of Florida, no significant differ-ence was noted in the outcome of inguinal hernias repaired simply on the basis of patient weight. Many patients who weighed more than 250 pounds have had inguinal hernia surgery performed without any unusual incidence of recurrence or other complications. However, our experience with incisional hernia repair in overweight patients parallels that reported by others, with increasing weight being associated with increased rates of failed repairs.

Patient age alone is not a reason to deny surgery. When older patients have been prepared properly for elective surgery, results are excellent. The difference in infection rates and seroma formation between older and younger patients is not unique to hernia surgery; it applies to all types of abdominal surgery. Surgery in elderly patients performed under emergency circumstances bodes high complication rates and significant mortality rates. Medical evaluation and patient preparation are the best hedges against disaster.

SPECIAL EQUIPMENT

In order of importance, the crucial surgical equipment elements are a qualified surgeon knowledgeable in anatomy of the groin, an adequate assistant, and prosthetic material for groin and incisional repairs. Use of local or regional anesthesia is extremely helpful in pre-

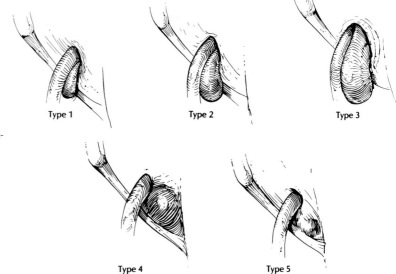

Figure 23–2. Five types of inguinal hernias.

venting failed groin hernia repairs. If a patient can cough or strain on the surgeon's request, then the soundness of the repair can be tested before the incision is closed. In our series, local or regional anesthesia was used in 99% of groin hernia repairs. Local anesthesia with intravenous sedation was used for most primary repairs. Regional (usually epidural) anesthesia was used for recurrent repairs or in very obese patients having primary repairs. Whereas general anesthesia was the most frequently applied technique for incisional herniorrhaphies, it was used in less than 1% of all groin hernia repairs.

Because 95% of all patients who underwent surgery were discharged within 2 hours, it was necessary for them to be driven home. Patients were prohibited from driving vehicles for 48 hours immediately after surgery to allow enough time for sedatives to be fully metabolized. The 5 percent of patients required to spend a night as "overnight outpatients" either had extensive scrotal hernias that required suction drainage or they lived more than 1 hour's drive outside of metropolitan Miami.

Perioperative antibiotics do not have routine application in hernia surgery except in patients who have reached their seventh decade.

RESULTS

From 1958 to 1976, the modified Bassini repair was used. Failure occurred in 10% of primary indirect, 20% of primary direct, and at least 25% of recurrent repairs. From 1976 to 1984, the four-layer classic Shouldice repair was done with local anesthesia. Failures were reduced to 1.8% for primary (indirect and direct) and 8% for recurrent repairs. Since 1984, prosthetic mesh repairs have been done in almost all primary and recurrent hernias in adults. Failure rates have been further reduced to 0.3% for primary and 3% for recurrent repairs. This series includes more than 10,000 hernia repairs with overall follow-up of 79% of patients seen 1 or more years after their repairs.

SCROTAL MASSES

More than 50% of patients whose chief complaint is based on groin pain or a scrotal mass do not have a hernia found on physical examination. Most have pain of vague musculoskeletal origin that usually resolves with time. Some have a painless mass or tender tissue in the scrotum.

Both history and physical examination are valuable in establishing the diagnosis as well as in the timing of diagnostic measures and in establishing the urgency of surgical treatment. Important considerations include trauma, infection (especially those of the urinary tract or prostate), chronicity, variability of the size of the mass, and association of the mass with pain. The character, radiation, and severity of the pain is important. Prior surgery for cryptorchidism is important in regard to the universal incidence of testicular tumors.

PHYSICAL EXAMINATION

The anatomy of the scrotal contents must be considered during the examination. The normal testicle is bordered anteriorly by the tunica vaginalis and posteriorly and superiorly by the epididymis, vas deferens, and pampiniform plexus of veins. Therefore, any mass can usually be categorized by its location and thereby its origin.

An anterior mass involving the tunica vaginalis is a hydrocele, communicating hydrocele, or hernia. A mass in the testis itself must be considered neoplastic until proven otherwise. A posterior mass that is painful generally involves an inflammatory process of the epididymis or torsion of the appendix testi. A nonpainful posterior mass is more likely to represent a varicocele or spermatocele. Distorted anatomy (i.e., changes in the axis of a testicle) suggests torsion of the cord. The more chronic any of these processes is, the more distorted is the structure. Epididymitis or torsion that is not treated promptly can cause progressive swelling of the entire contents of the scrotum.

CONFIRMATION OF ANATOMY

Two methods may be used to determine the presence and nature of a scrotal mass. These are ultrasound using high-frequency transducers (5–10 MHz) and technetium (99m) scanning. Ultrasound is faster and less invasive. It involves direct contact with the genitalia and its accuracy depends on technician experience. Technetium scanning takes longer to perform, does not require contact with the genitalia, and is easier to interpret. Scrotal sonography is helpful in determining structure and determining solid from fluid-filled masses. Technetium scanning determines the presence of blood flow to scrotal tissue. Color flow Doppler may eventually replace scanning. It is capable of differentiating the decreased blood flow in torsion from hyperemic inflammatory patterns associated with epididymitis.

Hydrocele

Hydrocele is a collection of fluid within the tunica vaginalis. The fluid may be confined to the area around the testicle, may be isolated in the cord, or may communicate with the peritoneal cavity. A communicating hydrocele reduces in size when the patient reclines. Clinically, it is no different from an indirect hernia with a small patency in the proximal portion of the processus vaginalis. A string of several distinct noncommunicating fluid collections may exist. Most hydroceles are idiopathic. They slowly enlarge in men aged 40 years or older. The cause of a hydrocele includes scrotal injury, radiotherapy, acute epididymitis, orchitis, or testicular neoplasm. In the case of an associated neoplasm, the fluid may be bloody and contain cancer cells. The mass is rounded, firm, nonreducible, usually nontender (unless an underlying inflammatory process exists), and it transluminates.

As a general rule, hydroceles are aspirated for temporary relief of symptoms but not to establish diagnosis. If necessary, ultrasound is helpful to confirm the diagnosis of hydrocele and to identify whether any solid mass exists in the testicle. Indications for treatment of hydrocele are bulk and discomfort. There also may be some testicular atrophy due to compression. A scrotal incision is the ideal operative approach for hydrocelectomy. The majority of the wall of the hydrocele is excised, leaving only the areas attached to the testicle and cord structures. The remaining edges of the hydrocele sac must be closely inspected for bleeders to avoid postoperative hematoma. A hydrocele found at the time of inguinal hernia surgery may be treated through the groin incision only if it can be done easily without mobilizing the testicle; otherwise, it is preferable to make a separate scrotal incision rather than elevating the testicle from the scrotal sac and interrupting collateral blood flow.

Spermatocele

Spermatocele usually is a small painless cystic mass above and posterior to the testis. Occasionally, a spermatocele grows large enough to mimic a second testicle in the ipsilateral hemiscrotum. It can be differentiated from a testicular tumor in that it is a separate mass, it is movable, and it transluminates. It consists of a cloudy white fluid containing dead spermatozoa, as opposed to the clear yellow fluid of a hydrocele. Treatment of a large symptomatic spermatocele is by excision through a scrotal incision.

Varicocele

Varicocele is the dilation of veins in the pampiniform plexus. The dilated mass of veins starts at the testis and extends up through the internal ring. Varicocele is usually found on the left side, it affects 10% of the male population, and it becomes apparent with the onset of sexual maturity. The cause is thought to be incompetent valves of the spermatic vein. Acute onset of a varicocele in an older man classically is a sign of a neoplasm blocking those veins in the pelvis. However, it is almost never the initial presenting sign of a malignancy. Varicocele has been observed in men with recurrent deep vein thrombophlebitis.

Varicocele is seen as tortuous veins that cause a dragging discomfort when the patient stands for long periods of time. Many patients are unaware of their scrotal venous abnormality. Dilatation of the veins decreases with recumbency and increases with Valsalva's maneuver or coughing. This may lend the examiner to think that the mass is a hernia. Hernia and varicocele frequently coexist. In such a case, at the time of hernia repair, it is recommended to leave the varicocele alone unless it has been symptomatic or there is a question of infertility. Even though spermatozoa counts and motility may be decreased in 75% of the patients with a varicocele, most patients are unaware of any abnormality in their fertility.

Treatment of varicocele is by ligation of the internal and external spermatic veins at or above the level of the internal ring. This treatment is permanently successful in 75% of cases. Dilatation of previously small collateral veins accounts for recurrence in the remaining 25%. If the patient chooses not to undergo surgery, primary and recurrent varicoceles can be treated by percutaneous radiologic venous occlusive methods. Adjunctive ligation of the spermatic veins at the time of hernia surgery increases the morbidity of hernia repair. It oftens results in a prolonged period before the patient returns to work and increased testicular sensitivity.

Testicular Tumors

Testicular tumors are rare; they occur in 1:50,000 males in the general population. In one purely hernia practice, the incidence of malignant testicular or spermatic cord tumors is 1:1500 patients. A thorough examination of both testicles is essential for any patient who complains of a scrotal mass. It is important to compare the testicle in question to its contralateral partner. The presence of a hernia or hydrocele does not preclude a neoplasm. If a hydrocele appears in a man in the 20 to 35-year age group, it may be the first clue that a tumor is present.

The usual presentation of a testicular tumor is in a young man who notices a painless mass in his scrotum. Thorough history may reveal mild discomfort, but severe pain is rare in the absence of trauma. Trauma is a presenting complaint in 20% of patients. The tumor usually is incidental rather than causative. If hem-

orrhage occurs into the tumor, it increases the patient's awareness that something is abnormal. Torsion, infection, or ischemic necrosis may also increase discomfort in the testicle. A history of cryptorchism is important in testicular tumors. An undescended testicle, as well as the contralateral testicle, both have an increased incidence of development of a malignancy. Orchiopexy makes examination of the testicle easier but may not reduce the incidence of malignancy. Atrophic testes from other causes, such as mumps, may also be associated with an increased incidence of tumor.

Physical examination reveals a mass within the testicle. If the mass can be separated from the testicle, it is assumed to be epididymal or a cord structure, not a testicular tumor. Cord tumors such as liposarcoma and rhabdomyosarcoma of the cremasteric muscle are typically found incidentally at the time of hernia surgery. In the ambiguous examination of a testis, ultrasound may be useful, but the ultimate confirmation or exclusion of a tumor is by direct examination.

Normal lymphatic drainage of the testicle follows the spermatic vessels up into the retroperitoneum. There is no communication of lymphatics into the surrounding scrotal structures. When the diagnosis of malignancy is suspected, surgical confirmation of tumor or orchiectomy should be done in a way to avoid contamination of adjacent structures. Lymphatics may have been altered in the case of previous orchiopexy or hernia repair. Aspiration of a hydrocele may also alter normal drainage. Surgery is done through an inguinal hernia-type incision. Initially, the cord structures are isolated and occluded with a noncrushing clamp. Then, the testicle is brought up into the protected wound and inspected. Suspicion of a malignancy warrants orchiectomy. Cord structures must be secured carefully and marked with clips because they will retract back into the retroperitoneum. The vas deferens should be secured separately.

Torsion of the Testicle and Epididymitis

Neither torsion of the testicle nor epididymitis is usually considered a mass lesion. The usual manifestation is pain. Torsion is typically seen in young boys, often occurring during sleep. It is more likely to occur in cryptorchid testes and is thought to be caused by spasm in the cremasteric muscle. The left testicle rotates counterclockwise and the right testicle clockwise.

Examination reveals a swollen testicle with red scrotal skin. The testicle is retracted upward from the twisted cord and the epididymis may be displaced from its normal posterior position. Epididymitis usually occurs after puberty. The epididymis is tender. Often—especially in early cases—the testicle itself is relatively pain free. Pyuria often accompanies the inflammation.

Difficulty occurs in differentiating torsion and epididymitis when the conditions become more chronic. It may also be difficult to differentiate these conditions from an incarcerated or strangulated scrotal hernia. Delay in treatment of torsion with strangulation of the spermatic cord is catastrophic, resulting in testicular loss. Surgical intervention for epididymitis is usually not necessary. Classically, the pain of epididymitis is alleviated by gently lifting the testicle over the symphysis pubis. This maneuver usually increases the pain of torsion. Once scrotal swelling and pain have occurred, it is difficult to differentiate between torsion and epididymitis. Color flow synography may be the best examination to differentiate the two, but it is often easier for technicians to perform technetium scanning. The testicle in torsion is typically avascular, whereas the inflamed epididymitis is hypervascular. When there is doubt about organ viability, immediate scrotal exploration is advised to confirm the diagnosis. If torsion is found, the testicle must be derotated and fixed in position. The contralateral testicle should also be explored and secured. Even a nonviable-appearing testicle should be treated and not removed because it may be capable of some residual hormonal function.

Torsion may involve the appendix testes also. These are embryologic remnants that lie in the upper pole of the testes. Torsion manifests as a painful mass in the upper pole of the testicle. Initially, the area of pain is confined and a small dark mass may be seen. As the condition becomes more chronic, the sur-rounding tissue also becomes inflamed and this condition becomes difficult to differentiate from epididymitis. Treatment for an appendix testis in torsion is excision.

Selected Readings

1. Altaffer LF III, Steele SM Jr. Torsion of testicular appendages in men. J Urol 1980;124:56.
2. Anson BJ, Morgan EH, McVay CB. The anatomy of the hernial regions. Surg Gynecol Obstet 1949;89:417,753.
3. Chan CK. Transversalis fascial replacement—an underlay. Postgrad General Surg 1992; (Apr):126–128.
4. Gilbert AI. Inguinal hernia repair: Biomaterials and suture repair. Perspect Gen Surg 1991;2:113–129.
5. Gilbert AI. Medical/legal aspects of hernia surgery: Personal risk management. Surg Clin North Am 1993;73:583–594.
6. Gilbert AI. An anatomic and functional classification for the diagnosis and treatment of inguinal hernias. Am J Surg 1989;157:331–333.
7. Gilbert AI. Infection in inguinal hernia repair considering biomaterials and antibiotics. Surgery 1993; 177:126–130.
8. Griffith CA. The Marcy repair revisited. Surg Clin North Am 1984;64:215–227.
9. Halsted WS. The cure of the more difficult as well as the simpler inguinal ruptures. Johns Hopkins Hosp Bull 1903;14:208–214.
10. Knight PS, Vossy LE. The diagnosis and treatment of the acute scrotum in children and adolescents. Ann Surg 1984;200:664.
11. McAninch JW. Disorders of the testis, scrotum and spermatic cord. In: Tonagho EA, McAninch JW, eds. Smith's General Urology. 12th ed. Norwalk, CT: Appleton & Lange, 1992:616–624.
12. Meares EM Jr. Prostatitis, orchitis and epididymitis: Acute and chronic. In: Schrier RW, Gottscholk CW, eds. Diseases of the Kidney. 4th ed. Boston: Little, Brown, 1988:815–833.
13. Middleton WD, Siegel BA, Nelson GL, Yates CK, Andriole GL. Acute scrotal disorders: Prospective comparison of color Doppler US and testicular scintigraphy. Radiology 1990;177:177–181.
14. Nyhus LM. Iliopubic tract repair of inguinal and femoral hernia. Surg Clin North Am 1993;73:487–499.
15. Pike MC, Chilkers C, Peckham MJ. Effect of age at orchiopexy on risk of testicular cancer. Lancet 1986;1:1246.
16. Presti JC Jr, Herr HW. Genital tumors. In: Tonagho EA, McAninch JW, eds. General Urology. 12th ed. Norwalk, CT: Appleton & Lange, 1992:413–425.
17. Ralphs DNL, Brain AJL, Grundy DJ, Hobsley M. How accurately can direct and indirect inguinal hernias be distinguished? BMJ 1980;12:1039–1040.
18. Ravitch MM, Hitzrot JM. The Operations for Inguinal Hernia. St. Louis: CV Mosby, 1960.
19. Russell RH. The saccular theory of hernia and the radical operation. Lancet 1906;2:1197–1203.
20. Seaman EK, Sawczvk I. Testis tumor in an adult presenting with torsion of testis. Urology 1993;42:453–454.
21. Stoppa R, Rives J, Warlaumont C. The use of Dacron in the repairs of hernias of the groin. Surg Clin North Am 1984;64:269–285.

22. Thomas AJ Jr, Geisinger MA. Current management of varicoceles. Urol Clin North Am 1990;17:893.
23. Usher FC, Hill JR, Oshner JL. Hernia repair with Marlex mesh, a comparison of technique. Surgery 1959;46:718–724.
24. Wantz GE. Giant prosthetic reinforcement of the visceral sac for repair of a re-recurrent inguinal hernia. Postgrad Gen Surg 1992;4:109–113.
25. Welsh DRJ, Alexander MAJ. The Shouldice repair. Surg Clin North Am 1993;73:451–469.

Chapter 24

Hernias: Prosthetic Material Repair

Joel S. Goodwin II • L. William Traverso

The whole concept and development of ambulatory surgery has paralleled the recent evolution of inguinal herniorrhaphy. At our institution, inguinal herniorrhaphy has been performed on a routine outpatient basis for nearly a decade. The goals of current outpatient hernia surgery are (1) overall effectiveness, (2) permanence, (3) safety, (4) minimization of pain, (5) absence of functional impairment, and (6) maintenance of low cost. These goals have remained essentially unchanged over time, but the capability to achieve these goals has improved significantly because of the continued evolution in medical science and socioeconomic impetus. Advances in anesthetic techniques (e.g., use of effective shorter-acting agents), increased use of local and regional techniques, and a "short stay" philosophy have been crucial in the transition from overnight hospital stays to same-day discharge. Likewise, use of improved surgical techniques such as "tension-free" repairs with prosthetic mesh and minimally invasive surgery has led surgeons to improve open herniorrhaphy procedures to be done cost effectively and to allow for safe discharge with easy home management. This chapter discusses prosthetic materials and their role in the evolution of inguinal herniorrhaphy in the ambulatory surgery setting.

INGUINAL HERNIAS

Inguinal hernias are a common problem. In approximately 5% to 10% of the U. S. population, a hernia develops spontaneously at some point. There are 500,000 hernia operations performed per year in the United States. The socioeconomic costs measured in dollars, work hours lost, and personal rehabilitation are enormous.

Inguinal hernias are basically of three types: indirect, direct, and femoral. (Combinations also occur.) The indirect and direct types are by far the most common. Their anatomic distinction is marked in the preperitoneal space by the inferior epigastric artery, with the indirect type being lateral and the direct type being medial to this landmark. Indirect hernias may enlarge and descend into the scrotum. Direct inguinal hernias occur through the inguinal floor because of a weakness or attenuation of the transversus abdominis aponeurosis, carrying with it the transversalis fascia. Ipsilateral direct and indirect hernias that are present at the same time are known as pantaloon hernias. Femoral hernias protrude through the femoral canal medial to the femoral vein. All three hernia spaces are within the myopectineal orifice, which is defined as the area bounded by the pubic tubercle, Cooper's ligament, transversus abdominis arch, and anterior inferior iliac spine (Fig. 24–1).

Inguinal hernias occur five times more frequently in men than in women. This is thought to be due to the presence of a patent processus vaginalis, but this clearly is not the primary cause of inguinal hernias. The current pathophysiologic explanation for development of indirect inguinal hernia is loss of the

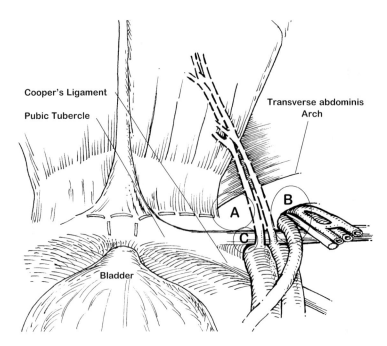

Cooper's Ligament

Pubic Tubercle

Transverse abdominis Arch

Bladder

Figure 24–1. A right-sided myopectineal orifice is shown in schematic form. The pubic tubercle (medial), Cooper's ligament (inferior), and transverse abdominis arch are the boundaries for this "orifice." The most lateral border is the anterior iliac spine (not pictured). Hernia spaces within the myopectineal orifice are direct *(A)*, indirect *(B)*, and femoral *(C)*.

"shutter-like effect," whereby the abdominal wall musculature contracts over the route of the vas deferens during increases in intra-abdominal pressure. The internal ring closes to prevent visceral or preperitoneal fat protrusion. Indirect hernias occur when a deficient shutter valve allows access into the internal ring of preperitoneal and then peritoneal contents.

Direct hernias occur when there is weakened or attenuated tissue. Biochemical explanations of hernia formation or recurrence point to a disequilibrium of collagen deposition and collagenolysis. Actions (e.g., aging, ischemia, infection, chronic injury, chronic pressure) or agents (e.g., antimetabolites, steroids) that decrease collagen deposition or increase collagenolysis may predispose a person to direct herniation.

INDICATIONS FOR REPAIR

Most surgeons recommend surgical repair for all hernias to relieve symptoms, prevent incarceration or strangulation, or avoid enlargement, which may make surgery technically more difficult. As is true for all operations, each case must be individualized. The primary goal of hernia repair is the effective repair of the anatomic abdominal wall defect while preserving the integrity of the vas deferens and testicular vessels.

PROSTHETIC MATERIALS

The primary goal in herniorrhaphy is anatomic closure of the abdominal wall defect. The controversy begins when discussing the best technique to achieve this goal. The theory behind herniorrhaphy invokes one of the foundations of surgery, namely, the principles of wound closure. The ideal closure requires the direct apposition, without tension, of strong musculoaponeurotic structures within a sterile field. In herniorrhaphy, tension-free primary closure is usually difficult to achieve. Large tissue defects often are present that make tension-free closure impossible. Incorrect technique, the most common of which is creating tension at the suture line, is the primary cause of early (less than 2 years) direct hernia recurrence. Other predisposing factors for failure include large or recurrent hernias, poor general condition of the patient, abdominal wall weakness, and obesity. Late hernia recurrence (over several years) is attributed to attenuated fascia secondary to the decreased amount or strength of collagen in the inguinal floor as a sequela to continued altered collagen metabolism, aging, or other factors.

A number of prosthetic materials have been used to repair abdominal wall defects in which the most tension-free herniorrhaphy is sought or a primary closure is impossible. These materials, as well as the indications for their use, have evolved over the last several decades. A prosthetic material used for repair of an abdominal defect must, at minimum, be strong and durable, yet be flexible, be easy to use, and permit the ingrowth of host tissues to fix it in place. The ideal biosynthetic material must, according to Lichtenstein, (1) be inert, (2) be resistant to infection, (3) stimulate tissue ingrowth, and (4) be rapidly fixed into place by the patient's "fibrin glue." Metal gauzes of stainless steel and tantalum have been used. Prosthetic materials (Fig. 24–2) commonly used today, however, include expanded polytetrafluoroethylene (PTFE) (Gore-Tex), multifilamented PTFE (Teflon), multifilamented polypropylene mesh (Surgipro), monofilamented polypropylene mesh (Marlex), double filamented polypropylene mesh (Prolene), and multifilamented polyester mesh (Mersilene). Materials with pores or spaces smaller than 10 μm can harbor 1-μm bacteria away from contact with 10- to 15-μm neutrophils. Theoretically, this could lead to an increased chance of infection and sinus tract formation. Expanded PTFE, polyester mesh, multifilamented polypropylene mesh, and PTFE mesh all have pores smaller than 10 μm and are theoretically at risk for removal in case of infection.

The development of prosthetics and the surgical techniques to use them evolved from the abdominal wall reconstruction required in the repair of massive ventral hernias. Mesh allowed the surgeon a practical, durable solution for abdominal wall repair when few alternatives existed. These procedures are not usually performed as ambulatory surgery. The knowledge gained from ventral hernia repairs has been crucial in the development of current materials and methods being routinely used for a tension-free inguinal hernia repair.

HISTORY OF MESH USE IN PERFORMANCE OF INGUINAL HERNIORRHAPHY

The use of polypropylene mesh in the performance of inguinal herniorrhaphy was first reported in 1958. Many authors reported the use of mesh subsequently with variations of technical placement. Rene Stoppa initially reported preperitoneal polyester mesh placement for recurrent inguinal hernias in 1975. The technique of giant, preperitoneally placed mesh for recurrent, bilateral herniation or groin eventration was so successful that it was enthusiastically accepted by many surgeons in Europe over the next decade. The outstanding results with mesh repairs for recurrent and complex inguinal hernias led to the use of mesh in the repair of primary hernias. Lichtenstein discussed the use of mesh in primary herniorrhaphy in the early 1970s, and he has used monofilament polypropylene mesh in all hernia repairs since 1984. His application of an onlay, tension-free mesh technique has resulted in only two recurrences and no infections in 1552 operations. Lichtenstein likewise reported on four other series that used mesh in primary herniorrhaphy and showed an overall recurrence rate of 0.2% and an infection rate of 0.03% in 3019 operations. Several

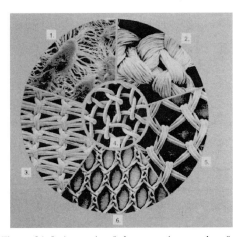

Figure 24–2. A mosaic of electron micrographs of commonly used prosthetic mesh are shown as follows: *(1.)* expanded polytetrafluoroethylene (Gore-Tex), *(2.)* multifilamented polytetrafluoroethylene (Teflon), *(3.)* multifilamented polypropylene (Surgipro), *(4.)* monofilamented polypropylene (Marlex), *(5.)* double filamented polypropylene (Prolene), and *(6.)* multifilamented polyester (Mersilene). (From Amid PK, Shulman AG, Lichtenstein IL, Itakaha M. Biomaterials for abdominal wall hernia surgery and principles of their applications. Langenbecks Arch Chir 1994;379:168–171.)

other surgeons have also reported their successful techniques and results using mesh in primary herniorrhaphy.

Mesh repairs appear to be durable. According to Stoppa, recurrences after mesh repair result exclusively from technical mistakes, and his series showed that, after tension-free repairs with mesh, no recurrences appeared after the first year.

LAPAROSCOPIC HERNIORRHAPHY

The increased use of mesh during open inguinal hernia repairs occurred just before laparoscopic surgery became popular, and both these techniques have been used in inguinal herniorrhaphy. In 1990, Schultz was the first to report on laparoscopic transabdominal preperitoneal placement of mesh for herniorrhaphy. Many subsequent reports have followed, detailing variations of the preperitoneal, as well as intraperitoneal and extraperitoneal, laparoscopic mesh herniorrhaphies. In addition, the outcome and cost analyses of these laparoscopic procedures have led surgeons to improve standard open repairs, which were previously undertaken as painful outpatient procedures.

For surgeons, choosing a specific technique of herniorrhaphy is a somewhat emotional and controversial decision. It perhaps stems from the prejudices learned during training and often from the perceived zealousness with which the designers of these techniques trumpet their successes. The recent application of laparoscopic technique to inguinal herniorrhaphy has revitalized the emotion and controversy while stimulating debate and interest in herniorrhaphy. The basic premises behind laparoscopic herniorrhaphy are that it must be as good as open repair and it must offer something beyond traditional herniorrhaphy, such as laparoscopic cholecystectomy did when compared with open cholecystectomy (e.g., enabling decreased hospital stay, decreased postoperative pain, and decreased length of convalescence).

Performing laparoscopic inguinal herniorrhaphy with mesh, as it is currently performed in North America, has certain basic techno-

logic requirements. These include using high-resolution digital video cameras and monitors, high-volume insufflation devices, specialized abdominal trocars, grasping and dissecting tools, and expensive specialized staplers. In addition, mesh is needed because tissues cannot be opposed easily during minimally invasive surgery. General anesthesia has also been used in most cases, but reports of success using regional or even local anesthesia are beginning to appear.

The many techniques described recently can be distilled into three basic types, two of which are still commonly used. The first is the transabdominal preperitoneal (TAPP) approach, in which the laparoscope and instruments are placed transabdominally into the peritoneal cavity. The repair is performed by first incising the peritoneum to enter the preperitoneal space over the myopectineal orifice. Mesh is then stapled over all existing and potential inguinal hernia defects.

The second method uses an intraperitoneal onlay mesh (IPOM) technique, in which mesh is placed over the indirect hernia defect and then stapled directly to the peritoneum. This technique has been recently abandoned because of problems with infection.

The third and most recent technique reported is the totally extraperitoneal laparoscopic inguinal herniorrhaphy (EXTRA), in which the peritoneal cavity is not entered. The preperitoneal space is entered and dissected from the infraumbilical area "transfascially" with laparoscopic instruments. The hernia defects are defined and the myopectineal orifice is patched with stapled mesh. This procedure is more difficult to learn than the TAPP repair; both are more difficult than a laparoscopic cholecystectomy.

Laparoscopic herniorrhaphy is usually performed with the patient under general endotracheal anesthesia. Prosthetic mesh is integral for the repair. Monofilament and woven polypropylene, polyester, PTFE, and Mersilene have all been used in laparoscopic herniorrhaphy. The materials that have been used successfully in open mesh repairs have been used in laparoscopic surgery.

Several series of laparoscopic hernia repairs have been reported with favorable results. Felix and associates reported 205 TAPP repairs in 183 patients without recurrence at a median follow-up of 12 months. Wheeler reported on 135 TAPP hernia repairs with mesh in 110 patients without recurrence at a median follow-up of 12 months. Ferzli and colleagues reported on 122 EXTRA procedures in 101 patients and showed no recurrence at a median follow-up of 12 months. It is clear from these reports and others that, in the hands of experienced laparoscopic surgeons, inguinal hernias can be technically repaired with a low recurrence rate.

Although only short-term follow-up is reported so far, recent larger series suggest that the recurrence rate for laparoscopic herniorrhaphy will not greatly increase as follow-up reaches the 3- to 4-year range. The question of recurrence after long-term follow-up remains to be answered for laparoscopic herniorrhaphy. However, recurrence after open herniorrhaphies with mesh is usually related to technical mistakes and therefore usually occurs within the first year. We feel that the laparoscopic series will have a similar outcome.

Recurrence is only one issue in laparoscopic mesh repair. Also of importance is the safety of the procedure. Several authors have reported low complication rates associated with laparoscopic herniorrhaphy. Likewise, complications are liable to be minor and temporary and to diminish with experience. However, a multicenter retrospective registry study reported a 1.2% intraoperative complication rate, with complications of bladder perforation, colon injury, spermatic and epigastric artery injuries, a lost intra-abdominal needle, and an anesthetic-induced arrhythmia, among others, being reported. Other individual studies report the occurrence of bowel injuries, trocar hernias, bowel obstruction, urinary retention, scrotal hematoma, nerve entrapment, seromas, subcutaneous emphysema, wound infection, and inguinal pain. We are not aware of any deaths.

The economics of laparoscopic hernia repair are complex. The increased expense of laparoscopy has been either ignored or justified on the grounds of earlier return to productive work. We have shown previously that charges for the unilateral TAPP procedure were twice that of conventional open repair but that individuals returned to out-of-house activity and to full activity twice as quickly after a TAPP procedure versus open repair. However, our comparison of a tension-free laparoscopic technique to a non–tension-free open repair was not a fair study to compare postoperative pain. In a prospective cost and outcome analysis, we recently compared the procedures of TAPP with an open tension-free preperitoneal (PPO) placement of mesh through the floor of the inguinal canal. The study involved 139 consecutive cases (TAPP, 98; PPO, 41). When just the unilateral TAPP cases (n = 59) were compared with unilateral PPO (n = 40), the initial return to activity and number of days taking postoperative pain medication were similar, but the cost of TAPP (not charges or reimbursement) was almost twice that of PPO ($2176 versus $1343). Operating times were significantly longer for TAPP (104 versus 70 minutes). This study indicates that the benefits of unilateral laparoscopic inguinal herniorrhaphy noted by surgeons in the immediate postoperative period could be duplicated by applying just the tension-free aspects of TAPP to an open repair. In our study, we observed a noticeable improvement in a simpler and less expensive technique. Other series have already reported techniques that used tension-free open repairs.

Whereas cost considerations may favor the use of tension-free open repair over TAPP for unilateral herniorrhaphy, the role of TAPP or EXTRA in repair of bilateral or recurrent inguinal hernia is still not well defined in terms of cost analysis. In these settings, the laparoscopic approach may offer advantages over open repair. As cost and outcome data become known, perhaps there will be less controversy regarding adoption of tension-free techniques and the use of prosthetic material in the performance of inguinal herniorrhaphy.

Selected Readings

1. Amid PL, Shulman AG, Lichtenstein IL, Hakakha M. Biomaterials of abdominal wall hernia surgery and principles of their application. Langenbecks Arch Chir 1994;379:168–171.
2. Felix EL, Michas CA, McKnight RL. Laparoscopic herniorrhaphy. Surg Endosc 1994;8:100–104.
3. Ferzli GS, Massad A, Dysarz FA, Kopatsis A. A study of 101 patients treated with extraperitoneal endoscopic

laparoscopic herniorrhaphy. Am Surgeon 1993;59:707–708.

4. Filipi CJ, Fitzgibbons RJ Jr, Salerno GM, Hart RO. Laparoscopic herniorrhaphy. Surg Clin North Am 1992;72:1109–1124.

5. Gill BD, Traverso LW. Continuous quality improvement: Open laparoscopic groin hernia repair. Surg Endosc 1993;7:116.

6. Goodwin JS, Traverso LW. A prospective outcome and cost analysis of laparoscopic transabdominal preperitoneal inguinal hernia repair to an open tension-free repair. Surg Endosc 1995;9:981–983.

7. Hoffman HC, Vinton-Traverso AL. Preperitoneal prosthetic herniorrhaphy. Arch Surg 1993;128:964–970.

8. Knoll JA, Eckhauser FE. Inguinal anatomy and abdominal wall hernias. In: Greenfield LJ, et al, eds. Surgery. Philadelphia: JB Lippincott, 1993:1081–1106.

9. Lichtenstein IL, Shulman MG, Amid PK. The cause, prevention, and treatment of recurrent groin hernias. Surg Clin North Am 1993;73:529–544.

10. McFadden BV, Arregui ME, Corbitt JD, Filipi CJ, Fitzgibbons RJ, Franklin ME. Complications of laparoscopic herniorrhaphy. Surg Endosc 1993;7:155–158.

11. McKernan JB, Laws HL. Laparoscopic repair of inguinal hernias using a totally extraperitoneal prosthetic approach. Surg Endosc 1993;7:26–28.

12. Phillips EH, Carroll BJ, Fallas MJ. Laparoscopic preperitoneal inguinal hernia repair without peritoneal incision. Surg Endosc 1993;7:159–162.

13. Read RC. Preperitoneal herniorrhaphy: A historical review. World J Surg 1989;13:532–540.

14. Shulman AG, Amid PK, Lichtenstein IL. The safety of mesh repair for primary inguinal hernias. Am Surg 1992;58:255–257.

15. Stoppa RE. The treatment of complicated groin and incisional hernias. World J Surg 1989;13:545–554.

16. Tetik C, Arregui ME, Duhier JL, et al. Complications and recurrence associated with laparoscopic repair of groin hernias. Surg Endosc 1994;8:1316–1323.

17. Wheeler KH. Laparoscopic inguinal herniorrhaphy with mesh: An 18 month experience. J Laparoendosc Surg 1993;4:345–350.

25

Cholecystectomy: Minilaparotomy

John W. Braasch

Standard cholecystectomy, minilaparotomy cholecystectomy, and laparoscopic cholecystectomy are three techniques for accomplishing the same purpose and whose relative merits have been debated hotly. The popularity of any procedure that might be followed by less pain and disability is understandable. In the competitive surgical environment, surgeons emphasize the success of their technique to increase their market share of patients. Thus, expectations of success are raised, and as a consequence, the difficulties of obtaining a true assessment comparing the three methods of cholecystectomy have increased. It seems self-evident that smaller incisions lead to less pain and disability, but proving this point has been difficult because pain and disability are hard to quantify. The new technique of laparoscopic cholecystectomy has leapfrogged minilaparotomy cholecystectomy and has been established as the procedure of choice without adequate evaluation of either minilaparotomy cholecystectomy or laparoscopic cholecystectomy.

LITERATURE REVIEW

In 1966, Zierold and Moos provided one of the first reports of a minicholecystectomy technique. They used an incision described approximately 40 years previously (a vertical midline incision into the rectus sheath with elevation of the right rectus muscle and a horizontal incision through the posterior rectus sheath) to perform cholecystectomy in 374 patients older than 60 years of age. Before this first report, no studies had been published on

length of hospital stay or postoperative disability after any type of cholecystectomy. However, most of the patients of Zierold and Moos did exceedingly well, with much less pain and discomfort than that associated with the usual large incision of a cholecystectomy (personal observation).

Another technique is that of Goco and Chambers, who used a 4-cm subcostal incision in 50 patients. They recorded an average hospital stay of 1.5 days with a mean off-the-job disability of 18.6 days. In another report, Morton stated that 96 patients had a 4- to 5-cm subcostal incision with retrograde dissection of the gallbladder followed by an average hospital stay of 2.5 days, and most patients were back to light work within 2 weeks. Merrill reported a series of 100 patients discharged within 24 hours of elective cholecystectomy using a midline incision and a minimal "no-touch" procedure in a "well." In yet another study by Ledet, 200 consecutive outpatient cholecystectomies were performed through a 5- to 10-cm transverse incision. In this report, patients were selected on the basis of the desire for ambulatory surgery and a lack of significant contraindicating medical problems. No patient was rejected because of age or weight. All were discharged from the hospital between 3 and 10 hours after operation.

These reports establish that a cholecystectomy can be performed safely through a very small incision, and the dissection can be accomplished by direct vision. A small incision presumes that less surgery is followed by lesser amounts of pain and disability. Even with a larger incision, patients can be discharged from the hospital on the same day as the operation.

COMPARING MINICHOLECYSTECTOMY WITH TRADITIONAL AND LAPAROSCOPIC CHOLECYSTECTOMY

There are limitations in retrospective and nonrandomized comparisons between different surgical techniques. A prospective, randomized trial comparing minicholecystectomy with conventional cholecystectomy was reported by Assalia and coworkers in 1993. Twenty-six patients underwent conventional cholecystectomy and 24 patients underwent minilaparotomy cholecystectomy. The latter procedure was performed through a right subcostal incision, which varied in length from 4 to 10 cm in the minicholecystectomy operation. A "fundus down" technique was used in all patients. The mean length of the incision was 14.4 cm in the conventional type and 5.4 cm in the minicholecystectomy type. The mean operative time was the same, but mean operative "difficulty" was greater for the minicholecystectomy. Less postoperative narcotics were used after the minicholecystectomy, and the mean duration of hospitalization was 4.7 days for the conventional operation and 3.0 days for the minicholecystectomy. In addition, overall patient satisfaction was greater for the minicholecystectomy.

On the other end of the spectrum, it is necessary to compare minilaparotomy cholecystectomy with laparoscopic cholecystectomy. Two series compared these two techniques on a randomized, prospective basis. The first, reported in 1992 by Barkun and colleagues, was carried out using 38 patients randomly allocated to laparoscopic cholecystectomy and 32 patients to a minicholecystectomy. Thirty-seven of 38 patients and 25 of 32 patients underwent the assigned procedures. The mean hospital stay was significantly shorter in the laparoscopic cholecystectomy group than in the minicholecystectomy group, as was the duration of convalescence.

The second trial, reported in 1994 by McMahon and coworkers, involved 302 patients ran-domized to laparoscopic or minilaparotomy cholecystectomy. A 5- to 10-cm subcostal incision was used for the minilaparotomy. The findings in this trial were that laparoscopic cholecystectomy took 15 minutes longer than minilaparotomy, the postoperative hospital stay was 2 days shorter, and the hospital costs were significantly greater. Patients having laparoscopic cholecystectomy were discharged to home and to work sooner, and had more rapid return to physical and social activities. In a similar study, the same authors noted better blood oxygen saturation and a smaller reduction in pulmonary function postoperatively in patients who underwent laparoscopic cholecystectomy.

Any comparison of morbidity and disability relative to minilaparotomy cholecystectomy and laparoscopic cholecystectomy must include a survey of complications. In Deziel and associates' analysis of 77,604 laparoscopic cholecystectomies, 33 postoperative deaths (or less than 0.05%) were reported. The rate of common or hepatic duct injury was 0.6%, which might be slightly higher than for open cholecystectomy, but comparison is difficult. Outcome data for minilaparotomy cholecystectomy are relatively sparse, with limited numbers and short follow-up times.

The two studies by McMahon and associates indicate that patients experience less pain and disability postoperatively after laparoscopic than minilaparotomy cholecystectomy. As discussed, a perfectly controlled, prospective, randomized trial is not possible in comparing these two operative procedures. All minilaparotomy cholecystectomies are not equal when a variety of surgeons are involved, whereas laparoscopic cholecystectomy is fairly standardized with regard to the numbers, position, and length of incisions. In these prospective trials, other variables, such as weight, age, inflammation around the gallbladder, and other technical impediments, were fairly well matched.

With careful selection and preparation, some patients with a standard large incision cholecystectomy can be discharged on the day of operation and do reasonably well. However, laparoscopic cholecystectomy is probably less painful and is associated with less disability. This does not denigrate the value of the small incision or minilaparotomy cholecystectomy. Minilaparotomy permits direct vision during

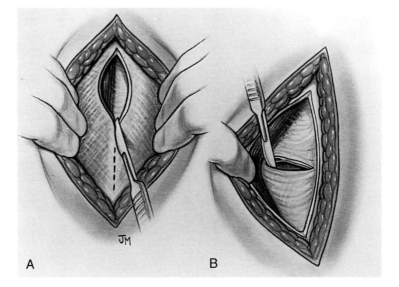

Figure 25–1. (A) A vertical midline incision is made slightly to the right, opening the right rectus sheath. (B) After the right rectus muscle is retracted laterally, a transverse incision is made through the posterior rectus sheath and peritoneum. (Courtesy of Lahey Clinic, Burlington, MA.)

A   B

the dissection of Calot's triangle and superior safety in certain instances.

Because open cholecystectomy is necessary in approximately 5% of laparoscopic procedures, minilaparotomy cholecystectomy could be the backup procedure to failed laparoscopic cholecystectomy. It is possible that surgeons might choose this alternative more readily, knowing that disability and morbidity from pain are not greatly increased. One caveat to this suggestion is that open minilaparotomy cholecystectomy in the morbidly obese and for the shrunken gallbladder can be extremely difficult and often requires a standard cholecystectomy incision.

TECHNIQUE OF MINILAPAROTOMY CHOLECYSTECTOMY

The best incision for minilaparotomy cholecystectomy, which gives adequate exposure and optimal strength after closure of the abdominal wall, is an upper midline incision that gives access to the right rectus compartment. This compartment is opened, and the rectus muscle is retracted laterally, thus permitting a horizontal incision through the posterior sheath and peritoneum (Fig. 25–1). The length of the skin incision should be adequate to permit a 2-inch horizontal incision in the

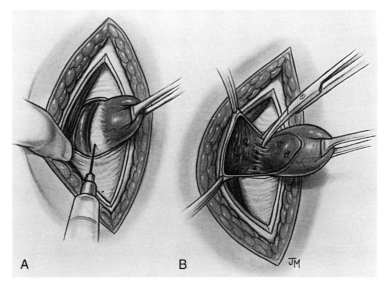

Figure 25–2. (A) The fundus of the gallbladder is grasped in a Pennington clamp, and the liver bed is infiltrated with saline solution or lidocaine with or without adrenaline. (B) Traction on the gallbladder and on the gallbladder serosa attached to the liver expedites downward traction of the fundus. (Courtesy of Lahey Clinic, Burlington, MA.)

A   B

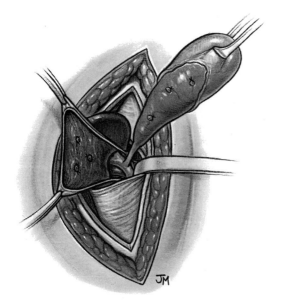

Figure 25–3. At the completion of dissection, the cystic duct–common duct junction is clearly seen. (Courtesy of Lahey Clinic, Burlington, MA.)

posterior sheath and peritoneum. This incision does not require that the rectus muscle be severed, and the sensory and motor nerves are not cut.

Guided by two fingers of the left hand, a Pennington clamp is placed on the fundus of the gallbladder, and the gallbladder and edge of the liver can be drawn into the posterior rectus sheath incision. Saline solution or lidocaine with or without adrenaline is injected into the base of the gallbladder to accentuate its attachment to the liver. The gallbladder is removed from the fundus downward by sharp dissection (Fig. 25–2). Bleeding is controlled by ligation of the small branches of the cystic artery. As dissection progresses, with smaller arterioles coagulated by the electrocautery, the gallbladder continues to rise out of the incision. Little by little, the triangle of Calot is approached. The cystic artery can be displaced superiorly and medially as the cystic duct–common duct junction is approached. This junction can be verified by direct inspection, and, often, the final portions of the cholecystectomy can be accomplished with the cystic duct–common duct junction at the skin level (Fig. 25–3). This procedure can give access to the common duct for cholangiography or even

for extraction of calculi and the insertion of a T-tube. The incision is closed in layers and results in a strong and relatively pain-free abdominal wall incision.

Each procedure—minilaparotomy cholecystectomy and laparoscopic cholecystectomy—requires special expertise for low morbidity and mortality. Data relative to these yardsticks of quality assume that special expertise is being used. In the final analysis, both procedures are useful, and they should complement one another.

Selected Readings

1. Assalia A, Schein M, Kopelman D, Hashmonai M. Minicholecystectomy vs conventional cholecystectomy: A prospective randomized trial—implications in the laparoscopic era. World J Surg 1993;17:755–759.
2. Barkun JS, Barkun AN, Sampalis JS, et al. Randomised controlled trial of laparoscopic versus mini cholecystectomy. Lancet 1992;340:1116–1119.
3. Cheslyn-Curtis S, Russell RCG. New trends in gallstone management. Br J Surg 1991;78:143–149.
4. Deziel DJ, Millikan KW, Economou SG, Doolas A, Ko S-T, Airan MC. Complications of laparoscopic cholecystectomy: A national survey of 4,292 hospitals and an analysis of 77,604 cases. Am J Surg 1993;165:9–14.
5. Goco IR, Chambers LG. "Mini-cholecystectomy" and operative cholangiography: A means of cost containment. Am Surg 1983;49:143–145.
6. Ledet WP Jr. Ambulatory cholecystectomy without disability. Arch Surg 1990;125:1434–1435.
7. McDermott EWM, McGregor JR, O'Dwyer PJ, Murphy JJ, O'Higgins NJ. Patient outcome following laparoscopic and minilaparotomy cholecystectomy (abstr). Br J Surg 1991;78:1503.
8. McMahon AJ, Russell IT, Baxter JN, et al. Laparoscopic versus minilaparotomy cholecystectomy: A randomised trial. Lancet 1994;343:135–138.
9. McMahon AJ, Russell IT, Ramsay G, et al. Laparoscopic and minilaparotomy cholecystectomy: A randomized trial comparing postoperative pain and pulmonary function. Surgery 1994;115:533–539.
10. Merrill JR. Minimal trauma cholecystectomy (a "no-touch" procedure in a "well"). Am Surg 1988;54:256–261.
11. Morton CE. Cost containment with the use of "mini-cholecystectomy" and intraoperative cholangiography. Am Surg 1985;51:168–169.
12. Moss G. Discharge within 24 hours of elective cholecystectomy: The first 100 patients. Arch Surg 1986;121:1159–1161.
13. O'Dwyer PJ, Murphy JJ, O'Higgins NJ. Cholecystectomy through a 5 cm subcostal incision. Br J Surg 1990;77:1189–1190.
14. Saltzstein EC, Mercer LC, Peacock JB, Dougherty SH. Outpatient open cholecystectomy. Surg Gynecol Obstet 1992;174:173–175.
15. Zierold AA, Moos DJ. A method for cholecystectomy in older patients. Surgery 1966;60:511–516.

LAPAROSCOPIC SURGERY

26

Special Considerations for Performing Laparoscopic Surgery: Personnel, Equipment, and Costs

C. Randle Voyles

In the broadest sense, the success of ambulatory surgery represents a major paradigm shift in U. S. health culture. Cost pressures have pushed more surgery to an outpatient setting, and patients and surgeons have accepted that major procedures can be accomplished without several days of in-hospital observation. The pace of change has increased with managed care. The future of ambulatory surgical care and all special considerations regarding personnel, equipment, and costs continue to be molded by the following three dominant influences under the new paradigm:

- Measurable outcomes
- Costs
- Safety and litigation

Anecdotal references of "goodness" will be replaced by a considerable database reflecting procedure-specific measurable outcomes under appropriately managed care. For example, measurable outcomes of quality after laparoscopic cholecystectomy might include conversion rates (corrected for degree of illness), the incidence of bile leak or ductal injury, the frequency of readmission and reoperation, and the frequency of totally uncomplicated cholecystectomy.

The new financial paradigm reflects a fixed reimbursement per procedure (or population base) compared to a previous system that based reimbursement on charges. Thus, the financial success of the ambulatory center will be based more on controlling costs than on generating charges. To control costs, special consideration must be given to the operational aspects of personnel and equipment.

The introduction of new laparoscopic procedures has been followed by an increased frequency of complications, which has led to increased health care costs and litigation expenses. Educational efforts have been initiated to improve the safety of specific laparoscopic techniques. Malpractice premiums have increased for general surgeons who perform laparoscopic surgery in many areas.

This chapter outlines specific details regarding personnel and equipment that are essential for providing the highest quality surgical care under the evolving paradigm. After defining expected outcomes in quality, the cost differentials between specific practices and techniques are readily measurable. For practical purposes, the primary procedure for the ambulatory laparoscopic setting is laparoscopic cholecystectomy. The lessons learned from scrutiny of cholecystectomy should apply to other laparoscopic procedures.

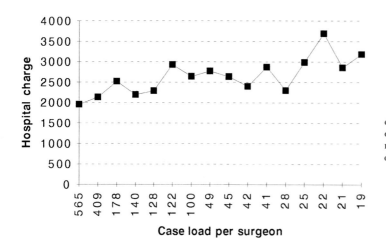

Figure 26–1. The mean hospital charge varies according to the operating experience of the surgeon, as determined by a review of more than 1500 cases in 3 years in one facility.

VARIANCE OF FACILITY COSTS WITH LAPAROSCOPIC PROCEDURES: THE EVOLUTION OF DATA FOR DECISION-MAKING

Under the previous system of conventional health insurance, charges varied markedly among centers due to cost-shifting from indigent patients, unreimbursed expenses, and mandated profit margins. A center's costs also vary due to a number of factors: "for-profit" or "not-for-profit" status, influencing the taxability for services, purchases, sales, and property; increased administrative expenses to comply with new regulations and changes in health care; debt service; educational function regarding the training of residents and other personnel; purchase agreements of hospital buyer groups; local economic factors, with variance in wages, union influence, and real estate expenditures; and litigation expenses.

Good data regarding true costs are not readily obtainable because most data relate to charges and not costs. Hospital charges for laparoscopic cholecystectomy dating from around 1991 ranged from $1817 to $7500. The data were not controlled for degree of illness of the patient or experience of the surgeon. Part of the variation in costs was attributed to the inappropriate use of lasers and disposable instruments. At that point in time, excesses were rewarded more handsomely than cost-responsible care, leaving insurers and hospitals with little financial incentive for encouraging

the outlined recommendations. Finally, some critics suggested that charges should not be compared between different states.

Good data regarding regional costs or charges also are difficult to obtain. Recently, a major insurer was asked to provide data on variation in costs for simple laparoscopic cholecystectomy in different centers within one state. Data were provided on insurance reimbursement to each center, rather than costs or charges. In the analysis, controls for degree of illness and complications were provided as age younger than 60 years and hospital stay of less than 48 hours. Marked variation existed in reimbursement for a definable study group in different cities within a single state (Table 26–1). Charges to the patient are higher than insurance reimbursement because the patient usually has a copayment. The use of disposable instruments likely contributed to some differences, although inhouse controls and full cooperation from sister cities were lacking.

Another study was initiated to determine the effect of the varying caseload of each surgeon on hospital charge and operating time within a single facility (Mississippi Baptist Hos-

Table 26–1. Hospital Reimbursement From Insurer for Cholecystectomy

Institution	Cost
Mississippi Baptist Hospital, Jackson, MS	$2472
St. Dominics, Jackson, St. Dom.	$2813
Hattiesburg, MS	$3963
Tupelo, MS	$4260

pital, Jackson, MS). The 3-year review included gross data without control for degree of illness or policy regarding operative cholangiograms; quality issues were not addressed. Although the study included only data on hospital charges, the argument regarding costs versus charges is less important in evaluating differences among surgeons within one hospital. Greater operating experience was associated with lesser charges (Fig. 26–1), and there was a variance of operating room time versus caseload of the surgeon. The operating room time included the period from when the patient entered the operating room until the patient exited, thus reflecting preparation and anesthesia induction time, the operating time, and the immediate postoperative period. Thus, these data reflect efficiency of the entire laparoscopic team and not just proficiency of the surgeon. With the more proficient surgeons, the mean operating time averaged 20 to 40 minutes in most cases. It appeared that greater operative experience as measured by caseload was associated with a reduced operative time (Fig. 26–2).

In another study from 1993, a number of variables were controlled, including a longer operating time by excluding the additional charges incurred beyond the first 60 minutes. Data were compiled on the operating room charges in more than 300 cases (Table 26–2). A marked variation in charges persisted and was attributed primarily to the surgeon's selection of disposable instruments. Other variables included the frequency of performance of op-

Table 26–2. Case Load Versus Charges Corrected for Operating Room Time

Surgeon	Time (min)	No. of Cases	Charge*
A	65	123	$1136
B	61	113	$1316
C, D	81	20–60	$1600
E–L	90	5–19	$1800
M	120	1	$3700

*Excluding changes incurred after first 60 minutes.

erative cholangiograms. It was apparent that experienced surgeons tended to prefer reusable instruments, whereas less experienced surgeons used disposable instruments. Surgeon M was the most prolific user of disposable instruments in the study group. The surgeon-specific variance in facility charges would probably persist in a cost-based analysis.

To provide a benchmark for other centers, the hospital administration provided cost–charge ratios by hospital department for 30 patients undergoing laparoscopic cholecystectomy for uncomplicated chronic calculous cholecystitis. All cases were performed by a single surgeon. As of June 1993, the estimated mean facility cost for the 30 patients was $2094.

In conclusion, there is considerable variance in costs, charges, and reimbursements for laparoscopic cholecystectomy. The lowest costs have been incurred at centers with high volume and shorter operating times. Other factors are discussed in subsequent paragraphs.

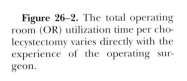

Figure 26–2. The total operating room (OR) utilization time per cholecystectomy varies directly with the experience of the operating surgeon.

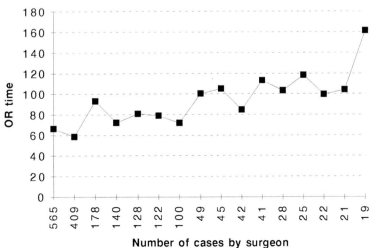

SAFETY AND LITIGATION CONSIDERATIONS

The successful laparoscopic procedure is associated with less pain, earlier return to preoperative activities, and potentially lower costs. The enthusiasm for laparoscopic successes has been tempered by the occasional complication—unique to laparoscopy—that can be devastating. Increasing litigation expenses have led to some malpractice premium increases for laparoscopic surgeons (e.g., a $9000 surcharge in Mississippi).

A recent analysis was completed by 31 insurance companies associated through Physician Insurers Association of America (PIAA). The PIAA study included data from 615 claims associated with laparoscopy. Significantly, *the majority of injuries were not recognized during the laparoscopic procedure.* Potential reasons for the unrecognized injuries include the inherent limitations of laparoscopy (poor visualization with incomplete surveillance as a result of minimal invasion), an incomplete understanding of energy sources used in laparoscopy, the inherent risks of blind insertion of sharp instruments into the abdomen, the learning curve, and variance in judgment or technical ability. Once an injury occurs, the problem is always compounded by delayed recognition and initiation of treatment.

Another observation of the PIAA study was that the *percentage of claims closed with an indemnity payment was higher with laparoscopy* than with former open procedures. As a matter of conjecture, delayed treatment of potentially preventable injuries is the leading explanation for this observation. It appears that the litigious nature of society, sharp skills of plaintiff attorneys, and higher expectations of patients are secondary factors. The complication rate in the early laparoscopic experience appears to be lower when surgeons are assisted by other surgeons rather than by nonphysicians, when surgeons practice in groups rather than solo, and when surgeons participate in ongoing continuing education.

SPECIAL PERSONNEL CONSIDERATIONS

To maximize quality and efficiency, a dedicated and committed laparoscopic team is essential. During open procedures, the inexperience of a technician or assistant can be more readily overcome by a skillful surgeon. Laparoscopic procedures, however, are somewhat "all or none," in that each member of the team must function well or else the operation cannot be performed.

To control costs, even more emphasis is placed on coordinated teamwork. Proficiency of the team must include attention to turnover between cases, because the facility costs of personnel are just as high between cases as during operations. Although use of reusable instruments is significantly less expensive than the cost of disposable instruments, they require some additional processing. Lack of commitment by any member of the team—surgeon, technician, nurse, or operating supervisor—will derail the transition to more cost-responsible care. Recently, improvements in instrument design have eliminated many of the problems with function and reprocessing of reusable instruments. Current data show that processing of reusable instruments causes no delay during or between cases with sophisticated laparoscopic teams.

An effort has been made to develop mechanical devices for holding retractors and cameras. With some devices, the surgeon manually readjusts the position of the instruments. If adjustments are infrequent, the manually controlled device works well. A robotic arm has been devised that can be adjusted by foot control of the surgeon. The utility of such devices increases when operations are longer, instruments stay in the same position for long periods of time, and constraints on personnel are high. The benefit is less with short operations performed by proficient teams.

A successful laparoscopic team has support from several other departments within the hospital. The role of the anesthesiologist is outlined in Chapter 16. A member of the biomedical engineering department may be helpful in sorting out occasional problems with laparoscopes, cameras, video monitors, and electrical interference. The radiology department must provide fluoroscopy units with storage capabilities.

The expertise of the surgeon is even more critical when efforts are made to reduce costs. As discussed, variance in facility costs is often surgeon specific. The surgeon must establish a leadership role in directing the team and selecting the most appropriate instruments and energy sources.

The structured educational programs for laparoscopic training have essentially been sponsored by the disposable instrument industry. Herein lies a conflict in that most surgeons initiated their experience using disposable instruments and may feel some commitment to use disposable instruments to maintain access to certain educational facilities. The reusable instrument companies, whose products will reduce costs and increase profits when reimbursements are fixed, do not generate ample revenue to provide the equivalent sales force and educational programs of the disposable instrument industry. Perhaps, financial pressures will encourage facilities and insurers to support ongoing educational efforts regarding cost-responsible care.

SPECIAL EQUIPMENT CONSIDERATIONS

Trocar-Cannula

The first instrument that the surgeon must choose is a trocar-cannula. There are basically three categories from which to choose. The completely disposable systems have the advantages of familiarity (most surgeons learned laparoscopy using disposable trocar-cannulas), uniformly sharp trocars, and kits that contain all the parts. The disadvantages of disposable systems relate primarily to increased costs. In addition, there are distinct ecologic concerns as well as potential electrosurgical hazards from the use of nonconductive plastic cannulas.

The completely reusable trocar-cannulas offer the greatest potential cost advantage, but varying sharpness of trocars can increase risks during insertion. In addition, the trumpet-valved cannulas contain many parts for processing and require two hands for instrument exchanges.

A combination of reusable cannulas with disposable trocars may represent the best combination for most centers. Disposable or limited-use trocars provide uniform sharpness.

Cannula valves are designed with trap doors that allow single-handed instrument exchanges. Two-part instrument design and special instrument trays facilitate reprocessing between cases. The metal cannulas are conductive, reducing some electrosurgical hazards.

Many surgeons prefer trocar-cannulas containing "safety-shield" devices that reduce the chance for bowel or major vessel puncture during trocar insertion. Safety-shields either have a shield that slides over the sharp trocar or have a trocar that retracts into the cannula after abdominal wall penetration. Despite the design, corroborating clinical data supporting their use are lacking. Furthermore, some injuries may have occurred due to a false sense of security associated with the safety-shield. A further contributing factor may be that some trocars "float" within the cannulas, even though the surgeon's hand may rotate. Accordingly, the only motion that allows entry is downward pressure rather than lateral displacement by a twisting motion. The significance of these issues is highlighted by one recent survey showing that almost half of the legal cases associated with laparoscopy were related to trocar-cannula insertion.

An open technique of trocar insertion has theoretic advantages over blind puncture insertion. The underlying principle is that no sharp instruments are blindly inserted into the abdomen. Our preferred technique for initial trocar-cannula insertion is as follows:

1. The umbilicus is elevated with lateral tension. Towel clips are placed in the lateral edges of the umbilicus. The umbilicus is everted and elevated, increasing the distance from retroperitoneal structures. (Lifting the lower abdominal wall by hand may not alter the distance between the umbilicus and the aorta.)

2. A vertical incision is made through the center of the umbilicus. The skin incision is extended through the fascia using tactile feedback as a guide. Lateral and upward tension on the towel clips facilitates this step. Commonly, an occult fascial defect allows direct access to the peritoneal cavity.

3. The hemostat tip is inserted into the peritoneal cavity and spread. In most patients, the skin, fascia, and peritoneum are fused cen-

trally. On occasion, the peritoneum must be penetrated with the hemostat.

4. A blunt pyramidal trocar-cannula is inserted and rotated until it is firmly seated within the fascial defect. The blunt trocar is removed while upward pressure is maintained on the towel clips and insufflation is begun. The rounded conical trocars are disadvantageous because they allow insertion only by downward pressure and not by the lateral displacement associated with the twisting motion of a pyramidal tip.

5. The laparoscope is advanced through the fascial defect under "direct vision."

There are several advantages of this technique. Conceptually, there is no blind insertion of a sharp instrument. Peritoneal access is obtained by "video vision." The chance for preperitoneal insufflation or carbon dioxide embolus is less compared with that associated with Veress techniques, and operating time is reduced.

Scissors

As with trocar-cannulas, scissors are available as disposable, reusable, and mixed disposable-reusable, or so-called reposable instruments. Scissors must be predictably sharp. In cholecystectomy, the only maneuver that requires mechanical cutting is transection of the cystic duct and artery. The skilled surgeon can use mechanical and electrosurgical dissection for the remainder of the operation. The surgeon's choice of scissors has most commonly been related to surgical preference. The per-procedure facility cost for a disposable scissors ($90–$100) allows considerable leeway for less expensive mechanical cutting. Disposable scissors are not designed for reprocessing and should be thrown away after each case. Reusable instruments can have a long life if surgeons are careful not to cut metal clips while transecting the cystic duct and artery. The reposable scissors allow replacement of the cutting edges and reuse of the handles.

Clip Appliers

Disposable clip appliers allow placement of several clips during one insertion. The reus-

able clip applier is "single action" and requires reloading for every clip; a set of two appliers increases proficiency if reusable clip appliers are used. When complex procedures are performed that require many clips, the role for the multiclip applier is greater. However, during a simple cholecystectomy, only six clips may be required and a disposable clip applier may have a patient charge exceeding $300. The reusable clip applier seems more appropriate for simple cholecystectomy.

Suction-Irrigators

Suction-irrigators are available as disposable and reusable instruments. The reusable instruments contain multiple parts, frequently leak, and often become clogged. However, they are adequate for simple cholecystectomy if the surgical team maintains good care of the instruments. Disposable suction-irrigators are more appropriate for complex cases and cost only $45 to $55 per procedure. Various sizes of reusable cannula tips can be exchanged on the disposable handles.

SPECIAL CONSIDERATIONS FOR ENERGY SOURCES

A wide variety of energy sources have been used in laparoscopy, although monopolar electrosurgery is considered the gold standard. Monopolar electrosurgery was used in tubal fulguration in the early 1970s, but its use was abandoned after a number of complications were not adequately explained. Rather than correcting the problems, gynecologic surgeons switched to using bipolar electrosurgery. As laparoscopic techniques became more advanced, a more effective energy source was required and gynecologists adopted laser technology. General surgeons began laparoscopic cholecystectomy with laser devices in the United States but quickly switched back to monopolar electrosurgery. Complications directly attributable to monopolar electrosurgery have been relatively infrequent with laparoscopic cholecystectomy, probably because the liver is so tolerant to inexact application of energy. More recently, the initial problems with monopolar electrosurgery have been formally addressed and resolved.

Art and Science of Monopolar Electrosurgery

The goal of electrosurgery is to develop a specific tissue effect (e.g., desiccation, cutting) by directing a variety of electrical currents through the target tissue without causing an ill effect to nontarget tissues. Most simply, the art and the science of electrosurgery are based on controlling tissue temperatures. Ideally, the surgeon should use the least energy to achieve the desired temperature change to accomplish a given laparoscopic task. The scientific basis of local tissue heating at the electrode–tissue interface is outlined in the following formula:

$$\text{temp change} = (l^2/r^4) \ R \ t$$

where l = current, r = radius of tissue–electrode contact, R = tissue resistance, and t = time.

The most important determinant of local tissue heating is the radius of electrode contact. The good technical surgeon is proficient at maintaining a high current density by controlling the radius of electrode contact through appropriate tension and countertension. Points in the circuit with a very low power density (i.e., the dispersive return pad, or, perhaps, the all-metal trocar-cannula with inadvertent electrode contact) have a minimal temperature change in tissue during electrode activation.

Monopolar electrosurgery is provided by an alternating current with a frequency of approximately 500,000 Hz; the high frequency minimizes neuromuscular stimulation, as was discovered by French researchers almost 100 years ago. Lower frequency currents can be caused by intermittent arcing to metal devices such as clips, instruments, cannulas, or the laparoscope.

The surgeon may select varying waveforms from the generator. The "coag" mode has a higher voltage than the "cut" mode. The higher voltage "drives" an electrical charge deeper into tissue or arcs for a longer distance to target tissue. With most modern generators, the surgeon selects the wattage, but the voltage varies during application of energy. The voltage increases automatically as tissue is desiccated (and current decreases) or if the generator is activated as an open circuit (i.e., the electrode does not touch tissue, a high-voltage condition). Wattage equals voltage times current.

Higher voltage conditions are desirable in certain situations because high voltage leads to longer arcs when noncontact techniques are used and to deeper penetration of the electrical charge when contact techniques are used. Although hemostasis may be improved with higher voltage, the higher voltage also increases the surrounding electromagnetic field and the risk of injury with insulation breakdown or induced currents around the electrodes. The coag mode also provides an interrupted or dampened waveform as opposed to the continuous waveform of the cut; thus, for a given wattage, the cut waveform provides higher amperage and lower voltage compared with the coag waveform.

The specific tissue effects with monopolar electrosurgery vary according to generator, generator settings, electrode design, and surgical techniques.

Fulguration

Fulguration is a technique that provides superficial desiccation of tissue by arcing current from the electrode to the nearby tissue. The most effective fulguration occurs with a high-voltage generator operated in the coag mode because higher voltages generate longer arcing to tissue. The maximum voltage of the coag mode varies by manufacturer as well as by generator. The superficial effect is created because tissue contact is not made and some of the energy is dissipated in the "lightning." After the first "bolt" strikes a specific tissue point, that tissue is desiccated and loses its conductivity. Thus, the next bolt strikes the next most conductive area. Fulguration is a high-voltage delivery and carries a higher potential for insulation failure and capacitive coupling.

Contact Desiccation

Contact desiccation occurs when the electrode is activated in contact with tissue, providing excellent hemostasis as successive layers of tissue are desiccated. As the superficial tissue is desiccated, the voltage of the generator increases to facilitate deeper tissue effects. Contact desiccation leads to the development of an eschar, which may be desirable in some settings but the eschar may distort anatomic planes. With broad enough contact between the electrode and tissue, desiccation without cutting occurs with either the cut or the coag mode. Desiccation in the cut mode takes somewhat longer than in the coag mode but is associated with a lower voltage (leading to a smaller electromagnetic field and less potential for insulation breakdown or induced currents) and, perhaps, a more superficial tissue effect. If the power density is high enough, a tissue cutting effect may be achieved with either the cut or coag mode.

Vaporization

The optimal cut (vaporization) tissue effect is provided by the cut mode with the electrode edge or needle near but not touching tissue. When there is ample power density, there is immediate heating and boiling of intracellular contents by the uninterrupted waveform. The "exploding" cells give a cutting effect seen as vaporization. When the electrode is held near but not contacting the tissue, hemostasis is poor because superficial cells are vaporized without significant desiccation of deeper tissue.

Coaptive Coagulation

Coaptive coagulation occurs when tissue is compressed within a grasper and current is applied; excellent desiccation occurs with the development of a "collagen weld" of the compressed tissue. This tissue effect can be obtained with either cut or coag mode. The benefit of the cut mode is that there is less voltage.

With any of the aforementioned electrosurgical techniques, good tension and countertension are essential. Appropriate tension reduces the radius of tissue–electrode contact and separates the treated tissue to reveal the next tissue plane.

Potential Problems With Monopolar Electrosurgery

The true incidence of electrosurgical injuries is unknown because injuries are typically not recognized during the procedure, treatment is often delayed, and surgeons are often reluctant to discuss the complications that frequently lead to litigation. Some bile duct injuries during laparoscopic cholecystectomy have been attributed to thermal injury from the energy source. Significant injuries related to monopolar electrosurgery are likely to increase as general surgeons pursue more aggressive laparoscopic procedures beyond the right upper quadrant.

Because of the difficulties in retrospectively studying the characteristics and mechanisms of bowel injury during laparoscopy, it is important to categorize potential mechanisms of energy transfer in order to prevent injuries. Most bowel injuries can be avoided with education and relatively simple engineering advances.

Electrosurgical injuries within the view of the laparoscope are related to surgical technique and, accordingly, could be reduced with increased vigilance. The surgeon's ability to apply science to achieve a specific tissue effect is an art form. With the fully developed art form, the anatomy is well defined with little injury to adjacent tissue. A lack of appreciation of the art form may be manifest by a higher incidence of subhepatic bile leaks or abscess, uncontrolled bleeding or need for transfusions, and ductal injury. Lesser manifestations may relate to prolonged operating time, more patient discomfort, and increased core costs of the procedure. The dissection of tissue planes around bowel or dissection of adhesions creates a much less forgiving scenario than freeing the gallbladder from its bed in the liver.

Electrosurgical injuries outside the view of the scope may occur because of three different types of "stray energy": insulation failure, capacitive coupling, and direct coupling. Burns at the return pad site (the most common electrosurgical injury 15 years ago) have been virtually eliminated by dynamic electronic monitoring of adequacy of the skin–return pad interface.

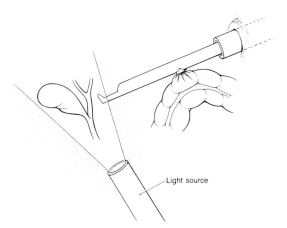

Figure 26–3. Defects in instrument insulation may be too small to visualize but still deliver 100% of the electrical current to tissues outside the view of the surgeon.

Insulation Failure

Insulation defects in the shaft of electrodes can be acquired from mechanical trauma, repeated heating through use or sterilization, manufacturing flaws, and capacitively coupled meltdown. Insulation failure is common and represents one of the most common reasons that instruments are returned to the manufacturer (Fig. 26–3).

The hazard of insulation failure depends on the location of the point of failure (Fig. 26–4). Defects in the handle of the electrode (zone 4) may burn the surgeon. The tips of most articulating electrodes (scissors and atraumatic grasper-dissectors) are incompletely insulated and have several centimeters of exposed metal that may cause injury to nontarget tissue (on the liver during laparoscopic cholecystectomy) with a loss of efficacy at the target tissue. A defect in the shaft of the electrode (zone 2)

may cause a nondetectable injury to bowel outside the view of the surgeon.

The signs of insulation failure within zone 3 (within the cannula) depend on whether a metal or plastic cannula is used. If a metal cannula is used, there is often current flow between the metal of the electrode and the metal of the cannula. The resulting arcing of the current creates a lower frequency current (referred to as a demodulated frequency), which can be as low as a few cycles per second. With this lower frequency, there may be neuromuscular stimulation, with jerking of the abdominal wall or diaphragm, but a distinct pattern of video interference ("lightning artifact") is common whenever the active electrode touches any metal within the abdomen. These indirect signs of insulation failure may suggest to the informed surgeon that insulation failure exists. Most surgeons, however, are not knowledgeable about the indirect signs of insulation failure. Because there are no clues to insulation failure if the electrode is within a plastic cannula, the utility of metal cannulas is apparent. Plastic anchoring devices over a metal cannula should not be used; they insulate the abdominal wall at the expense of the viscera.

All forms of conventional insulation are based on a passive system with layers of nonconductors around the electrode. Defects in insulation may deliver 100% of the current to biologic tissue outside the field of view of the surgeon and yet remain imperceptible to visual inspection. A new concept of insulation is based on dynamic electronic monitoring of insulation integrity during the operation (Electroscope, Boulder, CO). Continuous insulation monitoring with an overlying Electroshield or with new instruments constructed

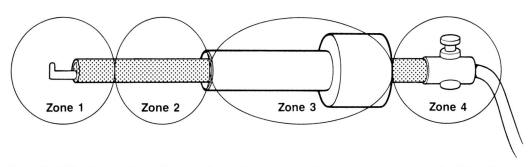

Figure 26–4. The risk associated with defective insulation varies with the location or zone of the defect. The zone 2 defects carry the greatest patient risk and are eliminated most effectively with active electrode monitoring.

with a fully integrated monitoring system guarantees that energy is being delivered only in zone 1.

Capacitive Coupling

Capacitive coupling is a mechanism whereby electrical current in the electrode induces a current in nearby conductors (unintended) despite otherwise intact insulation. Some degree of capacitive coupling occurs with all standard monopolar electrosurgical instruments. Whether the "stray energy" of capacitive coupling causes any clinical injury depends on (1) the total amount of current that is transferred and (2) the concentration of the current (i.e., the power density) as it makes its way back to the patient return electrode (inappropriately referred to as the "ground pad").

Capacitive coupling is increased by higher voltages. The low-voltage cut mode exhibits less coupling than the coag mode. The low-voltage generator (such as the Valleylab SSE2L) exhibits very little coupling compared with the higher voltage generators (Force 4B or 40). However, higher voltage generators offer better cutting and dessication. Surgeons must recognize that open-circuit activation (i.e., electrodes do not touch tissue) increases voltage and capacitive coupling dramatically. On one hand, noncontact activation of the generator should be limited and low wattage should be used. On the other hand, the use of high-voltage generators in the open-circuit coag mode provides a useful tissue effect (fulguration) if the potential hazards are recognized and controlled.

Four conditions exist when capacitive coupling can cause enough current to result in an injury:

1. Hybrid cannulas (a metal cannula sheath within a plastic tissue anchor) create a condition whereby current is induced in the metal cannula but the abdominal wall is insulated by the plastic anchor (Fig. 26–5).

2. Capacitive coupling also occurs when a conventionally insulated electrode is passed through a metal suction-irrigator. Approximately 70% of the current may be induced in the suction-irrigator. This instrument combination is particularly dangerous when a plastic cannula is used, because all of the stray cur-

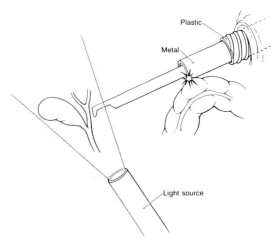

Figure 26–5. Capacitive coupling can lead to a burn to the bowel outside the view of the surgeon when a metal cannula is secured by a plastic anchoring device. All-metal cannulas and active electrode monitoring are recommended.

rent may be transmitted through a narrow contact with the bowel. An all-metal cannula at the abdominal wall "bleeds off" the stray current through the abdominal wall. Standard electrodes should not be passed through metal suction-irrigation devices.

3. Another significant capacitor is constructed when a surgical electrode is passed through the operating channel of an operating laparoscope.

4. Thin insulation increases capacitance. The extremely thin insulation of some instruments decreases the separation of the electrode from the surrounding conductor and increases the capacitance effect.

A partial-thickness defect in the insulation of an electrode increases capacitively coupled current. The potential for injury from capacitively coupled currents can be reduced with good electrosurgical technique and an understanding of the biophysics of that technique. The risks of capacitive coupling can be eliminated by recently designed electrosurgical instruments (Electroscope, Boulder, CO) that "collect" the stray current, remove it from the surgical site, and monitor the total amount of current before delivering it to the "return pad." This system confines capacitive coupling to the surgical instrument and monitoring circuit, thereby eliminating transmission to either the cannula or biologic tissues.

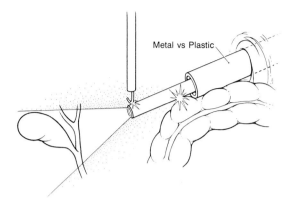

Figure 26–6. Inadvertent and easily unrecognized contact between the active electrode and the laparoscope can lead to a burn to the bowel if a plastic cannula is used at the abdominal wall. Metal cannulas are recommended to prevent this injury.

Direct Coupling

Direct coupling refers to the condition wherein the activated electrode touches other metal instruments (in particular, the laparoscope) within the abdomen, creating energy that can be unknowingly transferred to tissue outside the view of the laparoscope (Fig. 26–6). All cannulas housing conductive instruments (laparoscope and metal graspers) should be introduced through metal cannulas.

Summary of Energy Sources and Their Uses

In the relatively short history of laparoscopic surgery, many different energy sources have been used for tissue dissection. The laser had a rapid introduction but its use quickly diminished because of lack of efficacy and increased costs. Bipolar devices have limited application due to poor cutting capability, lack of efficacy, and increased costs. Although bipolar devices are considered to have inherent safety, the incidence of bowel and ureter injuries may be comparable to that of monopolar devices. Additional energy sources relying on ultrasonic tissue manipulation have been advocated, but they increase cost and their efficacy is questioned. It appears that the current gold standard energy source for both laparoscopy and laparotomy is monopolar electrosurgery.

The fully developed art of electrosurgery is reflected by the surgeon's ability to manipu-late fine electrodes and tissue to achieve results with an appropriate wattage. The informed surgeon understands the relative merits and disadvantages of both high- and low-voltage waveforms. If only cutting is needed, a low-voltage, pure "cut" waveform is appropriate using a light feathery motion in a noncontact mode. However, high voltage and high wattage are useful for deeper desiccation and especially for noncontact superficial arc fulguration. Safety is enhanced when bursts of current are used rather than continuous generator activation during laparoscopy.

The primary deficiency of laparoscopic monopolar electrosurgery is not technologic but rather relates to surgical education regarding the underlying biophysics of the technique. Injuries related to stray currents (insulation failure, capacitive coupling, and direct coupling) are most effectively eliminated with all-metal cannulas and actively monitored electrodes.

THE SURGEON AS AN INDUSTRIAL SCIENTIST

The complexity of the surgeon's task is increasing. After correcting for geographic or local socioeconomic factors, the bulk of variation in costs (and probably quality) between centers is surgeon specific, relating to judgment, technical proficiency, and selection of instruments and energy sources. Recommendations are as follows:

1. Maintain an absolute commitment to all aspects of technical proficiency. The fully developed surgical technique represents a nonquantifiable art form that leads to fewer complications, shorter operating room times, and reduced cost.

2. Eliminate the widespread use of disposable instruments. With the exception of limited-use trocars (within reusable cannulas) and an occasional disposable suction-irrigation device, the rest of the instruments should be reusable for routine laparoscopic cholecystectomy. Use of the Veress needle has been supplanted by open techniques.

3. Eliminate clumsy, inefficient, and unidirectional energy sources (laser, bipolar, and ultrasonic dissectors) that cannot deliver energy through favored dissecting instruments.

4. Learn more about the science of monopolar electrosurgery in order to improve the art of delivery and to reduce complications. An articulating grasper-dissector in the hands of a proficient electrosurgeon may be the only instrument that is required for most dissection. Limiting the number of instruments limits the number of instrument exchanges. However, use of articulating instruments requires a greater skill level than using hooks and spatulas.

5. Mandate a dedicated laparoscopic team for laparoscopic procedures. A minimum case load is essential for maximal efficiency and proficiency.

Selected Readings

1. Apelgren KN, Blank ML, Hadjis NS. Reusable instruments are more cost-effective than disposable instruments for laparoscopic cholecystectomy. Surg Endosc 1994;8:32–34.
2. Diathermy injury during laparoscopic surgery. Safety Action Bulletin (94) 38: September 1994.
3. ECRI. Monopolar electrosurgical safety during laparoscopy. Health Devices 1995;24(1):6–22.
4. Levy BS, Soderstrom RM, Dail DH. Bowel injuries during laparoscopy: Gross anatomy and histology. J Reprod Med 1985;30(3):168–172.
5. Luciano AA, Soderstrom RM, Martin DC. Essential principles of electrosurgery in operative laparoscopy. J Am Assoc Gynecol Lap 1994;1:189–195.
6. PIAA Laparoscopic Procedure Study. Washington, DC, Physician Insurers Association of America, 1994.
7. See WA, Cooper CS, Fisher RJ. Predictors of laparoscopic complications after formal training in laparoscopic surgery. JAMA 1993;270:2689–2692.
8. Soderstrom RM. Bowel injury litigation after laparoscopy. J Am Assoc Gynecol Lap 1993;1:74–77.
9. Voyles CR. The laparoscopic buck stops here! Am J Surg 1993;165:472–473.
10. Voyles CR, Petro AB, Meena AL, Haick AJ, Koury AM. A practical approach to laparoscopic cholecystectomy. Am J Surg 1991;161:365–370.
11. Voyles CR, Tucker RD. Education and engineering solutions for potential problems with laparoscopic monopolar electrosurgery. Am J Surg 1992;164:57–62.

Chapter 27

Laparoscopic Cholecystectomy

Nathaniel J. Soper

E. Mühe of Böblingen, Germany, performed the first laparoscopic-assisted cholecystectomy in 1985. However, most authors have assigned the credit to Phillipe Mouret of Lyon, France, who, in 1987, facilitated the procedure by rotating the entire right lobe of the liver in a cephalad direction with traction applied to the gallbladder itself. This maneuver allowed the gallbladder and porta hepatis to be viewed from a telescope placed at the umbilicus and directed cranially toward the undersurface of the liver. Surgeons in Paris and Bordeaux subsequently learned the procedure and performed the initial clinical series of laparoscopic cholecystectomies. This procedure was first performed in the United States in mid-1988 by surgeons in private practice. Because of the competitive, free-market medical system, patients' preference for "less invasive" procedures, and the marketing efforts by individuals and hospitals, laparoscopic cholecystectomy was adopted at a rate unprecedented in American surgery. Laparoscopic cholecystectomy rapidly became the new gold standard therapy for symptomatic cholelithiasis.

Laparoscopic cholecystectomy has many potential advantages over traditional open cholecystectomy (Table 27–1). Postoperative pain and intestinal ileus are diminished. The multiple small incisions are cosmetically more appealing than the large incision made during traditional cholecystectomy. The patient can usually be discharged from the hospital within 24 hours of operation and can return to full activity within a few days. The small size of the fascial incisions allows rapid return to heavy physical labor. These factors lead to a decreased overall cost of the procedure and ren-

der laparoscopic cholecystectomy an ideal procedure to be performed in an ambulatory setting. Laparoscopic cholecystectomy also has several disadvantages. Patients must be acceptable candidates for general anesthesia. Three-dimensional depth perception is limited by the monocular image of the video telescope, and the operative field being viewed is determined by an individual other than the surgeon. Some patients may be excluded from undergoing this therapy by virtue of their anatomy or intra-abdominal adhesions. The common bile duct is more difficult to visualize and instrument during laparoscopy than during traditional open surgery. It is technically difficult to remove the gallbladder from the fundus to the infundibulum, and control of brisk hemorrhage is diminished using laparoscopy compared with laparotomy.

Table 27–1. Comparison of Laparoscopic Cholecystectomy with Open Cholecystectomy

Advantages	Disadvantages
Smaller incisions	Technical limitations
Less pain	It is more difficult to control
Shorter	hemorrhage and explore
hospitalization	common bile duct.
More rapid return	Monocular vision is controlled by
to full activity	an assistant.
Decreased total	There is less tactile discrimination.
cost	Technologically advanced
	instruments are expensive.
	Anatomic limitations
	Inflammation and adhesions restrict
	application.
	Antegrade removal of gallbladder is
	difficult.
	Incidence of bile duct injury may be
	increased.

Many of the limitations of laparoscopy are under investigation. Three-dimensional video systems are being developed and marketed. Mechanical camera holders allow the surgeon to control the camera position remotely and to easily program the robotic arm to return to set positions. Pneumoperitoneum can be avoided altogether with use of various designs of abdominal retractors. Acquiring these technologic advances, however, is often costly. This chapter reviews the current status of laparoscopic cholecystectomy, focusing on preoperative, intraoperative, and postoperative considerations.

PREOPERATIVE CONSIDERATIONS

Indications

Two studies have documented an increased frequency of cholecystectomy since the introduction of laparoscopic cholecystectomy. It is unclear whether patients are simply more willing to undergo a minimally invasive procedure rather than suffer biliary pain or whether the indications for cholecystectomy have become more liberal with the advent of laparoscopy. In general, patients should have documented cholelithiasis and symptoms attributable to a diseased gallbladder. Gallbladder discomfort is typically severe recurrent upper abdominal pain, which often radiates to the back. Attacks frequently occur after large meals and pain may awaken the patient from sleep at night. Gallstone patients with porcelain gallbladder, immunosuppression, or no access to medical care may be considered for laparoscopic cholecystectomy despite a lack of biliary symptoms. Patients with no stones but typical biliary symptoms may also benefit from cholecystectomy. Recent studies suggest that symptoms develop in less than 20% of individuals with asymptomatic gallstones over a prolonged period and that the risk of "prophylactic" operation outweighs the potential benefit of surgery. In an individual with typical biliary colic, the only diagnostic test necessary is a high-quality ultrasound. This study demonstrates the stone size and number, the thickness of the gallbladder wall, pericholecystic fluid collections, sludge,

polyps, and the diameter of the common bile duct. It may also give clues to nonbiliary disorders, such as hepatic lesions or fatty infiltration, masses in the pancreas, or renal tumors. When ultrasound is negative and typical biliary symptoms persist, cholecystokinin (CCK)-stimulated biliary scintigraphy demonstrating a low gallbladder ejection fraction or reproducing pain after CCK administration is suggestive of acalculous cholecystitis. If atypical symptoms are present, a more extensive workup, including upper gastrointestinal contrast radiographs or endoscopy, computerized tomography, or cardiac evaluation, may be appropriate.

Contraindications

Preoperative evaluation should determine the presence of biliary and nonbiliary conditions that may adversely affect the outcome of laparoscopic cholecystectomy. Absolute contraindications include the inability to tolerate general anesthesia, uncorrectable coagulopathy, diffuse peritonitis, a "frozen" abdomen, cholecystoenteric fistula, and gallbladder cancer (Table 27–2). Numerous relative contraindications, which are primarily dictated by the surgeon's philosophy and experience, also exist. Many of the relative contraindications listed in Table 27–2 were previously considered absolute.

Morbidly obese patients are rarely denied the benefits of laparoscopic surgery. Longer trocars may be useful to transverse the anterior abdominal wall, and higher insufflation pressures may be required to obtain an adequate working space. Difficulty with closing trocar sites places these patients at a higher risk of cannulation site herniation.

Despite scattered reports of laparoscopic cholecystectomies having been performed during pregnancy, the effects of the prolonged carbon dioxide pneumoperitoneum on the fetus are unknown, and the position of the gravid uterus itself may present a problem. At my institution, five laparoscopic cholecystectomies were performed during the second trimester of gestation of pregnancy. Open insertion of the initial port is recommended to avoid accidental injury to the uterus. Patient hyperventilation and the monitoring of end-

Table 27–2. Contraindications to Laparoscopic Cholecystectomy

Absolute	Relative
Unable to tolerate general anesthesia	Acute cholecystitis with suspected empyema
Uncorrected coagulopathy	Morbid obesity
Peritonitis or cholangitis	Previous upper abdominal surgery
Biliary fistula	Cirrhosis or portal hypertension
Suspected carcinoma	Severe obstructive lung disease
Generalized peritonitis	Pregnancy
Other conditions requiring laparotomy	Possible malignancy
	Immunosuppression and hypercortisolism
	Uncertain diagnosis
	Unreducible abdominal or inguinal hernia
	Umbilical abnormalities
	Abdominal aortic or iliac aneurysm

tidal carbon dioxide prevent maternal and fetal acidosis. Insufflation pressures, kept below 12 mm Hg, obviate respiratory problems and compromised venous return. Monitoring fetal heart sounds is done in consultation with an obstetrician. To date, all pregnancies have resulted in normal deliveries of healthy infants. For the novice laparoscopic surgeon, it is wise to avoid such potentially difficult cases.

Operating Room Preparation

Performance of laparoscopic biliary surgery requires more personnel than do open operations. The surgeon stands to the left of the patient for cross-table access to the right upper quadrant (Fig. 27–1). (French surgeons prefer to operate in the lithotomy position, with the surgeon standing or sitting between the patient's legs.) The first assistant stands to the patient's right to manipulate the gallbladder and provide exposure. A laparoscopic video camera operator, who stands below the surgeon, assumes the important responsibility of being the surgeon's eyes. The camera operator must maintain the proper orientation of the camera and scope, particularly if an angled laparoscope is used, keep the surgeon's instruments in the center of the video monitor, follow (or guide) all instruments as they enter or exit the operative field, and assist with instruments or trocar valves as needed. No sharp or pointed instruments should be moved unless under direct vision. The camera operator must also take care of any obstruction to vision, such as wiping off condensation or blood that

may cloud the lens. Condensation on the lens itself can be minimized by heating the tip of the laparoscope in warm water or applying antifog solution to the lens before inserting the laparoscope into the abdominal cavity. A hot plate on the operating room table heats sterile water to 38°C and is readily available to rewarm the lens whenever the scope is outside the abdomen.

PREOPERATIVE CARE AND ANESTHESIA

As for any abdominal operation, patients are fasted from midnight before the operation and administered a preoperative sedative and histamine-2 receptor antagonist. All patients are given a single dose of intravenous antibiotics, usually a first-generation cephalosporin. Upon the patient's arrival in the operating room, sequential compression stockings are placed on both legs to avoid pooling of blood in the lower extremities caused by the reverse Trendelenburg position. Although minidose heparin is not routinely used, it can be used safely in patients at risk for venous thromboembolism. After induction of anesthesia, an orogastric tube is generally placed. At my institution, we no longer routinely place a Foley catheter in the urinary bladder. The abdomen is prepared in standard fashion, except that particular care is taken to clean the umbilicus of all detritus.

Although diagnostic laparoscopy can be performed with either local or regional anesthesia, laparoscopic cholecystectomy is generally

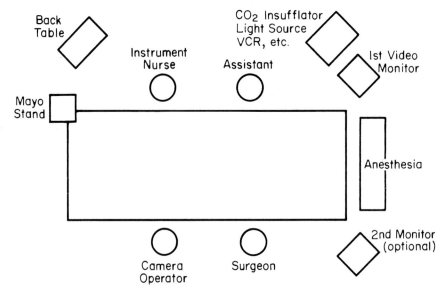

Figure 27–1. The organization of the operating room for laparoscopic biliary surgery. The patient's head is to the right, the surgeon stands at the patient's left and the first assistant is to the patient's right. The electronic laparoscopic equipment is placed on protective carts and the monitors are positioned to allow clear visualization by the entire surgical team. Irrigation, suction, and electrocautery originate at the head of the table on the left side. (From Soper NJ. Laparoscopic cholecystectomy. Curr Probl Surg 28:585–655, 1991.)

performed using inhalation anesthesia and controlled ventilation. Important considerations for optimal anesthetic management are adequate depth of anesthesia, complete muscle relaxation, administration of amnesics, and administration of antiemetics such as metoclopramide or a scopolamine patch before the conclusion of the operation. Patient monitoring during therapeutic laparoscopy using general anesthesia includes electrocardiography, blood pressure, precordial stethoscope, airway pressure, and capnography (specifically to assess end-tidal carbon dioxide). Invasive monitoring (arterial line, Swan-Ganz catheter) may be indicated in selected high-risk individuals (see Chapter 18).

There are scattered reports of laparoscopic cholecystectomy being performed using thoracic epidural (bupivacaine) anesthesia supplemented with intravenous sedation and local anesthetics. Referred shoulder pain may be troublesome with this technique, but it can be diminished by insufflating the peritoneal cavity slowly or by maintaining a lower abdominal pressure (<10 mm Hg). Regional anesthesia may be appropriate for high-risk patients or those who are highly motivated to avoid a general anesthetic. However, at my institution,

general anesthesia is used in all cases because of the potential need for rapid conversion to an open laparotomy. Postoperative pain is best avoided by preincisional subcutaneous injection at the cannulation sites with a long-acting local anesthetic. Usually, bupivacaine 0.5% is used to a maximum dose of 0.5 mL/kg.

Creation of Pneumoperitoneum and Trocar Insertion

A pneumoperitoneum, which is established by instilling gas, is usually used to allow visualization of the abdominal cavity. Recently, devices that elevate the abdominal wall by external retraction to create the working space have been described. This technique would potentially eliminate the adverse local and systemic effects of the pneumoperitoneum and would allow the use of instrumentation free of the design limitations imposed by maintenance of an airtight system. This novel instrumentation may ultimately replace peritoneal insufflation for abdominal wall lift during laparoscopy. Prospective randomized trials will be necessary to assess whether perioperative pain or morbidity is altered when these traction devices are used.

For diagnostic laparoscopy, both carbon dioxide and nitrous oxide are applicable. Nitrous oxide is not usually used to create the pneumoperitoneum for laparoscopic cholecystectomy; although noninflammable, it supports combustion. Carbon dioxide has the advantage of being noncombustible and of being eliminated rapidly from the body; most carbon dioxide disappears within 4 hours postoperatively. Absorption of carbon dioxide from the blood is ordinarily rapid and safe, without formation of gas emboli when infused into a systemic vein at a rate of less than 1 L/min. However, absorption may lead to hypercarbia in patients with chronic obstructive pulmonary disease. Also, carbon dioxide is converted to carbonic acid on the moist peritoneal surfaces and may therefore cause mild postoperative discomfort. Because of these adverse effects, studies are ongoing to establish whether other gases (such as helium or argon) may be preferable for use during laparoscopic surgery.

The pneumoperitoneum can be established by either a closed or an open technique. In the closed technique, carbon dioxide is insufflated into the peritoneal cavity through a needle. The initial laparoscopic trocar and sheath are placed blindly into the abdominal cavity. Using the open technique, a small incision is made, and a laparoscopic sheath without the sharp trocar or Hasson is inserted under direct vision into the peritoneal cavity. The pneumoperitoneum is established only after ensuring safe peritoneal entry. There are advantages and disadvantages to both techniques, and surgeons performing laparoscopy should learn both and use them on a selective basis.

When using the closed technique, carbon dioxide is insufflated through a Veress needle or one of its disposable counterparts. Before insertion, the pneumoperitoneum needle should be checked to ensure that the spring-loaded stylet is functioning properly and that the lumen is patent to the injection of water. The patient is then placed in a 10° to 15° Trendelenburg position, and a small incision is made into the subcutaneous tissue of the infraumbilical skinfold. The surgeon stands to the left of the patient and grasps the lower abdomen, elevating and stabilizing the abdominal wall. The Veress needle is then inserted at a right angle to the abdominal wall, usually at a 45° angle off the vertical axis toward the pelvis. The surgeon hears one or two "clicks" of the obturator as the needle passes through fascial layers into the peritoneal cavity. Various tests confirm the correct needle position. A syringe containing 5 mL of normal saline solution is attached to the Luer lock connector to aspirate and demonstrate the absence of blood, urine, or stool. If the aspiration is negative, it is repeated after injecting a few milliliters of saline. If blood-stained fluid or frank blood is recovered, the needle should be removed and its position changed. If after needle or trocar insertion there is brisk return of blood and associated hemodynamic compromise, the surgeon should proceed immediately to an open laparotomy. If no fluid is aspirated, an assessment is made of the ease with which saline flows by gravity into the relatively negative pressure of the peritoneal cavity. Manually elevating the lower abdominal wall decreases intra-abdominal pressure and enhances free flow. The fluid flows much slower if the needle is in the preperitoneal space.

In patients who have had previous abdominal surgery, an alternative site for initial puncture may be required. With an upper midline scar, the insertion should be in the right or left lower quadrant, two thirds of the distance from the umbilicus to the iliac crest. A lower midline scar favors an initial puncture in the right or left upper abdomen at the lateral edge of the rectus muscle. If this approach is used, the position of the liver and spleen must be ascertained before needle insertion. Alternatively, a supraumbilical insertion or open infraumbilical insertion may be used.

The tubing from the insufflator is connected to the Veress needle, and insufflation of carbon dioxide is initiated at a flow rate of 1 L/min. The abdomen is percussed to confirm symmetrical tympany associated with the intraperitoneal gas. The abdomen is then inflated with the upper pressure limit of the insufflator set at 15 mm Hg pressure, which usually requires 3.5 to 6 L of carbon dioxide, depending on the size of the abdominal cavity and the weight of the abdominal wall. Obese or muscular patients tend to have heavier abdominal walls and higher abdominal pressures, and sometimes the pressure limit needs to be raised to allow for an adequate pneumoperitoneum.

During insufflation, the patient must be monitored closely for signs of gas embolism (e.g., hypotension, "millwheel" heart murmur), vagal reaction (e.g., hypotension or bradycardia), ventricular arrhythmias, and hypercarbia with acidosis. Most of these complications require immediate treatment by allowing the carbon dioxide to escape and then gradually reestablishing the pneumoperitoneum after the patient's condition has stabilized. Gas embolism results in an "air-lock" right ventricular outflow obstruction with a dramatic decrease in end-tidal carbon dioxide. When suspected, this entity should be treated by placing the patient in Trendelenburg position with the left side down and inserting a central venous catheter to aspirate the carbon dioxide. When the intra-abdominal pressure exceeds 20 mm Hg, central venous pressure and blood pressure decline because of decreased venous return and diminished cardiac output. Adequate muscle relaxation helps minimize the increase in intra-abdominal pressure.

After the pneumoperitoneum has been established, the Veress needle is removed. The initial large (10–11 mm) trocar and sheath are placed in the infraumbilical incision. This is inserted with a gentle "drilling" motion for controlled entry into the peritoneal cavity. The sheath is inserted at the same angle as that of the Veress needle while the lower abdominal wall is stabilized manually. With practice, it is generally apparent when the resistance of the fascia and peritoneum is overcome and the sheath enters the abdominal cavity. With a nondisposable trocar, the hissing noise of escaping carbon dioxide indicates that the trocar tip is correctly positioned in the pneumoperitoneal space. With a disposable sheath, the safety shield can be heard springing into place over the trocar tip. Cannulas may be secured in place with screw threads, internal balloons, or suture. The trocar is then removed, and the laparoscope is inserted.

Creation of the pneumoperitoneum by the open technique is performed similarly to open diagnostic peritoneal lavage. A 1.5-cm skin incision (either vertical or horizontal) is made in the infraumbilical skinfold (Fig. 27–2A). Dissection of the subcutaneous tissue should be performed deep to the skin of the umbilicus to reach the fascia quickly, even in obese patients, because this is the thinnest part of the abdominal wall. Kocher clamps are then applied to both sides of the midline of the linea alba, and a small vertical incision is made into the peritoneal cavity. A finger or curved Kelly clamp is placed into the incision to ensure that the free peritoneal cavity has been entered and to sweep away any adhesions.

If Hasson trocars (Weck & Co., Research Triangle Park, NC) are available, two heavy absorbable sutures are placed on both sides of the fascial incision and are tied to the "wings" of the olive-tipped trocar after it is inserted into the peritoneal cavity under direct vision (see Fig. 27–2B). Alternatively, standard laparoscopic sheaths can be used after placing two concentric purse-string stitches of heavy monofilament suture around the fascial incision (see Fig. 27–2C and D). The laparoscopic sleeve without its sharp trocar is then inserted into the peritoneal cavity, and the purse-string sutures are tightened down by using a section of red rubber catheter similar to a vascular tourniquet. At the conclusion of the case, after removing the sheath, the outer purse-string suture is removed and the inner one is tied down. Open insertion of the initial port takes a few minutes longer than its closed counterpart. However, extraction of the gallbladder at the conclusion of the operation is easier. At my institution, open insertion is performed on a routine basis. This technique is particularly helpful in patients with previous periumbilical incisions, patients in whom insertion of the Veress needle is not performed satisfactorily, and in those with large (>2.5 cm) gallstones or acute cholecystitis.

TECHNIQUE OF LAPAROSCOPIC CHOLECYSTECTOMY

A 10.5-mm laparoscope is inserted into the abdomen. The retroperitoneum immediately posterior to the umbilicus and the pelvis are first viewed to ensure that there is no injury as a result of insertion of the trocar or sheath.

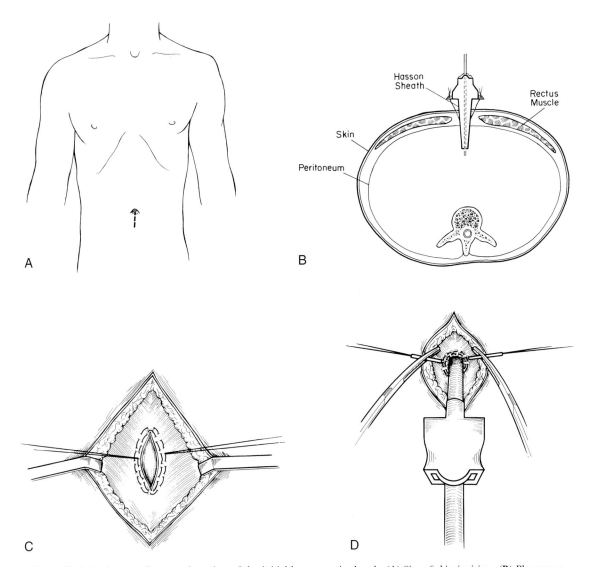

Figure 27-2. Techniques for open insertion of the initial laparoscopic sheath. **(A)** Site of skin incision. **(B)** Placement of Hasson sheath through the abdominal wall, which is secured in place with sutures between the fascia and the wings of the sheath. **(C and D)** An alternative technique using a standard laparoscopic sheath and two concentric purse-string sutures placed in the abdominal fascia. (From Soper NJ. Laparoscopic cholecystectomy. Curr Prob Surg 28:585–655, 1991.)

The pelvic viscera are examined for other pathologic abnormalities before the upper abdomen is evaluated. The anterior surface of the intestines, omentum, and stomach are examined for abnormalities. The patient is then placed in a reverse Trendelenburg position of 30° to 40° and the table is rotated to the patient's left by 15° to 20°. Repositioning the patient intraoperatively is facilitated with a motorized surgical table. This maneuver generally allows the colon and duodenum to fall away from the liver edge. The falciform ligament and both lobes of the liver are closely examined for disease. The inferior margin of the liver is then visualized to determine the location of the gallbladder; usually, the gallbladder can be seen protruding beyond the edge of the liver, but sometimes the gallbladder is not visible without carefully elevating the liver or taking down adhesions.

The two small accessory subcostal ports in the right upper quadrant are then placed under direct vision. The first trocar is placed in the anterior to middle axillary line between the twelfth rib and the iliac crest. This sheath should be placed inferior (caudad) to the gallbladder fundus and liver edge. A second 5-mm port is then inserted under direct vision approximately midway between the axillary sheath and the xiphoid process. It should be possible to avoid major abdominal wall blood vessels during trocar insertion by exercising a combination of transillumination of the abdominal wall and direct examination of the parietal peritoneum. Grasping forceps are then placed through these two sheaths, and the gallbladder is secured. The assistant (standing on the right side of the table) manipulates the lateral grasping forceps, which are used to elevate the liver edge to expose the fundus of the gallbladder. The surgeon (standing to the left of the patient) uses a dissecting forceps to raise a serosal "fold" of the most dependent portion of the fundus. The assistant's heavy grasping forceps are then locked onto this fold using either a spring or ratchet device. Using this axillary grasping forceps, the fundus of the gallbladder is then pushed in a lateral and cephalad direction so that the entire right lobe of the liver rolls cephalad. The successful performance of this maneuver facilitates exposure of the porta hepatis and gallbladder neck.

In patients with few adhesions to the gallbladder, pushing the fundus cephalad exposes the entire gallbladder, cystic duct, and porta hepatis. Most patients, however, have adhesions between the gallbladder and the omentum, hepatic flexure, or duodenum. These adhesions are generally avascular and may be lysed bluntly by grasping them with a dissecting forceps at their site of attachment to the gallbladder wall and gently "stripping" them down toward the infundibulum. Vascular adhesions may be divided with a hook cautery. After exposing the infundibulum, blunt grasping forceps are placed through the midclavicular trocar for traction on the neck of the gallbladder. The operative field is thereby established, and the final working port is then inserted.

The last 10- to 11-mm trocar is placed through a transverse skin incision in the midline of the epigastrium. In general, this is placed 5 cm below the xiphoid process, but the position depends on the location of the

gallbladder as well as on the size of the medial segment of the left liver lobe. When the surgeon is uncertain about the appropriate position for this trocar, a Veress needle may first be placed at the proposed site to ascertain whether its location and angle of insertion are optimal. The trocar is then inserted with a drilling motion; the surgeon angles its tip just to the right of the falciform ligament while aiming toward the gallbladder.

The basic positions for placement of the various ports are shown in Figure 27–3. The accessory sheaths should be separated as far as possible so that the external portions of the instruments do not cross or interfere with one another. The orientation of the laparoscope is generally parallel to that of the cystic duct when the fundus is elevated, whereas the instruments placed through the axillary and epigastric sheaths enter the abdomen at right angles to this plane. Finally, the midclavicular sheath is anterior to the gallbladder, thereby making the instruments passing through it perpendicular to the cystic duct. Thus, all of the accessory sheaths are placed at right angles to the axis of the cystic duct and the surgeon's vision is directed parallel to its axis. French surgeons prefer to elevate the liver lobe with

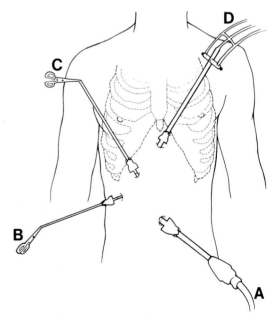

Figure 27–3. Positions for insertion of the initial (**A**) and accessory (**B** through **D**) sheaths for biliary surgery. (From Soper NJ. Laparoscopic cholecystectomy. Curr Prob Surg 28:585–655, 1991.)

a rod placed in a medial right subcostal position and to operate through a left paramedian port.

Having established the positions of all sheaths, the first assistant places the fundus and infundibulum of the gallbladder under tension away from the common bile duct in a superior and lateral direction. Then either a "one-handed" or "two-handed" dissection technique may be used, depending on whether the surgeon or the assistant manipulates the gallbladder infundibulum. With the fundus and neck of the gallbladder under tension, fine-tipped dissecting forceps are used to tease away the overlying fibroareolar structures from the gallbladder infundibulum and Hartmann's pouch. This is done with a blunt stripping action, always starting on the gallbladder and pulling the tissue toward the porta hepatis.

During this initial dissection around the gallbladder neck, the peritoneum is lysed with the blunt dissector similar to the technique by which the peritoneum is incised and pushed bluntly with a Kittner dissector during a traditional open cholecystectomy. With the laparoscopic dissection performed under two-dimensional optics, it is vital to identify clearly the structures contained within two triangles: Calot's triangle and its reverse side. Calot's triangle is the ventral aspect of the area bounded by the cystic duct, hepatic duct, and liver edge. The reverse side of Calot's triangle

is the dorsal aspect of this space. Calot's triangle is placed on tension and maximally exposed by retracting the gallbladder infundibulum inferiorly and laterally while pushing the fundus superiorly and medially (Fig. 27–4A). A lymph node usually overlies the cystic artery, and, occasionally, a brief application of electrical current is required to obtain hemostasis as the lymph node is swept away. The assistant then places the infundibulum of the gallbladder on stretch in a superior and medial direction while pushing the fundus superiorly and laterally, thereby exposing the reverse of Calot's triangle, an area defined by the cystic duct, the inferior lateral border of the gallbladder, and the right lobe of the liver (see Fig. 27–4B).

Further blunt dissection is used to identify precisely the junction between the infundibulum and the origin of the cystic duct. Identification of this junction is the critical maneuver in the operation; no structure should be sharply divided until the cystic duct is clearly identified. The strands of peritoneal, lymphatic, neural, and vascular tissue are stripped away from the cystic duct to gain as much length as possible. Curved dissecting forceps are helpful in creating a "window" around the posterior aspect of the cystic duct to skeletonize the duct (see Fig. 27–4). Alternatively, the tip of a hook-shaped cautery probe can be used to encircle and expose the duct. The cystic artery may be separated from the sur-

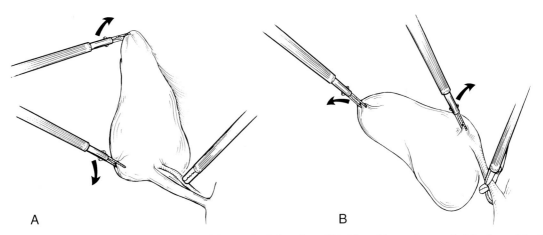

Figure 27–4. (A) Calot's triangle is exposed by manipulating the gallbladder with traction applied by the assistant's grasping forceps. The surgeon's curved instrument is encircling the cystic artery; the cystic duct is anterior. Arrows indicate vector of forceps movement. (B) The reverse (dorsal aspect) of Calot's triangle is displayed. Arrows indicate vector of forceps movement. (From Soper NJ. Laparoscopic cholecystectomy. Curr Prob Surg 28:585–655, 1991.)

rounding tissue by similar blunt dissection either at this time or later, depending on its anatomic location. In the usual position, the cystic duct is dissected and divided first, because it is the structure presenting most anteriorly in the field. If the cystic artery crosses anterior to the duct, the artery may require dissection and division before the cystic duct can be approached. An additional maneuver, which is often helpful during dissection of the duct, is to use the blunt concave blade of the spatula-tipped cautery. Enacting gentle irrigation through its central lumen while pushing away the periductal structures aids precise visualization.

After initial dissection of the cystic duct, a cholangiogram or intracorporeal ultrasound may be performed. At my institution, laparoscopic ultrasound is routinely performed to teach surgical residents ultrasound interpretation and as part of an ongoing investigational study. Besides accurately locating stones in the gallbladder and common bile duct, ultrasound delineates anatomic structures and pathologic disease. Cholangiography may also be performed selectively or routinely. Before a catheter is inserted in the cystic duct, a dissecting forceps is used to squeeze the cystic duct gently in the direction of the gallbladder, thereby "milking" cystic duct stones back into the gallbladder. A clip applier placed through the epigastric sheath is used to apply a single clip at the junction of the cystic duct with the gallbladder. An incision is made in the anterolateral wall of the cystic duct, and a 4- or 5-French catheter is inserted into the duct and fixed in place. The cholangiogram should be scrutinized to ascertain the following: (1) the size of the common bile duct, (2) the location of the junction between the cystic duct and common bile duct, (3) the presence of intraluminal filling defects, (4) free flow of contrast media into the duodenum, (5) the anatomy of the proximal biliary tree, and (6) aberrant biliary radicles entering the gallbladder directly.

After the cholangiocatheter is removed, the cystic duct is doubly clipped near its junction with the common bile duct and divided. The posterior jaw of the clip applier must be visualized before each clip is applied to avoid injury to surrounding structures. Great care should

be taken so that the common bile duct is not tented up into the clip. If the cystic duct is particularly large or friable, it may be preferable to replace one of the clips with a performed loop ligature or suture.

Attention is then directed to the cystic artery. The assistant places the infundibulum of the gallbladder on tension, and the surgeon dissects the cystic artery bluntly from the surrounding tissue. The surgeon must ascertain that the structure is the cystic artery and not the right hepatic artery looping up onto the neck of the gallbladder. After an appropriate length of cystic artery has been separated from the surrounding tissue, it is doubly clipped both proximally and distally and divided sharply. Clips should be fastened at right angles to the artery and should clearly include the whole structure to avoid later slippage. Electrocautery should not be used for this division, because the current may be transmitted to the proximal clips, leading to subsequent necrosis and hemorrhage. A common error is to dissect and divide the anterior branch of the cystic artery, mistaking it for the main cystic artery. This may result in hemorrhage from the posterior branch during dissection of the gallbladder fossa.

The ligated stumps of the duct and cystic artery are then examined to ensure that neither bile nor blood has leaked, that the clips are securely placed, and that the clips compress the entire lumen of the structures without impinging on adjacent tissue. To avoid injury to structures in the porta hepatis, no dissection is undertaken medial to the stumps. A suction-irrigation catheter is used to remove any debris or blood that has accumulated during the dissection of the duct and artery. The heavy grasping forceps traversing the midclavicular trocar are repositioned on the proximal end of the gallbladder at Hartmann's pouch. The infundibulum is retracted superiorly and laterally, and is distracted anteriorly away from its hepatic bed. The surgeon uses the dissecting forceps to thin out the tissue that tethers the neck of the gallbladder and to ensure that no other sizable tubular structures are traversing the space. Dissection of the hepatic fossa is then initiated using a thermal source to divide and coagulate small vessels and lymphatics. Occasionally, a larger blood vessel or aberrant small bile duct requires placement of a clip for control.

Once the appropriate plane has been identified, the separation of the gallbladder from its bed is performed with electrocautery (Fig. 27–5). Extensive cauterization often generates smoke, which must be periodically released through a port valve. With the tissue connecting the gallbladder to its fossa placed under tension, the surgeon uses an electrocautery spatula or hook in a gentle sweeping motion with low-power wattage (25 to 30 W) to coagulate and divide this tissue. Using the cautery probe, the surgeon can also perform blunt dissection, pushing the tissue to facilitate exposure of the proper plane. Occasionally, hemorrhage from the liver bed or gallbladder obscures precise identification of anatomic structures. Tears in the gallbladder wall may be clipped or loop ligated to prevent further bile leak. Small liver lacerations frequently stop with direct pressure, further electrocauterization, or application of a topical hemostatic agent. Frequent irrigation through the port of the electrocautery instrument during this dissection clarifies visualization of the plane.

Dissection of the gallbladder fossa continues from the infundibulum to the fundus, with intermittent movement of the midclavicular grasping forceps to a position closer to the

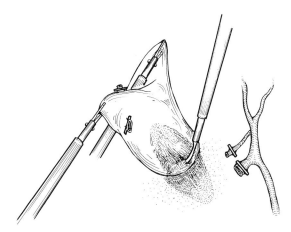

Figure 27–5. Separation of the gallbladder from its bed by dissection with a blunt-tipped thermal-energy probe. The neck of the gallbladder is placed on traction in a superior direction and then twisted to the left and right to place tension on the junction between the gallbladder and hepatic fossa. (From Soper NJ. Laparoscopic cholecystectomy. Curr Prob Surg 28:585–655, 1991.)

plane of dissection to allow maximal countertraction. The dissection proceeds until the gallbladder is attached by only a thin bridge of tissue. At this point, before losing visualization of the operative field afforded by cephalad traction applied to the gallbladder, the hepatic fossa and porta hepatis are once again inspected for hemostasis and bile leakage. The clips are reinspected to ensure that they did not inadvertently dislodge during dissection of the gallbladder fossa. Small bleeding points are coagulated with the electrocautery. The right upper quadrant is then liberally irrigated and aspirated dry.

The final attachments of the gallbladder are lysed, and the liver edge is once again examined for hemostasis. After cholecystectomy is performed, the gallbladder is removed from the abdominal cavity. Although costly and usually unnecessary, placing the gallbladder in a plastic pouch may assist in extraction. We recommend placing the gallbladder in a specimen bag if the gallbladder is purulent, fragmented, perforated with multiple small stones, or suspicious for carcinoma. The gallbladder is usually removed through the umbilicus, as there are no muscle layers and only one fascial plane to traverse. Also, if the fascial opening needs to be enlarged because of large or numerous stones, extending the umbilical incision causes less postoperative pain than enlarging the subxiphoid trocar site.

The laparoscope is removed from the umbilical port and placed into the epigastric sheath. The pelvis and lower abdomen are inspected for evidence of unappreciated injury to the bowel, bladder, or retroperitoneal blood vessels. The umbilical trocar insertion site is examined for hemorrhage. Large "claw" grasping forceps are introduced through the umbilical sheath and guided to the right upper quadrant. The assistant presents the gallbladder neck into the jaws of the grasper so that it is lined up parallel to the axis of the forceps. The assistant then releases the gallbladder, and its infundibulum is pulled up into the umbilical sheath. The forceps, sheath, and gallbladder neck are then retracted as a unit through the umbilical incision. The neck of the gallbladder is thus exposed on the anterior abdominal wall, with the distended fundus remaining within the abdominal cavity (Fig. 27–6).

If the gallbladder is not distended with bile or stones, it can be simply withdrawn with gentle traction. In most cases, a suction catheter is introduced into the gallbladder to aspirate bile and small stones. A stone forceps can be placed into the gallbladder to extract or crush calculi if necessary. Occasionally, the fascial incision must be dilated or extended to deliver larger stones. The laparoscopic sheaths are opened to deflate the abdomen. Otherwise, a partial vacuum is formed, which may carry omentum or small intestine into the cannulation site during removal of the sheath, thereby increasing the risk of herniation and intestinal injury. Placing the patient in a slight Trendelenburg position and providing high-volume manual ventilation may facilitate escape of carbon dioxide trapped under the diaphragm. The sheaths are then removed.

Each incision is infiltrated with 0.5% bupiva-

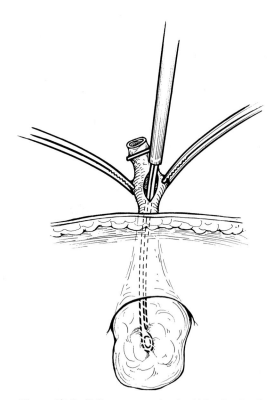

Figure 27–6. Gallstones contained within the fundus may be crushed or removed after delivering the neck of the gallbladder through the umbilical incision. (From Soper NJ. Laparoscopic cholecystectomy. Curr Prob Surg 28:585–655, 1991.)

caine and irrigated with saline solution. The fascia of the umbilical incision is closed with one or two large absorbable sutures. Failure to adequately approximate fascial edges has resulted in incisional hernia. The skin of the subxiphoid and umbilical incisions is closed with subcuticular absorbable sutures, and Steri-strips (3M Health Care, St. Paul, MN) are applied to each incision. Ideally, 30 minutes before both extubation and skin closure, an intramuscular or intravenous nonsteroidal anti-inflammatory such as ketorolac tromethamine is given to alleviate diaphragmatic irritation and postoperative discomfort. A loading dose of 30 to 60 mg followed by 15 to 30 mg every 6 hours is effective.

Anatomic Hazards

The surgeon performing laparoscopic cholecystectomy must be aware of anatomic hazards that may lead to complications. The common bile duct may be "tented up" because of the vigorous superolateral traction placed on the gallbladder, making it susceptible to injury during placement of clips. Likewise, dissection in the region of the lateral wall of the common bile duct may cause bleeding from its nutrient vessels. Application of electrocautery in this area must be avoided, because subsequent devascularization and stricture may occur. Absent or extremely short cystic ducts may lead to two potential problems. The surgeon must recognize this anomaly and not mistake the common bile duct for the cystic duct. Also, it may be extremely difficult to occlude the cystic duct with a clip of insufficient length. The surgeon may need to convert to an open cholecystectomy in these circumstances, or possibly close a small portion of gallbladder infundibulum with a laparoscopic suture.

Aberrant bile ducts may also be present. If they are not recognized and ligated, direct communications between the biliary system and the gallbladder bed may lead to postoperative bile collections. Aberrant origin of the right hepatic duct is not uncommon and must be ruled out in every case. Anomalous hepatic and cystic arteries may also be present. The most frequent anomaly found at my institution has been a right hepatic artery that loops up onto the infundibulum of the gallbladder. In this situation, the cystic artery must be dissected up onto the gallbladder wall, clipped, and divided to allow the hepatic artery to retract away from the operative field. Finally, patients with a large left hepatic lobe may pose special problems. The epigastric trocar must be placed in an appropriate location so that instruments enter the operative field from an angle that does not lacerate the left liver lobe. If needed, an extra 5-mm port can be placed for insertion of a blunt probe to retract the left hepatic lobe during the operation.

Conversion to Open Operation

Surgeons performing laparoscopic cholecystectomy should not hesitate to convert to a traditional open cholecystectomy if anatomic structures are unclear or if complications arise (Table 27–3). It is better to "open one too many (patients) than to open one too few." Some complications requiring laparotomy are massive hemorrhage, bowel perforation, and major injury to the bile duct. An additional indication for open laparotomy is when anatomic structures, because of inflammation, adhesions, or anomalies, cannot be delineated. Fistulas between the biliary system and bowel are rare, but generally require laparotomy for optimal management. Finally, the demonstration of potentially resectable carcinoma necessitates open exploration.

Acute Cholecystitis

Acute cholecystitis may be treated within the first 72 hours of presentation or may be al-

Table 27–3. Reasons to Convert to Open Cholecystectomy

Known or suspected injury to major blood vessel, viscus, or bile duct
Unclear anatomy
Unexpected pathology not amenable to laparoscopic management
Common bile duct stone not removable laparoscopically with little chance of subsequent endoscopic extraction (e.g., Billroth II anastomosis, duodenal diverticulum, previously failed ERCP)

lowed to "cool down" and an elective laparoscopic cholecystectomy performed 6 to 8 weeks after the acute attack. Intervention during the early phase reveals an inflamed, thick-walled, tensely distended organ. To gain purchase for the grasping forceps, it may be necessary to decompress the gallbladder by aspirating it with a large-gauge needle. As long as the inflammation is limited to the gallbladder, laparoscopic cholecystectomy is usually technically feasible. However, if inflammation extends to the porta hepatis, great care must be taken in proceeding with the operation. The normally thin, minimally adherent tissue that invests the cystic duct and artery is markedly thickened and edematous and may not readily separate from these structures with the usual blunt dissection techniques. The duct wall also may be edematous, thus making its external diameter similar to that of the gallbladder neck and common bile duct. If anatomic structures are unclear, a cholangiogram must be performed before clipping or dividing tissue. When acute inflammation has been present for several days or weeks before operation, the pericholecystic tissue planes may be obliterated by thick, "woody" tissue that is impossible to dissect bluntly. The surgeon may therefore need to convert to open cholecystectomy if laparoscopic surgery is initiated during this subacute phase.

The ability to perform laparoscopic cholecystectomy should not influence the management of patients with acute cholecystitis. Antibiotics and bowel rest are initiated on patient admission to the hospital, and operation is undertaken within 24 to 48 hours. There is no harm in inserting the laparoscope and assessing the right upper quadrant. The subcostal working ports are placed, and the initial dissection performed. If the anatomy is obliterated, a laparotomy is performed; if laparoscopic dissection is possible, the operation is completed. The decision to convert to an open operation is a matter of judgment, based on existing anatomic structures and surgeon experience. Several authors have reported performing laparoscopic cholecystectomy in the face of acute inflammation. Sometimes, the edema of the tissue planes may actually aid in the dissection of the gallbladder from its fossa. Despite a greater incidence of conversion to open surgery, the procedure may be completed safely in most patients.

POSTOPERATIVE CARE

Patients may be observed in the hospital or discharged later the same day following laparoscopic cholecystectomy. It is reasonable to perform this operation on an outpatient basis for responsible individuals who live near the hospital with another person and for those without evidence of acute cholecystitis, urinary retention, or persistent nausea. Orders are written for antiemetics and analgesics as needed. The patient is allowed clear liquids in the immediate postoperative period and the diet is advanced as tolerated. Nausea and shoulder pain due to diaphragmatic irritation may occur in the early postoperative period. No activity restrictions are placed on the patient, because functional status depends entirely on the degree of abdominal tenderness, which usually subsides by the second or third postoperative day. The patient may return to work as soon as the abdominal discomfort is tolerable, but is encouraged to do so within 1 week. At my institution, we routinely evaluate the patients in the office at 1 month after the operation, or sooner if they have cause for concern.

RESULTS OF LAPAROSCOPIC CHOLECYSTECTOMY

Author's Personal Series

Since November 1989, more than 2250 laparoscopic cholecystectomies have been performed at Washington University's affiliated hospitals. In my series of 1000 laparoscopic cholecystectomies, there has been a conversion rate of 2.6% and one perioperative death (0.1%). Cumulatively, major morbidity has occurred in 0.69% of patients. The postoperative course in most patients has been uneventful, with 95% of patients being discharged from the hospital within 24 hours of surgery and only 10% requiring parenteral narcotics after leaving the recovery room. Similarly, the duration of disability is minimal; the average post-

operative interval to return to full activity is 9 days. These results are superior to those of traditional open cholecystectomy, after which hospitalization for 3 to 5 days and return to work 1 month after surgery are standard.

Other Reported Series

Data from my series reflect those of most series of laparoscopic cholecystectomies. Mortality is rare after this procedure, usually being attributed to unrelated events. However, death due to bile duct or intestinal injury has been reported. The rate of conversion from laparoscopy to an open operation ranges from 1.8% to 8.5% and is generally greater early in the surgeon's experience with the procedure. Major complications, such as bile duct injury, are relatively rare in these series of cases performed by surgeons who have been performing laparoscopic cholecystectomy since its description. However, if bile duct injury occurs, a coordinated effort by radiologists, endoscopists, and surgeons is necessary to optimize management.

SUMMARY

Laparoscopic management of gallstones has rapidly become the new gold standard therapy in the United States and throughout the world. Most cases of symptomatic gallstones can be treated laparoscopically. Occasionally, anatomic or physiologic considerations preclude the laparoscopic approach, and conversion from an open operation reflects sound surgical judgment and should not be considered a complication. Many patients can undergo laparoscopic cholecystectomy in an ambulatory setting.

Selected Readings

1. Bass EB, Pitt HA, Lillemoe KD. Cost-effectiveness of laparoscopic cholecystectomy versus open cholecystectomy. Am J Surg 1993;165:466–471.
2. Gracie WA, Ransohoff DF. The natural history of silent gallstones: The innocent gallstone is not a myth. N Engl J Med 1982;307:798–800.

3. McMahon AJ, Russell IT, Baxter JN, et al. Laparoscopic versus minilaparotomy cholecystectomy: A randomized trial. Lancet 1994;343:135–138.

4. Rattner DW, Ferguson C, Warshaw AL. Factors associated with successful laparoscopic cholecystectomy for acute cholecystitis. Ann Surg 1993;217:233–236.

5. Soper NJ, Barteau JA, Clayman RV, et al. Laparoscopic vs. standard open cholecystectomy: Comparison of early results. Surg Gynecol Obstet 1992;174:114–118.

6. Soper NJ, Stockmann PT, Dunnegan DL, et al. Laparoscopic cholecystectomy: The new "gold standard"? Arch Surg 1992;127:917–921.

7. Strasberg SM, Hertl M, Soper NJ. An analysis of the problem of biliary injury during laparoscopic cholecystectomy. J Am Coll Surg 1995;180:101–125.

8. The Southern Surgeons Club. A prospective analysis of 1518 laparoscopic cholecystectomies. N Engl J Med 1991;324:1073–1078.

9. Unger SW, Scott JS, Edelman DS. Laparoscopic approach to gallstones in the morbidly obese patient. Surg Endosc 1991;5:116–117.

10. Unger SW, Edelman DS, Scott JS, et al. Laparoscopic treatment of acute cholecystitis. Surg Laparosc Endosc 1991;1:14–16.

Chapter 28

Laparoscopy for Acute Abdominal Pain and the Acute Abdomen

Gene D. Branum • Aaron S. Fink

Whereas laparoscopy is preferred for the treatment of symptomatic cholelithiasis and is increasingly used for the treatment of gastroesophageal reflux disease, inguinal hernia, and colorectal disorders, the role of laparoscopy in urgent and emergent abdominal conditions remains undefined. Of urgent procedures studied, laparoscopic appendectomy is the most feasible and most widely applied use. Laparoscopic evaluation of the acute abdomen and the patient with blunt or penetrating abdominal trauma has yet to be fully evaluated. This chapter discuss these topics, emphasizing laparoscopic intervention in the ambulatory setting.

The diagnostic accuracy in patients with acute abdominal pain has been closely scrutinized in the past two decades. Numerous studies have shown that the clinical diagnosis of abdominal pain is no more than 75% accurate. This figure is significantly worse when lower abdominal pain is evaluated in women in their childbearing years. As general surgeons have gained more facility with the use of laparoscopy, interest in extending the use of this technique to the evaluation and treatment of acute abdominal pain has increased.

A recent study of nearly 1200 patients admitted to the hospital with acute abdominal pain revealed an in-hospital mortality rate of 4%. This figure increased dramatically to 23% in patients with perforated peptic ulcers and to 71% in patients with leaking abdominal aneurysms. Similarly, high mortality figures of 15% to 20% are reported for ruptured appendicitis in children and elderly patients, prompting surgeons to accept a 15% to 25% "negative" appendicitis rate in explorations for this condition. Through the use of video endoscopic techniques, this negative exploration rate can be dramatically lessened without increased morbidity. Timely laparoscopic diagnosis and treatment of pelvic disease (particularly appendicitis and pelvic inflammatory disease) routinely lead to patient discharge within 24 to 48 hours.

APPENDECTOMY

Although the diagnosis of appendicitis in the young male with fever, anorexia, right lower quadrant pain, and leukocytosis poses little diagnostic dilemma, clinical evaluation of many patients with right lower quadrant pain can be challenging. This is especially true of women in their childbearing years and of elderly patients. At exploration, pelvic disease may be overlooked because of the inability to adequately explore the lower abdomen or pelvis through a McBurney incision.

Numerous diagnoses are possible when right lower quadrant pain is the presenting sign or symptom. Cox and coworkers reported a diagnosis other than acute appendicitis in 35% of 107 women who underwent diagnostic laparoscopy for right lower quadrant pain.

Table 28–1. Diagnoses Found in Three Recent Series of Laparoscopy for Suspected Appendicitis

	Number	Percent
Acute appendicitis (with or without rupture)	175	55
Tubo-ovarian disease	80	25
Adenitis, enteritis, unknown	32	10
Miscellaneous	24	7.5
Small bowel disease (Crohn's, Meckel's)	7	2.5
TOTAL	318	100

Twenty-seven of these women had tubo-ovarian conditions. Taylor and colleagues reported a 37% alternative diagnosis rate in women with right lower quadrant pain. Connor and associates reported a 13% incidence of tubo-ovarian disease in a series of 87 patients. These data clearly demonstrate the relatively high incidence of misdiagnosis of appendicitis in young women. Moreover, tubo-ovarian disease can be difficult to diagnose through the McBurney incision, especially in an obese patient. Laparoscopic exploration allows visualization of the pelvic organs bilaterally. In addition, other common diagnoses such as Meckel's diverticulum and inflammatory bowel disease may be made laparoscopically.

The first laparoscopic appendectomy was performed in 1982 by Semm. However, despite the explosion of laparoscopic technology and its application to numerous intra-abdominal problems, general surgeons have been reluctant to use diagnostic laparoscopy for acute lower abdominal pain. Diagnostic laparoscopy for acute lower abdominal pain can decrease the incidence of negative laparotomy by 15% to 20% and is particularly valuable in evaluating female patients with right lower quadrant pain.

Findings in patients explored laparoscopically for presumed appendicitis are highly variable. The combined results of three recent series revealed that a preoperative diagnosis of appendicitis was confirmed in only 55% of patients. Furthermore, despite the excellent visualization and the ability to manipulate the abdominal viscera, 10% had no source of abdominal pain identified (Table 28–1).

Several advantages have been proposed for laparoscopic versus open exploration when appendicitis is suspected (Table 28–2). The three most commonly cited advantages are a lower incidence of wound infection, more accurate diagnosis of other pelvic conditions, and more rapid recovery (Table 28–3).

Rates of all complications after laparoscopic appendectomy are low. Numerous studies have revealed that abdominal wound infection rate is lessened by laparoscopic appendectomy. Ortega and colleagues observed a wound infection rate of 2.3% in laparoscopic procedures versus 13% in open appendectomy in a prospective randomized trial. Similarly, McAnena and coworkers reported a wound infection rate of 4% for laparoscopic versus 11% for open procedures. Pier and Gotez reported 2% wound infection rate in 625 cases. Clearly, wound infection rate is lower following laparoscopic versus open appendectomy, which averages approximately 8.5%. The lower rate is possibly attributable to the removal of the infected appendix through an abdominal trocar or retrieval bag instead of through the abdominal wound. Even though wound infection may be considered a relatively minor complication by the surgeon, it can lead to an extended period of disability for the patient.

Although shortened hospital stay and more rapid return to normal activity are claimed for laparoscopic appendectomy, these potential advantages remain controversial. Schirmer and colleagues reported no statistical difference in length of postoperative stay (3.5 ± 0.5 vs. 5.9 ± 1.6 days) in laparoscopic versus open procedures. The prospective randomized study

Table 28–2. Advantages of Laparoscopic Appendectomy

Diagnosis and treatment of conditions other than appendicitis
Improved visualization in obese patients
Reduced wound infection rate
Shorter average hospitalization
Decreased postoperative pain (probable)
Earlier return to normal activity

Table 28–3. Comparisons of Laparoscopic and Open Appendectomy in Prospective Randomized Trials

Study	Operative Time (Mean)		Hospital Stay (Days)		Return to Normal Activity		Wound Infection (%)		All Complications (%)	
	Lap	Open	Lap	Open	Lap	Open	Lap	Open	Lap	Open
Attwood (1992)	61	51	2.5	3.8*	21	38	0	3*	0	13*
Frazee (1994)	87	65*	2	2.8	14	25*	—	—	8	5
Kum (1993)	43	40	3.2	4.2	17	30	0	9*	—	—
Ortega (1995)	68	58*	2.1	2.8*	9	14*	2.3	13*	—	—
Tate (1993)	70	47*	3.5	3.6	No difference		10	14	21	25

*$P < 0.05$
Lap = laparoscopy; Open = open procedure.

of Ortega and colleagues reported a significantly shorter postoperative stay in laparoscopic versus open procedure patients. Williams and coworkers reported a mean postoperative stay of 40 hours with open appendectomy versus 27 hours for laparo scopic patients. Probably the greatest savings result from the prevention of unnecessary laparotomies, which would otherwise require extended hospitalization and recovery time.

Whether laparoscopic appendectomy allowed earlier return to normal activity was addressed in four prospective randomized studies. Ortega and colleagues reported a mean return to full activity at 9 days after laparoscopic procedures versus 14 days after laparoscopic procedures. Frazee and associates reported return to full activity at 14 days for laparoscopic appendectomy versus 25 for open appendectomy. Tate and associates reported "no difference" in return to normal activity, whereas Atwood reported a decrease of 17 days for laparoscopic versus open appendectomy. Similar differences have been observed for postoperative analgesic use.

In the Ortega study, patients were blinded to the operative technique; level of pain and the administration of medication were scored on an analog scale. In this study, both groups required analgesia for the same length of time, but the laparoscopic group had significantly less severe pain at 24 and 48 hours. These results were confirmed by the Frazee study, although the Tate and Kum studies found no difference in pain.

OPERATIVE TECHNIQUE

Patients should be placed on the operating table in the supine position. In most cases,

three trocars are optimal for dissection and removal of the inflamed appendix (Fig. 28–1). Monitors should be placed near the patient's feet at the center and right of the operating table. The trocars should be positioned to allow for a two-handed dissection technique. Standard trocar insertion techniques are used with visual examination to ensure absence of trocar injury. The pelvis should be visualized

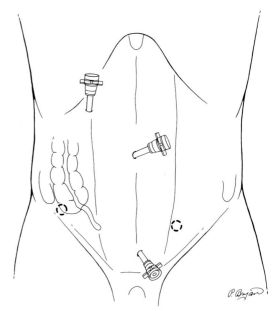

Figure 28–1. Three 11- to 12-mm trocar sites are usually sufficient for laparoscopic appendectomy. The umbilical trocar site is typically used for the camera, with the right upper quadrant and superpubic or left lower quadrant sites used for dissection and stapling. (Optional sites are denoted as hatched circles.) Alternatively, the right upper quadrant site may be used for the camera, with the surgeon operating from the two other sites. The optional site over the cecum is rarely necessary but can allow for blunt dissection in the right paracolic gutter or division of the lateral colonic peritoneum.

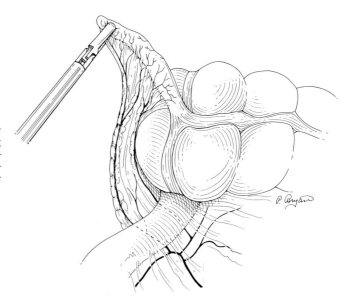

Figure 28–2. Appendectomy is begun by grasping the appendiceal tip and identifying the base of the appendix at the cecum. Mobilization of the appendiceal tip may require lateral elevation of the colonic peritoneum if the appendix is retrocecal.

with the patient in the Trendelenburg position to rule out other causes of abdominal pain.

If the appendix is to be removed, the patient should be placed in a moderate Trendelenburg position with the right side slightly elevated. The first step is to identify the appendix and its cecal base (Fig. 28–2). This is best accomplished by grasping the appendix with an atraumatic Babcock or grasping forceps and retracting medially. In cases of severe inflammation or retrocecal appendix, the entire cecum and part of the right colon should be mobilized. This is accomplished by dividing the lateral peritoneal reflection using scissors or hook electrocautery, while elevating the cecum medially. With the surgeon using a two-handed technique, the appendix is elevated and a loop of suture material is placed around its tip, allowing for repeated grasping and retraction without the risk of tearing or perforation (Fig. 28–3). A window in the mesoappendix can usually be made using an atraumatic dissecting forceps (Fig. 28–4). In such cases, the appendix may then be removed with two

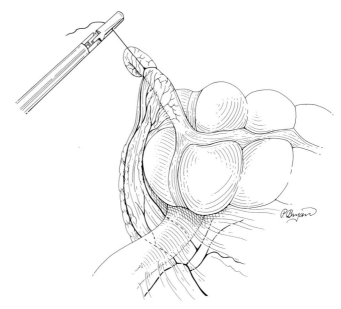

Figure 28–3. A loop of suture material may be passed over the tip of an appendix that is too inflamed or friable to be grasped with a clamp. The suture then may be used to manipulate the appendix, giving better visualization medially, laterally, and inferiorly. The suture is also useful for guiding the transected appendix into a bag for removal.

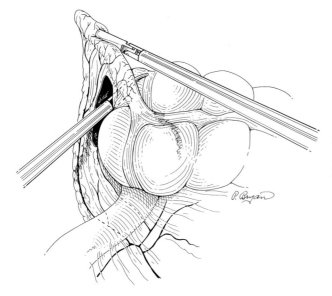

Figure 28–4. A combination of blunt, cautery, and sharp dissection is used to form a window through the mesoappendix. This window is enlarged using careful blunt or cautery dissection under direct visualization.

sequential firings of a laparoscopic stapling device (Fig. 28–5). Some surgeons prefer to bluntly dissect the mesoappendix, ligating the appendiceal artery and its branches with clips. When there is severe inflammation at the appendiceal base, the laparoscopic stapling device can be used to divide the base of the appendix by elevating a small portion of the cecum into the jaws of the stapling device (Fig. 28–6). The tips of the stapler must always be clearly visualized before firing to ensure that no other structure has been inadvertently trapped.

Surgeons performing laparoscopic appendectomies should be experienced with endoscopic suturing techniques, because the endoscopic staple line on the mesoappendix occasionally bleeds and requires oversewing. Moreover, if an endoscopic stapling device is not available, intracorporeal or extracorporeal suturing techniques allow the appendectomy to be performed in the same manner as an open procedure. Ortega and colleagues observed that there were higher rates of intra-abdominal abscess and ileus when the appendix was divided between loops than when the

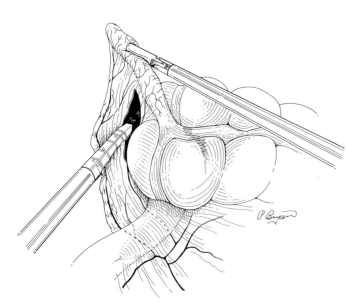

Figure 28–5. Once an adequate window has been prepared, a stapling device is fired across the appendiceal mesentery. This staple line is typically hemostatic, but suture ligation of bleeding points may be necessary. Care must be taken to visualize both tips of the stapling device before firing; otherwise, structures such as the ureter, fallopian tube, or a loop of intestine may be inadvertently stapled.

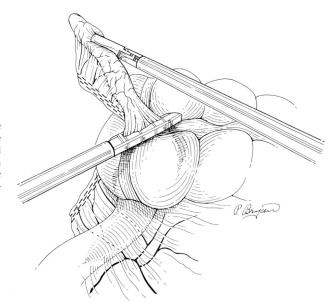

Figure 28–6. The stapler is fired across the base of the appendix. Even if the base of the appendix is friable, the stapling device may still be used by elevating a cuff of normal cecum into the jaws of the stapler. Once again, care must be taken to visualize both tips of the stapling device before firing.

appendix was divided with the stapler. This is probably due to the larger appendiceal stump left exposed to the abdominal cavity after the loop division.

In laparoscopic appendectomy, the inflamed appendix should never come into direct contact with abdominal wall. Many severely inflamed appendices can be removed through a 12-mm trocar. The appendix should be retracted completely within the trocar and a new sheath placed after the extraction. A second method involves placing the appendix in one of several bag devices introduced through one of the trocars (Fig. 28–7). If the appendix has been looped with a suture, the tail of the suture may be introduced into the bag, pulling the appendix along with it. The bag may then be removed through the trocar site. The trocar incision may need to be stretched slightly to allow for the removal of the bag. Irrigation of the right lower quadrant and pelvis may then be accomplished through the remaining trocar site. Examination for bleeding should be performed. The placement of drains should be based on the same principles as in open appendectomy. Finally, the fascia at any trocar site that is 10 mm or greater in size should be closed.

THE ACUTE ABDOMEN

In adults, acute generalized or upper abdominal pain is usually caused by visceral inflammation such as cholecystitis or pancreatitis, perforation of hollow viscera, or mesenteric ischemia. For most of these conditions, radiographic or ultrasonographic evaluation usually yields a correct diagnosis. As many as 30% of gastroduodenal perforations may occur without the typical finding of free air un-

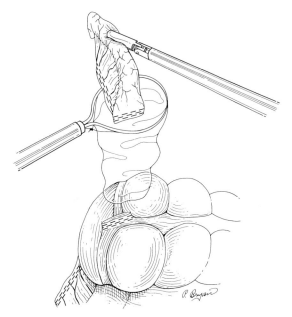

Figure 28–7. The appendix may then be placed into one of numerous bag devices that allow for removal of the inflamed appendix through a trocar without exposing the trocar site to the infected organ. Once the appendix is removed, the area of dissection can be irrigated and both staple lines inspected for hemostasis.

der the diaphragm on an upright chest or abdominal roentgenogram. When a diagnosis cannot be confirmed radiographically, laparoscopy is an excellent technique for confirming or discovering the source of acute abdominal pain.

Patients with gastric or duodenal perforation have been treated successfully using laparoscopic techniques. Acute perforations may be closed or patched, if appropriate. Definitive ulcer procedures including highly selective or truncal vagotomy with pyloroplasty or a gastroenterostomy have been performed laparoscopically. These procedures necessitate hospitalization beyond that of the "ambulatory" setting.

Most surgeons consider laparoscopic procedures to be contraindicated in patients with colonic perforation, diverticulitis or its complications, or small bowel obstruction. Small bowel obstruction is usually not approached laparoscopically because of the risk of enteric perforation. Patients with a single or limited number of bands causing adhesive intestinal obstruction with a clear transition zone identifiable laparoscopically are uncommon. Recovery and resolution of ileus in such patients typically removes them from the ambulatory population.

ABDOMINAL TRAUMA

Diagnostic evaluation of patients with blunt and penetrating abdominal trauma seeks to determine the need for surgical intervention in a timely fashion. Operative exploration is the obvious treatment of choice for unstable patients or those with obvious signs of internal abdominal injury. However, the stable patient with an equivocal examination or altered mental state may be difficult to evaluate. There is extensive experience and literature describing the evaluation of such patients using physical examination supplemented by ultrasonography, computed tomography (CT) scanning, or peritoneal lavage. Despite these methods, negative or nontherapeutic laparotomies continue to be performed in patients with abdominal trauma. Thus, over the past 5 years there have been numerous investigations of the ability of laparoscopy to decrease negative laparotomy rates in such patients. Investigators have evalu-

ated both emergency department laparoscopy using small scopes under local and intravenous analgesia and operating room laparoscopy using standard 10-mm scopes and general anesthesia.

Laparoscopy has been compared with peritoneal lavage and CT scanning in the evaluation of patients with blunt abdominal trauma. Townsend and colleagues performed laparoscopy in a series of patients with solid organ injury documented by CT scan. Hemoperitoneum was confirmed in 93% of the patients and occult bowel injuries were found in two patients. Spleen or liver injury was upgraded in eight patients and downgraded in one patient. Seven patients underwent laparotomy including two for enteral injury. This study highlights the inaccuracy of CT scanning in the evaluation of enteral trauma.

The use of diagnostic peritoneal lavage (DPL) in blunt trauma has been extensively studied. Henneman and associates documented a 13% unnecessary laparotomy rate in patients who suffered blunt trauma when the operative decision was based on DPL. Other researchers have documented nontherapeutic laparotomy rates as high as 39% when the standard criteria of 100,000 RBC/mm^3 is used. Salvino and coworkers compared emergency department laparoscopy under local anesthesia with medazolam supplementation to DPL in 59 patients who suffered blunt abdominal trauma. Forty-two patients had negative DPL and laparoscopy findings and four had positive findings on DPL. Two of the four patients had insignificant findings on laparoscopy and two had injuries in need of operative repair. The authors concluded that, although feasible, the routine use of laparoscopy had no advantage over DPL in the primary evaluation of blunt abdominal trauma.

Diagnostic laparoscopy in penetrating trauma has been evaluated by several groups. Livingston and colleagues identified peritoneal penetration, or lack thereof, in all patients examined. Significantly, four missed small bowel injuries were found on subsequent laparotomy. However, patients with these injuries had been identified at laparoscopy as needing laparotomy. The authors observed that the main difficulties with laparoscopic exploration were examining the entire small intestine, visualizing the spleen and, in some cases, evacuating hemoperitoneum.

Fabian and colleagues studied 165 patients with penetrating abdominal trauma. No peritoneal penetration was found in 90 patients and they did not undergo laparotomy. There were no missed abdominal injuries in this group. In the patients in whom peritoneal penetration was identified, the subsequent laparotomy was negative or nontherapeutic in 25 of 75 patients. The authors reported only four complications related to the laparoscopy, including a missed splenic injury, pneumopreperitoneum, a tension pneumothorax, and an enterotomy. The authors concluded that diagnostic laparoscopy appeared most applicable to penetrating trauma with a low likelihood of significant injury, and they concluded that the technique was safe but expensive. Finally, they suggested that improved optics and laparoscopes that are smaller in diameter would make laparoscopy under local anesthesia more feasible and practical and that improved instrumentation would allow for more therapeutic applications during laparoscopic exploration.

Ivatury and coworkers studied 100 stable patients with penetrating trauma. Peritoneal penetration was found in 57 patients, 54 of whom underwent laparotomy. Laparotomy confirmed the laparoscopic findings in all 54 patients, although seven bowel injuries had been missed. The authors concluded that laparoscopy was an excellent method for determining peritoneal penetration and for evaluating solid organ injury. The authors agreed with Fabian and others that laparoscopic evaluation of the small bowel and colon was currently suboptimal.

To be performed optimally, emergency laparoscopy for penetrating or blunt abdominal trauma requires an experienced laparoscopist and general anesthesia in the operating room. Moreover, identification of injuries to the retroperitoneum, pancreas, and small intestine is difficult. The technique is useful, however, in the stable patient when findings with CT and DPL are equivocal or if there is a question of peritoneal penetration.

SUMMARY

Laparoscopic evaluation of suspected appendicitis is safe and accurate, and it allows for both diagnosis and treatment. The main advantages of laparoscopic appendectomy are a lower rate of wound infection, shorter hospital stay, and earlier return to normal activity. Laparoscopic evaluation of acute right lower quadrant or pelvic pain is clearly the approach of choice in women in their childbearing years and in obese patients. The procedure is more expensive than open appendectomy. Whether the procedural costs are balanced by savings achieved by shorter hospitalization varies among different locales.

The utility of laparoscopy in the setting of abdominal trauma is less clear. Laparoscopy seems to add little to CT scan combined with DPL in the setting of blunt trauma. Evaluation of small bowel injury remains difficult. Laparoscopy accurately identifies peritoneal penetration in stable patients with penetrating trauma and an equivocal examination. This may be beneficial in lowering the negative laparotomy success rate.

Selected Readings

1. Fabian TC, Croce MA, Stewart RM, et al. A prospective analysis of diagnostic laparoscopy in trauma. Ann Surg 1993;217:557–565.
2. Frazee RC, Roberts JW, Symmonds RE, et al. A prospective randomized trial comparing open versus laparoscopic appendectomy. Ann Surg 1994;219:725–731.
3. Henneman PL, Marx JA, Moore EE, et al. Diagnostic peritoneal lavage: Accuracy in predicting necessary laparotomy following blunt and penetrating trauma. J Trauma 1990;30:1345–1355.
4. Ivatury RR, Simon RJ, Stahl WM. A critical evaluation of laparoscopy in penetrating abdominal trauma. J Trauma 1993;34:822–828.
5. Kum CK, Ngoi SS, Goh PMY, et al. Randomized controlled trial comparing laparoscopic and open appendectomy. Br J Surg 1993;80:1599–1600.
6. Livingston DH, Tortella BJ, Blackwood J, et al. The role of laparoscopy in abdominal trauma. J Trauma 1992;3:471–475.
7. McAnena OJ, Austin O, O'Connor PR, et al. Laparoscopic versus open appendectomy: A prospective evaluation. Br J Surg 1992;79:818–820.
8. Ortega AE, Hunter JG, Peters JH, et al. A prospective randomized comparison of laparoscopic appendectomy with open appendectomy. Am J Surg 1995;169:208–213.
9. Salvino CK, Esposito TJ, Marshall WJ, et al. The role of diagnostic laparoscopy in the management of trauma patients: A preliminary assessment. J Trauma 1993;34:506–515.
10. Schirmer BD, Schmieg RE, Dix J, et al. Laparoscopic versus traditional appendectomy for suspected appendicitis. Am J Surg 1993;165:670–675.

11. Tate JJT, Chung SCS, Dawson J, et al. Conventional versus laparoscopic surgery for acute appendicitis. Br J Surg 1993;80:761–764.
12. Townsend MC, Flancbaum L, Choban PS, et al. Diagnostic laparoscopy as an adjunct to selective conservative management of solid organ injuries after blunt abdominal trauma. J Trauma 1993;35:647–653.

29

Laparoscopy for Chronic Abdominal Pain

Henry L. Laws

Pain stimulates people to seek surgical attention more frequently than any other symptom. One third of Americans suffer with chronic painful conditions. If one considers lost time from work, health care costs, compensation, litigation, and quackery, Bonica estimates the annual costs of chronic pain to exceed $79 billion. Back pain is most common, probably followed by other musculoskeletal complaints, but many people suffer with chronic abdominal pain. Some authorities divide pain into two groups, acute and chronic, the latter being that which lasts more than 6 months. A more useful division would be to further divide chronic pain into two subgroups: pain that is present for weeks and pain that is present for months. This chapter primarily discusses patients who have been experiencing pain for months.

The organism's perception of chronic pain differs from that of acute pain. Visceral chronic pain travels over the small unmyelinated nerve fibers, tends to be less localized, and may be modulated by many factors. Afferent impulses transmitted in the peripheral nerves over A delta and C fibers may be modified, dampened, or augmented in the dorsal horns of the spinal cord by many factors, both from within and external to the organism. These include the individual's general health, comorbid conditions, personal expectations, and social environment, among others. The surgeon must consider all these factors before deciding on the propriety of surgical intervention. The careful surgeon should approach the patient with chronic pain with the attitude that there may be much to offer. In addition to the possibility that many painful conditions can be relieved, the surgeon can assist the patient in understanding the problem, can avoid unnecessary operations, and can guide the patient to the most reasonable and feasible management. Often, this requires the services of an anesthesiologist, psychologist, psychiatrist, physical therapist, social worker, or other professional.

When consulted by a patient with chronic abdominal pain, the surgeon must take a careful history, review the records and laboratory data, and seek appropriate consultation to select those problems for which there may be a surgical solution. Additional testing should be done only after careful deliberation. Operative intervention must be judiciously used to avoid adding another bad operative result to the patient's problem list.

MECHANISMS OF PAIN

Threatened or actual tissue damage stimulates nociceptive activation. Nociceptive stimulation travels via A delta and C nerve fibers. The former rapidly carry the initial signals to the dorsal horn of the cord and then to the brain, affording rapid and fairly precise localization of actual or threatened injury. The unmyelinated C fibers are responsible for afterpain—the dull, uncomfortable sensation that persists after the initial stimulus. Visceral pain is transmitted by C fibers. This pain signal continues from the dorsal horn up the paleospinal tract to the thalamus and then to the cortex, including areas other than the specific sensory cortex (Fig. 29–1). Areas in the periaqueductal region that are under descending cortical control transmit signals down the cord that modulate the afferent messages in the dorsal horn of the cord. Thus, central pain states (e.g., phantom limb pain), psychogenic pain, and behavioral pain (environmentally influenced pain) may affect the incoming signals through this mechanism. For instance, the overly solicitous spouse may reinforce "pain behavior."

Somatic (i.e., cutaneous, muscular, skeletal) pain and visceral pain travel through different pathways. The former ascends via the peripheral nerves, providing rather accurate localization of the source. The latter courses via the autonomic system with less precise localization of the origin. Pain of gastrointestinal origin tends to be perceived in the midline; pain originating from the kidneys, ureters, oviducts, and ovaries tends to be lateralized.

SOMATIZATION OF ILLNESS

An illness consists of both a disease and the individual's experience of it. Somatization often occurs in the absence of detectable disturbances in organ system or cellular function. In primary care, many visits are due to psychosocial stress manifested by somatic complaints. As many as 60% of primary care patients are recurrently seen with somatic symptoms that are an expression of psychosocial distress. Although many of these may be musculoskeletal, many patients experience abdominal complaints.

Approximately 70% of patients with primary or secondary diagnoses of emotional disorders give a somatic complaint as a reason for their visits to physicians. Among the most common complaints are constitutional symptoms, headache, dizziness, *abdominal or* extremity pain, and requests for checkups. Primary care physicians find that these patients constitute approximately 25% of their practices. Somatization is most frequently associated with depression, anxiety reactions, and somatiform disorders, which include somatization disorder, conversion disorder, hypochondriasis, and psychogenic pain. Patients with classic somatization disorder have a history of multiple physical symptoms of several years' duration beginning before the age of 30 years for which they have taken medications, seen physicians, or altered their life pattern. Conversion symptoms are defined as alteration in physical functioning or symptoms suggestive of a physical disorder without a pathophysiologic explanation. Hypochondriasis is an abnormal response to a normal sensation, assuming it is pathologic, or an amplified response to a minor abnormal sensation. Psychogenic pain is severe and prolonged pain that is inconsistent with or out of proportion to objective findings and that interferes with activities of life. The surgeon may attempt to classify patients with inappropriate responses into one of these categories.

Kaplan and colleagues said, "Diagnosing somatization is not a process of ruling out other organic etiologies, rather it is a positive pro-

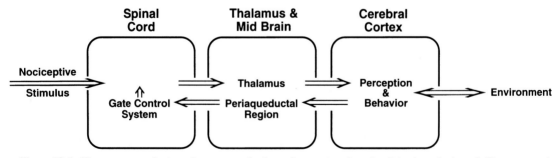

Figure 29–1. The gate control system impacts on the incoming nociceptive stimuli in the spinal cord. The message is then transmitted to the thalamus and thence to the cerebral cortex. Messages are sent down from the cortex with or without interaction with the environment via the periaqueductal region down to the dorsal horn in the spinal cord. Thus, many incoming stimuli may be altered dramatically before their perception at the cortex.

cess achieved by carefully listening to symptoms and discovering their place in the patient's life, and learning of the patient's cultural and personal habits of sensory perception." The physician should first determine whether the patient is suffering from unexplained complaints or is preoccupied with fear or conviction of disease. The part the symptoms play in the patient's life should be evaluated. Interpersonal relations with family, use of medical services, and the extent to which the patient uses illness to cope in the environment should be investigated. Positive criteria useful in the diagnosis of psychogenic symptoms include a hysterical personality; illness beginning in a psychologically meaningful setting; a symbolic meaning to the patient of the illness; a vague, inconsistent, bizarre description of symptoms; symptoms persisting despite allegedly specific medical treatment, much doctoring and little curing; denial of psychological role in the symptoms; associated psychological illness, polysurgery, and pain that is a mechanism to allow the patient to communicate with the doctor about psychological problems. The surgeon must weigh all these factors in making a decision about the propriety of operation for a specific pathologic problem in the abdomen.

If the pain is chronic, patients are usually referred by their primary physician. Ordinarily, there have been repeated evaluations and testings and, often, prior abdominal operations. If the patient is self-referred after visiting other physicians, the surgeon should be cautious to avoid operating when the presumed surgical condition is not (or is only a facet of) the patient's real problem.

PLACEBO EFFECT

The placebo remains a powerful force. More than 1000 articles have been written about placebos, with all recognizing a significant effect. A placebo is effective 30% to 35% of the time. I believe the effect often lasts 15 to 18 months. An operation may serve as a placebo. Such a powerful tool has two important messages for the surgeon. First, mature surgeons should do all within their power to invoke a placebo effect in every patient. If an operation is 70% effective, then 30% of the time it is ineffective. If one third of the poor results can be converted into good results by the placebo effect, then the surgeon should invoke this response in the patients. Second, an unfounded treatment may be effective more than 30% of the time and outcomes should be interpreted with this in mind. The results of a presumed beneficial intervention should be scrutinized most cautiously in the management of chronic pain. "Adhesiolysis" or adhesiotomy for chronic pelvic pain fits this category. Some writers purport great benefit, but many find substantial benefit in only 50% or less of patients.

APPROACH TO THE PATIENT WITH ABDOMINAL PAIN

The surgeon should accept the pain as being real. Great care should be taken to separate real organic pain from "unreal" psychosomatic pain. Often, the patient should be made to realize that the cause of the pain has not been established and that the surgeon does understand the patient is suffering and he or she will earnestly try to use the most effective management, whether it is surgery or something else. What the patient wants is relief from the cause (which is often multifactorial), not necessarily an operation. Surgery seems to be a wonderful solution because it is a one-time event, it officially legitimizes the pain for the patient's work and social environment, and it appears to require only cooperation as opposed to active, continuing effort on the part of the patient. Usually, there is a real source of nociceptive pain that is being aggravated by other factors. A good example is posthernior-rhaphy ilioinguinal neuralgia. Transection of the nerve proximal to the groin does not necessarily ablate the pain. The surgeon well may not be the person to seek out and mollify the impacting problems, which may require a multidisciplinary approach. He or she should avoid compounding the issue by applying unnecessary tests or inappropriate operative intervention.

A careful and thorough history is essential and may require more than one office visit. The examiner should listen carefully to the patient's perception of the cause, the onset, and the relation of the pain to other life events. Patients with a psychogenic illness usually do not consider this possibility as an option, whereas patients with organic illness do. A vague and inconsistent description of the pain suggests a nonorganic cause. Continued symptoms after specific treatment, previous poor results, and polysurgery all tend to imply a psychogenic source for all or part of the pain. Depression or anxiety may be overt or covert. Careful scrutiny for these conditions is often beneficial. Several specific questions must be asked. What is the effect of various bodily functions (e.g., eating, defecating, voiding, menstruation) on the pain? Is there weight loss? Is the pain worse at night or in the day? What is the sleep pattern? Why were previous operations done and what was the outcome? What does the patient expect to achieve by surgery? Lack of weight loss suggests a nonorganic cause; however, depressed patients may lose weight from not eating. Sleep pattern disturbances, especially in patients who awaken more tired than when going to sleep, suggest depression.

In taking the history, assiduous investigation of the pain is important. Continuous pain—day and night—without other associated symptoms is not organic. Organic pain is worse at night. Pain aggravated by twisting, bending, and moving tends to be musculoskeletal in origin. Lancinating, momentary pains

that shoot across the abdomen or down the legs stem from a source that does not require surgery. Catamenial abdominal, pelvic, perineal, or even right chest pain suggests endometriosis. Frequent intermittent pain that is poorly localized to the midline with associated nausea suggests partial small bowel obstruction. Pain that is intermittent and localized to a specific point in the lower abdominal wall, particularly with associated nausea, suggests underlying adhesions. Those patients usually have a history of prior operation. In some persons, an incisional hernia or even a groin hernia that is not detectable on physical examination or computed tomography scan may be readily apparent by laparoscopy and can cause this type of pain (Fig. 29–2). When persistent nausea or a "bloated feeling" without weight loss dominates over pain, the cause is rarely corrected by surgery.

An often vexing situation occurs when the patient has chronic pain and an unassociated intra-abdominal condition such as cholelithiasis. If the surgeon is convinced that the demonstrated condition is not the cause of the pain, usually it is better to resist attacking the defined condition until there is some resolution of the chronic pain, even if this takes a protracted period.

The surgeon's responsibilities for patients thought to have nonorganic conditions include the following:

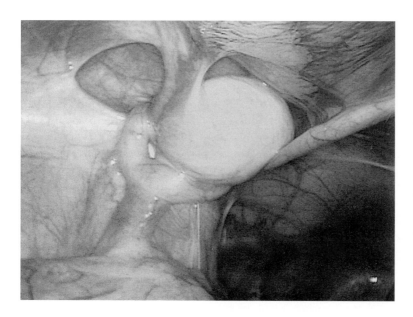

Figure 29–2. An intra-abdominal view of the left groin in a 21-year-old man with recurrent abdominal pain since age 13. The pain seemed to be worse with the need to void. An indirect inguinal hernia can be seen at the internal ring, and an undescended testicle, which is intra-abdominal, is seen lying medial to the inferior epigastric vessels and lateral to the obliterated umbilical ligament.

- Acceptance that the pain is real
- Careful evaluation followed by clear assurance in the presence of the patient's spouse or other family member of the surgeon's opinion
- Resistance to excessive, repetitive testing, especially if it is invasive
- Clear communication to the primary physician of the surgeon's findings and opinions
- Willingness to reevaluate the patient after a period if the primary physician thinks it is in the patient's best interest

Potential reasons for diagnostic or therapeutic laparoscopy for protracted complaints include the following:

- Suspected liver disease for which biopsy may be helpful
- Idiopathic ascites
- Suspicion of neoplasm
- Suspected peritoneal inflammatory process such as tuberculosis
- Partial small bowel obstruction from adhesions or hernia
- Pelvic inflammatory disease or parametrial disease
- Lower abdominal adhesions causing intermittent pain

THERAPY

Diagnostic laparoscopy as a general inspection without a specific diagnosis in mind tends to be futile and unrewarding. The laparoscopic approach to acute surgical problems and concerns are discussed in other chapters (see Chapters 27, 28, and 30). Other diseases causing long-standing pain can and should be managed by operation, specifically laparoscopy. Usually, laparoscopic surgery is indicated for the following:

- Recurrent pain, worse at night, with weight loss
- Sporadic or recurrent pain with associated nausea (not nausea with minor associated pain)
- Pain that is intermittent and localized to a specific area of the abdominal wall or pelvis
- Catamenial pain with associated physical findings suggesting endometriosis

Purely diagnostic laparoscopy and therapeutic laparoscopy for gynecologic–pelvic disease may be successfully and cost-effectively done in an ambulatory surgical unit. If there is a likelihood of a therapeutic endeavor such as adhesion lysis of the small intestine, the procedure is probably best performed in a facility where open laparotomy and in-hospital stay, if necessary, are options. Probably 15% or more of patients undergoing lysis of intestinal adhesions will require a laparotomy. The operator should be prepared to repair the intestine if necessary.

The patient should have a clear understanding of the surgeon's plans, the objectives of the operation, and the possibility that a laparotomy may become necessary. This is particularly important because most patients already have had more than one previous operation.

OPERATION

The surgeon should have at the ready: the usual 0° telescope, a 5-mm telescope, an angled telescope (45° or 30°), and an operating telescope with the necessary long instruments. It is important for the operating room table to be capable of rotating in various directions to aid with exposure.

The colon should be cleansed and a Hibiclens bath should be prescribed the evening before operation. I routinely give prophylactic antibiotics (cephalosporin).

Although local anesthesia is an option for simple diagnostic laparoscopy, general anesthesia is used routinely. The patient should be placed on the table with the arms tucked and should be carefully strapped in place. When pelvic disease is suspected in a woman, the low lithotomy position with the legs spread to allow placement and use of a cervical manipulator should be selected (Fig. 29–3). It is important not to elevate the thighs excessively because this may limit instrument manipulation toward the upper abdomen. Some surgeons also use an 81-French rectal probe when performing extensive surgery in the cul-de-sac of Douglas.

Ordinarily, the camera port is placed in the infraumbilical position by the open technique. If there have been previous operations (the

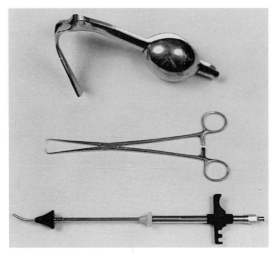

Figure 29–3. Cohen's uterine manipulator may be used with a cervical tenaculum and a weighted vaginal speculum to allow intraoperative uterine manipulation.

usual situation), then initial entry should be gained in an upper quadrant—usually the left—in a subcostal position near the ninth rib (Fig. 29–4). The open technique is still preferred. Additional ports should be placed under direct vision to allow inspection and division of adhesions underlying prior surgical scars. Sometimes the operating telescope is helpful for this task. The camera may be changed to the infraumbilical position when this becomes feasible. Upper abdominal exposure is best done with two ports at or above the umbilicus.

To inspect the small intestine, I use two ports: one in the middle of the right abdomen and one in the left lower quadrant (Fig. 29–5). These can be used to inspect the pelvis, and additional cannulas can be inserted as necessary under direct vision.

A systematic approach should be used for adhesions. If one adhesion is clearly the cause of pain, only that adhesion should be divided and the operation should be discontinued; however, this is uncommonly the case.

First, adhesions to the anterior abdominal wall are cleared to allow adequate exposure. Sometimes, adhesions may tether the colon upward, aiding inspection of the small intestine. When present, these should be left undisturbed. After the cecum is identified, the small bowel is examined beginning at the ileocecal valve and moving proximal with two graspers.

It is very important to work from the distal ileum toward the jejunum if proximal intestine is distended. The surgeon may prefer to stand initially at the patient's left and switch to the patient's right to see the proximal jejunum. The table should be rotated from side to side to facilitate exposure.

Offending adhesions are rarely in the upper abdomen; rather, they are usually in the pelvis or lower abdomen, or they may be posterior. If there has been a localized area of persistent pain, this should be carefully inspected for an underlying adhesion or a hernia. With the patient in the Trendelenburg position—angled 20° to 30° or more—the pelvic viscera and cul-de-sac are inspected for abnormalities: adhesions, inflammation, ovarian or oviduct disease, and endometriosis. The last may appear as small fibrotic nodules near the uterosacral ligaments, in the cul-de-sac, or on the broad ligaments. Uterine manipulation

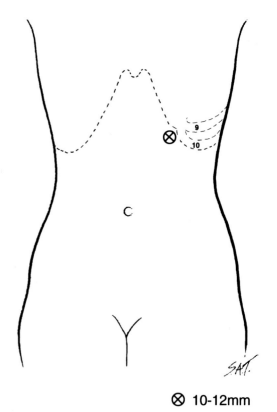

Figure 29–4. If initial entry is not feasible in the mid abdomen, a cannula may be placed in an upper quadrant by open technique. Additional cannulas may be placed to allow dissection of omentum and intestine away from the midline so that more cannulas can be placed.

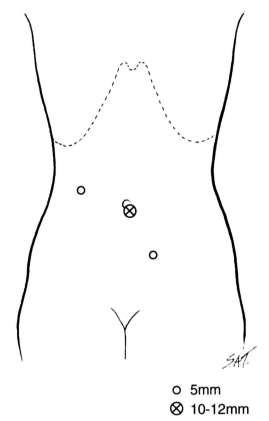

○ 5mm
⊗ 10-12mm

Figure 29–5. To inspect the small bowel, two 5-mm trocars may be used, with the camera inserted at the umbilicus. Additional cannulas should be placed as needed.

through the cervix may be helpful. It may be wise to photograph evident disease.

Filmy adhesions can be swept away. Most adhesions should be placed under tension and cut with the scissors. I prefer scissors with bipolar cautery to transect vascular adhesions. Monopolar cautery or lasers should be used very cautiously near the intestine. Generally, the safest point at which to divide an adhesion is near its insertion. Interloop adhesions require precise division to avoid bowel entry.

After the offending adhesions, or all adhesions (when there is no obvious culprit), are addressed, the intestine should be carefully examined for intraoperative injury. The abdomen should be copiously irrigated with electrolyte solution. I attempt to aspirate all intra-abdominal fluid before final closure. Any entry port site in the lower or mid abdomen greater than 5 mm in size should be closed with suture before ending the procedure.

If no intraperitoneal source of pain is identified, it is worthwhile to examine the pancreas. In thin patients, the pancreas is often visible through the lesser omentum. Inferior traction on the stomach often reveals a clear space in the gastrohepatic ligament. This can be incised to allow direct inspection and palpation of the pancreas. In patients with chronic pancreatitis, the gland is generally firm and thickened in contrast to the soft, thin, normal gland. The supragastric approach to the lesser sac does not allow examination of the head of the gland. Therefore, it is often necessary to open the gastrocolic ligament to more thoroughly examine the pancreas. If laparoscopic ultrasound is available, the presence of pancreatic duct dilation, small pseudocysts, or tumors may be ascertained that might be overlooked by conventional preoperative imaging studies.

AFTERCARE

Patients may be discharged as soon as they can take liquids and void spontaneously. This may be on the day of the procedure or the next day. However, if there has been extensive small bowel manipulation, the patient should be kept in the hospital 1 or 2 days until the surgeon is confident there has been no occult small bowel perforation. Full-thickness cautery injury of the bowel may not be evident for 4 to 7 days. Consequently, the patient should be instructed to call or return if there is any ensuing problem.

Selected Readings

1. Baker PU, Symonells EM. The resolution of chronic pelvic pain after normal laparoscopic findings. Am J Obstet Gynecol 1992;166:835–836.
2. Beecher HK. Surgery as a placebo. JAMA 1961; 176(13):1102–1107.
3. Bonica JJ ed. The Management of Pain. 2nd ed. Philadelphia: Lea & Febiger, 1990.
4. Bonica JJ. Neurophysiologic and pathologic aspects of acute and chronic pain. Arch Surg 1977;112:750–761.
5. Guyton AC, Hall JE. Textbook of Medical Physiology. Philadelphia: WB Saunders, 1996.
6. Howard FM. The role of laparoscopy in chronic pelvic pain: Promise and pitfalls. Obstet Gynecol Surg 1993;48:357–387.

7. Kaplan C, Lipkin M Jr, Gordon GH. Somatization in primary care: Patients with unexplained and vexing medical complaints. J Gen Intern Med 1990;(3)177–190.
8. Murphy TM. Chronic pain. In: Miller RD, ed. Anesthesia. Vol. 2. New York: Churchill Livingstone, 1994.
9. Reich H. Laparoscopic surgery for adhesions. In: Arregui ME, et al, eds. Principles of Laparoscopic Surgery. New York: Springer-Verlag, 1995;283–308.
10. Van der Velpin GC, Shimi SM, Cuscheri A. Diagnostic yield and management benefit of laparoscopy: A prospective audit. Gut 1994;35:1617–1621.

30

Laparoscopic Treatment of Gynecologic Emergencies

Bruce G. Bateman

During the past decade, laparoscopy has replaced laparotomy for the diagnosis and management of many gynecologic conditions. This chapter discusses the application of laparoscopic technique for management of ectopic pregnancy, ovarian cysts, adnexal torsion, and tubo-ovarian abscess.

SURGICAL SETUP FOR GYNECOLOGIC LAPAROSCOPY

Gynecologic laparoscopy procedures may be performed with the patient in the supine or lithotomy position. A "low" lithotomy, with the patient's thighs at a 30° angle, is preferred to allow operating space for the surgical team and access to the cervix for uterine manipulation. The bladder is drained by an indwelling Foley catheter. Diagnostic procedures require a 10-mm subumbilical trochar for the laparoscope and a 5-mm midline trochar placed 4 to 5 cm above the pubic symphysis. Higher midline accessory trochar placement results in collisions with the laparoscope and lower placement adds the risk of bladder injury. A steep Trendelenburg position for the patient facilitates displacement of the small bowel out of the pelvis.

If operative laparoscopy is required, the lower midline accessory trochar may be converted to a 10-mm port and two additional 5-mm trochars may be placed in the lateral lower abdomen. The superficial and inferior epigastric vessels are at risk with lateral trochar insertion. Transillumination of the abdominal wall usually aids in identifying the superficial epigastric vessels. In all but the thinnest patients, the inferior epigastric vessels cannot be transilluminated. The inferior epigastric artery and vein course lateral to the obliterated umbilical arteries, which may be seen as bands of tissue along the anterior peritoneum in a V configuration. In most patients, the inferior epigastric vessels can be directly visualized through the peritoneum.

There are two options for lateral trochar placement. Trochars may be placed medial to the epigastric vessels (at the same level as the midline accessory trochar). Although this usually avoids vascular injury, hematomas in the rectus muscle have been reported and the resultant proximity of multiple trochars may not be convenient. Alternatively, and preferably, these trochars may be placed lateral to the epigastric vessels. With this approach, the incision is more cephalad—typically 3 to 4 cm medial to the anterior superior iliac spine. The angle of trochar insertion is medial and inferior. This approach involves the risk of injury to the ascending branch of the deep circumflex iliac vessels as they course into the anterior abdominal wall. The external iliac vessels are also at risk of injury from insertion at an improper angle.

ECTOPIC PREGNANCY

Diagnosis

Reproductive-age women with pelvic pain or abnormal uterine bleeding are initially divided into pregnant and nonpregnant categories based on serum human chorionic gonadotropin (hCG) levels. Tubal pregnancies characteristically result in amenorrhea followed by abnormal bleeding and lateralizing pelvic pain. The signs and symptoms vary from minimal to extreme. Patients are usually afebrile with a normal white blood cell count or mild leukocytosis. The hematocrit varies on the basis of the extent of intraperitoneal bleeding. Incomplete abortion may mimic these signs and symptoms. The pain of incomplete abortion is midline and crampy in nature.

Patients with hypotension due to intraperitoneal hemorrhage are not a diagnostic dilemma, and they are not candidates for laparoscopy. The presence of mild to moderate pelvic discomfort associated with a positive serum hCG is the diagnostic challenge of this condition. Transvaginal sonography identifies an intrauterine gestational sac when serum hCG is greater than 2000 mIU/mL. Absence of a sac establishes the diagnosis of ectopic pregnancy. Twenty percent to 30% of women with tubal pregnancies come to surgery because of symptoms and physical findings with hCG of less than 2000 mIU/mL. In 9% of tubal pregnancies, fetal cardiac motion is present in the adnexa as a pathognomonic sonographic sign. Rarely, tubal pregnancies are bilateral or heterotopic (coexistent with an intrauterine implantation).

Surgical Technique

In some cases, it may be appropriate to perform a dilatation and curettage (D & C) with frozen section as an initial maneuver. The presence of chorionic villi establishes the diagnosis of incomplete abortion and essentially rules out tubal pregnancy. Occasionally, frozen section misses the chorionic villi and subsequent permanent sections are positive. The surgeon should be mindful of this possibility when laparoscopy does not clearly reveal a tubal pregnancy. In addition, there may be trace amounts of bleeding from the tubes after a D & C. Bilateral bleeding is the key sign of this phenomenon.

Ninety percent of tubal pregnancies can be managed by operative laparoscopy. The criteria for laparotomy are rapidly changing. Publications from only 5 years ago typically noted that size greater than 5 cm, presence of tubal rupture, location other than the tubal isthmus or ampulla, and presence of adhesions were indications for laparotomy. These criteria are highly restrictive. Size limitation is generally unnecessary except in interligamentous pregnancies (tubal rupture into the broad ligament). Interligamentous pregnancies become unmanageable by laparoscopy with only modest dimensions (>4 cm diameter). The mass of large ampullary pregnancies is accounted for by blood clot in the tubal lumen; therefore, even large ampullary ectopic pregnancies can be handled by decompression-salpingostomy, whatever the ultimate surgical plan. Tubal rupture relates to criteria for laparotomy only in terms of blood loss. Hypovolemic shock is a clear indication for laparotomy. Ovarian and even interstitial ectopic pregnancies can be managed by operative laparoscopy in selected cases. With regard to adhesions, in the absence of rapid blood loss, lysis of adhesions is a basic laparoscopic maneuver.

In general, salpingectomy is the appropriate management for ruptured tubal pregnancies and for patients who do not want to preserve their fertility. Ampullary or isthmic pregnancies can be recognized as a hemorrhagic bulge in the tube and can be excised by division of the tube proximal to the pregnancy (on the uterine side) using a burn and cut sequence with electrosurgery or thermocoagulation. After division of the tube, the mesosalpinx is divided by the burn and cut technique, with care taken that the mesosalpinx remains just beneath the tube and parallel to its course. If large vessels are encountered in the mesosalpinx or if the surgeon prefers, endoloop pretied ligatures may be used. Two ligatures of 0 chromic gut are sufficient and backbleeding is not a significant problem (Fig. 30–1). Endoloop ligatures must be applied perpendicular to the course of vessels to be ligated. The Endo GIA (United States Surgical Corp., Norwalk, CT) stapler may also be used.

If the pregnancy is in the distal ampulla or the fimbria, endoloop ligatures or the stapler may be used to simply amputate the affected region of the tube. When salpingectomy is

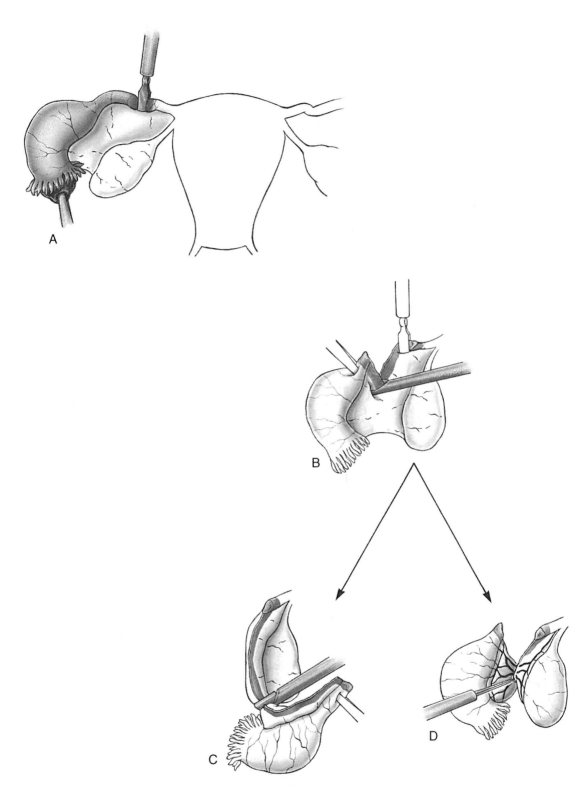

Figure 30–1. Salpingectomy for ectopic pregnancy. (A) The fallopian tube is desiccated by electrosurgery proximal to the tubal pregnancy. **(B)** Salpingectomy progresses with a burn and cut sequence through the mesosalpinx. **(C)** Final removal of the tube after burn and cut sequence salpingectomy. **(D)** Alternatively, loop ligature application for final tubal removal.

performed, care must be taken to avoid injury to the ovarian vessels. The usual course of the ureter makes ureteral injury unlikely unless lysis of adhesions to the pelvic sidewall is required.

In patients wanting to preserve their fertility, tubal conservation is appropriate. Ninety percent of tubal pregnancies are in the ampulla. A salpingotomy or salpingostomy may be performed with unruptured tubal pregnancies in this region. The antimesenteric portion of the tube overlying the pregnancy is injected with 3 to 5 mL of dilute vasopressin (1 U per 10 mL). This may be accomplished with a 22-gauge spinal needle passed freehand through the abdominal wall. Vasopressin injection tends to separate the tubal serosa and muscularis layers.

The tubal serosa is then cauterized along the intended incision line by electrosurgery and incised with microscissors. The muscularis layer is incised to reveal the lumen (Fig. 30–2A through C). Alternatively, the tube may be incised by laser. When properly performed, both techniques provide equivalent outcomes. The length of the incision is approximately one half the length of the ampullary bulge.

After opening the tube, ampullary ectopic pregnancies usually appear as a blood clot cast. The trophoblast is mixed in with the clot and is not visually distinct. Active ectopic pregnancies, with high hCG levels or fetal cardiac motion on ultrasound, may contain a distinct sac and a recognizable fetus. The trophoblastic tissue is typically fluffy and white, and has a buoyant character. The tubal contents are gently teased out of the tube with 5-mm forceps or 10-mm spoon forceps (see Fig. 30–2D). The suction-irrigator may be helpful to dislodge clots. The 10-mm spoon forceps is useful for final removal of the tubal contents. Complete removal of the tubal contents is essential.

Bleeding from the implantation site or the tubal incision is localized by irrigation and controlled by gentle electrosurgery or endocoagulation. At times, hemostasis is difficult. Bleeding from the implantation site may fill the tubal incision with blood, obscuring the bleeding point. Extension of the tubal incision, injection of the mesosalpinx with dilute vasopressin, ligation of the underlying mesosalpingeal vessels, or "inversion" of the tube are management options. The tube may be "inverted" by gently grasping the mesenteric wall, through the salpingotomy site, and pulling that part of the tube out through the tubal incision (see Fig. 30–2E). Irrigation identifies the point of bleeding. Rarely, salpingectomy is necessary to control bleeding.

The fallopian tube may be left open to heal by secondary intention or it may be sutured. In most publications the former is favored. Subsequent tubal function as judged by pregnancy rate is similar with each approach. If suture closure is used, two or three sutures of 4-0 polyglactin 910 or polyglycolic acid are sufficient (see Fig. 30–2F and G). The closure may be confined to the serosa or it may include the muscularis. A one-layer closure is adequate. Ampullary fistulas have been observed to develop after salpingostomy; although their functional significance is unknown, it is believed that they are undesirable.

Unruptured isthmic pregnancies are generally not amenable to salpingotomy or salpingostomy. The muscularis of the isthmus is significantly thicker than in the ampulla, the serosa is tightly adherent to the muscularis, and the tubal lumen is quite small. The trophoblast tends to invade the muscularis earlier in this region, and attempted salpingostomy causes damage to the involved tubal segment. Alternatively, tubal conservation in the isthmus may be accomplished by segmental resection with subsequent reanastomosis. Microsurgical reanastomosis is generally performed as an interval procedure because of the increased vascularity caused by pregnancy.

Fimbrial ectopic pregnancies typically are seen as a bloody mass between the fimbria and the ovary or other adjacent tissue. If appropriate, tubal conservation is usually feasible. The pregnancy tissue and blood clot are "picked" off of the affected organs, and hemostasis is rarely a problem. Implantation in the distal ampulla may be difficult to distinguish from a fimbrial ectopic pregnancy. Aspiration of the ectopic trophoblastic tissue from the distal ampulla runs an unusually high risk of persistent trophoblast; therefore, if tubal conservation is the goal, a salpingotomy may be preferable.

Although ruptured ampullary ectopic pregnancies generally require a salpingectomy, if

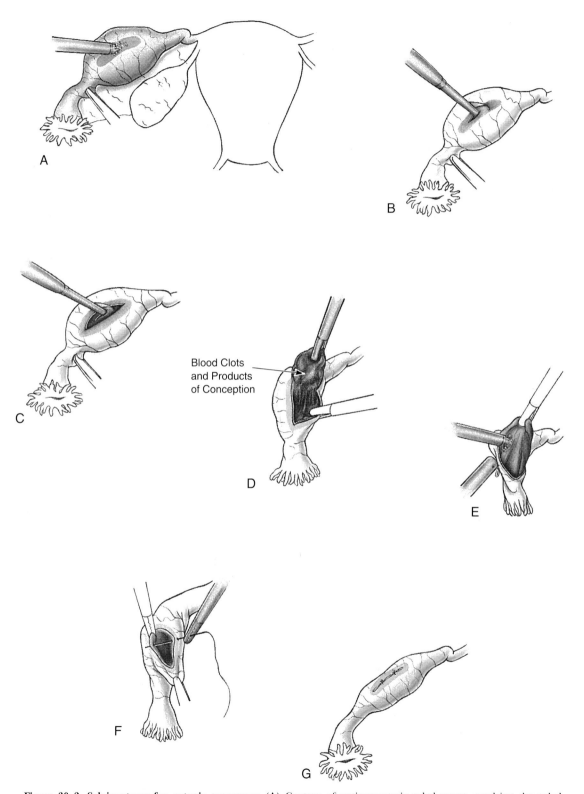

Figure 30–2. Salpingotomy for ectopic pregnancy. (A) Cautery of antimesenteric tubal serosa overlying the tubal pregnancy. **(B)** Incision of the tubal serosa using microscissors. **(C)** Incision of the tubal muscularis using hooked scissors. **(D)** Removal of blood clot and products of conception. **(E)** Inversion of tubal ampulla for hemostasis. **(F)** Suture closure of salpingotomy site. **(G)** Final appearance after suture closure.

the site of rupture is antimesenteric and relatively small, tubal conservation may be possible. Ruptured isthmic ectopic pregnancies may be managed by segmental resection as described. Rarely, a tubal pregnancy penetrates into the mesosalpinx or the broad ligament (interligamentous pregnancy). In this case, tubal conservation is not possible and attempted laparoscopic salpingostomy or salpingostomy usually results in bleeding, necessitating laparotomy.

Interstitial ectopic pregnancies are rare and present a surgical challenge. Interstitial pregnancies typically reach 14 to 16 weeks' gestation without significant symptoms. Rupture results in life-threatening hemorrhage. Uterine reconstruction is generally not possible and a hysterectomy is required. Early interstitial ectopic pregnancies are often missed at the time of diagnostic laparoscopy. Small, inactive interstitial pregnancies have been managed by laparoscopic surgery with electrosurgical excision of the cornual region of the uterus.

Retained Trophoblastic Tissue

With conservative tubal surgery there is the risk of retained trophoblastic tissue. The rate of retained trophoblast after salpingotomy or salpingostomy varies from 3% to 18%. Studies have shown a higher incidence of persistent trophoblast after laparoscopic surgery compared with laparotomy. Interestingly, failure of the histologic permanent sections to show trophoblastic tissue does not correlate with persistent trophoblastic activity. The risk of persistent trophoblast is higher in smaller ectopic pregnancies (2 vs. 3 cm diameter) and "earlier" ectopic pregnancies (shorter period of amenorrhea). The hCG level on the day of surgery is useful for comparison with postoperative levels. HCG level shows a biphasic decay pattern, with a rapid initial component (48–72 hours) and a slower secondary rate of decline. The initial follow-up level is most useful on postoperative day 6, with subsequent testing done every 3 days. If hCG plateaus or increases, further treatment is required.

Management options for retained trophoblast include repeat surgery or methotrexate therapy. Trophoblastic tissue is more difficult to recognize at repeat surgery and tends to be proximal to the initial incision site. Salpingectomy may be the best course of action if the contralateral tube is normal. If repeat surgery for retained trophoblast is performed, careful attention must be directed to the pelvic peritoneum, especially if the tubes are normal in appearance. Implants of active trophoblastic tissue have been documented on the vesicouterine peritoneum, pelvic sidewall, and in the cul-de-sac, presumably from spillage at the time of salpingostomy.

Methotrexate Treatment of Ectopic Pregnancy

There has been recent interest in methotrexate as primary treatment for ectopic pregnancy. Most protocols rely on a nonsurgical diagnosis of tubal pregnancy and systemic treatment. Methotrexate may also be injected directly into the tube at the time of laparoscopy.

Results in terms of resolution and subsequent fertility are similar to those of salpingotomy and salpingostomy. However, in half of patients given methotrexate, troublesome pelvic pain develops during resolution. Resolution may take 4 to 8 weeks, and a small but not insignificant percentage of patients ultimately require surgery because of bleeding.

Ovarian Pregnancy

Trophoblastic implantation within the ovary is rare, occurring in approximately 1 per 7000 conceptions. The history and findings in ovarian pregnancies do not differ significantly from those in tubal ectopic pregnancies. Ovarian pregnancies present as a hemorrhagic ovarian mass with normal-appearing fallopian tubes. In most cases, the pregnancy tissue can be dissected free from the ovary, and ovarian preservation is the rule. Because of the rarity of this condition, laparoscopy experience is limited, although successful laparoscopic management has been reported.

OVARIAN CYSTS

Diagnosis

Ovarian conditions most likely to occur as a surgical emergency include cyst rupture and ovarian (adnexal) torsion. (Adnexal torsion is discussed later as a separate topic.) The pelvic pain caused by ovarian cysts—ruptured or intact—varies from extreme to mild and may be unilateral or bilateral. Types of cysts and frequency are listed in Table 30–1. Pelvic examination findings of an adnexal mass with lateralizing tenderness are consistent with this diagnosis. Affected patients are typically afebrile with negative serum hCG and normal white blood cell count. The hematocrit varies depending on intraperitoneal bleeding. In the presence of ruptured ovarian cysts, transvaginal sonography shows free fluid in the pelvis, and identification of the cyst is generally not possible. Within intact cysts, transvaginal sonography provides precise dimensions and sonographic characteristics of the mass.

Varying size parameters have been proposed as limits with regard to laparoscopic management of ovarian cysts. With drainage being a part of the laparoscopic approach, cysts that are 10 cm and larger have been managed successfully.

Laparoscopic surgery for intact ovarian cysts is controversial because of the risk of spillage if the cyst is malignant. Sonographic findings predictive of benign cysts include their being unilocular, echo free, and free of septations or papillary excrescences. Findings suggestive of malignancy include septations, and a complex mass with solid components or excrescences. Color Doppler sonography may provide more accurate prediction by differentiating the neovascularity of tumors from normal arteries. Doppler waveforms show "low impedance" flow predictive of malignancy. In a recent study, the negative predictive value of this technique was 98% and the positive predictive value was 83%. Color Doppler information is more accurate in postmenopausal than in premenopausal women.

Surgical Technique

Operative technique for management of ovarian cysts varies with the cyst type and size. On the basis of size alone, cysts as large as 5 cm in diameter can be removed intact, but larger cysts require initial drainage.

Functional Cysts

Persistent, inactive follicular cysts are characterized by sonographic findings of unilocular, echo-free cystic masses with a simple, smooth internal wall. Corpora luteum cysts are more difficult to diagnose due to internal echoes. At the time of surgery, functional cysts are typically free of adhesions.

Intact removal is seldom successful with functional cysts. Incision of the ovarian capsule overlying the cyst with microscissors or laser usually results in immediate rupture. The interior of the cyst is typically smooth without papillary excrescences. Although it may be possible to develop a plane of dissection between the cyst wall and normal ovarian tissue, follicular cysts are fragile and tear easily. Complete removal by stripping is seldom possible. Cyst wall destruction by electrosurgery or thermocoagulation is an alternative. Fresh corpora luteum cysts are quite vascular, and persistence in attempted removal can result in significant blood loss and damage to the ovary. Persistent corpora luteum cysts are less vascular, making cyst wall removal more feasible.

Suspected functional cysts may be sampled for biopsy and the cyst wall fenestrated by electrosurgery. With this technique, persistent corpora luteum cysts are more likely to recur than follicular cysts. Biopsy and fenestration may result in incomplete surgery for benign ovarian tumors, which are grossly indistinguishable from functional cysts.

Table 30–1. Cyst Type by Histologic Frequency*

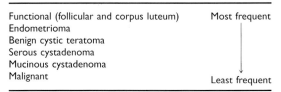

Functional (follicular and corpus luteum)	Most frequent
Endometrioma	
Benign cystic teratoma	
Serous cystadenoma	
Mucinous cystadenoma	
Malignant	Least frequent

*Types by histologic frequency of 809 cysts from premenopausal women.

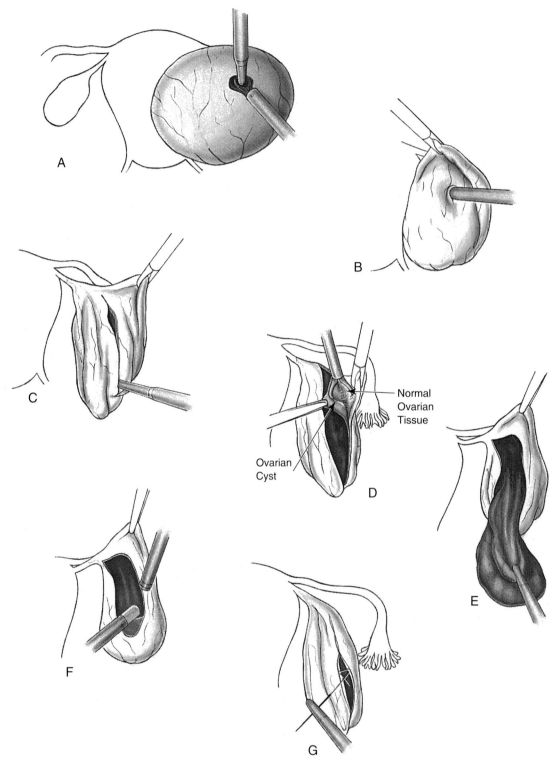

Figure 30–3. Oophorocystectomy for ovarian endometrioma. (A) Incision of ovarian endometrioma. **(B)** Drainage of ovarian endometrioma. **(C)** Extension of incision in ovarian capsule and cyst wall. **(D)** Development of tissue plane, dissecting ovarian cyst wall from normal ovarian tissue. **(E)** Final removal of cyst wall. **(F)** Establishing hemostasis. **(G)** Suture repair of the ovary.

Endometriomas

Endometriomas may be echo free but more typically they exhibit diffusely echogenic (ground-glass) appearance on ultrasound. At laparoscopy, ovarian endometriomas are usually associated with implants of endometriosis on the pelvic peritoneum and adhesions on the involved ovary. Because of their content, endometriomas have a typically dark hue. Intact removal of endometriomas is virtually impossible (even at laparotomy). Attempts to identify a tissue plane result in rupture and drainage. When this diagnosis is evident, initial intentional puncture and drainage is appropriate (Fig. 30–3A and B). The interior of endometriomas is rough and hemosiderin stained but lacking in papillary excrescences. There are three effective management strategies: removal of the cyst wall, destruction of the cyst wall, or oophorectomy.

Aggressive ovarian conservation is appropriate for women who want to preserve their fertility. The endometrioma cyst wall is tough and rind-like owing to extensive fibrosis. After drainage the tissue plane between endometrioma cyst wall and remaining normal ovary can be developed by gentle blunt dissection (see Fig. 30–3D and E). The endometrioma cyst wall can be easily stripped from normal ovarian tissue in most cases. Electrosurgery or laser destruction of the interior of endometriomas is also effective and is the approach of choice in most surgical series. I prefer surgical cystectomy to provide tissue for pathologic analysis and to ensure complete removal. Ovarian conservation is possible even in large endometriomas measuring 8 to 10 cm. The risk of recurrence is low. Aggressive ovarian preservation is less appropriate in patients who are not concerned with future fertility, assuming that the contralateral ovary is intact.

There are two techniques for laparoscopic oophorectomy. The ovary may be mobilized by division of the utero-ovarian ligament and the meso-ovarium using a burn and cut sequence. This results in isolation of the ovarian vascular pedicle near the pelvic brim. The ovarian vessels may be ligated by two endoloop ligatures of 0 chromic gut, desiccated by electrosurgery or stapled with an Endo GIA (United States Surgical Corp., Norwalk, CT).

Care must be taken to avoid ureteral injury. Traction on the ovary and ovarian vessels may elevate the ureter. The second approach is initial isolation and division of the ovarian vessels. With this technique, the retroperitoneal space is opened lateral to the ovarian vessels just below the pelvic brim. The course of the ureter is noted, and the vessels can be stapled or desiccated by electrosurgery. Removal then proceeds in a prouterine direction.

Benign Cystic Teratomas

Ovarian dermoids have a complex appearance on ultrasound and may contain densely echogenic areas due to calcification. Dermoids are typically free of adhesions and have a yellow-tan appearance due to their sebaceous content. Laparoscopic removal of recognized dermoids is controversial because their liquid contents may cause intense peritonitis. With careful dissection, intact laparoscopic removal of tumors of 5 cm or less in diameter is possible in most cases. Incision of the ovarian capsule to identify the cyst wall and careful dissection to separate the wall from the normal ovary require gentle tissue handling and patience (Fig. 30–4). Small perforations with minimal leakage can still be managed by laparoscopic technique. Gross rupture and spillage, especially early in the dissection, make laparotomy an appropriate consideration. On the other hand, with copious irrigation, the risk of peritonitis following spill is low (2.1%). Thorough removal of hair by laparoscopy is possible but tedious. Oophorectomy is seldom necessary in the management of ovarian dermoids. Intact dermoids or their contents are conveniently removed by an endoscopic plastic pouch.

Serous Cystadenoma and Mucinous Cystadenoma

Serous and mucinous cystadenomas lack a characteristic ultrasound or laparoscopic appearance. Tissue planes between these benign cysts and normal ovarian tissue are of intermediate clarity—better than a functional cyst but not as clear as an endometrioma or dermoid. Mucinous cystadenomas are evident at the time of drainage (intentional or uninten-

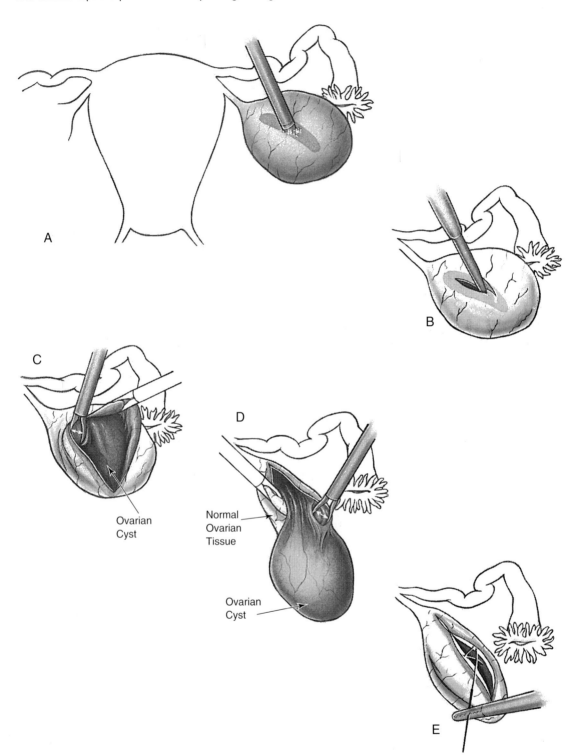

Figure 30–4. Oophorocystectomy for benign cystic teratoma. (A) Electrosurgery of ovarian capsule overlying a benign cystic teratoma. **(B)** Incision of ovarian capsule with microscissors. **(C)** Developing tissue plane. **(D)** Identification of blood supply in final step of cyst removal. **(E)** Suture repair of the ovary.

tional) related to their mucoid content. The risk of pseudomyxoma peritonei secondary to spill of benign mucinous tumors is controversial; it is probably quite low. Oophorocystectomy is usually possible with either tumor, depending on size.

Ovarian Cancer

Contamination of the peritoneal cavity by spillage of a malignant ovarian cyst is a subject of controversy in gynecology. The risk of rupture during surgery is increased by endoscopic approach.

Laparoscopic findings consistent with malignancy are obvious in cases with metastatic disease. Spill of cystic ovarian malignancies may worsen prognosis if definitive surgery is delayed. If definitive surgery is immediate, spill is probably not detrimental to overall prognosis. In two recent laparoscopy series of 819 and 809 ovarian cysts, the risk of cystic malignancy spill was 0.9% and 0.6%, respectively.

Suture Repair of the Ovary After Oophorocystectomy

Suture repair of the ovary after endoscopic oophorocystectomy is controversial. In most series, the ovary is allowed to heal by secondary intention. Endoscopic suture closure of the ovary has been linked to an increased risk of adhesions. Typical ovarian closure has used 3-0 or 2-0 suture with interrupted technique (through the cortex). This is a paradigm for adhesion formation. Before the advent of endoscopic ovarian surgery, ovarian closure at the time of laparotomy was typically subcortical, using 4-0 or 5-0 suture. This type of closure is tedious but possible by laparoscopy, and one wonders whether the trend away from endoscopic ovarian repair is a decision of convenience.

ADNEXAL TORSION

Diagnosis

Torsion of the fallopian tube and ovary is an uncommon cause of pelvic pain, account-

ing for 2.7% of emergency gynecologic operations in a recent series of 3772 cases. Most cases are associated with ovarian or paratubal cysts, and torsion involves both the tube and the ovary. Adnexal torsion is seen predominantly in reproductive-age women, occasionally in postmenopausal women, and rarely in children. Torsion involves the right adnexa more frequently than the left, perhaps due to a stabilizing effect of the sigmoid colon in the left pelvis. Torsion is typically caused by ovarian cysts, which are not associated with adhesions (e.g., functional cysts, benign cystic teratomas, paratubal cysts).

Symptoms of adnexal torsion are sudden in onset and unilateral. Pain may radiate from the flank to the groin and into the anterior or lateral thigh. Pain characteristics and severity vary widely. When pain is intense, nausea and vomiting are common features. In some cases, the symptoms are intermittent. Pelvic examination reveals unilateral tenderness usually associated with a mass. Thirty percent of patients exhibit leukocytosis and 13% have low-grade fever. Transvaginal ultrasound shows unilateral ovarian enlargement, which, taken together with the presence of multiple follicular cysts around the periphery of the ovary, has been suggested as a sign of torsion. Color flow Doppler assessment of the ovarian vessels may demonstrate decreased arterial blood flow. There are no large series documenting the usefulness of this finding.

Surgical Management

In 1946, Stanley Way described and promoted conservation of the adnexa in cases of torsion by detorsion of the adnexa, application of "hot packs," and observation for 10 minutes to document color change suggestive of perfusion. However, in a series of 128 cases compiled from 1974 to 1984, only 7% had conservation of the affected adnexa. More recently, aggressive conservation has been reported, even with adnexas that are severely ischemic. Mage and colleagues reported conservation in 29 of 35 cases with 77% performed by laparoscopy. Adnexas that failed to show perfusion after detorsion were removed. Oelsner and coworkers reported an even more aggressive conservation of 40 consecutive cases, all showing "edema and black-blue color." Fourteen of the 40 were managed by laparoscopy. Long-term follow-up in 37 of the 40 suggested normal ovarian function on the affected side in 35 patients.

Venous embolism is consistently mentioned as a risk of detorsion. The frequency of this complication is unknown, and it does not appear in the English literature over the past 20 years. Oophoropexy to stabilize the adnexa is another management option. The ovary may be fixed to the lateral pelvic sidewall by a single nonabsorbable suture. There are no clear data on the value of this maneuver.

Detorsion can usually be accomplished by laparoscopy. Mild or moderate ischemia of the involved structure does not present a management dilemma in patients wanting to preserve ovarian function. Detorsion of "blue-black" adnexa requires careful observation for evidence of perfusion. Intravenous fluorescein may be a helpful adjunct. If an ovarian cyst is present, laparoscopic cystectomy is performed as a part of most series. Depending on the cyst type, tissue planes are variable, as previously discussed. If a solid ovarian tumor is present, oophorectomy is usually necessary. As with all ovarian masses, if there is evidence of malignancy, laparotomy is appropriate. The relative frequencies of ovarian and tubal conditions in a series of 135 cases are listed in Table 30–2.

If, after detorsion, salpingo-oophorectomy is indicated, the area of torsion may provide a convenient pedicle for ligation. The course of the ureter should be observed, and if necessary the lateral pelvic peritoneum can be opened. Endoloop ligatures, 0 chromic gut, bipolar coagulation, and automatic staplers are equally effective for ovarian vessel ligation.

Final removal of the ovarian specimen may

be accomplished by cutting the ovarian cyst wall into strips for removal through a 10-mm trochar sleeve. Removal of intact ovaries or larger amounts of tissue may be done by means of a plastic pouch.

ACUTE SALPINGITIS AND TUBO-OVARIAN ABSCESS

Diagnosis

Acute salpingitis is typically associated with bilateral lower abdominal pain, tenderness on pelvic examination, and leukocytosis. There is a growing tendency in gynecologic practice to confirm this diagnosis by laparoscopy initially or if patients fail to show prompt defervescence with parenteral antibiotic therapy. In some series, there is a surprisingly high discordance in admitting diagnosis and laparoscopic findings. Many patients have endometriosis or negative laparoscopy. In this setting, laparoscopy is diagnostic only.

Tubo-ovarian abscess (TOA) is suggested by the presence of a pelvic mass. Symptoms of pain are highly variable. Leukocytosis is present in 70% and temperature greater than 38.5°C in 76% of patients. Acute-phase C-reactive protein has been found to be elevated in association with TOAs. Pelvic ultrasound, computed tomography, and gallium scans are useful and show comparable sensitivity and specificity for the diagnosis of abdominal abscess. Of these, transvaginal sonography is the most convenient and cost effective. Ultrasound typically shows a cystic or complex mass. TOAs are frequently unilateral (70%).

Laparoscopic Management

The management of TOAs has evolved from extirpative surgery by laparotomy to medical or laparoscopic therapy. Early laparoscopy has become a frequent diagnostic maneuver. Depending on the philosophy of the surgeon, the procedure may be purely diagnostic and used to collect material for culture or laparoscopic drainage may be performed.

Spontaneous rupture of TOA is morbid and potentially lethal. Laparoscopic management

Table 30–2. Frequency of Ovarian and Tubal Disease Associated With Adnexal Torsion

Condition	Frequency
Benign ovarian tumors	40%
Functional ovarian cysts	27%
Ovarian malignancy	15%
Tubal disease	13%
Normal ovary	3%
Normal tube	2%

of this situation has not been addressed in the literature and is probably ill advised. In the 1980s, Reich and McGlynn promoted lysis of recently formed adhesions and abscess drainage by gentle blunt dissection. Electrosurgery and sharp dissection were avoided. Also in the 1980s, Henry-Suchet and colleagues promoted a similar technique in recent TOAs. They were, however, more aggressive in chronic TOAs. Areas of dense adhesion were needle aspirated and irrigated. Overall, 10% of 50 patients required "early" laparotomy, apparently during the same hospitalization, and 6% had laparotomy later for chronic pain. More recent studies of this issue are conspicuously absent from the literature.

There is no clear comparative data to document improved outcome or shortened hospitalization with laparoscopic drainage versus medical treatment alone. The key facet of medical management, whatever the overall situation, is appropriate antibiotic selection. *Neisseria gonorrhoeae* and *Chlamydia trachomatis* are seldom isolated from TOAs. Anaerobes and facultative bacteria predominate in this process.

SUMMARY

In general, gynecologists have eagerly embraced operative laparoscopy, in advance of controlled comparisons to laparotomy. Comparative studies have since clearly verified the effectiveness of laparoscopic management for tubal pregnancies and there is growing data to support the use of this technique for endometriomas. The appropriateness of other applications is less clear.

Assuming that treatment is adequate, the advantages of laparoscopic surgery for gynecologic emergencies are easily cited—less pa-tient discomfort, improved cosmetic effect, decreased recovery time, and a monetary savings for the health care system. Based on 88,000 cases per year, with $600 to $1200 savings per case, the annual savings for management of ectopic pregnancy alone are estimated to be $50,000,000 to $100,000,000.

Selected Readings

Bateman B, Kolp L, Mills S. Endoscopic versus laparotomy management of endometriomas. Fertil Steril 1994; 62:690–695.

Canis M, Mage G, Pouly J, et al. Laparoscopic diagnosis of adnexal cystic masses: A 12-year experience with long-term follow-up. Obstet Gynecol 1994;83(5 Pt 1):707–712.

Henry-Suchet J, Soler A, Loffredo V. Laparoscopic treatment of tuboovarian abscesses. J Reprod Med 1984; 29:579–582.

Hibbard L. Adnexal torsion. Am J Obstet Gynecol 1985;152:456–461.

Mage G, Canis M, Manhes H, et al. Laparoscopic management of adnexal torsion: A review of 35 cases. J Reprod Med 1989;34:520–524.

Manyonda I, Baggish M, Bower S, et al. Combined laparoscopic and microlaparotomy removal of benign cystic teratomata. Br J Obstet Gynaecol 1993;100(3):284–286.

Mecke H, Lehmann-Willenbrock E, Ibrahim M, et al. Pelviscopic treatment of ovarian cysts in premenopausal women. Gynecol Obstet Invest 1992;34:36–42.

Murphy A, Nager C, Wujek J, et al. Operative laparoscopy versus laparotomy for the management of ectopic pregnancy: A prospective trial. Fertil Steril 1992;57:1180–1185.

Oelsner G, Bider D, Goldenberg M, et al. Long-term follow-up of the twisted ischemic adnexa managed by detorsion. Fertil Steril 1993;60:976–979.

Pouly J, Mahnes H, Mage G, et al. Conservative laparoscopic treatment of 321 ectopic pregnancies. Fertil Steril 1986;46:1093–1097.

Reich H, McGlynn F. Laparoscopic treatment of tuboovarian and pelvic abscess. J Reprod Med 1987;32:747.

Seifer D, Gutmann J, Doyle M, et al. Persistent ectopic pregnancy following laparoscopic linear salpingostomy. Obstet Gynecol 1990;76:1121–1125.

Vermesh M, Silva P, Rosen G, et al. Management of unruptured ectopic gestation by linear salpingostomy: A prospective, randomized clinical trial of laparoscopy versus laparotomy. Obstet Gynecol 1989;73:400–404.

VASCULAR SURGERY

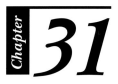

Pitfalls in Ambulatory Vascular Access Surgery

Worthington G. Schenk III

The trend toward outpatient therapy of increasingly complex disorders has increased the demand for chronic vascular access in support of treatment modalities including chemotherapy, home parenteral nutrition, home intravenous (IV) therapy for long-term antibiotics, and maintenance hemodialysis. Most vascular access procedures in support of these treatments can be conducted safely and effectively on an ambulatory basis. The cost of vascular access is substantially reduced by avoiding inpatient status; this is best demonstrated in the approximately 180,000 dialysis patients in the United States, for whom cost of vascular access maintenance exceeds that for treatment of all nonrenal medical conditions. Of the $10 billion annual cost of chronic renal failure, $7 billion of which is paid by Medicare, almost half goes to placement, revision, and maintenance of vascular access. The average reimbursement for each dialysis access placement can be reduced from $10,557 to $2990 by conducting the procedure on an outpatient basis, with similar savings possible with access revision and maintenance procedures. If use of outpatient surgery for dialysis access were increased from 25% to 75%, a taxpayer savings of almost $1 billion annually could be realized.

Vascular access surgery is not generally difficult or complex; this chapter focuses on avoiding the pitfalls that, nonetheless, have the potential to cause serious morbidity.

Pitfall: Inadequately Prepared Facility

Any day-surgery unit or freestanding surgery center can be adequately equipped for vascular access surgery, but it does require preparedness for common contingencies. Any surgically installed central venous device beyond a simple percutaneous (uncuffed, untunnelled, small bore) catheter requires fluoroscopic capability. A simple percutaneous catheter could be placed using the portable chest radiograph alone for position confirmation, but placement of other devices, especially any catheter greater than 9 French (F), requires fluoroscopy for optimal success and safety. It is the initial and ongoing cost of high-quality enhanced-video fluoroscopy equipment (and the licensed technician to operate it) that is the largest obstacle to overcome for a freestanding unit. I also make liberal use of duplex ultrasound, but this is not an absolute requirement. The facility must stock, in addition to all catheter lengths and sizes likely to be used, a complete range of vascular dilators from 8 to 18 F, vascular guide wires from 0.021- to 0.038-inch diameter in varying lengths and stiffness, extra tear-away introducer kits in addition to those that come with catheter kits, and injectable vascular contrast agents.

Placement of arteriovenous (A-V) dialysis conduits can also be done in freestanding surgery units; in some cases, it has been incorporated into the dialysis unit facilities. The unit must stock an assortment of polytetrafluoroethylene (PTFE) grafts, but a small inventory of four or five choices, plus patch material, is sufficient. Standard vascular instruments and sutures are easily maintained. No blood banking facility is needed.

Pitfall: Selecting the Wrong Access Device

The installation of the wrong access device is usually the result of inadequate communication. "PermCath" sounds very similar to "Port-a-Cath," and access requests frequently specify the wrong device for a specific indication. In addition, it is common for the individual who requests access for a patient not to be the individual or agency who will actually use it. For example, it is common for an internist to request a device for chemotherapy, whereas a different oncologist will be using it and be more knowledgeable regarding the pattern and timing of therapy, and thus the most appropriate device. Table 31–1 gives examples of preferred devices for specific indications. The individual who installs the access device must determine who will actually use it and communicate directly with that person regarding choice of the best device. The referring physician may not be completely knowledgeable regarding the choices, but the consultant surgeon should be. This communication should be done before the patient's arrival.

CENTRAL VENOUS ACCESS

Preoperative Evaluation

In addition to accurate determination of the indication and appropriate device, a history of prior devices used—and difficulties with them—should be elicited from the patient. Preoperative imaging studies are not necessary except in circumstances of multiple prior central accesses, particularly if it is known that difficulties were encountered. Whereas duplex ultrasound can offer some anatomic information regarding patency and size of internal jugular and subclavian veins, contrast venography is usually needed if continuity of intrathoracic central veins is in question. A prior sternotomy, particularly for reoperative cardiac surgery, may result in stenosis or interruption of the left innominate vein. Even though a preoperative chest radiograph may not be mandatory, films already available should be brought to the operating suite. Extensive laboratory surveillance is not necessary; I require only a prothrombin time and platelet count. A history of contrast allergy should be specifically elicited; iodinated contrast may occasionally be used intraoperatively.

Table 31–1. Choice of Ambulatory Vascular Access Device

Indication	Device (in Approximate Order of Preference)
Antibiotics 4–6 weeks	Home intravenous therapy (no special device) Peripherally inserted central catheter line Valve-end catheter*
Long-term home total parenteral nutrition	Valve-end catheter* Open-end catheter†
Frequent blood products (Hemophilia, acquired immunodeficiency syndrome)§	Open-end catheter† Port‡
Intermittent ChemoRx	Port‡ Valve-end catheter*
Immediate Hemodialysis (also plasma or cell pheresis)	"Surgical" dialysis catheter** "Percutaneous" dialysis catheter††
Permanent Hemodialysis	Autologous A-V fistula Prosthetic A-V shunt

*Groshong and others.
†Hickman, Leonard, Broviac, and others.
‡Lifeport, Port-a-Cath, and others.
§Avoiding blood-borne transmission: avoiding the organism (blood) is better with a buried port; avoiding the vector (needle) is better with an external catheter. The best policy is to discuss the specific device with the staff or agency who will actually use it.
**PermCath and others.
††Sorensen and others.

Intraoperative Techniques

For central venous devices entering either the subclavian or internal jugular vein, a Seldinger technique is used wherein the vessel lumen is entered with an 18-gauge thin-wall needle; the intravascular position is confirmed by free aspiration of blood into the syringe; a vascular flexible J-tip guide wire, typically 0.035 or 0.038 inch, is passed through the needle; and the course and central location of the tip (in the right atrium not right ventricle, or preferably down the inferior vena cava [IVC]) are confirmed by fluoroscopy. A simple percutaneous catheter can then be passed over the wire. Any catheter that does not have a tapered tip, and particularly one that is very soft and flexible, must be carried into the central position. This is done by enlarging the skin entry site, passing a long vascular dilator over the wire to enlarge the tract, then passing an introducer sheath of sufficient diameter to allow unimpeded passage of the catheter through the sheath, which is subsequently removed. Tunnelled catheters or port devices must also have the other end of the device brought through a remote exit site or into a pocket developed for the subcutaneous port. Final position is documented by plain chest radiograph. Each of these steps has its own pitfalls.

Pitfall: Incomplete Knowledge of Subclavian Vein Anatomy

For subclavian venipuncture, knowledge of the precise relationship between the subclavian vein and artery, first rib, clavicle, and scalenes anterior muscle is crucial, yet this relationship is not always accurately depicted in teaching materials (Fig. 31–1). The common serious complications of pneumothorax and arterial puncture are largely preventable by precise knowledge of the anatomic relationships. B-mode ultrasound can also be used successfully to puncture the axillary/subclavian vein junction under real-time imaging.

Pitfall: The Errant Dilator

The "errant dilator" hazard derives from the common but dangerous assumption that a properly located guide wire will guarantee that the dilator will follow a safe course. It is crucial to understand that a relatively stiff dilator passed over a more flexible guide wire does not reliably follow the same course as the wire and can easily lacerate or perforate the great vessels. This phenomenon is shown in Figure 31–2. The risk of this complication is highest

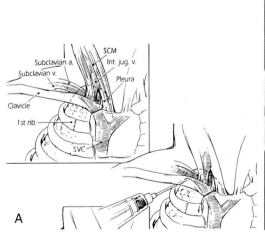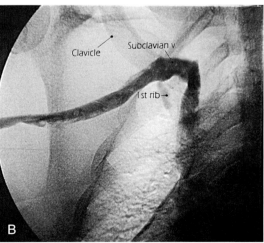

Figure 31–1. An accurate knowledge of the precise anatomic relationships between the subclavian vein and surrounding structures is essential for safe subclavian venipuncture. These relationships are not always accurately depicted. **(A)** A composite drawing adapted from several popular house staff manuals shows a large gap between clavicle and first rib, the subclavian vein does not pass through this window, the vein is parallel to the middle third of the clavicle, and is completely cephalad to the clavicle. Also illustrated is the "cephalad angulation" technique of needle insertion—an excellent technique for temporary or bedside line placement, but one that can make subsequent placement of a large-bore catheter more difficult (see Fig. 31–2). **(B)** A subclavian venogram illustrates the small window between clavicle and first rib; the vein is draped over the first rib, and is roughly perpendicular to the middle third of the clavicle.

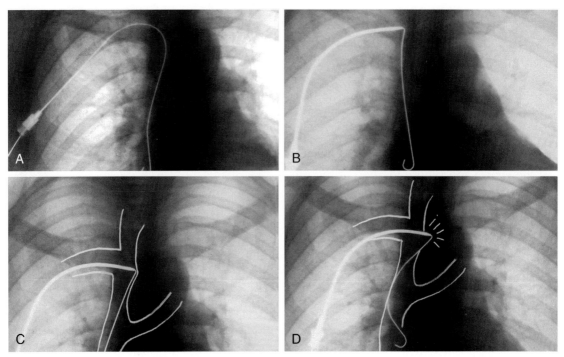

Figure 31–2. The "errant dilator" phenomenon. A guide wire that passes from puncture site to the right atrium does not guarantee that a dilator passed over the wire will do the same. The phenomenon is most common from a right subclavian approach, particularly when the initial entry into the vein uses a "cephalad angulation" technique as shown in Figure 31–1A. **(A)** The guide wire negotiates a fairly tight radius curve at the junction of right subclavian and brachiocephalic veins. **(B)** Whether a dilator passed over the wire will negotiate the same curve depends on the relative bending resistance or "stiffness" of the dilator with respect to the wire. If the dilator has a greater bending resistance, the wire bends, not the dilator. Bending resistance increases with increasing diameter of the dilator. **(C)** Once the wire has been bent, the wire trails, rather than leads, the dilator. **(D)** Serious vascular injury can result. (Computer reconstructed and enhanced images.)

when a large-bore catheter, requiring a large-bore and thus stiff introducer, is placed from a site requiring an acute curve in its intravascular course. A list of recommendations for avoiding this complication is given in Table 31–2, and even though every technique is not used every time, the principles should be understood. The two hints that are always useful are as follow: (1) move the guide wire in and out 1 cm after each 1- to 2-cm advance of the dilator to recognize "binding" of the wire at the tip, and (2) make liberal use of fluoroscopy to visually confirm that the dilator is following the wire. The phenomenon can also be avoided altogether by using a cutdown rather than Seldinger technique.

Pitfall: The S-Curve Phenomenon

The "S-curve phenomenon" is closely associated with the errant dilator phenomenon in

that it can be difficult for a stiffer catheter or dilator to follow a flexible guide wire over a tortuous course. Figure 31–3 shows a left internal jugular vein approach, in which a stiff

Table 31–2. Techniques for Avoiding the Errant Dilator Hazard

Use right IJ or left subclavian approach.
Avoid the "cephalad angulation" technique of subclavian venipuncture (illustrated in Fig. 31–1A).
Make liberal use of intraoperative fluoroscopy.
Use a wire of adequate length, preferably with tip manipulated well into IVC.
Never advance dilator further than tip of wire.
Make initial dilatation with small dilator and progressively increase size.
If dilator does not follow wire, switch to a stiffer wire (see Fig. 31–3).
Use contrast injection if necessary to image anatomy.
Avoid any force. Stop immediately if the wire is pinched by dilator tip and no longer moves freely in and out.
Be willing to stop, obtain diagnostic data, change approach, or abort altogether if the procedure is not going well.

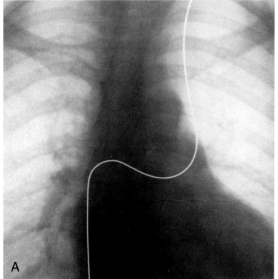

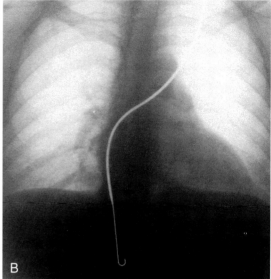

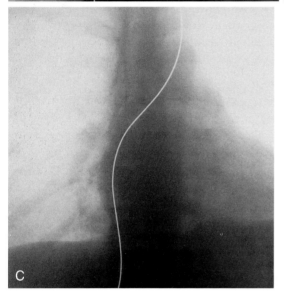

Figure 31–3. The S-curve phenomenon. **(A)** Shown from a left internal jugular approach, the guide wire follows an S-curve route to the right heart. The phenomenon is exaggerated by aortic ectasia and uncoiling. The wire is shown in the preferred location well down the IVC. A relatively stiff dilator or catheter advanced over this wire could preferentially perforate the left brachiocephalic vein rather than follow the S curve to the right heart. **(B)** A small flexible dilator or exchange catheter is passed over the wire first. The flexible catheter more safely negotiates the S curve. **(C)** A stiffer guide wire is then exchanged through the catheter, under fluoroscopic observation, to straighten the S curve. A stiffer dilator or introducer can then be safely advanced to the right heart from the left internal jugular approach. (Computer reconstructed and enhanced images.)

dilator passing downward over the wire is more likely to perforate the left innominate vein than it is to follow the wire to the right atrium. The solution is to substitute a wire that is stiffer than the dilator or introducer that must follow it. The stiffer wire, such as an Amplatz "super stiff" more safely directs the dilator, but it must not be used for the initial negotiation of the curve. After a flexible wire is used for the initial passage to the right heart and down the IVC, a flexible exchange catheter, or small vascular dilator, such as 6 or 8 F, is manipulated over the wire. That wire is then removed and the stiffer wire passed through the catheter or dilator. When a stiff wire is used to negotiate the S-curve phenomenon, there is a tendency to leave the final catheter position too short. After the wire and any sheath are removed, the vessels resume the S curve and the tip of a more flexible soft catheter is drawn into too high a position in the superior vena cava. It is advisable to intentionally place the catheter too long until the curve relaxes, then slowly and incrementally, under fluoroscopic control, withdraw the catheter into the correct position.

Pitfall: Costoclavicular Scissors

When a subclavian venipuncture is made at a point where the subclavian vein crosses the first rib, the catheter is tethered at that point, whereas entry into the vein more peripherally, so that the catheter is mobile within the lumen as it crosses the first rib, is preferable. When a catheter is tethered in the "scissors" between clavicle and first rib (Fig. 31–4), repeated trauma to the vein from movement of neck, shoulder, and thorax increases the risk of injury, fibrosis, and stenosis of the vein at this point, which can complicate future access, even eliminate the availability of the extremity completely. Furthermore, although catheter fracture is rare, it usually occurs at the "costoclavicular scissors," probably from the same mechanism: repeated flexing at a tethered point causing fatigue fracture and possible intravascular fragment embolization. Classic subclavian venipuncture techniques intentionally target this zone for vascular entry because the anatomy is fixed, predictable, and constant with respect to surface landmarks at this point. The only consistent way to avoid it is to enter the vein more peripherally where the landmarks are less constant using imaging techniques such as real-time ultrasound or to avoid the subclavian approach altogether.

Pitfall: The Tectonic Shift Phenomenon

Tectonic shift occurs primarily with subcutaneous ports, wherein movement of the port results in undesirable movement of the attached intravascular catheter (Fig. 31–5). Risk factors for this problem are (1) the subclavian approach, (2) a shallow subcutaneous port pocket, (3) women with abundant breast tissue in the infraclavicular fossa, and (4) obesity. The biomechanics of the tectonic shift depend on redundant soft tissue applied to the thorax which can move caudally (away from the subclavian puncture site) in response to gravity in the upright posture. If the port is placed within this tissue plane, it too moves caudally, and the catheter tip migrates peripherally. Suture attachment of the port to the pectoral fascia, while protecting the port from overlying tissue shift, may also render the port difficult or impossible to use because it cannot be palpated. Intentionally leaving the catheter too long (while in the operating room with the patient in the supine position) is not foolproof, because repeated up-and-down shifting tends to incrementally deliver a loop of cathe-

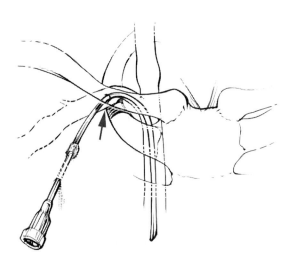

Figure 31–4. The costoclavicular scissors phenomenon. The entry into the subclavian vein is precisely at the crossing zone between the clavicle and first rib, tethering the catheter at this point. Repetitive motion of the arm, shoulder, and thorax can produce trauma to the vein at this point, resulting in sclerosis, complete occlusion, or, rarely, fracture of the catheter from repeated flexion.

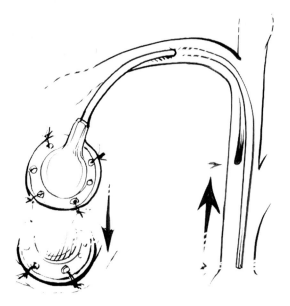

Figure 31–5. The tectonic shift phenomenon. If the catheter, its exit site, or subcutaneous port is attached to mobile tissue, the attached catheter, and thus the internal end, migrates outward with the patient in an upright posture. A device that looks perfectly placed in a supine position in the operating room may prove substantially too short on the upright chest film.

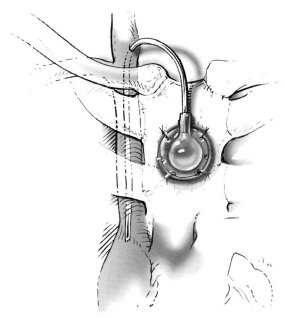

Figure 31–6. The midline position for a subcutaneous infusion port, with the port sutured to the pectoral fascia over the manubrium. This is an effective solution to the problem of tectonic shift because the pectoral fascia is quite immobile in this area, and the overlying soft tissues are relatively thin, facilitating palpation and access of the port. The catheter enters the right internal jugular vein.

ter out of the intravascular space, into the subcutaneous infraclavicular fossa. It may be helpful to place the port as close as possible to the clavicle in at-risk patients. It is also advisable, in any device that is tunnelled away from the entry site, to make an adequately deep subcutaneous enlargement of the entry site. Otherwise, the catheter becomes tethered to the dermis near the original puncture site and, no matter how securely the device is attached at the port or exit site, it still migrates out of the vessel because it is tethered to the dermis, which shifts away from the clavicle with change in posture. The best defense against the tectonic shift is probably to avoid the subclavian approach altogether, place the device from a jugular approach, and place exit site or port in the midline (Fig. 31–6). A subcutaneous port can be firmly attached to the pectoral fascia over the sternum where the device is both fixed in location and easily palpated. This location is preferred by many patients because of improved comfort, convenience, and cosmetics.

Pitfall: Variability of Jugular Anatomy

There are advantages of the internal jugular (IJ) approach for semipermanent vascular access, several of which are described in this section. Additional advantages include reduced pneumothorax risk, straighter course to the right heart, less difficulty with symptomatic venous obstruction, and, most important for the dialysis population, elimination of the long-term problem of subclavian stenosis or obstruction, which can interfere with future A-V access. When a temporary subclavian dialysis catheter is in place longer than 6 weeks, there is approximately a 30% risk that the ipsilateral extremity will be permanently excluded as a site for A-V access because of complete obstruction or significant stenosis of the subclavian vein. The most significant drawback to routine use of the jugular approach is that the orientation of the relevant anatomy with respect to surface landmarks is less reliable, making it a more "blind" procedure. For example, an anatomic survey of the relationship of IJ to ipsilateral common carotid artery showed that it lies in the expected anterolateral orientation only 70% of the time. It is directly overlying the carotid pulse 14% to 18% of the time and is occasionally even deep to the artery.

The solution to anatomic variability is the use of intraoperative ultrasound imaging. There are several advantages to the use of ultrasound in central venous access surgery (Table 31–3). It is a skill that requires some training and practice, but is easily within the capability of any motivated surgeon. It does require an initial capital outlay, but as an essentially noninvasive imaging technology, in-

Table 31–3. Value of Duplex Ultrasound in Central Line Placement

Perform preliminary diagnostic survey to select best approach.
Assess patency, continuity, course, valves.
Assess adequacy of size of central vein for intended catheter.
Identify anatomic anomalies and relationship to adjacent structures.
Determine best patient position and degree of Trendelenburg position.
Puncture under real-time observation.
Advance guide wire partially with real-time ultrasound; does not eliminate need for fluoroscopy.

cremental cost is its only disadvantage. The few minutes required for setup are offset by the time savings of reliable first-pass vascular entry. The amortization of the instrument itself is another issue, but that is at least partially offset by the savings in wasted catheter and guide wire sets from unsuccessful entry attempts. The ultimate major benefit to the patient is safety. Particularly with large-bore catheters (such as 18 F dialysis lines), it is helpful to survey the central veins first for adequate size for percutaneous placement; in marginal cases, it is still safer to perform a direct cutdown than to risk uncontrolled internal bleeding from trying to advance a large dilator through a small vein.

Pitfall: The Skew Plane Phenomenon

B-mode ultrasound imaging has its own pitfalls, but they are easily overcome if recognized. When real-time imaging is used for direct observation, a longitudinal image, along the course of the vein, is generally used. The "slice" width of the ultrasound image is only 2 to 3 mm thick in most instances, so if the needle is in a skew intersecting plane to that of the slice, only that portion of the needle traversing the plane is visualized, while the tip may be invisibly threatening an adjacent structure (Fig. 31–7). The phenomenon can only be avoided by keeping the needle precisely within the image plane throughout its course. Outrigger guides can be obtained for many ultrasound probes to facilitate this. Furthermore, the operator learns to recognize the characteristic ultrasound signature of the beveled needle tip.

Pitfall: The Systolic Fling Phenomenon

As shown in Figure 31–8, the anatomic configuration of the internal jugular vein is not always static. Its size, shape, and orientation change with Trendelenburg position and with head and neck rotation, and, in this case, with cardiac cycle. The tortuous common carotid artery displaces and effaces the IJ with each systole, such that even if the needle tip is rigidly held in the lumen of the vein (in diastole), the next systole punctures the artery, leading to hematoma formation or accidental

arterial entry. The phenomenon is easily recognized during real-time imaging. It can then be treated by changing the location or angle of venipuncture, or even by coordinating vascular entry with the cardiac cycle.

Pitfall: The Flattened Introducer

The flattened introducer is a problem encountered in the subclavian approach, more frequently on the right side, during the use of a tear-away sheath-type introducer. The introducer and accompanying dilator are passed intravascularly, but when the internally supporting dilator is withdrawn, the thin-walled introducer collapses or kinks from one of the following: angulation beneath the clavicle, angulation within a turn in the vessel, or both. The catheter to be installed then cannot be advanced through the flattened introducer. The common reaction to this problem is to try a larger introducer; however, a larger diameter thin-walled tube is more kink-prone than one of smaller diameter. Several other techniques may be more useful. Particularly if the angulation is outside the vascular space, typically between clavicle and first rib, it may be useful to dilate the tract one or two French sizes larger than the introducer (e.g., to 12 F for a 10 F introducer), then return to the smallest introducer that will pass the catheter. For intravascular angulation, occasionally success is achieved by fluoroscopically withdrawing the sheath to a minimum intravascular intrusion, although subsequent catheter passage may fail to make the same turn toward the right heart. The phenomenon can be ameliorated by puncturing further from the clavicle and more peripherally and more parallel to the vein; it can be avoided completely by using a jugular approach.

Postoperative and Predischarge Care

After (or during) recovery from any sedative medication, a plain chest film is obtained to exclude any complication, mostly pneumothorax, and document catheter position. Even when an ultrasound-directed jugular approach is used (all but eliminating any pneumothorax

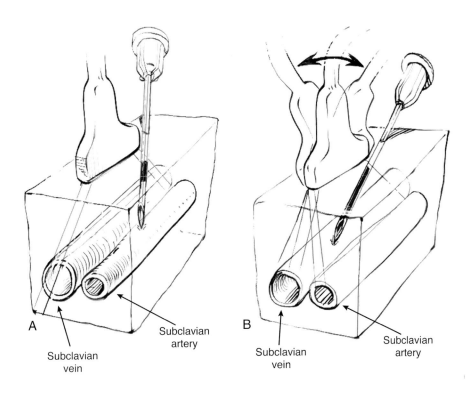

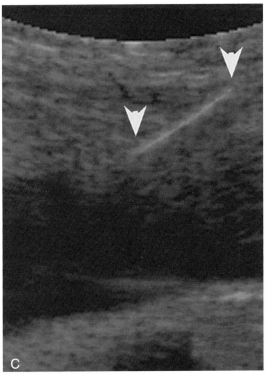

Figure 31–7. The skew plane phenomenon. **(A)** If the needle penetration is not in precisely the same plane as the ultrasound image, the shaft of the needle can appear to be approaching the target when the tip of the needle has actually passed out of the plane and may be invisibly threatening an adjacent structure. **(B)** When the entire needle remains within the ultrasound image plane, needle-tip penetration of the desired lumen can be observed. **(C)** Visualization of part of the needle shaft by ultrasound *(arrows)*, corresponding to the drawing in **A**, must be avoided.

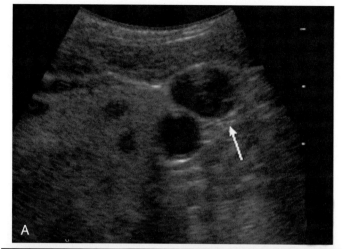
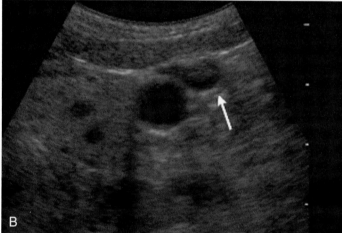

Figure 31–8. Transverse images of the left internal jugular vein *(arrow)* in diastole **(A)** and systole **(B)**. The common carotid artery displaces significantly anteriorly with each systole, compressing and effacing the internal jugular vein. A needle placed into the center of the vein during diastole, held rigidly in place, can puncture the artery and result in hematoma formation or inadvertent arterial entry. (Coincidental note is made of several small thyroid cysts.)

risk) and the catheter position is confirmed under fluoroscopy, it is essential to obtain, and personally examine, the radiographic confirmation.

Pitfall: Errant Catheter Course

Malposition of a catheter into a jugular vein or across the contralateral innominate vein is usually obvious, but other more subtle errors can also be picked up by careful evaluation of the film. In the case illustrated in Figure 31–9, it was several months following port placement before an intra-arterial placement was discovered. More careful scrutiny of the postoperative film should have identified the error sooner. (Intraoperative confirmation of guide wire passage to the right heart, not the descending aorta, should have identified the error.) Figure 31–10 illustrates a case in which a catheter functioned for chemotherapy infusion but not for blood withdrawal. The catheter tip appears to pass beyond the border of the SVC and, indeed, was wedged into the azygous vein. This problem usually occurs from a left subclavian approach when the catheter is left too short. It should have been recognized on the postoperative film.

Pitfall: Reverse Orientation of Dialysis Catheter

Central venous catheters must permit high blood flow rates, 300 mL/min or more, in each of two lumina and are thus less tolerant of minor imperfections in final position. In addition to the other pitfalls of central lines, the catheters with side-by-side offset lumina

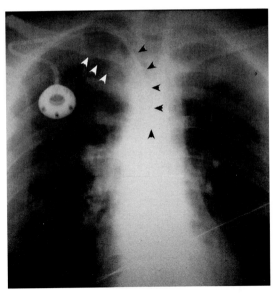

Figure 31–9. Arterial port placement. This port remained in place for 5 months before its arterial placement was recognized. The catheter does not pass through the window over the first rib, behind the clavicle, and anterior to scalenus anterior *(white arrows)* and the tip crosses the midline *(black arrows)*. It is also doubtful that an intraoperative fluoroscopic check confirmed the guide wire in the right heart.

are subject to the reverse orientation phenomenon. Blood is aspirated into the shorter "red" shoulder orifice and returned via the longer "blue" port. If the catheter lies against the atrial-caval junction, the long blue side should be oriented toward that side, so that the red port lies in the freest part of the vessel lumen (Fig. 31–11). Otherwise, with attempts at adequate flow aspiration, the red shoulder sucks up against the endothelial surface, obstructing the catheter. It is often useful to observe the position of the guide wire before catheter insertion. If the wire tends to lie against the medial side of the atrial-caval junction, it is likely that the catheter will do the same and should be oriented with the longer blue lumen in that direction.

Before concluding placement of a dialysis catheter, adequate flow tolerance in both lumina should be checked. The mere ability to aspirate blood is not sufficient, as it is for other central lines. However, the ability to quickly "flash" a full 10 mL into a syringe without hesitation or chatter is fairly good assurance of adequate position and orientation.

ARTERIOVENOUS ACCESS CREATION

Permanent hemodialysis access is usually achieved by creation of either an autologous or prosthetic A-V conduit. When an autologous fistula is planned, local anesthesia is adequate and discharge on an ambulatory same-day basis is routine. For insertion of a subcutaneously tunnelled PTFE graft in the upper extremity, an axillary block provides good anesthesia, and a single overnight stay may sometimes be necessary. In my experience, approximately two thirds of PTFE graft patients can be discharged the same day, a fraction that has progressively increased over several years. The conditions that must be met for discharge are adequate pain control (following resolution of any nerve block) and adequate extremity perfusion without excessive edema. Unless there is another specific concern or excessive comorbidity, the patient may be discharged whenever these conditions are met. An arrangement for individual accommodation of ambulatory discharge versus short inpatient stay, depending on a brief period of observation, is most useful and cost effective.

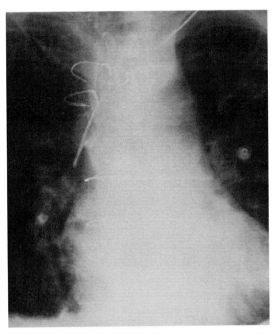

Figure 31–10. Postoperative chest film of a catheter that would not aspirate. On the film, the catheter appears to extend beyond the border of the superior vena cava. The catheter is wedged in the azygous vein.

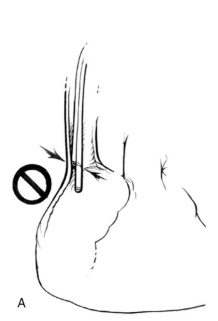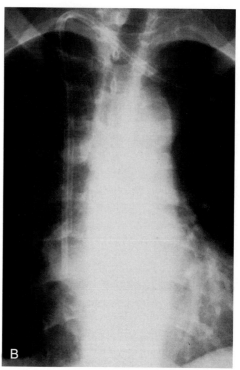

Figure 31–11. Double lumen central venous catheters for dialysis access must sustain fairly high flow rates. If an "offset lumen" catheter, such as the one illustrated, tends to lie along one side of the atrial-caval junction, the shorter red port should be oriented toward the center of the lumen of the superior vena cava (SVC). **A,** If the red port is toward the caval sidewall, it tends to occlude with increasing flow rates, preventing effective dialysis. **B,** The red port is oriented toward the freest part of the atrial-caval junction, permitting better flow rates. The tunnel to the entry site into the vein (in both *A* and *B*) is shown coming from the patient's left, which often tends to direct the catheter along the right side of the SVC. This is not an entirely predictable phenomenon, and reversal of the orientation under fluoroscopy may be required.

This strategy is increasingly being used for many ambulatory procedures.

Pitfall: Inadequate Venous Conduit for Fistula

A Brescia-Cimino fistula or similar arterialized cephalic vein conduit is an excellent first choice for permanent dialysis access. The anesthetic impact is less, and postoperative morbidity is usually minimal. However, the commonly held belief that it has better long-term patency than a prosthetic PTFE conduit has been disproven in several series. Even though autologous dialysis conduits appear to have lower maintenance requirements (and cost) while in use, a cohort of fistula patients does not appear to enjoy longer secondary patency, on average, than a PTFE conduit cohort. The single greatest factor lowering the average fistula long-term patency is inclusion of those that

never developed adequate size or flow to be usable (i.e., long-term patency of zero). The frustrating situation of a fistula that is a technical success (remains patent) yet a practical failure (not useful for dialysis) usually stems from use of an inadequate venous conduit. Because the advantage of an autologous fistula over a prosthetic graft is marginal at best, there is no compelling reason to construct a fistula using a marginal or inadequate cephalic vein. A vein smaller than 3 mm is unlikely to develop adequately. The fistula itself, the A-V anastomosis, is not used for dialysis access; rather, the venous conduit leading away from the fistula is the crucial area to examine preoperatively for adequacy. The determination of vascular adequacy, both arterial and venous, should be made preoperatively; attempting to decide on an autologous conduit after arrival in the operating room is notoriously inaccurate.

Pitfall: Inadequate Long-Range Planning

The prosthetic PTFE dialysis conduit has good early reliability, generally approximately 1 year of primary patency and 4 to 6 years of useful secondary patency. None of these vascular grafts, however, when subjected to intentional repeated violation and trauma, lasts forever. Therefore, for each patient a contingency plan should be developed for access salvage when the conduit fails and for the next new access when the conduit is no longer salvageable. It is shortsighted, for example, to place an A-V access in a location that precludes future options in the same extremity, especially in the younger patient. Because venous intimal hyperplasia is the most common final pathway of graft failure, it is advisable to begin as peripheral as possible, so that subsequent revision or replacement can progress central to the venous obstruction. In contrast, if an A-V graft is placed initially in the upper arm (brachial artery above the elbow to the brachial/axillary vein), the development of intimal hyperplasia in the axillary vein will likely preclude any subsequent A-V access in that extremity. I recommend a forearm loop (brachial artery bifurcation to either brachial or antecubital vein) in the nondominant extremity first if an autologous fistula is not possible, with subsequent revisions and replacements in the same extremity being possible for as long as is feasible. Using this strategy, a revision to a more central vein and eventually a de novo upper arm conduit are still possible. I rarely use the forearm straight graft (radial artery to antecubital vein) because it has less usable length of conduit, uses the same venous outflow as a loop, and is more likely to have inadequate arterial inflow.

Pitfall: Incorrectly Fashioned Anastomosis

The importance of proper technique to avoid narrowing of a vascular anastomosis is ubiquitous in vascular surgery, but it is of particular technical importance in the A-V graft, especially at the venous end where stenosis on the native side of the anastomosis quickly becomes critical. Figure 31–12 shows the subtle but critical effect of a pointed "toe" on an end-to-side anastomosis. Even perfectly placed sutures must occupy some margin of both ves-

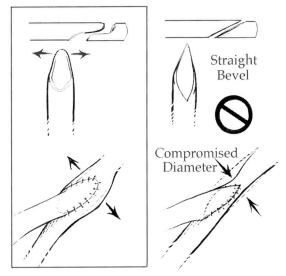

Figure 31–12. The proper technique for graft fashioning for an end-to-side anastomosis. The correct "cobra head" configuration requires that the graft be cut in an S curve, which terminates perpendicular to the graft at the heel and toe, so that there is a patch effect that widens the native vessel. If the graft is cut to a sharp point, it is very difficult to avoid an "hourglass" stenosis at the toe. This is particularly important in A-V access grafts in which intimal hyperplasia at the venous end is accelerated by any degree of iatrogenic stenosis.

sel and graft. Along the sides of the anastomosis, this creates no problem because the graft hood creates a patch effect, resulting in a larger luminal diameter than the unopened vessel. If the graft is fashioned with an angled or pointed toe rather than the recommended "cobra head" configuration, however, some luminal narrowing at the toe is inevitable. The cobra-head graft end, with a flat toe of sufficient width to encompass at least three sutures, that is, at least one on either side of center, permits the patch effect of the graft to widen rather than narrow the toe of the anastomosis. The same principle applies to the heel.

Pitfall: Using Arteriovenous Access Too Soon

Both autologous and prosthetic A-V fistulas serve the patient better and longer if not used immediately, although the reason for the delay is different in the two circumstances. Following an autologous fistula, the usable venous conduit increases in size and flow rate over several weeks. The delay of several weeks is advisable to avoid irreversible traumatic injury to the vein by laceration of a relatively small vein with a large needle. In the case of the prosthetic conduit, the dimension of the graft is constant from the beginning. The delay of 4 to 6 weeks permits tissue encapsulation of the graft so that, following removal of needles, there is improved hemostasis and reduced risk of tunnel hematoma formation, which can threaten the longevity of the graft by further interfering with tissue ingrowth into the graft surface. Thus, although the postoperative delay is similar in the two circumstances, the first use of a prosthetic graft is determined by the calendar; the usability of the autologous fistula is best determined by examination of the patient. When the vein is quite large preoperatively, little delay is necessary.

There are modified PTFE conduits marketed for their ability to be used earlier postoperatively for dialysis access. The material is designed to be more hemostatic for needle sticks, thus possibly obviating the need for delay, without risking complications from needle pulls. Although this is an appealing concept, studies have not yet shown superiority of the modified conduits, and concerns have been raised regarding increased complication rates and decreased long-term patency.

SALVAGE OF FAILED ARTERIOVENOUS ACCESS

Restoration of patency in clotted A-V access is conceptually simple, but there are actually three objectives when faced with the failed fistula: (1) restore flow, (2) determine and correct the underlying cause of failure, and (3) avoid the use of temporary access. There are surgical and nonsurgical techniques for both the thrombectomy and the correction and modification stages, and thus also numerous permutations possible for access restoration strategies.

Restoring patency can be accomplished by surgical thrombectomy under local anesthesia or by interventional radiology. Both have good efficacy for restoration of flow. I prefer surgical thrombectomy for reasons of cost, time, and safety. Surgical thrombectomy is safely conducted on an ambulatory outpatient basis, al-

though the timing of surgery may require coordination with vascular radiology personnel.

The vascular radiologist can also restore graft patency without surgery, using either thrombolytic therapy or a thromboemulsification catheter. Interventional thrombolysis may be preferable to surgical thrombectomy for real-time observed acute thrombosis, partial thrombosis, or autologous venous conduits that may respond better to thrombolysis than thrombectomy. The radiologic approach also has the intellectual appeal of immediate availability for performance of diagnostic angiography.

Pitfall: Inadequate Diagnosis of Access Failure

Correcting the underlying cause of access thrombosis, the second phase of access resuscitation, is crucial to long-term success. There is an underlying condition in almost all instances of graft thrombosis, thus thrombectomy alone is usually not a durable solution. During thrombectomy, it is often possible to determine the likely problem, and stenosis at the venous anastomosis is the most common cause. In 15% to 20% of cases, there is a different or, more commonly, an additional lesion from that predicted intraoperatively. Figure 31–13 illustrates such a case. There is an unexpected tight subclavian vein stenosis in tandem with the expected outflow stenosis. For this reason, I do not recommend correction of the presumed lesion without complete angiographic imaging. Unless the operating suite is equipped with dedicated digital contrast imaging capability, postoperative transfer to the angiography suite is necessary within a fairly short period, before graft rethrombosis. Interventional balloon angioplasty then becomes a good alternative to surgical repair or bypass of stenoses. The only study to randomize between surgical repair and interventional angioplasty showed moderately better patency with balloon angioplasty, and I have had approximately 70% 1-year salvage patency using this strategy. If a stenosis recurs rapidly after transluminal angioplasty or if an occlusion cannot be ballooned, then direct surgical repair is required. Jump grafting to an unobstructed vein, usually more centrally, generally

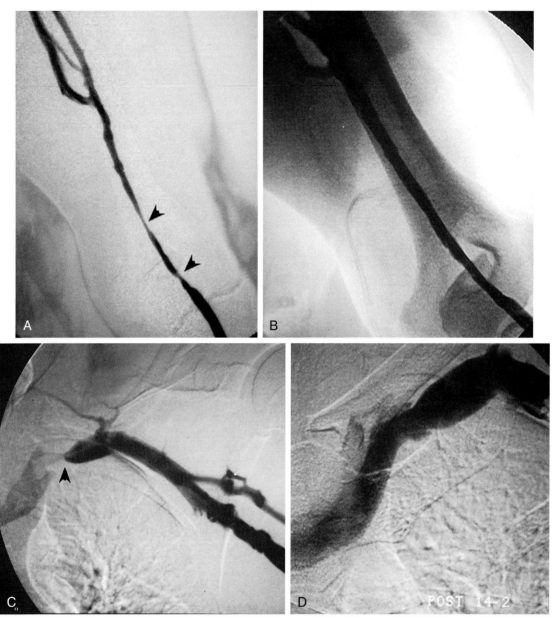

Figure 31–13. The value of complete angiographic surveillance before correction of a distressed A-V graft. **(A)** There is a tight stenosis at the venous end of the A-V graft. This lesion was accurately predicted at the time of surgical thrombectomy. **(B)** The lesion in *A* responded well to balloon angioplasty. **(C)** There was an unexpected second critical lesion, a tight stenosis in the subclavian vein. **(D)** This second lesion, unexpected at the time of surgical thrombectomy, was also treated with balloon angioplasty. Treatment of the anastomotic stenosis alone, at the time of original surgery, would probably result in early refailure because of the missed tandem lesion.

has better long-term success than patch angioplasty.

Effective coordination and communication between nephrologist, surgeon, and vascular radiologist are necessary for optimal salvage of the failed vascular access.

Selected Readings

1. Beathard GA. Mechanical vs. pharmacomechanical thrombolysis for the treatment of thrombosed dialysis access grafts. Kidney Int 1994;45(5):1401–1406.
2. Bleyer AJ, Rosso MV, Burkart JM. The cost of hospitalizations due to hemodialysis access management. Nephrol News Issues January 1995:19–22.
3. Brescia MJ, Cimino JE, Appel K, Hurwich BJ. Chronic hemodialysis using venipuncture and a surgically created arteriovenous fistula. N Engl J Med 1966;275:1089–1092.
4. Dapunt O, Feurstein M, Rendl KH, Prenner K. Transluminal angioplasty vs. conventional operation in the treatment of haemodialysis fistula stenosis: results from a five-year study. Br J Surg 1987;74:104–105.
5. Dickson CS, Roth SM, Russell JM, et al. Placement of internal jugular veins central venous catheters: anatomic ultrasound assessment and literature review. Surg Rounds 1996;19(3):102–107.
6. Didlake R, Curry E, Bower J. Composite dialysis access grafts. J Am Coll Surg 1994;178(1):24–28.
7. Katz SG, Kohl RD. The percutaneous treatment of angioaccess graft complications. Am J Surg 1995; 170:238–242.
8. Leapman SB, Boyle M, Pescovitz MD, et al. The arterial venous fistula for hemodialysis access: gold standard or archaic relic? Am Surg 1996;62(8):652–657.
9. Lohr JM, James KV, Hearn AT, Ogden SA. Lessons learned from the DIASTAT vascular access graft. Am J Surg 1996;172:205–209.
10. Palder SB, Kirkman RL, Whittemore AD, et al. Vascular access for hemodialysis: patency rates and results of revision. Ann Surg 1986;202(5):235–239.
11. Roberts AC, Valji K, Bookstein JJ, Hye RJ. Pulse-spray pharmacomechanical thrombolysis for treatment of thrombosed dialysis access grafts. Am J Surg 1993; 166(2):221–225.
12. USRDS 1995 Annual Data Report. Chapter X. The cost-effectiveness of alternative types of vascular access and the economic cost of ESRD. Am J Kidney Dis 1995;28(3):S1–S166.
13. Vanherweghem JL, Yassine T, Goldman M, et al. Subclavian vein thrombosis: a frequent complication of subclavian vein cannulation for hemodialysis. Clin Nephrol 1986;26(5):235–238.

32

Venous Diseases

Jonathan P. Gertler

Venous disease has many manifestations ranging from the significant disability and life-threatening aspects of deep venous thrombosis to the benign aesthetic concerns of individuals afflicted with minor varicose veins. Yet, treatment of the latter is predicated on as thorough an understanding of the pathophysiology of venous hemodynamics as is treatment of the former. Misunderstanding of physical findings and noninvasive venous testing can seriously hinder the ability to achieve excellent results.

The diagnoses most commonly encountered in the outpatient setting are superficial varicose veins with or without superficial phlebitis, venous insufficiency without associated deep venous thrombosis, and postphlebitic syndrome. The management issues that these problems pose range from prophylactic measures against ulcer formation to optimal means of improving the cosmetic appearance and physical discomfort associated with superficial varicosities. This chapter reviews the pathophysiology of these diseases, appropriate physical examination and laboratory diagnostic maneuvers, and optimal treatment in the outpatient setting.

PATHOPHYSIOLOGY OF VENOUS INSUFFICIENCY

The venous system of the lower extremity is divided into deep, superficial, and perforating veins. The vast majority of blood is carried back to the central circulation by the deep veins in a passive fashion. The deep veins are contained within the fascia investing the leg musculature and are emptied by action of the muscular pump. Valves prevent reversal of flow due to the hydrostatic pressure that the upright human brings to bear on the lower extremities. Without these valves, the hypostatic force at the lowest part of the legs would exceed 100 mm Hg. Venous insufficiency in the deep venous system occurs when the calf muscle pump and the valvular prevention of reflux fail to work. This may be caused by primary valve failure, or it may be due to venous thrombosis causing redistribution of pressure to remaining veins or destruction of valve apposition after recanalization of the affected veins.

The superficial venous system is composed of the greater and lesser saphenous systems. These veins run in the subcutaneous portion of the leg and do not have the benefit of the calf musculature to serve as a peripheral pump. The veins in the superficial compartments are more elastic than the deeper veins, perhaps acting as an aid to venous return; however, intact valve function remains the primary method of preventing reflux and deterioration.

Bridging the fascia separating the superficial and deep veins are the perforating veins. These veins are numerous and usually of little clinical consequence. Primary valvular incompetence occasionally occurs. However, in the setting of deep valvular incompetence for any reason, the perforating veins assume a greater volume of blood flow and subsequently may develop incompetent valves as well. In this scenario, the significant deep venous pressure is transmitted to the superficial veins, which, in turn, become distended and are rendered incompetent with regard to proper valvular function.

Recent work by several groups has emphasized the importance of the calf muscle pump in contrast to the standard interpretations of venous hypertension and ulcer formation as a passive phenomenon. In the current concept, the calf muscle pump is likened to a heart. Venous insufficiency with nonobliterated channels is similar to a dilated heart with preserved ejection fraction, the "preload" in this case being due to enlarged venous capacitance because of overfilled veins in either the superficial or deep system. In the patient with postphlebitic syndrome in which destruction of the outflow capacity predominates, "afterload" increase diminishes the efficacy of the calf pump, with excessive preload due to venous insufficiency being an exacerbating factor. The chronic venous hypertension that ensues leads to fluid extravasation, fibrin deposition, lipodermatosclerosis, and ultimately ulcer formation.

The challenge for the surgeon is differentiating the relative impact of these three contributing venous systems on each case of venous disease. Physical examination can reveal a great deal, and information may be supplemented by noninvasive testing. The latter, in recent years, has increased in sophistication due to the addition of duplex scanning and air plethysmography. For the diagnoses and treatments considered in this chapter, invasive testing of the venous system usually is unnecessary.

HISTORY AND PHYSICAL EXAMINATION

Symptoms of venous disease can range from aesthetic awareness to tissue loss, depending on the severity of hemodynamic abnormalities and the anatomic system involved. Superficial varicosities are rarely associated with skin changes, tissue discoloration, edema, or ulceration. In severe cases, superficial varicosities can be associated with ulceration if the calf muscle pump function is sufficiently defective.

The onset of venous insufficiency findings should be carefully noted and related to any periods of immobility, trauma, pregnancy, or episodes that might represent undiagnosed deep venous involvement. The identification of these more commonly deep venous symptoms should lead the examiner to precisely define the deep and perforating system hemodynamics.

Any history of phlebitic changes in the superficial system should be recorded as should a family history suggestive of an inherited hypercoagulable state. The latter usually is seen as venous rather than arterial thrombosis and manifests in the second to fourth decades of life. Sensations of fullness or discomfort after exercise or long periods of standing are common in both superficial and deep venous disorders. True venous claudication, the onset of significant leg fatigue after exercise, is suggestive of deep venous insufficiency. Finally, any history of previous interventions—surgical therapy, sclerotherapy, or conservative therapy—and the patient's previous compliance with and relief from a compressive dressing regimen or support stockings are important.

On physical examination, the pattern of disease should be carefully noted. Careful mapping of externally identifiable varicosities, measurement of calf and thigh girths, and inspection of the skin of the lower leg to identify discoloration, lipodermatosclerosis, and nascent or erupted ulceration help differentiate deep, perforator, and superficial problems. The approved categorization for chronic venous insufficiency is detailed in Table 32–1. The presence of bony or soft-tissue abnormalities can alert the examiner to congenital problems of venous drainage, lymphatic abnormalities, arteriovenous malformations, or structural tumors extrinsically blocking venous drainage. These scenarios are all uncommon. Attention should be paid to pulse status because arterial insufficiency can occasionally hinder the healing of venous ulcers. When the leg is swollen, pulses may be difficult to feel. There should be no hesitation in documenting arterial perfusion with arterial noninvasive testing. Similarly, chronic infection, especially in immunocompromised patients, may contribute to poor healing as much as hemodynamic issues, and culture of the involved area can reveal significant pathogens. Finally, ulceration can be due to skin malignancy such as squamous cell carcinoma and can be treated inappropriately as venous in origin. The presence of any refractory ulcer that does not re-

Table 32–1. Classification of Chronic Venous Insufficiency

Class	Current Symptoms	Prior Symptoms	Anatomic Location	Origin
0	None	Same	Unknown	Unknown
1	Mild	Same	Superficial veins	Congenital
2	Moderate	Same	Perforators	Postthrombotic
3	Severe (ulceration)	Same	Deep calf	
			Deep thigh	
			Deep iliofemoral	
			Deep caval combination	

From Porter J, Rutherford R, Clagett GP, et al: Reporting standards in venous disease. J Vasc Surgery 1988;8:172–181.

spond in part to simple topical dressings combined with external compression, such as with an Ace wrap or Unna's boot, should alert the examiner to malignant possibilities.

The use of the Trendelenburg test is helpful and provides similar information to venous noninvasive testing. Tourniquets are applied at the saphenofemoral junction and at the knee level after the leg has been elevated and fully depleted of as much venous blood as possible. The leg is returned to dependent position, usually with the patient standing, and the lower and upper tourniquets are removed sequentially. Filling of the veins before tourniquets are removed implies deep or perforator incompetence, whereas filling of the lesser saphenous vessels after the lower tourniquet is removed implies isolated lesser saphenous incompetence. Filling of the saphenous vessels after the upper tourniquet is removed implies saphenofemoral junction valvular incompetence. Variations, including the use of additional tourniquets at the ankle and above knee level, to more precisely identify the level of perforator incompetence have also been espoused.

NONINVASIVE VENOUS VASCULAR LABORATORY TESTING

Noninvasive testing is not routinely ordered in all patients undergoing varicose vein excision procedures but is advisable for several categories of patients. Patients who lack history suggestive of deep venous thrombosis, with no physical evidence of deep venous or perforator incompetence, and with either aesthetic concerns only or complaints referable to a distribution of superficial varicose veins may proceed directly to surgical treatment or sclerotherapy as long as the Trendelenburg test is normal. Patients with evidence of deep venous abnormalities (excluding those with acute deep vein thrombosis) are well served by a baseline hemodynamic assessment of the deep venous system. Because limb hemodynamics can change with recanalization of obliterated pathways and formation of collaterals, the long-term therapy of patients with venous hypertension due to deep system abnormalities can be guided by noninvasive patterns.

Traditionally, the two tests used were photoplethysmography (PPG) and triplex examination of the deep veins. Air plethysmography has gained increasing acceptance, both as a diagnostic measure and as a means of elucidating the pathophysiology of the process.

The basis of PPG is that venous refilling after exercise-induced emptying of the leg is accelerated in the presence of valvular incompetence. Compression of the offending systems of veins should eradicate the accelerated refilling time. The test is performed by placing a PPG sensor on the medial aspect of the patient's leg followed by plantar and dorsal flexion of the subject's foot five times. The limb is relaxed and the time to plateauing of the curve is noted. If the venous refilling time (VRT), in triplicate, is greater than 25 seconds, the test is terminated and interpreted as normal. When the VRT is less than 25 seconds, the test is repeated sequentially with a tourniquet placed on the thigh at 40 mm Hg to exclude saphenous incompetence and an external pneumatic compression (EPC) boot placed at the ankle. If either of these maneuvers normalizes the VRT, the test is terminated. Interpretation rests with either saphenous incompetence (thigh tourniquet normalization), perforator incompetence (EPC normalization), or incompetence in both systems. PPG is a qualitative test, however, that is being supplanted and replaced by air plethysmography.

Air plethysmography is a recently designed noninvasive test that differentiates the type of venous incompetence present and quantitates the degree of venous insufficiency. As it became clearer that the degree of reflux rather than the site of reflux predicted ulceration and venous insufficiency symptoms, air plethysmography assumed a more prominent role in venous noninvasive testing.

In this procedure, the entire calf is fitted in a long tubular air chamber that is inflated to 6 mm Hg and connected to a pressure transducer, amplifier, and recorder. Measurements are made after emptying the leg of blood by elevation and allowing a time period for temperature equilibration (room temperature) and arterial flow stabilization.

The patient then stands on the opposite leg while pressure is transduced in the measured leg until a plateau is reached. The increase from baseline to plateau is the functional venous volume (VV). The time to reach 90% of VV is referred to as venous filling time 90 (VFT90). The venous filling index (VFI) = 90% VV/VFT90 and expresses in milliliters per second the average rate of venous filling. The test is repeated with a tourniquet at the knee level to occlude the superficial venous system.

As techniques for venous valve repair evolve, it becomes crucial to differentiate those individuals with superficial varicosities as the source of edema and progressive chronic venous changes from those whose varicosities are secondary to significant deep venous reflux or insufficiency. Table 32–2 summarizes data from work done by Christopoulos and Nicolaides differentiating these patients by VFI.

The ejection fraction (EF) of the calf muscle pump has been calculated using a similar technique and has been used to identify further those patients with reflux who are particularly prone to ulceration. The EF is calculated by having the subject perform one toe stand, with the change in calf volume recorded as ejection volume (EV). The EF = EV/VV × 100. Using this technique, it was determined that, for a similar index of reflux as measured by VFI, an EF of less than 40% was associated with a greater incidence of ulceration. However, recent investigations have suggested that duplex examination should be included in venous assessment to maximize sensitivity and specificity for these patients.

Duplex examination, simultaneous ultrasonic imaging and Doppler insonation are the mainstay of the noninvasive diagnosis of venous disease in both the acute and chronic setting. The entire venous tree can be visualized, and the quality of Doppler signals (e.g., spontaneous, phasic, augmented, competence of valves) can be assessed. Vein wall characteristics and compressibility are cardinal signs to observe when acute occlusion is suspected. Calf vein assessment is much more difficult and less reliable than assessment of the upper structures in either acute thrombosis or chronic insufficiency.

For functional evaluation of venous hemodynamics, as opposed to the diagnosis of acute venous thrombosis, duplex examination must be carried out in combination with rapid cuff inflation at the thigh, calf, and foot levels as

Table 32–2. Venous Filling Index

PVV and PVV/S			Popliteal Reflux	
VFI (mL/sec)	Chronic Swelling (%)	Ulcer (%)	Chronic Swelling (%)	Ulcer (%)
<3	0	0	—	—
3–5	12.5	0	—	—
5–10	42	38	57	49
>10	71	68	70	76

PVV = primary varicose veins; S = with swelling.

well as evaluation of outflow obstruction at the level of the calf. By visualizing reflux at these points, in combination with outflow assessment and identification of significant perforators around the knee, investigators have provided a more complete evaluation of the leg with venous insufficiency and a more sensitive predictor of those limbs prone to ulceration and severe stasis changes.

Routine ascending and descending venography is used rarely for patients with venous problems that are able to be cared for in the ambulatory setting. Although many efforts are being made to devise reconstructions for deep venous incompetence, these must still be viewed as evolving. The frequent adjunctive need for anticoagulation and the absolute need for proper postoperative follow-up and hemodynamic assessment of results should preclude these procedures from being performed in a casual fashion. The occasional patient with isolated perforator incompetence or refractory ulceration due to deep and perforator incompetence may be well served by exact venographic identification of the perforating veins contributing to the high-pressure zone in an ulcer crater (Fig. 32–1). However, most of these patients also have wound care and immobilization issues that preclude outpatient procedures.

SURGERY FOR VARICOSE VEINS IN AN OUTPATIENT SETTING

Numerous techniques have been espoused for the primary therapy of varicose veins. The issues related to varicose vein treatment are reduction of symptoms, prevention of stasis changes, and relief of aesthetic concerns. The primary patient complaint and the anatomic distribution of the varicosities dictate the most effective therapy. This section describes the approaches and outcomes in each of these settings.

Varicose veins of the superficial system can be divided into several categories. There are patients with primary saphenofemoral junction reflux with primary greater saphenous vein hypertension, tortuousity, and varicose degeneration, possibly accompanied by varicosities in branch groups. There are patients with

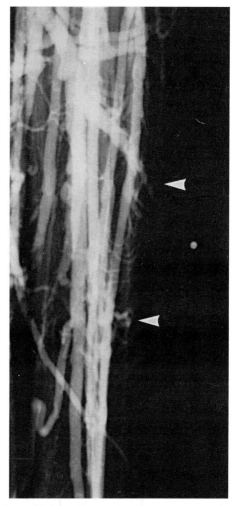

Figure 32–1. Perforators in area of a venous ulcer. A metallic BB marks the site of the ulcer. White arrows mark perforating veins penetrating near the ulcer.

greater saphenofemoral junction reflux but no noticeable abnormalities in the greater saphenous vein main trunk with extensive branch varicosities emanating from the greater saphenous vein or from its perforators at multiple levels. Lastly, there are patients without any evidence of main trunk reflux but with branch varicosities due to incompetent valves at the level of the accessory branch veins. These three conditions should be treated in markedly different ways (Fig. 32–2).

The issues facing the surgeon in the treatment of varicose vein problems stem from several considerations. Immediate cosmetic and symptom result must be balanced against long-term recurrence rate, potential complications

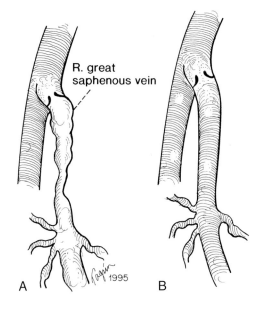

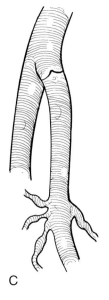

Figure 32–2. (A) Incompetent saphenofemoral junction with dilated greater saphenous vein and branch varicosities. (B) Incompetent saphenofemoral junction with normal-caliber spaphenous vein and branch varicosities. (C) Competent saphenofemoral junction with branch varicosities.

from surgery, and the potential need later in life for the greater saphenous vein as a conduit for coronary or lower extremity bypass surgery.

Greater Saphenous Vein Stripping and Ligation With Removal of Branch Varicosities

Greater saphenous vein stripping and ligation with removal of branch varicosities is a technique that mandates complete separation of the saphenofemoral junction and stripping of the long saphenous trunk, either from ankle to groin or from just below the knee to the groin (Fig. 32–3). The emphasis is placed on complete division of all saphenofemoral junction branches and tributaries because, if these are left in place, they are associated with recurrent varicosities both in the region of the groin and further down the leg. Stripping from groin to calf versus groin to ankle remains controversial; however, it is clear that the incidence of saphenous nerve injury is markedly increased when the ankle to calf saphenous vein is removed. In addition, the lower portion of the saphenous vein is infrequently varicose and, therefore, removal to midcalf only may be advantageous in preventing saphenous nerve injury and in preserving a conduit for later use if bypass is

necessary. In addition to the stripping of the greater saphenous vein and complete separation of the saphenofemoral junction, multiple stab avulsions for branch varicosities are necessary both to achieve a proper cosmetic and functional result.

Greater Saphenous Vein High Ligation and Stab Avulsion or Ligation of Varicosities

Greater saphenous vein high ligation and stab avulsion or ligation of varicosities is a technique that is predicated on the observation that ligation of the saphenofemoral junction prevents the reflux associated with valvular abnormalities at this level while preserving the main trunk of the saphenous vein (Fig. 32–4). This is not useful as a technique in the setting of severe greater saphenous trunk varicosities, but, in patients in whom reflux of the greater saphenous vein and common femoral junction is seen on preoperative evaluation and in whom multiple branch varicosities exist, proponents believe that high ligation prevents further deterioration and minimizes recurrence rates. The greater saphenous vein–common femoral junction is again skeletonized, with care taken to ligate all tributaries, and the ligatures are placed just at the junction of the greater saphenous and com-

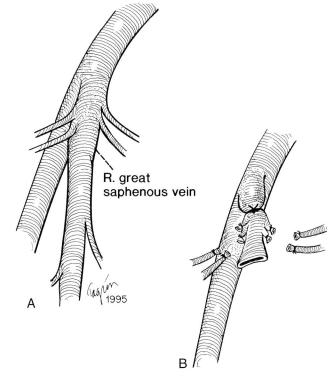

Figure 32–3. Technique for complete saphenofemoral disconnection for either high ligation or stripping used in conjunction with stab avulsion or berry picking approach.

R. great
saphenous vein

A

B

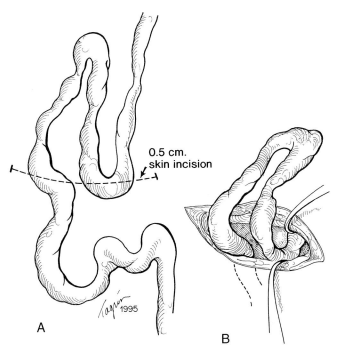

0.5 cm.
skin incision

Figure 32–4. Technique for dissection of branch varicosities through a stab incision approach.

A

B

mon femoral veins. This can be done through a small transverse groin incision under local anesthesia, and branch varicosities can be dealt with either by stab avulsion technique or with sclerotherapy.

Isolated Varicose Vein Excision (Berry Picking)

Isolated varicose vein excision is a technique that is reserved for patients without significant greater saphenous vein abnormalities. Patients with isolated varicosities not involving the saphenofemoral junction in the main saphenous trunk may have these varicosities either treated with sclerotherapy or excision. Although excellent results have been associated with sclerotherapy, it is clear that the larger the vein, the higher the chance of postinjection thrombophlebitis. In addition, due to the need for 4 to 6 weeks of compression therapy for large varicose veins, many patients tolerate stab avulsion techniques, which can be done on an outpatient basis using repetitive injections and long-term compressive therapy. The technique for local excision of varicose veins involves very small incisions over the previously marked varicose veins. The veins are isolated between snaps and, with appropriate traction and countertraction on the skin, can be teased out from surrounding subcutaneous investing tissue. Perforating branches extending deep into the leg may be ligated with 3-0 or 4-0 chromic ties, which produce little postoperative reactivity. The branches that may not be reached through the small stab incisions may be dissected out continually until they are avulsed at their perforating level, with compression held for just a few moments while the patient is in Trendelenburg position. This achieves hemostasis readily and veins are completely extirpated in this fashion, with any residual veins slated for sclerotherapy. It is essential that excellent compressive therapy be used postoperatively for 1 week to minimize hematoma formation and to improve cosmetic appearance of the leg. Closure for this technique may be simple interrupted subcuticular sutures of 5-0 absorbable suture with Steri-Strips and compressive dressings applied (Fig. 32–5).

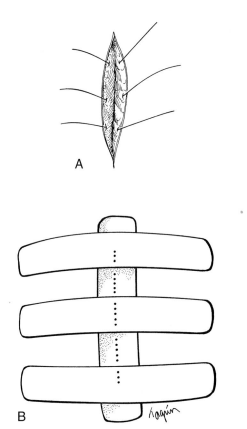

Figure 32–5. Subcuticular closure for stab incision. (**A**) Subarticular layer of 5-0 absorbable suture; (**B**) Steri-Strips approximate the epidermis.

Technique for Sclerotherapy

Sclerotherapy (Fig. 32–6) has been advocated as a panacea for varicose veins; however, the best result appears to be achieved when it is used for appropriately small reticular veins rather than for extensive varicosities, which include greater saphenous degenerative changes. The technique of sclerotherapy that I practice is done in the outpatient office setting. The patient stands for several minutes until the varicosities reach their maximum dimension. Butterfly needles (25 gauge) or 30-gauge straight needles are inserted into the varicosities and the vein is allowed to backbleed into the butterfly, which is then taped in place in the leg. Each session is usually limited to three vein injections. The patient then assumes a supine position and elevates the leg. A 1-mL tuberculin syringe with 0.25 mL of air and 0.75 mL of sclerosing solution, either hypertonic saline or 1% sodium tetradecyl sulfate injection, is prepared. With the patient's leg elevated and the vein emptied, the inferior portion of the vein is compressed to prevent continued flow into the vein, and the air is gently injected. This clears the vein and minimizes staining before the sclerosing solution is injected. Immediately upon injection, if extravasation is observed, the needle should be withdrawn and the vein compressed. In the absence of extravasation, the injection is completed with the vein blanched, then a compressive dressing is placed over the vein. After completion of the session of vein injections, the leg is bandaged and Ace wrapped. For small veins, 1 week of Ace wrapping is sufficient to achieve an appropriate cosmetic

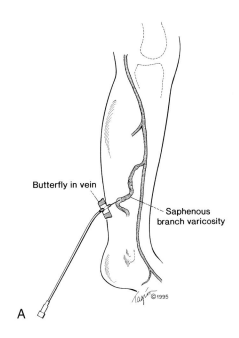

Figure 32–6. **(A)** Insertion of butterfly needle into branch varicosity. **(B)** Injection of agent with leg compressed and clearing of vein with small amount of air before sclerosing agent is introduced.

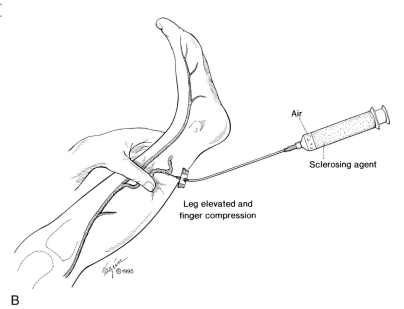

result. The patient should be advised that staining, superficial thrombophlebitis, and excoriations from extravasation may occur, although all these events are rare.

Venous Valve Banding

Recently, because of the interest in preserving a saphenous vein for later use in cardiovascular reconstructions, saphenofemoral banding valvuloplasty has been proposed and studied. The vein is appropriate for this procedure when the main axial portion is grossly normal without dilatation or tortuousity as determined by physical examination, palpation, and ultrasonic imaging. The approach to valvuloplasty is similar to that of high ligation in that dissection and division of the uppermost branches of the saphenofemoral junction are necessary. The uppermost valve, after 3 to 4 cm of saphenous vein is mobilized, is reinforced with a Dacron-reinforced silicone cuff. The cuff functions by narrowing the portion of the saphenous vein in which the incompetent valve is present, thereby bringing the valve leaflets into apposition. The vein is determined as competent by milking blood from the distal into the proximal segment of the vein, with release of the proximal segment and demonstration that no backfilling occurs with compression distally.

RESULTS OF CURRENT APPROACHES TO SUPERFICIAL VENOUS DISEASE

The issues facing the surgeon in treating varicosities of the lower extremity are primarily related to recurrence of varicosities, relief of symptoms or tissue changes, potential for injury to the saphenous nerve, and cosmetic results. Although the data are increasingly clear on the impact of different procedures on these endpoints, the endpoints that are desirable for one patient may not be so for another.

With regard to recurrence of varicosities, types A and B in Figure 32–2 are the relevant subtypes in exploration of the controversies of surgical therapy. Retrospective data document that recurrence rates after varicose vein excision range from 5% to 65%. These reports are not uniform with regard to follow-up, mode of surgical venous extirpation, and means of assessment of recurrence. Recent interest in the role of saphenofemoral venous ligation versus stripping of the long saphenous vein has resulted in several reports showing a clear superiority of long saphenous vein stripping over ligation alone. In Sarin and colleagues' series of prospectively randomized patients assessed for venous reflux and recurrences by physical examination, PPG, and duplex examination, 9 of 49 limbs developed persistent venous abnormalities after vein stripping versus 25 of 56 limbs in which saphenofemoral junction ligation alone was performed. The risk of saphenous nerve injury was lower in the stripped than in the ligated group. The technique used was the stripping of the vein only to midcalf, therefore avoiding the portion of the vein where the saphenous nerve is in closest proximity. A study of stripping and ligation versus sclerotherapy and ligation alone demonstrated similar results with respect to recurrences.

Despite the superior results of venous stripping with regard to recurrences, there are many individuals in whom the greater saphenous vein is incompetent yet neither dilated nor symptomatic. Because of the desire to preserve the saphenous vein for later use as a vascular conduit if needed, efforts have been made to study means of preserving the saphenous vein while limiting recurrence rates in patients with type B varicosities. Saphenofemoral junction ligation, as described, is encouraged for this reason; however, there is a finite incidence of postoperative phlebitis that undermines the intent of the procedure and can lead to significant morbidity. The development of the saphenofemoral banding technique has been studied with the specific intent of preserving the saphenous vein and minimizing the incidence of postligation phlebitis. A consecutive, nonrandomized series by Schanzer and Skladany comparing saphenofemoral banding with a high ligation technique demonstrated a 50% reduction in postoperative complete saphenous vein loss in banded patients. More impressively, any degree of vein thrombosis was present in 87% of ligated veins versus only 13% of banded veins. Reflux in the banded veins occurred only 5% of the time.

ADVANCES IN THE TREATMENT OF VENOUS INSUFFICIENCY

Although significant progress has been made in the diagnosis and understanding of the pathophysiology of venous disease, there has been little definitive advance in the treatment of venous ulcers and the symptoms of venous stasis. Two recent concepts, one nonoperative and one surgical, deserve mention as ambulatory therapies that hold significant promise.

The mainstay of outpatient therapy for venous ulcer disease has been the application of Unna's boot in addition to the use of compression stockings in the healing period. Increasing efforts to document the pathophysiology of ulcer formation have produced theories ranging from leukocyte trapping with subsequent release of free radicals and proteolytic enzymes to formation of capillary fibrin cuffs due to deranged fibrinolysis resulting in localized tissue hypoxia. Research is accelerating in the field and is producing interesting results; however, a clinical corollary has not been found. Various topical agents (e.g., silver sulfadiazine, tripeptide copper complex cream, platelet-derived healing factors, hydrocolloid gel with compression) have also been investigated and reported in the dermatologic and surgical literature; however, there are no convincing data to support any of the agents over traditional methods.

The application of pneumatic compression in addition to standard topical agents and support can accelerate healing in the patient with chronic venous insufficiency. Although trials have been few, the statistically increased rates of healing, as measured by time to healing and daily rate of healing and as assessed by ulcer size, suggest that pneumatic compression as an adjunct holds promise. The effect of pneumatic compression on local healing is not well understood; however, the changes in fibrinolytic potential that are systemically produced by pneumatic compression devices are an intriguing finding because it is theorized that localized abnormalities in the fibrinolytic system contribute to venous ulcer formation.

The other potential advance receiving increased attention is the modification of the Linton procedure for interruption of perforator veins and division of the paratibial fascia using the laparoscope. The Linton procedure is predicated on the theory that high pressure transmitted to the skin via the perforators of the lower leg and high compartment pressures in the superficial and deep posterior compartments are responsible for the symptoms and the breakdown of skin seen in chronic venous insufficiency. Historic difficulties with the Linton procedure are the need for extensive skin incisions, flap formation in the already diseased lower leg, and traversal of the ulcer bed to reach the perforating veins. The laparoscopic approach, as espoused in the United States by Bergan, Gloviczki, Hobson, and others, has been to use a modification of standard laparoscopic equipment to traverse the superficial and deep compartments, ligating the perforators and dividing the paratibial fascia through a small incision remote from the area of significant disease. Although experience is only beginning to accumulate, in the properly selected patient, the technique holds promise as a minimally invasive partial solution to the pathophysiology of venous insufficiency and ulceration.

SUMMARY

The treatment of venous insufficiency is predicated on a thorough knowledge of its pathophysiology. Noninvasive testing, primarily duplex and air plethysmography coupled with complete vascular examination, offers the best chance for diagnosis and selection of appropriate intervention. The treatment of varicose veins in the outpatient setting is based on type and cause of varicosity, as well as a balance between recurrence rates and need for preservation of the greater saphenous vein for use later in life. Sclerotherapy has a limited role but may be useful as a primary treatment for smaller veins or as an adjunct to extirpative procedures.

Selected Readings

1. Bergan J. Endoscopic subfascial perforator vein interruption for chronic venous insufficiency. Venous Digest 1995; Tape #1 ZDZZ2.
2. Christopolous D, Nicolaides AN, Cook A, et al. Pathogenesis of venous ulceration in relation to calf muscle pump function. Surgery 1989;106:829–835.
3. Christopoulos D, Nicolaides AN. Noninvasive diagnosis and quantitation of popliteal reflux in the swollen and ulcerated leg. J Cardiovasc Surg 1988;29:535–539.
4. Christopolous D, Nicolaides AN, Szendro G. Venous reflux: Quantification and correlation with the clinical severity of venous disease. Br J Surg 1988;75:352–356.
5. Cordts PR, Hanrahan LM, Rodriguez AA, et al. A prospective trial of Unna's boot versus Duoderm CGF hydroactive dressing plus compression in management of venous leg ulcers. J Vasc Surg 1992;15:480–486.
6. Fligelstone L, Carolan G, Pugh N, et al. An assessment of the long saphenous vein for potential use as a vascular conduit after varicose vein surgery. J Vasc Surg 1993;18:836–840.
7. Neglen P, Einarsson E, Eklof B. The functional long term value of different types of treatment for saphenous vein incompetence. J Cardiovasc Surg 1993; 34:295–301.
8. Neglen P, Raju S. A rational approach to detection of significant reflux with duplex Doppler scanning and air plethysmography. J Vasc Surg 1993;17:590–595.
9. Raju S, Fredericks R, Lishman P, et al. Observations on the calf venous pump mechanism: Determinants of post-exercise pressure. J Vasc Surg 1993;17:459–469.
10. Sarin S, Scurr JH, Coleridge-Smith PD. Assessment of stripping the long saphenous vein in the treatment of primary varicose veins. Br J Surg 1992;79:889–893.
11. Sarin S, Scurr JH, Coleridge-Smith PD. Stripping of the long saphenous vein in the treatment of primary varicose veins. Br J Surg 1994;81:455–458.
12. Schanzer H, Skladany M. Varicose vein surgery with preservation of the saphenous vein: A comparison between high ligation-avulsion versus saphenofemoral banding. J Vasc Surg 1994;20:684–687.
13. van Bemmelen PS, Matos MA, Hodgson KJ, et al. Does air plethysmography correlate with duplex scanning in patients with chronic venous insufficiency? J Vasc Surg 1993;18:796–807.

PLASTIC SURGERY

Chapter 33

Surgical Management of Difficult Wounds

Richard F. Edlich • Nguyen D. Nguyen
Raymond F. Morgan

Difficult wounds have long puzzled and fascinated surgeons. Broadly defined, difficult wounds are those that appear to be refractory to repair and are associated with a high incidence of complications. Dissatisfied with the results of surgery, many surgeons assume ownership of the disappointing results and do not rightfully attribute this failure to heal to an unknown disorder in wound repair. The dissatisfied patient begins the search for another surgeon, which may be the beginning of a lifelong disappointing journey. For the past 25 years, we have actively sought referral of patients with these difficult wounds, which has led to a partnership with our patients that has allowed us to identify the disorder in wound repair and achieve a satisfactory result. Our experiences with Gardner's syndrome (GS), pseudofolliculitis barbae, nasal septal perforation, factitious wounds, and hidradenitis suppurativa (HS) provide new insights toward achieving a satisfactory result.

MULTIPLE EPIDERMAL CYSTS IN GARDNER'S SYNDROME

The term familial polyposis coli (FPC) has been questioned in recent years because it has become apparent that this disease is much more than colonic disease. Use of alternative terms such as familial polyposis, hereditary adenomatosis, and adenomatosis polyposis enhances this point. FPC is recognized as a genetically determined and generalized growth disorder with manifestations of both a benign and malignant nature throughout the body. FPC was first reported in 1882 in two members of the same family. Over subsequent decades, the genetic and premalignant aspects of the condition became clear. In 1951, Gardner described a family with FPC in which seven members suffered from adenomas of the large intestines, osteomas of the skull and mandible, and multiple epidermoid cysts. This complex of manifestations is known as Gardner's syndrome, or GS. Many investigators have thought that FPC and GS are different conditions, but, as the number of extracolonic manifestations of the disease becomes apparent, it seems reasonable to believe that FPC can manifest itself with varying degrees of genetic expressions and that all of these lesions are part of the same disease complex.

The various manifestations of FPC appear to be controlled by a single genetic locus, which is inherited as an autosomal dominant trait. The wide spectrum of extracolonic manifestations represents varied penetrance of the same genotypic abnormality. GS represents a more complete phenotypic expression of the same genotype than does familial polyposis. Apart from the large bowel adenomas, which are always present, a common extracolonic symptom of GS is the occurrence of epidermal cysts. In the report by Weary and coworkers, the cysts were often small and not noticed by the patients. Leppard and Bussey reported that only 1 of their 74 patients with familial polyposis had 20 cysts that were large and disfiguring. Their experience is in sharp contrast with that of others, who have found numerous large cysts.

Treatment

Skin cysts in GS are epidermal. These cysts can be seen long before intestinal polyps develop, but they do not necessarily occur in all affected members of a family with the syndrome. In planning elective excision of these benign cysts, the surgeon's primary responsibility is to identify a site through which the operative procedure can be successfully and safely completed. If a variety of plans can achieve the same result without sacrificing the goals of the surgical procedure, then the surgeon's selection of an incision should result in the least possible cosmetic and physical deformity. Because epidermal cysts in patients with GS are always benign and incisions through skin overlying the cyst result in conspicuous and aesthetically displeasing scars, preferential locations for incisions should be those that give a superior cosmetic result. With facial cysts, we use incisions that are used commonly for rhytidectomy (Fig. 33–1). These incisions allow us to undermine the superficial subcutaneous tissue of the facial skin to visualize and excise completely the epidermal cysts. After wound closure, the narrow preauricular scar is the only noticeable deformity, because the other incisions are hidden in the scalp or covered by the patient's hair. An additional benefit of this approach is that it permits excision of the redundant skin that has formed over the disfiguring cysts. The alternative to this approach of excision of benign cysts from a distance would be to make approximately 20 skin incisions overlying the multiple cysts, resulting in conspicuous and disfiguring scars. This dramatic surgical deformity, in addition to the burden of the more life-threatening

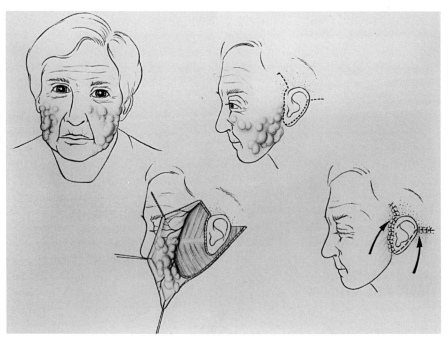

Figure 33–1. (Top, left) Multiple epidermal inclusion cysts in a patient with Gardner's syndrome. **(Top, right)** Outline of rhytidectomy incisions. **(Bottom, left)** Undermining of skin flaps permits visualization and complete excision of epidermal cysts. **(Bottom, right)** Closure of wound after excision of excess skin.

colonic and extracolonic complications of this disease, contributes significantly to the patient's social isolation. The principle of excision from a distance has been advocated by surgeons for other benign tumors to achieve an inconspicuous scar.

PSEUDOFOLLICULITIS BARBAE WITH KELOIDS

Pseudofolliculitis barbae affects 85% of blacks who shave their beards. The disease is a pseudofolliculitis, not a folliculitis, caused by ingrown hairs. Its predilection for blacks is due to the shape of their hairs, which assume a spiral or helical configuration. Ingrown hair occurs rarely in whites because their straight hairs are not prone to penetrate the skin.

This disease characteristically begins on the chin, anterolateral lower neck, and cheeks, although it may eventually appear all over the bearded area, except on the upper lip. It usually spares the posterior neck, even when it has been shaved. Because this is essentially a foreign body reaction to ingrown hair, the best initial treatment is to pull out the individual hair that penetrates the skin. Although numerous nostrums and shaving techniques have been recommended to prevent pseudofolliculitis barbae, it is generally recognized that the most effective form of therapy is abstinence from shaving. Curiously, this disease may be the only medical condition for which the most effective method of treatment (growing a beard) results in more social ostracism than the condition itself. Indeed, military and civilian personnel with pseudofolliculitis barbae who have been advised not to shave by physicians have become the victims of harassment, less than honorable discharges, and various forms of employment discrimination. If shaving abstinence is not a consideration, a variety of hair removal techniques have been specifically developed to reduce the likelihood of development of this disease. These include use of chemical depilatories, an electric razor designed for black men, and the double-edged foil-guarded blade.

When this disease is allowed to progress to keloid formation, we use a surgical approach that includes excision of the keloidal scar, meticulous debridement of all residual ingrown hairs in the underlying wound, and coverage of the defect with a thin split-thickness skin graft. Postoperative care of these patients must be directed at preventing recurrence of pseudofolliculitis barbae by either shaving abstinence or the use of a specially designed hair removal technique that reduces the likelihood of disease development.

Our surgical approach is to first excise the infected keloids with a 0.5-cm margin of uninvolved skin (Fig. 33–2A). The excision is extended downward to underlying subcutaneous tissue that is enmeshed with hair follicles. Using an operating room microscope to facilitate identification of the ingrown hairs, the surgeon meticulously excises each hair follicle using fine-toothed forceps and a number 67 Beaver blade (Beaver Surgical Products, Waltham, MA). After debridement of all residual hair follicles, the excised defect is covered without tension with a split-thickness skin graft harvested from the lateral aspect of the patient's thigh (see Fig. 33–2B). Because strong skin tensions are a contributing factor to keloid formation, primary closure of the defect is not used because it enhances skin tension. Thin split-thickness skin grafts, measuring 0.0008 inches thick, are used for wound coverage because they display the following distinct advantages over thicker skin grafts for this patient. First, thin split-thickness skin grafts usually do not support growth of their own hairs as do thicker grafts. Growth of the skin graft hairs may be a precipitating factor for recurrence of pseudofolliculitis barbae. Second, the donor site for a thin split-thickness skin graft reepithelializes more rapidly than that for a thick split-thickness graft, limiting patient discomfort at the donor site. Third, wounds with thin split-thickness skin grafts undergo more contraction than wounds with thicker grafts, reducing the graft size and improving the aesthetic result (see Fig. 33–2C). Although split-thickness skin grafts taken from the scalp provide a better color match for facial skin than does thigh skin, we are hesitant to use scalp as the skin graft donor site because the transected ends of the pilosebaceous units may be stimuli for keloid formation in the scalp donor site. A bolus tie-over stent dressing is used to immobilize the grafts

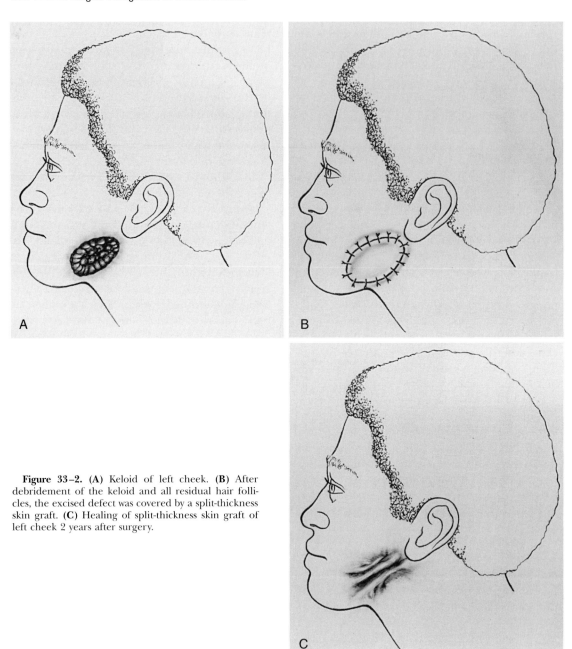

Figure 33–2. (A) Keloid of left cheek. **(B)** After debridement of the keloid and all residual hair follicles, the excised defect was covered by a split-thickness skin graft. **(C)** Healing of split-thickness skin graft of left cheek 2 years after surgery.

to the donor site. After being discharged from the hospital, the patient shaves his beard with a double-edged foil-guarded blade (American Safety Razor, Verona, VA). The purposes of this guard are to prevent nicking of the skin and to leave residual short hairs that cannot hook back and penetrate the skin, thereby resulting in recurrence of pseudofolliculitis barbae.

NASAL SEPTAL PERFORATION

Nasal septal perforation is a well-recognized complication of septal surgery. Other iatrogenic causes of perforation include cryosurgery, electrocoagulation for epistaxis, or nasotracheal intubation. In recent years, drugs, such as cocaine and methamphetamine, account for an increasing number of septal perforations. These perforations are usually large in size. Recently, beclomethasone dipropionate nasal spray has been implicated as a cause of nasal septal perforations. Wegener's granulomatosis as well as neoplasms are other causes of this deformity.

The frequency of septal perforations has declined over the past several decades because the major cause of the defect, submucous resection, is performed less frequently. Because nasal septal surgery is the most frequent cause of the perforation, the best treatment is prevention. The septum receives its blood supply from the overlying mucosa, which become necrotic in the presence of bilateral corresponding tears. Consequently, bilateral corresponding mucosal tears are best repaired at the time of injury. Not all unilateral tears need repair, but they should be immobilized and splinted or packed in position under no tension. Operative damage to the septum also can be prevented by avoiding tight suturing of septal splints and tight nasal packing.

The position and size of the perforation are important factors in producing symptoms. The more anterior and the larger the perforation, the greater is the likelihood that it will cause symptoms. Posterior perforations cause fewer symptoms because of the rapid humidification of the inspired air by the nasal lining and turbinates. In addition, posterior perforations are less common because of the inaccessibility of the septum to mechanical and chemical irritants and because of the support of the bony septum in this area. However, posterior perforations are often the result of a more serious disease process, such as tumors, infections, and granulomatous disease, and they may warrant a biopsy.

Treatment of septal perforations may be nonoperative, using nasal irrigations and Silastic prosthesis. Results with this symptomatic approach are disappointing. Obturators themselves may cause increased mucus, crusting, and obstruction. Moreover, with the modern success rate of surgical repair, most patients welcome a more permanent surgical solution to their perforations rather than a lifetime of obturators and nasal irrigations.

The literature is replete with surgical techniques for the closure of septal perforation. Additional intranasal flaps include the mucosa from the inferior turbinate with a 3.5-cm-wide flap. Further improvement in the technique of perforation closure occurred with the introduction of an intraseptal connective-tissue autograft (e.g., temporalis fascia, mastoid periosteum). These grafts have a low metabolic requirement and serve as a framework for ingrowth of fibroblasts, sustaining the growth of the mucosal edges toward each other. They also lend strength and durability to the repair. The advantage of the fascial and periosteal grafts is that they do not need to be covered on both sides by the intranasal flaps. Closure of the perforation on one side supports the connective-tissue graft and allows the mucosa on the opposite side to use the graft as a scaffold for migration.

Even with reliable intranasal flaps and use of the intraseptal connective-tissue autograft, the technical difficulty of closing septal perforations by means of the endonasal approach still resulted in a limited success rate. The reasons for failure included suboptimal exposure, inadequate mobilization, and poor flap approximation. It was only with use of the external approach that the repair became technically easier and more reliable. The external approach allows for greater surgical exposure and enables the surgeon to use both hands with the aid of binocular vision to mobilize and suture local mucosal advancement flaps and the intraseptal connective-tissue grafts. Some surgeons also have described a sublabial or midfacial degloving approach with this technique.

Treatment

The local mucosal flaps used depend on the location and size of the septal perforation. We use superior and inferior bipedicled flaps with a contralateral, posteriorly based mucoperiosteal flap in posterior septal perforations. In patients whose defect is in the caudal 1.5 cm of the septum, however, an anteriorly based flap is used. Both anteriorly and posteriorly based flaps are designed to exceed the anteroposterior dimensions of the perforation to allow for a tension-free closure. In perforations of less than 0.5 cm, the defect can be closed primarily over a connective-tissue auto-

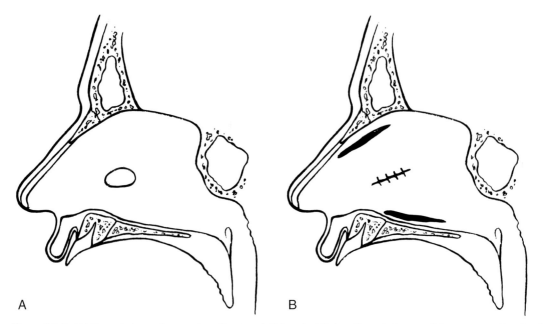

Figure 33–3. (A) Lateral views of a septal perforation (<0.5 cm). **(B)** A unilateral closure of the septal perforation is accomplished with a bipedicle flap.

graft after the perforated septal mucosal flaps from opposite sides of the nasal cavity have been mobilized (Fig. 33–3). In larger perforations (0.5–2.5 cm), bilateral septal mucoperichondrial flaps are elevated over the connective-tissue autograft (Fig. 33–4). In perforation

larger than 2.5 cm, mobilization of the turbinate and mucosa as a part of the advancement and rotation flap is often required. Possible complications from these repairs include epiphora as a result of obstruction of the nasal lacrimal duct, rhinitis sicca, granuloma forma-

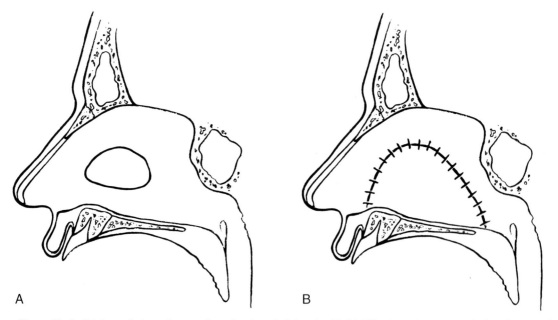

Figure 33–4. (A) Lateral view of a septal perforation (>0.5 cm). **(B)** Mobilization of a posteriorly based mucosal rotation flap allows closure of septal perforation.

tion, and nasal synechiae or stenosis of the nasal vestibule or sill. The high rate of success with this technique leads us to recommend surgical closure rather than a conservative nonoperative treatment of symptomatic septal perforations.

Not all patients with symptomatic septal perforations who are surgical candidates should undergo septal perforation repair. Those with very large perforations (greater than 3 cm) and those who have a severe saddle nose or nasal valve stenosis deformity with no underlying cartilaginous support, benefit from nasal reconstruction alone. An attempted closure in these patients is difficult and may accentuate their dorsal deformity. In these patients, simply correcting the caudal and retrodisplacement of the nasal tip and elevating the nasal dorsum often renders them asymptomatic.

FACTITIOUS SKIN WOUNDS

Because of its availability, visibility, and deep emotional significance, the skin is a common site for self-destructive behavior. The incidence of self-inflicted (factitious) cutaneous wounds is probably greater than is appreciated. Factitious skin wounds may constitute a formidable diagnostic challenge for several reasons. First, they frequently appear subsequent to treatment of a skin wound or performance of a surgery, and they can be perpetuated by a variety of cunning techniques that disguise the self-infliction. The denial of responsibility makes diagnosis of factitious disease even more difficult. Most important, patients strain the doctor–patient relationship that is based on trust and honesty. Physicians dealing with these patients often become frustrated, discouraged, or even angry when this patient–doctor covenant is broken. Diagnosis of self-infliction is essential to prevent ineffective, expensive, and time-consuming treatment.

History

The surgeon must take a detailed history that supports detection of gaps, contradictions, or anatomic anachronisms. Careful attention to chronology, logic, and consistency, as well as scrutiny of previous records, often reveals one blatantly false piece of data sufficient to alert the surgeon to consider this diagnosis. The patient may recount a history of numerous contacts with medical personnel as well as multiple admissions to different hospitals. Despite careful attention to details, the physician may never get a clear idea of how the lesions develop from what the patient tells. There are seldom any prominent signs. In persisting in obtaining a history, the physician may meet an undefinable wall of resistance that has been called a shallow history. When inconsistencies are detected, the patient rarely admits the truth, but gradually changes the story to increase its plausibility. When inconsistencies of the story are too great to be denied, the patient typically becomes angry. Demanding to be told the truth seldom succeeds and antagonizes the patient and relatives to such an extent that the physician is unable to help the patient. Many of these patients enjoy mystifying physicians by predicting the exact areas in which the new lesions will appear, claiming that they experience in these areas a sense of heat and burning and other abnormal sensations before the onset of the lesion.

Many patients with factitious skin wounds exhibit a special affect and behavior. Some patients have a Mona Lisa smile of artful innocence. While relating history, the patient may inadvertently pick, scratch, or rub the lesions. The patient may exhibit a sincere interest in, and almost dedication to, the care of the skin wounds. Along with the verbal expression of interest in the wounds, the patient often displays a readiness to show off the wounds. Self-inflicted skin wounds can also occur by proxy, which is a form of child abuse. The act of abuse is motivated by the parent's psychopathology.

Physical Examination

Women are especially prone to self-inflicted skin wounds. Rank, education, intelligence, devotion, and exemplary character do not exclude the possibility of self-infliction. The self-inflicted skin lesions have a classic appearance, with sharp geometric outlines, surrounded by skin that is normal. These lesions usually occur at sites accessible to the dominant hand of the patient. Another important feature is that wounds are unilateral. A right-handed person tends to inflict wounds on the left side of the body and to spare the right side. Factitious wounds are usually found at any site accessible to the hand, such as the face, neck, dorsum of the hand, and exposed part of the legs. Inaccessible sites, such as the interscapular area, are rarely involved. When multiple factitious skin wounds are evident, they show a variable progression of healing. A bleeding ulcer may be present in the midst of well-healed scars. Other clinical manifestations of self-inflicted skin wounds include blisters, bruises, purpura, erythema, edema, sinuses, nodules, and subcutaneous emphysema. Many patients are intelligent and creative and learn how to improve their technique of self-infliction (e.g., with phenol, acid, alkaline burns) and to use new methods (e.g., with a hypodermic needle).

Diagnosis

There are two reasons to make the diagnosis. First, psychiatric care can proceed without any doubt about the psychogenic nature of the illness. Second, the ulcer can then be healed by appropriate treatment designed to prevent the patient from tampering with the wound. The diagnosis is usually made by exclusion after an unproductive evaluation of the wound and a search for systemic factors that interfere with wound defenses and repair. Relevant personal, emotional, and psychosocial data that may contribute to or complicate the skin lesion must also be considered.

When the skin lesion is considered to be self-inflicted, several approaches have been used to confirm the diagnosis. First, the demonstration that the lesion will heal under efficient covering is an indirect confirmation of the diagnosis. This provision is easier to require than to obtain, because knitting needles, for example, go a long way under occlusive bandages. Encasing the wound in a plaster cast is one method to limit the patient's access to the wound. In such cases, the wound heals despite the development of infection. This

treatment commonly provokes bitter complaints of the imposed confinement.

Tetracycline fluorescence has been used to confirm the diagnosis. With this technique, the surgeon first covers the wound with a plaster cast to prevent patient manipulation of the wound. The cast is allowed to dry and a window is cut into it over the wound. A gauze dressing saturated with 2 mL of tetracycline hydrochloride solution is placed over the entire ulcer. The patient is told that the tetracycline is being used for its antibiotic properties and it is virtually certain that the ulcer could be healed with proper protection and immobilization. The window is then replaced and is held in place with one secure Velcro strap. The patient is left alone in the hospital room overnight, allowing convenient access to the wound. Early the following morning, ultraviolet examination is performed. The presence of fluorescence beneath the nail or in the nail folds indicates that the moist dressing has been handled by the patient's hands. The finding of a small amount of fluorescence on the volar pads of the fingertips is inconclusive, particularly if there has been any diffusion of tetracycline through the plaster cast.

Another diagnostic technique is patient isolation with constant surveillance. The patient is admitted to the hospital, stripped naked, placed in a bath, and watched constantly. A more humane and successful method of surveillance is to view the patient through a one-way mirror. Finding the tools that the patient uses to inflict the wound is extremely helpful. Sometimes, the weapon comes to light accidentally, such as a syringe or bottle of phenol being found in the bed, or it is discovered by a deliberate search.

Psychosocial Findings

Certain psychosocial factors occur with more than a casual frequency. Most of the patients with self-inflicted skin disease have two or more apparent neurotic symptoms. The most frequent of these is depression. Almost three fourths of the patients have prominent obsessive-compulsive personality traits. Virtually all of the patients whose skin lesions are severe and long-standing fall into this category. Relatively few of the patients are psychotic.

Most of the patients are incredibly unaware of the cause–effect relationship between their behavior and disease; the patients denied any and all responsibility for the self-inflicted damage. This denial may be conscious or unconscious. In every case, the painfully injured skin is a ticket for admission to the hospital.

The psychosocial factors of prisoners with factitious skin wounds also appear to play an important role in self-infliction. The most expressed reason for this behavior among prisoners is to gain immediate attention and to transfer out of the current prison environment. By adopting a sick role, particularly by gaining admission to a hospital, prisoners can satisfy a number of personal desires that would not otherwise be provided: personal attention and a sense of being cared for, isolation from a real or perceived danger, increased availability of drugs, more comfortable accommodations, and the chance to develop and maintain personal social contacts.

Treatment

Perhaps the only approach that might be successful is a method Hollender and Hersh introduced in 1970. They emphasized that the original surgeon should avoid playing the dual roles of detective/accuser and therapist/helper. If the surgeon tries to do both, there is little chance that a therapeutic rapport can be established after that surgeon has confronted the patient. Rather, the original surgeon should confront the patient and a psychiatrist should be available to provide therapy.

Because patients with factitious skin diseases have a wide spectrum of psychopathologic conditions ranging from malingering to neuroses to psychoses, the psychiatric intervention must be individualized for each patient. Although there are few specific recommendations, there is consensus on certain common guidelines. Support is widely advocated, whether it is in the form of social and practical measures, in a more superficial therapeutic relationship, or in the context of intensive therapy. In the latter, the patient–therapist relationship is of prime importance, providing the patient with a reality-oriented object. The achievement of insight should not be the goal of treatment. It does not help and can even be contraindicated because it can weaken the patient's defenses. When the patient's defenses are threatened, the patient may exhibit more factitious illness or break contact with the therapist.

In the psychotic patient, treatment is centered around controlling symptoms with antipsychotic medication and support counseling. Insight psychotherapy or confrontation of self-mutilation delusional thinking should be avoided, because these techniques lead to escalation of the psychotic illness. This counseling should be supported by other efforts to gain wound closure that include a protective dressing and symptom substitution. However, it is unlikely that these latter techniques will have any lasting benefit without counseling.

The ultimate fate of patients with self-inflicted skin wounds has been the subject of several investigations. On the basis of these studies, it appears that some patients go through a phase of self-infliction, whereas, for others, it becomes a way of life.

HIDRADENITIS SUPPURATIVA

Hidradenitis suppurativa (HS) is an inflammatory disease of the skin and subcutaneous tissue that occurs in apocrine gland–bearing areas distributed in the axilla, mammary nipple areola, mons pubis, groin, scrotum, perineum, perianal region, and umbilicus. HS generally occurs only after puberty, and most often in the third to fourth decade of life. It tends to be more common in women and blacks. Obesity or exposure to tropical climates is associated with HS. There also appears to be a genetic form of the disease with a single gene transmission. HS involves primarily the axilla or the inguinal region. Perianal and perineal HS are especially debilitating and less common forms of this disease.

The condition typically has an insidious onset, with pruritus and hyperhidrosis being the earliest symptoms. As time progresses, the inflammatory process spreads to adjacent skin, eventually resulting in extensive epithelialized sinus tracts within fibrotic dermal tissue. Recurrent infections result in a putrid, foul-smelling drainage that causes affected patients to limit their social contacts to the immediate family and security of their homes. Over the past 15 years, our team of scientists has documented that there are several important determinants in the pathogenesis of HS: (1) the bacterial concentration of the apocrine gland–bearing skin, (2) method of hair removal, (3) moisture content of apocrine gland–bearing skin, and (4) pyogenic infections.

Bacterial Concentration of the Apocrine Gland–Bearing Skin

The development of infection is determined, in part, by a delicate balance between the number of bacteria present and the resistance of the tissue to infection. Studies performed in our laboratory demonstrated that the critical infective dose of pure cultures of obligate and facultative aerobic bacteria was 1 million bacteria or greater per gram of tissue. The type of aerobic bacteria was less important in the development of infection than the number.

Host defenses of HS patients are usually normal. Nevertheless, the apocrine gland–bearing skin is warm and moist, and it contains abundant secretions; it is a veritable haven for microorganisms sufficient in number to cause infection if the integument is disrupted. The axillary microbial flora in healthy individuals consists of gram-positive, coagulase-negative staphylococci and coryneform bacteria. The latter bacteria are gram-positive, non–spore-forming pleomorphic rods. The aerobic coryneform bacteria of the skin are commonly known as diphtheroids, a name coined to indicate a close association with the diphtheria bacillus. The general term coryneform is more appropriate to these skin bacteria, because they resemble *Corynebacterium diphtheriae* in little but morphology. Staphylococci were present in nearly 100% of axillae; coryneform bacteria were found in more than 75%. The resident flora of these healthy subjects also included the gram-negative *Aerobacter* species and *Alcaligenes faecalis* in almost one half and one third of the individuals, respectively.

On average, persons with a predominance of diphtheroids in their axilla harbor total populations of several million bacteria per square centimeter, whereas those with more than 50% staphylococci average several hundred thousands total bacteria per square centimeter. If the diphtheroids are selectively suppressed by antibiotic treatment, the staphylococci resistant to the antibiotic increase proportionately. Thus, diphtheroids appear to limit the growth of staphylococci in the normal axilla.

Method of Hair Removal

The susceptibility of a woman's axillary skin to HS may be related, in part, to the practice of axillary hair removal with a safety razor. Removal of axillary hair is aesthetically pleasing to women and is helpful in preventing axillary odor. The presence of hair greatly increases axillary odor, because the hair acts as a collecting site for axillary secretions, debris, keratin, and bacteria. Shaving and careful washing of the axilla reduces odor for more than 24 hours.

Shaving the skin with a safety razor is associated with well-documented deleterious effects. A safety razor consists of a blade held in a fixed geometry. The razor blade transects the infundibulum of the hair follicle so that the wounded hair follicle provides access and substrate for bacteria. In addition, the impermeable corneal layer is damaged, resulting in an exudate that supports bacterial proliferation. In our experimental animals, bacterial inoculation of shaved skin resulted in dermatitis. In contrast, skin whose hair was removed by either an electric clipper or electric razor was refractory to bacterial contamination and dermatitis did not develop. The implications of the damaging effects of hair removal on the skin are being recognized by surgeons. The wound infection rate of patients whose hair is removed by a safety razor is significantly greater than that of patients whose hair is removed by electric clippers; consequently, electric clippers should be used to remove hair from the skin at the operative site and hair removal by a safety razor is potentially dangerous, inviting the development of infection. Prior to the development of axillary HS, many of our patients complained of nicking or cutting of axillary skin by a safety razor. This interruption of the skin allows access to the millions of microorganisms that reside on axillary skin. As in the case of the surgical patient, the razor compromises the local tissue defenses and appears to invite the development of HS. These deleterious effects of the safety razor could be prevented by using an electric razor for hair removal.

Moisture Content of Axillary Skin

The number of bacteria in the axilla is probably enhanced further by the increased moisture of the axillary skin. Experimental and clinical observations consistently emphasize the importance of moisture in colonization of skin by potential pathogens. The relative dryness of normal skin in most parts of the body contributes to the marked limitation of growth of bacteria, especially gram-negative bacilli with their greater moisture requirements (e.g., *Escherichia coli, Pseudomonas aeruginosa*).

A variety of factors that can potentially enhance the moisture content of axilla has been identified in patients with HS. Anderson and Perry reported that 20 (77%) of their 26 patients with HS were overweight. The excess weight ranged from 2.3 to 40.7 kg, with an average of 12.7 kg. Obesity was evident also in all women with axillary HS in our study. Obesity is prone to increase the moisture on axillary skin by maintaining an occlusive skin cover over the axillary skin. In the obese patient, the axilla is buried between the enlarged lateral thoracic wall and the upper arm. In the individual of normal body weight, the arm does not gain intimate contact with the thoracic cage in a resting position, thus allowing exposure of the axilla and permitting transepidermal water loss (TEWL). Excessive sweating, itching, and burning may be the first symptoms of axillary HS. These symptoms are followed by the development of a firm nodule that subsequently drains thick purulent material.

The inflammation of HS can be exacerbated by the use of aluminum-containing deodorants. Many HS patients believe that the application of antiperspirant preparations predisposes them to the development of HS. They note that topical application of these agents results in burning, itching, dermatitis, and infection, causing them to discontinue their use. Several mechanisms may account for the deleterious effects of these products on axillary skin. Some antiperspirants may produce an occlusive film over the axillary skin, impairing transepidermal water loss and increasing the moisture content on the underlying skin. Antiperspirants may also predispose patients to HS through chemical irritation, inducing pore closure, or changing axillary flora. The warning labels on antiperspirants lend credence to this belief that antiperspirants may indeed be chemical irritants. These labels indicate to the consumer that antiperspirants should not be used on broken or irritated skin.

Pyogenic Infection

Long-standing pyogenic infections have also been associated with the development of HS. Evidence suggests that occlusion of the follicular orifice (which also conducts apocrine sweat to the surface) is important in the pathogenesis of axillary HS.

Treatment

The method of treatment varies with the stage of the disease. The acute phase should be treated early and intensively to avoid progression into the chronic phase. Incision and drainage are usually needed to treat the localized disease. Specific attention must be paid to each factor that predisposes the patient to axillary HS. A strict weight reduction program must be instituted for all obese patients. Axillary hair must be removed with an electric razor rather than a safety razor. Antiperspirant and deodorants should be avoided. Local pyogenic infection (e.g., acne vulgaris) must be aggressively treated.

Treatment of the chronic stage of axillary HS is primarily surgical. Almost all surgeons agree that the only chance for a lasting cure is complete removal of the hair-bearing area and the underlying diseased deep dermal tis-

34

Excisional Biopsy of Skin Tumors

Richard F. Edlich • Scott E. Langenburg
David B. Drake

Skin neoplasms vary from those that are benign to others that are highly malignant. They are so common that every person will develop at least one or more skin tumors. More than 600,000 new cases of malignant skin tumors are diagnosed in the United States each year. Basal cell carcinoma (BCC) accounts for 65% to 80% of the cases. Squamous cell cancer (SCC) is the second most common malignant skin tumor and comprises 10% to 20% of the cases. Approximately 32,000 new cases of malignant melanoma are diagnosed annually in the United States. At the current rate, 1 of every 105 Americans will develop malignant melanoma.

The treatment of skin tumors is based either on their complete removal or destruction. One standard method of treatment is excisional biopsy. Because the definitive diagnosis of the skin tumor, especially precancerous ones, depends on histopathologic examination complemented by clinical data, the surgeon must provide the pathologist with as much clinical data as possible. This chapter describes a systematic approach to the excisional biopsy of skin tumors, allowing complete removal of the tumor with the most aesthetically pleasing result. This technique is designed to excise a circular specimen of skin and underlying adipose, whose diameter is 8 mm or less, after which the defect is closed primarily. This excisional biopsy is ideally suited for most skin tumors, including benign lesions and small superficial basal cell or squamous cell carcinomas. There are seven technical considerations involved in the excisional biopsy of skin tumors: aseptic technique, examination and demarcation of skin lesion, skin biomechanical properties, anesthesia, excisional biopsy, wound closure, and postoperative care.

ASEPTIC TECHNIQUE

The surgeon must use aseptic technique and wear a cap, mask, and powder-free gloves. Powder-free gloves are recommended because the glove powders (e.g., cornstarch) are foreign bodies that damage the host's resistance to infection. We use powder-free gloves coated by a hydrogel polymer (Regent Hospital Products, Ltd., Greenville, SC). The polymer facilitates donning of the gloves with either dry or wet hands. The hydrogel lining provides a barrier between the skin and the latex, which is especially important to individuals with sensitivities to latex proteins or accelerators.

Hair is a source of wound contamination, and removal of hair prevents it from becoming entangled in suture and the wound during closure. However, the infection rate in surgical wounds following razor preparation of the skin is significantly greater than that after hair removal by electric clippers. The increased incidence of infection following razor preparation is probably related to the trauma inflicted by the razor. As a result of the shave, wounded hair follicles provide access to and substrate for bacteria. Surgical electric clippers cut hair close to the skin surface without nicking the skin, and we now use only electric clippers to remove hair. Recent advances in the design of electric clippers have eliminated sharp edges that can abrade the skin. A new surgical clipper has a disposable clipper blade assembly that does not require cleaning, assembly, or disassembly (3M Center, St. Paul, MN).

After hair removal, the skin is then cleansed with a fine, pore-cell–sized sponge soaked in poloxamer 188 (Calgon Vestal Lab, St. Louis, MO). This nontoxic surfactant is an excellent skin-wound cleanser that can be safely poured into the patient's eye.

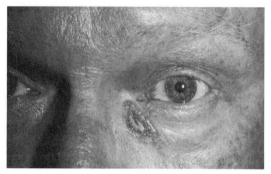

Figure 34–1. Basal cell carcinoma of the left lower eyelid. Note the pearly border with central ulceration and telangiectasia at the inferior margin.

EXAMINATION AND DEMARCATION OF SKIN LESION

The physician's visualization of the wound can be enhanced by magnification (2.5X) loupes. Physicians uniformly prefer keplerian loupes over the galilean lens system. The advantages of the keplerian lens system are its increased field of view and clearer peripheral view. This system allows the physician to visualize the exquisite details of the skin tumor and to perform wound closure using meticulous surgical technique.

Basal cell carcinoma occurs usually in sun-exposed skin sites and is seen as pearly papules, frequently containing prominent, dilated subepidermal blood vessels (telangiectasias). Some lesions contain melanin pigment. Despite the low potential for metastasis, advanced lesions have the capability of local invasion with ulceration and subsequent destruction of underlying bone. BCC frequently extends beyond its visible borders. For tumors with a diameter of less than 2 cm, a minimum margin of 4 mm is necessary to remove completely the tumor in more than 95% of the cases. Sclerosis or morpheaform variants of this tumor require more than a 7-mm margin from clinical evident tumor (Fig. 34–1).

Squamous cell cancer is also found in sun-exposed skin sites. Although these tumors usually remain locally confined, they exhibit a low, but significant propensity to metastasize. When this tumor does not advance through the basement membrane of the dermatoepidermal juncture (in situ carcinoma), it ap-

pears macroscopically as a sharply defined, red scaling plaque (Fig. 34–2). Advanced invasive lesions are nodular with a variable amount of keratin production (hyperkeratosis) and ulceration. Four-millimeter margins are adequate for removal of most SCC. However, certain tumor characteristics are associated with a greater risk of tumor invasion and include size of 2 cm or larger, invasion of the subcutaneous tissue, location in high-risk areas (e.g., scalp, ears, eyelids, nose, lips), and high histologic grades (2, 3, 4).

The clinical characteristics of early malignant melanoma are remarkably similar, regardless of the anatomic site. It is important that physicians recognize four characteristic features of these tumors. First, the shape of early malignant melanoma is often asymmetric, unlike benign pigmented lesions whose shapes

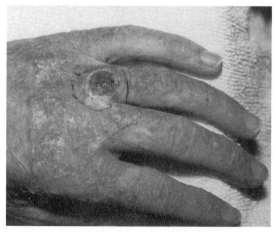

Figure 34–2. Squamous cell carcinoma of the hand. Note the advanced nature of this lesion with carotin of production and ulceration.

are generally round and symmetric. Second, the borders of early malignant melanoma are often irregular, whereas benign pigmented lesions tend to have regular margins. Third, macular malignant melanomas are usually variegated, ranging from hues of tan and brown to black, sometimes intermingled with red and white; benign pigmented lesions are more uniform in color (Fig. 34–3). Fourth, the diameter of malignant melanomas is frequently 6 mm or larger, whereas most benign pigmented lesions generally have diameters of less than 6 mm.

Until 1977, a 3- to 5-cm skin margin of normal skin in all directions from the visible borders of the primary melanoma was considered to be optimal for removal of all cutaneous melanomas. This dictum was questioned when no adverse effects were reported in a small series of melanomas not thicker than 0.76 mm that underwent limited excision, in some instances, of 2 mm of normal skin. The absence of local recurrence in a group of patients with primary melanomas thinner than 1 mm and the very low rate of recurrence for thicker melanomas (>1 mm) indicate that a narrow 1-cm margin excision is a safe and effective procedure. Narrow excision of malignant melanoma must be performed as follows: the skin must be cut 1 cm from the visible margins of the primary melanoma and the excision must be 1 or 2 cm wider in subcutaneous fat, extending through to muscular fascia.

Consequently, the physician's plan for excisional biopsy is dictated by the suspected pathology of the skin lesion. A margin of excision must be identified that allows the lesion to be completely excised. Outlining the extent of the lesions is essential for planning excisions. Its edges are marked with a fine pen filled with gentian violet. A safe, excisional margin of normal skin is then measured and outlined with gentian violet around the tumor, which usually has a circular configuration. Once the wound margins have been defined and the skin defect created after excision of the tumor, the configuration of the resulting defect is determined.

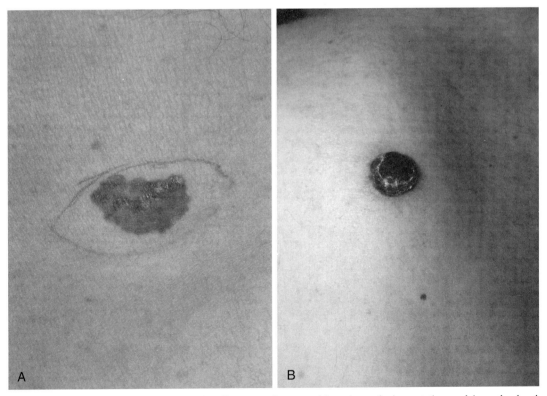

Figure 34–3. (A) Superficial spreading of malignant melanoma with variegated pigmentation and irregular border. **(B)** Nodular melanoma with blue-black pigmentation.

SKIN BIOMECHANICAL PROPERTIES

The ultimate appearance and function of a scar after closure of excisional biopsy can be predicted by the static and dynamic skin tensions on the surrounding skin. The static skin tensions are the forces that stretch the skin over the underlying bony framework when the body remains motionless (Fig. 34–4). These inherent forces are dependent partly on the natural characteristics of dermal collagen fibers and partially on the pattern in which they are woven. Clinical evidence of these tensions is the retraction of the edges of the wounds, permitting visualization of the underlying tissue.

Static skin forces differ considerably in their magnitude and direction within the same person and between individuals. Large differences are noted between various anatomic sites. The skin in one region may be relatively taut; in others, it is lax. In one human volunteer, the static skin tensions were fivefold greater in his extremities than in his abdominal skin. In some regions of the body, there is a directional orientation of static skin tensions. This was first appreciated by Dupuytren in 1834 when he examined a suicide victim who sustained three self-inflicted puncture wounds made by an awl. He noted that the wounds assumed an elliptical shape similar to the shape of skin wounds caused by a knife. He concluded that

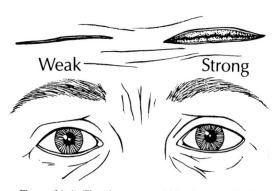

Figure 34–4. The degree to which the wound edges retract can be correlated with the magnitude of static skin tensions. The wound on the right side of the patient's forehead, being subjected to strong static skin tensions, exhibits marked retraction of its edges. The minimal separation of the edges of the wound on the left side of the patient's forehead is consistent with the presence of weak static skin tensions.

skin tensions in the long axis of the defect were substantially greater than in its short axis, distorting the wound accordingly.

In 1861, Langer published a more comprehensive study on the biomechanical properties of human skin. His observations were made on the skin of cadavers, which were lying in the normal anatomic position, by inserting an awl 2.0 mm in diameter to a depth of 2.5 mm. As Dupuytren reported, the circular defect was drawn into an ellipse. By drawing lines between the major axes of the ellipses, Langer identified the direction in which the tension predominated. These static lines of maximal skin tensions are known as "Langer's lines." In 1892, Kocher advocated that surgical incisions should follow Langer's lines. For nearly 100 years, surgeons referred to Langer's lines as the most appropriate guides for incisions that would heal with minimal scarring. It is currently realized that the charts of Langer's lines appearing in textbooks and articles have little practical application because they are erroneous in most cases and do not consider the highly important effect of the dynamic skin tensions on the healing scar.

The static skin tensions continually pull on the wound edges, resulting in the development of a visible scar. The width of this scar is proportional to the magnitude of skin tensions. Excisions made in skin subjected to strong skin tensions usually heal with wide, unattractive scars. In contrast, narrow, fine scars often result from the repair of excisions made in skin with weak static skin tensions.

Dynamic skin tensions also have considerable impact on the magnitude and extent of scar formation. These changing tensions are caused by a combination of forces that are associated with either joint movement or mimetic muscle contraction (Fig. 34–5). In the face, the dynamic skin tensions are perpendicular to natural skin wrinkles and parallel to the direction of contraction of the underlying mimetic muscles. Similarly, the dynamic skin tensions are perpendicular to the transverse axis of the joint. The clinical significance of dynamic tensions is apparent in skin of changing dimensions where elasticity is needed for normal function. In general, a linear scar intersecting the wrinkle lines, transverse axis of a joint, or lying parallel to the dynamic skin

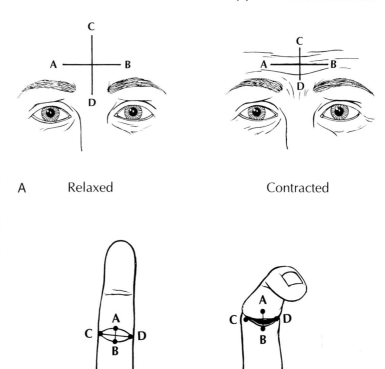

Figure 34–5. (A) Contraction of the frontalis muscle considerably shortens the skin in the direction of dynamic skin tensions *(line CD).* **(B)** As the proximal interphalangeal joint flexes, the distance along the longitudinal axis of the joint shortens considerably in the same direction as the dynamic skin tension *(line CD).*

tensions can result in a serious contracture because the scar does not stretch or recoil like uninjured skin.

ANESTHESIA

Infiltration anesthesia is preferred over regional nerve block because it does not interfere with muscle movement that causes dynamic tensions, which elongate the configuration of the defect. Regional nerve block affects the nerve supply to the muscles that account for dynamic skin tensions and prevents evaluation of the effect of muscle contraction on the distortion of defect resulting from excisional biopsy. Infiltration anesthesia is accomplished with a 1-inch long 30-gauge needle attached to a 5-mL syringe. Because the amide type of local anesthetic agents appear to be relatively free of causing sensitivity and allergic reactions characteristic of the ester-type derivative, physicians usually use amide-type agents (e.g., lidocaine, bupivacaine) for

infiltration anesthesia. These anesthetic agents do not damage tissue defenses or potentiate infection. In addition, the pain of subdermal injection, the onset of anesthesia, and the frequency of satisfactory anesthesia are similar. The pain of administration of local anesthetics can be reduced dramatically by pH buffering of the local anesthetic agents before injection. However, this is not recommended for bupivacaine because a precipitate forms. Because the duration of local anesthesia induced by bupivacaine is nearly four times longer than that by lidocaine, bupivacaine may be preferred for infiltration anesthesia. The duration of the anesthetic activity of these agents can be further enhanced by the addition of the vasoconstrictor epinephrine, which slows the clearance of the anesthetic agent from the tissue (0.5% bupivacaine with 1:200,000 epinephrine).

An understanding of the directional orientation of the dynamic skin tensions at the biopsy site provides insight into the sites of needle placement for infiltration anesthesia. After the patient contracts the muscles of facial expression or flexes the joint, the physician can visualize the outlined circular biopsy site change its shape from a circle to an ellipse. At a site approximately 1 cm from the midportion of the end of the ellipse, the point of the bevel of the needle is passed through the skin into the subcutaneous tissue (Fig. 34–6). The point of the needle lying in the subcutaneous tissue is first directed to one side of the elliptically shaped biopsy site. Before injecting the local anesthetic agent, the syringe barrel is withdrawn to aspirate blood if the needle is positioned in a vessel. Aspiration of blood is a forewarning of the danger of intravascular injection, which can be avoided by repositioning the needle in another site in the subcutaneous tissue. When syringe aspiration is accomplished without visualization of blood, the needle is slowly (≥10 seconds) withdrawn as approximately 1.5 mL of the local anesthetic agent is injected into tissue. As the needle nears its entry position, the direction of the needle is changed so that it can be positioned on the contralateral side of the wound, after which the technique for introducing the local anesthetic agent is repeated. Five to six minutes after injecting the anesthetic agent, the needle is reintroduced in the anesthetized skin that borders one lateral edge of the excisional biopsy site after it is advanced to a site opposite the original injection site. The technique for introducing the anesthetic agent is then repeated. Through anesthetized skin bordering the contralateral side of the biopsy site, the needle is passed and advanced toward the site

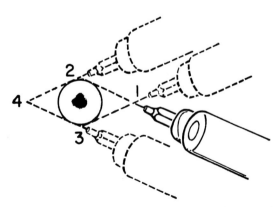

Figure 34–6. Anesthesia sites. Site 1 is the first site of needle penetration. Sites 2 and 3 are anesthetized sites through which the needle penetrates skin. After which, anesthesia is directed to site 4.

previously described. After waiting 5 to 6 more minutes, the circular excisional biopsy can be started in the anesthetized site.

The depth and speed of injection are important determinants of the magnitude of discomfort experienced by the patient. Placement of the needle into the superficial dermis is more uncomfortable than needle passage into the subdermal area. Moreover, intradermal injections resulting in superficial wheals are significantly more painful than injections into the subdermal region and cause distortion of the skin. Rapid injection (<2 seconds) of a local anesthetic agent always causes more pain than when the same volume of anesthetic agent is instilled over 10 seconds. Intracutaneous instillation of lidocaine at 37°C (98.6°F) is no less painful than injection at 21°C (69.8°F). Full anesthesia to pinprick is produced immediately with intradermal injections and is present 5 to 6 min after subdermal injection. A reliable method of minimizing the discomfort of infiltration anesthesia is to use a syringe fitted with a number 30 needle and to inject the smallest amount of anesthetic agent slowly (≥10 seconds) into the deep dermal–subcutaneous tissue as the needle is slowly withdrawn.

A new alternative to the use of infiltration anesthesia for excisional skin biopsies is the topical anesthesia containing a eutectic mixture of lidocaine and prilocaine in a water emulsion cream base (Astra Pharmaceuticals, Westborough, MA). The emulsion is applied to the tumor site, which is covered by an occlusive dressing. It can take up to 1 hour before the anesthesia is complete. A slight blanching of the skin in the areas that have been in contact with the cream is noticed in most cases. This effect is a useful marker for complete anesthesia, which persists for 1 to 2 hours.

EXCISIONAL BIOPSY

Most skin lesions are amenable to a circular excision. In these instances, it is worthwhile to use circular-shaped excisions. Circular excisional biopsy had its beginning less than a century ago when a new use for the ancient trephine was discovered. Small (≤4 mm) cutaneous reusable metal trephines or punches with sharp edges were used. The metal trephines were placed on the surface of the skin and then rotated, cutting out a circular piece of skin corresponding to the internal diameter of the lumen of the trephine. This technique of excision biopsy has several advantages over scalpel incision. The circular biopsy of the skin can be performed considerably faster using trephines than using scalpel excisions. More importantly, the trephine biopsy of the skin results in a circular defect whose shape is changed by the predominant local static and dynamic tensions. The defect elongates in the direction of maximal skin tensions, revealing the long axis of the defect. Closure of the elliptically shaped defect in the direction of its long axis results in a narrow scar.

The reusable metal trephines have been replaced by disposable trephines that have ribbed plastic handles attached to 316 stainless steel circular cutting blades. Because disposable trephines have been used predominantly for incision biopsies, the diameters of the circular cutting blades have been relatively small (≤4 mm). Use of disposable trephines for excision biopsy has been limited by the small size because they frequently do not provide adequate margins of uninvolved tissue surrounding the skin lesion. Consequently, disposable trephines (Acuderm, Inc., Fort Lauderdale, FL) with wider diameter circular cutting blades, either 6 or 8 mm, have been specially developed for excisional biopsy. The

height of the cutting blades is 6 mm to provide adequate and controlled depth of the specimen taken at excisional biopsy. Our extensive clinical experience with these disposable large skin trephines (more than 500 patients) has resulted in a reliable surgical technique that can be replicated in both the office and the medical center.

A disposable trephine whose diameter corresponds to that of the outline of the margins of the skin tumor is selected. If the margins do not have a circular configuration, the margins of the skin are incised by a number 15 stainless steel scalpel.

The plastic handle of the disposable dermatome is held between the thumb and the index finger (Fig. 34–7). The skin lesion should be in the central portion of the circular specimen taken at biopsy. The site of the excisional biopsy can be predicted by first positioning and then pressing the appropriate trephine against the skin, which results in a temporary indentation of the skin (see Fig. 34–7A). Once the lesion is appropriately centered in the circular biopsy site, the trephine is rotated back and forth between the fingers, cutting the circular specimen depth, which is 6 mm. The trephine is then removed from the biopsy site.

When the circular biopsy site is separated from the surrounding skin, the site as well as the surrounding skin undergo deformation in shape (see Fig. 37–7B). The skin lesion reduces considerably in size, while maintaining its circular configuration. In contrast, the skin

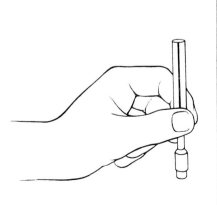

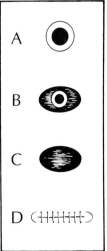

Figure 34–7. The disposable large-diameter trephine is held between the thumb and index finger. (A) The site of the circular excision is determined by pressing the appropriate trephine against the skin, producing a temporary indentation of the skin. (B) The circular skin lesion reduces considerably in size, while the resulting surrounding skin defect assumes an elliptic shape. (C) The skin lesion and underlying subcutaneous tissue are excised down to the underlying muscle. (D) The elliptic defect is approximated in the direction of its long axis by an interrupted braided absorbable synthetic suture and interrupted monofilament nonabsorbable percutaneous sutures.

surrounding the circular biopsy site assumes an elliptical shape. In our experience, the direction of the long axis of the elliptical defect often does not coincide with either Langer's lines or relaxed skin tension lines, indicating that these lines frequently do not accurately predict the orientation of the resulting defect. Consequently, preplanning the orientation of the lenticular shaped excision with length to width ratio of 4:1 has several disadvantages. The direction of the wound closure may be less than ideal. In addition, the length of the closed wound after excisional biopsy is unnecessarily long because it does not account for the elliptical wound deformation.

The skin lesion and the underlying subcutaneous tissue are then excised from the underlying muscle using a number 15 scalpel (see Fig. 34–7C). Each biopsy specimen is fixed separately in a bottle containing 10% formalin solution and is sent for histopathologic examination. Most bleeding can be controlled by applying gentle pressure to gauze sponges on the surface of the wound. Pinpoint electrocoagulation of bleeding vessels by use of bipolar tissue forceps is recommended.

WOUND CLOSURE

After circular excisional biopsy, we routinely undermine the peripheral margins of the defect (Fig. 34–8). With the skin edges elevated by a single hook, the skin margin of the biopsy site is undermined approximately 5 mm using a number 15 knife. Undermining the skin edges of defects resulting from circular skin biopsies decreases the forces required for wound closure, which should limit the ultimate width of the scar.

Wound closure is accomplished in the same direction as the long axis of the elliptical defect by first approximating the midportion of the defect with a 4-0 braided synthetic absorbable suture attached to the swage of the laser-drilled, compound-curved reverse cutting edge needle. Additional interrupted dermal (subcuticular) sutures are placed in each wound quadrant to approximate further the divided edges of the dermis. The dermal suture reduces tension on the wound edges, permitting early removal of the percutaneous su-

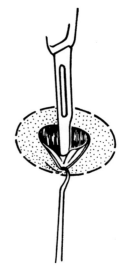

Figure 34–8. While retracting the skin edges of the defect with a skin hook, the surgeon undermines a 5-mm margin of the defect with a number 15 knife blade.

tures before the sixth postoperative day and thereby preventing the development of needle puncture scars. Sutural closure of the dead space beneath the dermis is contraindicated because these sutures potentiate the development of infection without enhancing wound security.

Compound-curved reverse cutting edge needles have been specifically designed for dermal closure. The compound-curved needle has two distinct radii of curvature, whereas the standard reverse cutting edge needle has only one (Fig. 34–9). The compound-curved needle has a relatively straight sharpened point with a reverse cutting edge, followed by a

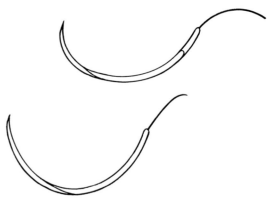

Figure 34–9. (Top) Compound curved needle with two distinct radii of curvature. **(Bottom)** Standard curved needle with one radius of curvature.

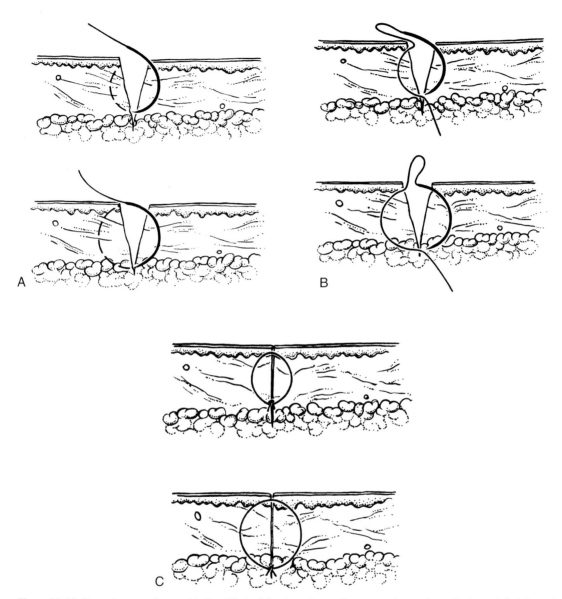

Figure 34–10. Dermal suture closure. **(A, Top)** Dashed line is pathway of compound curved needle through left dermal wound margin. **(Bottom)** Dashed line is pathway of standard needle with one radius of curvature through the left dermal wound margin. Note that the diameter of the pathway through tissue of the compound curved needle is smaller than that of the standard needle **(B, Top)** The pathway of the compound curved needle through the right dermal wound margin. **(Bottom)** The pathway of the standard needle with one radius of curvature through the right dermal wound margin. Note that the diameter of the pathway of the compound curved needle through tissue is smaller than that of the standard needle. **(C, Top)** Tied suture loop following the tissue passage of the compound curved needle. **(Bottom)** Tied suture loop following the tissue passage of the standard needle. Note that the diameter of the tied suture loop constructed by a compound curved needle is smaller than that of one constructed by a standard needle with a single radius of curvature.

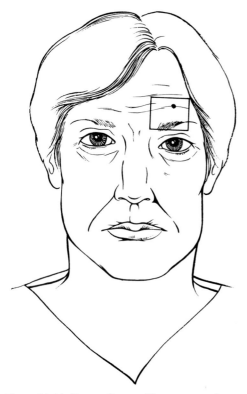

Figure 34–11. Box outlines a skin tumor on the transverse frontal line of the left forehead.

nonabsorbable sutures are then used to close the divided skin edge. We place the first percutaneous suture in the midportion of the wound, after which an interrupted percutaneous suture approximates the skin edges of each wound quadrant ("divide and conquer technique"). One more interrupted percutaneous suture usually is passed through the midportion of each wound quadrant, providing meticulous approximation of the skin edges. Each monofilament synthetic suture is swaged to a laser-drilled cutting edge needle. Excess skin or "dog ears" can be encountered at the ends of the approximated wound and should be excised as necessary in the direction of the long axis of the closed wound.

Our approach to the circular excision of a skin tumor near the transverse frontal line of the left forehead and closure of the defect are illustrated in Figures 34–11 and 34–12. Similarly, circular excision of a skin tumor near the left nasolabial groove and closure of the defect are depicted in Figures 34–13 and 34–14.

Skin tensions at the wound margins of large defects (>8 mm diameter) may be so great

curved distal section. The compound-curved needle can be passed through the dermis with greater accuracy to a controlled depth and length of bite than the standard cutting edge needle.

The passage of the reverse cutting edge needle with a single radius of curvature through dermal tissue is not predictable, and its point of emergence through the dermis is difficult to predict (Fig. 34–10). In some cases, the point of the needle remains buried in the dermis, becoming a technical challenge to retrieve. These difficulties encountered in the use of a standard needle are overcome by use of the compound-curved needle. The geometric design of the needle allows the physician to position it accurately and repeatedly from the point of needle entry into the dermis and to its exit. The physician can easily predict the site at which its relatively straight point will emerge, allowing the needle to be regrasped by the needle holder for repeated passage through the opposite dermal wound edge.

Interrupted 6-0 monofilament synthetic

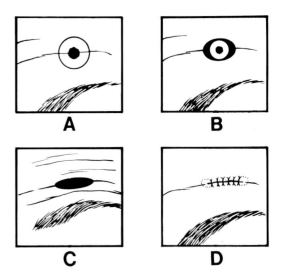

Figure 34–12. Enlargement of left forehead. **(A)** Margin of tumor and site of excision outlined by fine pen using gentian violet. **(B)** Circular incision of margin using trephine. Note the elongation of the incision with its long axis in the direction of the transverse frontal line. **(C)** After excision of the skin tumor, contraction of the frontalis muscle further elongates the elliptical defect. **(D)** Closure of the elliptical-shaped defect by interrupted dermal synthetic braided absorbable sutures followed by interrupted synthetic nonabsorbable monofilament sutures.

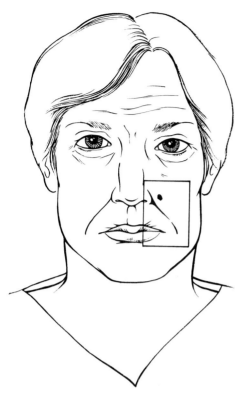

Figure 34–13. Box outlines a skin tumor adjacent to the left nasolabial fold.

than the potential dangers of surface contamination. These clots are replaced by a healing scar that can be easily avoided by swabbing the wound with half-strength hydrogen peroxide every 6 hours until the wound edge is free of blood. Because hydrogen peroxide causes the sutures to lose their color, the decolorized suture becomes a sign of patient compliance with the postoperative wound care regimen. These percutaneous sutures must be removed before the sixth postoperative day because needle puncture scars can develop. The wound edges then should be supported by sterile tape skin closures until their adhesive tape bond weakens.

Rigorous follow-up examination is essential for any patient with a history of a skin cancer

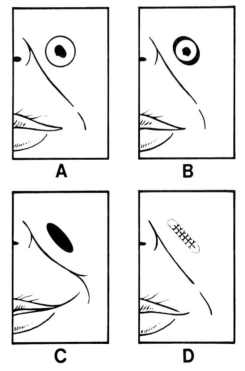

Figure 34–14. Enlargement of the left nasolabial fold and adjacent skin tumor. **(A)** Margin of tumor and site of excision outlined by fine pen with gentian violet. **(B)** Circular incision of the margin using trephine. Note the elongation of the incision with its long axis in the direction of the left nasolabial fold. **(C)** After excision of the tumor, smiling occurs by contraction of levator labii superior is muscle, levator anguli oris, zygomaticus major and minor, and risorius muscle and results in elongation of the elliptical-shaped defect. **(D)** Closure of elliptical shape defect by interrupted braided synthetic absorbable dermal skin sutures and interrupted percutaneous monofilament nonabsorbable skin sutures.

that the skin edges cannot be approximated by dermal and percutaneous sutures. In such cases, coverage of the defect by either a skin graft or local skin flap may be needed. In patients with low skin tensions, it is important to emphasize that sizable wounds, even in the face, have been allowed to heal by contraction (secondary intention) with surprisingly good results. However, most surgeons, especially those with training in reconstructive surgery, close the defect by a graft or local flap without the development of infection or hypertrophic scar formation.

POSTOPERATIVE CARE

In our clinical service, primarily closed wounds (except those on the face) are covered by nonwoven microporous polypropylene dressings attached to surrounding skin by wide strips of microporous tape. In facial lacerations, the development of blood clots between the edges of the wounds are of more concern to detect recurrence and prevent further actinic damage. Much of the morbidity from actinic damage can be prevented by limiting sun exposure and by photoprotection with a sun-blocking agent. Photoprotection against ultraviolet A in the past has been limited by the restricted range of ultraviolet A wavelengths absorbed by available sunscreen agents. With the introduction of Parsol 1789 in combination with padimate O (Photoplex, Herbert Laboratories, Santa Ana, CA), there is a full-spectrum absorbent sunscreen effect against the ultraviolet A and B wavebands. This sunscreen should prove to be valuable in helping to prevent further actinic damage.

Selected Readings

1. Abidin MR, Becker DG, Paley RD, et al. A new compound curved needle for intradermal suture closure. J Emerg Med 1989;7:441–444.
2. Breslow A, Macht SD. Optimal size of resection margin for thin cutaneous melanoma. Surg Gynecol Obstet 1977;145:691–692.
3. Brodland DG, Zitelli JA. Surgical margins for excision of primary cutaneous squamous cell carcinoma. J Am Acad Dermatol 1992;27:241–248.
4. Doctor A, Cutler PV, Westwater JJ, et al. Emergency medicine magnifying loupes. J Emerg Med 1989;7:321–327.
5. Dupuytren JF. Traite theorique et practique des blessure par armes de guerre. Vol 1. Paris: JB Bailliére, 1834.
6. Edlich RF, Stamp CV, Rodeheaver GT, Birk KA, Morgan RF. Large disposable trephines for circular excision biopsy of the skin. Surg Gynecol Obstet 1988;166:71–72.
7. Friedman RJ, Rigel DS, Silverman MK, Kopf AW, Vossaert KA. Malignant melanoma in the 1990s: The continued importance of early detection and the role of physician examination and self-examination of the skin. CA Cancer J Clin 1991;41:201–228.
8. Juhlin L, Evers H, Broberg F. A lidocaine–prilocaine cream for superficial skin surgery and painful lesions. Acta Derm Venereol (Stockh) 1980;60:544–546.
9. Keyes EL. The cutaneous punch. J Cutan Genitourin Dis 1887;5:98–101.
10. Kocher T. Chirurgische Operationslehr. Jena, Germany: Gustav Fisher, 1907.
11. Langer K. On the anatomy and physiology of the skin. I: The cleavability of the cutis. Br J Plast Surg 1978;31:3–8.
12. Masterson TM, Rodeheaver GT, Morgan RF, Edlich RF. Bacteriologic evaluation of electric clippers for surgical hair removal. Am J Surg 1984;148:301–302.
13. Olbricht SM. Treatment of malignant cutaneous tumors. Clin Plast Surg 1993;20:171–172.
14. Pinkus H. Skin biopsy: A field of interaction between clinician and pathologist. Cutis 1977;20:609–614.
15. Ruhl CM, Urbancic JH, Foresman PA, et al. A new hazard of cornstarch, an absorbable dusting powder. J Emerg Med 1994;12:11–14.
16. Salasche SJ, Amonette RA. Morpheaform basal-cell epitheliomas: A study of subclinical extension in a series of 51 cases. J Dermatol Surg Oncol 1981;7:387–394.
17. Thacker JG, Iachetta FA, Allaire PE, et al. Biomechanical properties of skin—Their influence on planning surgical incision. In: JJ Krizek, JE Hoopes, eds. Symposium on Basic Science in Plastic Surgery. St Louis: CV Mosby, 1975:72–79.
18. Veronesi V, Cascinelli N. Narrow excision (1-cm margin). A safe procedure for thin cutaneous melanoma. Arch Surg 1991;126:438–441.
19. Wolf DJ, Zitelli JA. Surgical margins for basal cell carcinoma. Arch Dermatol 1987;123:340–344.

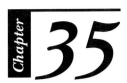

Subcutaneous Nodules

Leslie Ottinger

This chapter discusses soft-tissue nodules that lie in the subcutaneous fat layer. Some are attached to the overlying skin, arising from it or its appendages. Generally, though, on physical examination, they are found to be attached neither to the skin nor the underlying deep fascia. They are often of concern to the patient because of worry about malignancy but may also be painful, the site of infection, or large enough to be unsightly. Either reassurance or excision in a minor surgery setting is usually all that is needed in their management. Nodules in the axillary and femoral areas and the breast are discussed in other chapters.

NODULES ARISING FROM THE SKIN AND ITS APPENDAGES

"Sebaceous cysts" are seen with greater frequency in older patients. They may occur in any area but most commonly occur on the scalp, face, and chest wall. By careful examination, they may be shown to be attached to the overlying skin with a small dimple at the site. Patients are aware of the generally harmless nature of these lesions and often do not seek assistance until they become large or infected. Some are true sebaceous cysts, but most are dermal inclusion cysts that perhaps develop at a site of prior trauma. They contain a waxy, foul smelling material and have a distinct wall.

With infection, there is a painful increase in size and overlying redness. Antibiotics are neither useful nor necessary unless there is surrounding cellulitis. The proper treatment is surgical drainage with evacuation of the cyst contents. Intradermal injection of lidocaine

over the lesion is a simple way to obtain local anesthesia. Approximately 1 mL of lidocaine is slowly infused through a fine needle. It is not necessary to carry out further injections unless the cyst is to be removed. Through a short incision, the infected contents are removed. Because of the superficial location, packing is seldom necessary. Excision of an infected cyst is feasible but often requires a relatively large incision and is quite painful under local anesthesia. Thus, it is usually preferable to have the patient return for excision when the inflammation has cleared. Failure to eventually remove the cyst is usually followed by recurrent infection.

Elective excision is best accomplished through a short, double-elliptical incision to include the point of skin attachment. Entering the wall of the cyst is unpleasant but does not compromise the excision. Leaving part of the wall, especially prone to occur when there is an infection, results in recurrence. Closure with a single deep vertical mattress stitch often suffices. Closure of the subcutaneous space is difficult and unnecessary.

Scalp cysts may be single but are often multiple and some have a familial occurrence. Most times they can be easily removed through a short incision which is closed with a single nylon stitch. Local anesthesia is easily induced. Because infection after excision is rare, preparation of the skin by shaving is not necessary and, further, may lead to a permanent bald spot.

Generally, all lesions removed should be submitted for microscopic examination. Rare instances of unusual and even malignant appendage tumors and metastases from remote malignancies have been recorded. Conversely, the possibility of malignancy is so low that it does not serve as an indication for the removal of just any typical "sebaceous cyst."

LIPOMAS

Lipomas are benign tumors that are microscopically indistinguishable from mature subcutaneous fat. Liposarcomas in the subcutaneous area are rare. When they do occur, they are large, bulky tumors, usually located in the buttocks or medial thighs. Subcutaneous lipomas lie in the fat layer between the superficial fascia and the investing fascia of the underlying muscle. The typical lipoma is seen as a soft, rounded, freely moveable nodule. When they are asymptomatic, the choice of removal may be left to the patient. Fear of malignancy, local pain from pressure, and cosmetic considerations are the usual indications for excision.

These typical lipomas lie within a capsule of compressed adjacent tissue deep to the superficial fascia and are easily removed under local anesthesia. A short incision is made to expose the surface and then, with limited blunt dissection and pressure, they may be extruded. Most have such a meager blood supply that ligation of vessels can be confined to the initial incision unless the operator has dissected out into the surrounding tissues.

Angiolipomas are simple lipomas that contain an increased number of small blood vessels. They are firm and sometimes painful. They require no special handling.

Some lipomas are configured like a cluster of grapes. They are especially likely to be found in the posterior neck and upper back near the midline. Complete removal is tedious and may be very difficult under local anesthesia when they are large. After removal is thought to be complete, residual nodules can often be detected by careful palpation around the incision. With this configuration, recurrence is frequent.

Intramuscular lipomas, usually found in the posterior axilla or around the inferior border of the scapula, may feel like subcutaneous lipomas. They are easily removed. A row of one to three lipomas, sometimes bilateral, is occasionally present in the lumbosacral paraspinous

area. These actually are sites of herniation of fat through defects in the fascia and are often the source of pain. They are removed through short transverse incisions. Especially over the buttocks and thighs, lipomas may break through the superficial fascia and become adherent to the skin, forming a characteristic thin-skinned soft bubble. For an optimal scar, the skin should be excised with the lipoma.

Fat pads, not true lipomas, may develop over the lower cervical spinous processes and in the region of the knee and elbow. With those on the extremities, the presence of a symmetrical lesion on the other side may point to the diagnosis. They are diffuse rather than localized. It is difficult to remove them with a good cosmetic result, and sometimes they are best referred to a cosmetic surgeon.

Patients with familial lipomatosis sometimes have almost countless lesions. They are not difficult to remove, and the best policy is just to remove the troublesome ones under local anesthesia.

Infections are rare after excision of lipomas, but hematomas are not. Some hematomas may be aspirated through a large needle, but most are just left to reabsorb, a process that takes several weeks.

UNUSUAL SUBCUTANEOUS NODULES

A host of other subcutaneous nodules are encountered in a general surgical practice. Fibromas form at the site of hematomas or fat necroses. Enlarged lymph nodes are found especially in the lower axillary area and upper arm and thighs. Nerve sheath tumors form hard nodules characteristically moveable only in the lateral–medial axis. Ganglions are found especially around the wrist, and fascia nodules and tendon sheath tumors are not uncommon in the palm and plantar surface of the foot. Small traumatic aneurysms of the branches of the temporal arteries occur in the lateral–frontal regions. Because isolated malignant subcutaneous nodules are so rare, most of these lesions can be safely observed unless they are symptomatic.

Acute thrombosis of a segment of vein, often the result of trauma or a needle, can lead to a characteristic tubular lesion whose configuration is often obscured by inflammation. When in the region of the breast or anterior axilla, a tumor nodule may be suspected. This particular lesion, when of unknown cause, has been referred to as Mondor's disease. On resolution of phlebitis, there may be a residual firm nodule. These are harmless, but biopsy is sometimes necessary to reassure an overly anxious patient or primary care physician.

Selected Readings

1. Sakai Y, Okazaki M, Kobayashi S, Ohmori K. Endoscopic excision of large capsulated lipomas. Br J Plastic Surg 1996;49:228–232.
2. Kenawi MM. "Squeeze delivery" excision of subcutaneous lipoma related to anatomic site. Br J Surg 1995;82:1649–1650.
3. Reinking GF, Parsa FD. Extraction of lipomas: A simple technique. Hawaii Med J 1993;52:96.
4. Hallock GG. Endoscope-assisted suction extraction of lipomas. Ann Plastic Surg 1995;34:32–34.
5. Moore C, Greer DM Jr. Sebaceous cyst extraction through mini-incisons. Br J Plastic Surg 1975;28:307–309.
6. Albom MJ. Surgery of sebaceous cysts. J Dermatol Surg 1975;1:73–74.
7. Khafif RA, Attie JN. One-stage excision of infected sebaceous cysts. Arch Surg 1969;98:117–118.
8. Vivakananthan C. Minimal incision for removing sebaceous cysts. Br J Plastic Surg 1972;254:60–62.

36

Pigmented Skin Lesions

Craig L. Slingluff, Jr.

Almost all patients have pigmented skin lesions. Most are simple nevi or, in older patients, keratoses. The focus of this chapter is (1) on pigmented skin lesions for which the principal concern is to rule out the presence of malignant melanoma and (2) on outpatient surgical procedures that are useful in the management of melanoma.

INCIDENCE AND ETIOLOGY OF MELANOMA

Malignant melanoma is not the most common skin neoplasm. It accounts for only 4% of skin cancers, or 30,000 to 35,000 new cases annually in the United States. The most prevalent skin cancer is basal cell cancer, and the second most prevalent is squamous cell cancer. Less prevalent than melanoma are unusual cancers of the skin such as adenocarcinomas of sweat glands and epithelioid schwannomas. Whereas cancer deaths from basal cell and squamous cell cancers are uncommon, melanoma accounts for approximately 7000 deaths annually in the United States.

Melanoma is a malignancy arising from melanocytes, pigment-producing cells of the skin, usually but not always in sun-exposed areas. Commonly, melanomas in women arise on the lower extremities. In men, they commonly arise on the trunk, especially the back. It is believed that the primary cause of melanoma is related to exposure to ultraviolet (UV) radiation from the sun. However, the etiologic role of UV light is not entirely understood, and some melanomas arise in areas not exposed to the sun. The association between melanoma

and sun exposure is based on a number of observations, including studies showing that persons who had severe burns in childhood seem to be at higher risk for development of melanoma later in life. Persons who have been exposed to the sun on a regular basis, however, such as farmers and maritime workers, appear not to be at increased risk for melanoma. Persons at highest risk for melanoma are those with fair complexions whose skin burns easily. In particular, persons whose skin type is most associated with melanoma have a "Celtic" complexion, that is, pale skin, freckles, blond or reddish hair, and light-colored eyes. Melanoma is uncommon in Caucasians with dark skin and is even more uncommon in people of Asian or African-American background.

SIGNS OF MELANOMA

Many melanomas arise from preexisting nevi, but most probably arise de novo. Usually they have irregular borders and variations in color. Often they are raised above the skin surface. Occasionally they are very dark black without any other coloration. Although many skin changes may have these appearances, any with these characteristics should be evaluated by a physician and most should be biopsied. The mnemonic useful for identifying melanomas is A (asymmetry), B (border irregularity), C (color variation), with additional features being D (diameter >6 mm) and E (elevated) (Table 36–1). All these features are evident in the melanoma shown in Figure 36–1. This lesion on the skin of the anterior chest was 4.3 mm thick. To diagnose melanoma early, small

Table 36–1. Physical Features of Melanomas

1. Asymmetry
2. Irregularity of borders
3. Color variation
4. Diameter >6 mm
5. Elevation

and flat lesions that satisfy the A-B-C criteria or are totally black should be considered suspicious. The lesion in Figure 36–2 is quite extensive but almost totally flat. Excision revealed the lesion to be almost entirely a dysplastic nevus with only a 3-mm wide area of melanoma, only 0.8 mm thick. The patient's prognosis is good, which is credited to his physicians, who identified and excised this lesion at this stage.

If a melanoma is diagnosed and removed when it is very thin, cure may be possible. If it is diagnosed when it is much thicker, metastasis may have occurred and cure is less likely. Signs that are particularly worrisome in a primary lesion are itching, bleeding, ulceration, or the presence of satellite lesions. Some melanomas do not have brown or black pigment and appear very much like normal skin. These can be difficult to diagnose, even by an experienced physician. Among these amelanotic melanomas, there is a disproportionate number of melanomas that fit into an uncommon histologic group—the desmoplastic melanomas. Because of the variable presentations of melanoma, any pigmented skin lesion that has changed should be evaluated for possible biopsy.

BIOPSY TECHNIQUES

The diagnosis of a pigmented skin lesion can be made easily with a simple biopsy. There can be a difference between removing a skin lesion and making a diagnosis. Shave biopsies are often performed for the easy removal of benign skin lesions such as keratoses, but significant diagnostic and prognostic information can be lost if a shave biopsy is performed for a melanoma. The goals, if melanoma is suspected, should be to make a diagnosis, to collect the most prognostic information possible, and not to interfere with subsequent ther-

apy. The principles that ensure success of these goals are to always take full-thickness biopsy samples, include normal skin in the biopsy, and orient the incision longitudinally on extremities. A full-thickness biopsy includes all layers of the skin, so that the subcutaneous fat is entered during the biopsy. This is usually done by excising a small ellipse of skin with a scalpel. The amount of normal skin included in the biopsy need not be extensive. A 1- to 2-mm margin of normal skin allows the pathologist to examine the junctional changes that are crucial to identifying melanoma and to determine whether it is a primary or a metastatic lesion.

These biopsies are easily performed in the outpatient or ambulatory setting. No preoperative laboratory studies need to be performed. The skin should be prepped with an antiseptic solution and draped with a sterile fenestrated drape. A small wheal of 1% lidocaine may be injected through a 27-g needle under and around the skin lesion. The lesion is then excised with a number 15 blade, maintaining a 1- to 2-mm margin, lifting the skin up with Adson forceps. Hemostasis can usually be achieved without electrocautery by a combination of gentle pressure and suture closure. The incision is closed, in many cases, with a subcuticular 4-0 absorbable suture and Steri-Strips. If there is significant tension, a few interrupted vertical mattress sutures of 4-0 monofilament suture material will suffice. The wound can be covered with a sterile simple dry dressing for 2 to 3 days. Antibiotics are not required.

In some cases, the lesion is extensive enough that even simple excision would leave a large wound, giving concern for functional and cosmetic implications. In those cases, excision of the portion of the lesion of greatest concern will suffice. Again, some normal skin should be included. Partial excision of a melanoma does not compromise subsequent therapy and does not alter prognosis, as long as the full thickness of the lesion can be evaluated.

A punch biopsy technique may be useful, such as for small nevi that are suspicious. A punch biopsy instrument is a disposable circular blade on a handle that can be used to excise a small circle of full-thickness skin. Punch biopsy instruments that excise circles

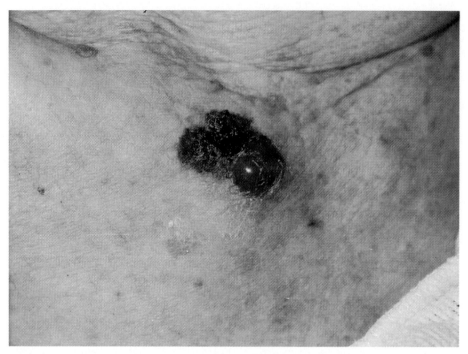

Figure 36–1. A thick melanoma is characterized by asymmetry, border irregularity, color variations, diameter greater than 6 mm, and marked elevation. The black, flatter portion measured 11 × 14 mm across. The raised reddish nodule was 1 cm across and 4 mm high. The Breslow thickness was 4.3 mm.

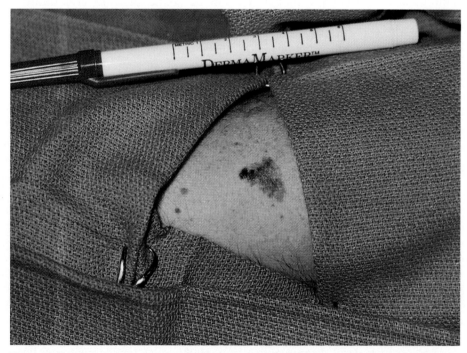

Figure 36–2. The melanoma arising in this large dysplastic nevus was in the more darkly pigmented portion and was only 3 mm across and 0.8 mm deep. The remainder of the lesion was benign. The entire lesion was excised with a 1-cm margin.

of skin 4, 5, or 6 mm in diameter are useful for quick excisions of small nevi, but, when using the instruments, the clinician must be certain that the lesion can be completely excised with a 1- to 2-mm margin and that the lesion is not crushed during excision. After punching out the skin, the circle of skin containing the lesion must be excised with scissors below the dermis. A fine forceps can be used to elevate the skin circle while scissors are used to cut underneath it. After excision, the lesion should be placed in formalin and sent for histologic evaluation.

At least as important as the biopsy technique is the choice of skin incision. Especially on extremities, the orientation of the initial skin biopsy is a crucial determinant of the subsequent therapy. If the pigmented lesion is melanoma, a wide excision will be needed, the orientation of which is determined largely by the orientation of the initial excision. It is difficult to close a transverse incision on an extremity; thus, a transverse incision is more likely to require a skin graft. Also, because the innervation to skin surfaces runs longitudinally, a transversely oriented excision interrupts more of the innervation to skin distal to the lesion. On the other hand, if an incision crosses a joint, it may lead to a contracture that limits range of motion, so extremity excisions near a joint may need to be oriented transversely or be closed with a Z-plasty across the joint.

These and other concerns of a cosmetic and functional nature should be considered in making incisions on extremities and elsewhere. For example, on the back, a transverse incision results in a smaller area of numbness laterally and is usually under less tension during normal movements of the arms in an anterior direction. Ultimately, it is far preferable to close a wide excision site primarily, and selection of the optimal orientation for the original biopsy has a significant impact on that outcome and on functional results after definitive surgical therapy. Thus, the effects of the possible incisions should be considered before an excisional biopsy is performed.

PROGNOSIS

When a primary melanoma is diagnosed in a skin biopsy, several characteristics of it are noted by the pathologist. The most important of these is thickness, which is measured in millimeters. Melanomas that are less than three fourths of a millimeter (<0.76 mm) thick are considered thin melanomas and are unlikely to recur once they are removed. Melanomas thicker than 4 mm are considered thick melanomas and have more than a 50% chance of recurring or metastasizing to other organs. Melanomas intermediate in thickness have a likelihood of recurrence that averages roughly 30% to 40%. For example, right axillary nodal metastases developed in the patient with the melanoma shown in Figure 36–1 within 2 years of initial diagnosis, a finding not surprising given the thickness of that primary lesion.

SURGICAL TREATMENT OF A PRIMARY MELANOMA: WIDE LOCAL EXCISION

The initial treatment of melanoma of the skin requires wide excision after the initial biopsy. The goal is to remove an area of normal skin around the melanoma to remove dermal or subcutaneous micrometastases that often occur as a result of lymphatic spread. By doing so, the chance that the melanoma will recur locally is reduced. For melanomas in situ (Clark level I melanoma, confined to the epidermis and epidermal–dermal junction), a 5-mm margin is adequate. Thin melanomas, up to 1 mm thick, should be excised with a 1-cm margin. Thicker melanomas require a 2- to 3-cm margin. In many locations on the body, this can be accomplished with an elliptical skin incision, and the wound can be closed primarily. In some locations, a skin graft may be required. This is particularly true on the face, the hands, and the feet but may be true on other parts of the body as well. In some of these locations, concern for appearance or function may necessitate that smaller margins be taken to permit primary closure.

Wide excisions can generally be performed easily in the outpatient or ambulatory setting but require more time than a simple skin biopsy. The goals of the wide excision are to obtain an adequate margin of normal tissue radially, to resect full-thickness skin and subcutaneous tissue in the area of concern, and to minimize morbidity. This is usually best performed in an operating room using local anesthetic (lidocaine 1%, with epinephrine 1:100,000 to slow systemic distribution, and sodium bicarbonate 0.084% to decrease patient discomfort) and intravenous sedation. An incision is planned, first by measuring the appropriate margin of excision around the initial scar and extending the ellipse in the direction that will best permit primary closure under the least tension. Again, for extremity melanomas, the excision scar is best oriented longitudinally. Once the planned ellipse of skin has been marked out, a field block can be performed with the lidocaine, anesthetizing deeply through the full thickness of the subcutaneous tissue. The incision is then made with a scalpel and deepened through the full thickness of subcutis, down to the muscle fascia with electrocautery in all directions. The attachments to the fascia are divided with electrocautery as the specimen is lifted from the wound. An Allis clamp is useful for grasping one end of the skin as the dissection progresses. When large cutaneous nerves are encountered deep in the subcutis, they can be preserved. When they run through the superficial subcutaneous tissue or innervate the excised skin, they should be sacrificed.

Closure of the wide excision can usually be accomplished, under some tension, in two layers, using interrupted 3-0 absorbable sutures to reapproximate the subcutaneous fascia, then using 3-0 nonabsorbable monofilament sutures in a full-thickness vertical mattress pattern to reapproximate the skin and to reinforce the subcutaneous closure. The closure usually heals well and the skin and scar stretch with time, much as is observed with tissue expanders, so the tension resolves over a few weeks to months.

Where the wide excision wound does not close initially, some limited undermining of the skin permits raising of skin flaps under less tension. If this fails or is not feasible, a skin graft may be needed. Bulky flaps are not usually recommended because of the difficulty of evaluating for early local recurrences in that setting. However, split-thickness skin grafts that are harvested from skin distant from, or contralateral to, the primary site can be used to cover a defect. In certain more sensitive patients or in more sensitive locations, a full-thickness graft may be harvested from the inguinal area, the neck, or the abdominal wall and used similarly, but with better cosmesis expected than with a split-thickness graft. In either case, if the graft is placed on deep tissue that may move, such as on the calf, the limb should be immobilized (e.g., in a cast or splint) to facilitate healing. The graft can then be exposed after 5 days and cared for in a routine manner. In general, a skin graft can be harvested after injection of local anesthetic, but, in some patients, this is more difficult and a brief general anesthetic is advisable.

METASTATIC PATTERNS AND NATURAL HISTORY OF MELANOMA

Although wide excision of melanoma is curative in some cases, all invasive melanomas have some risk of metastasis, with that risk correlating well with the maximal thickness (Breslow thickness) of the primary melanoma. Although other factors, including the level of invasion (Clark level), ulceration, and site of the melanoma, also have prognostic significance, thickness is the principal prognostic factor. Thus, it is important to know the stage accurately. This requires full-thickness skin excisions at the time of original biopsy.

Melanomas typically metastasize through lymphatic channels, usually to the regional nodes draining the primary melanoma. If a melanoma arises on an arm, the most common place for metastases to be found is in the axillary nodes. However, when a melanoma arises on the trunk or on the head and neck, lymphatic drainage patterns can be less predictable.

A total of 80% to 90% of first metastases of melanoma can be found on physical examination, either in the skin or in lymph nodes. Metastases in the skin typically appear as nodules that are either black or dark blue, but they may appear without any color. When melanoma metastasizes to lymph nodes, the nodes usually appear large, round, and very hard, much like marbles. Usually, there is no tenderness or pain associated with them. Suspicious-appearing nodes can usually be evaluated easily, accurately, and rapidly by fine-needle biopsy in the outpatient setting. Surgery often permits complete removal of cutaneous and isolated nodal metastases, and some patients treated surgically for nodal or cutaneous metastases survive for years without distant disease.

Melanoma is also prone to metastasize to visceral sites through hematogenous dissemination. There is often little that can be done to effect cure in those cases, but some treatments may be helpful, including chemotherapy and cytokine therapy. There are novel experimental immunotherapy approaches available in certain circumstances, including several melanoma vaccine approaches.

MELANOMA FROM AN UNKNOWN PRIMARY

It is uncommon but possible for metastatic melanoma to be identified in lymph nodes or in viscera without an apparent primary melanoma. It is believed that in these situations the immune system may have destroyed the original, or primary, melanoma, while failing to destroy the melanoma cells that spread to other sites.

EVALUATION OF REGIONAL NODAL BASINS

One of the most controversial issues in the management of melanoma has been the appropriate surgical management of clinically negative regional lymph node basins. Evidence is accumulating that elective lymph node dissections (ELND) do not provide a survival advantage over selective dissections of nodal basins when palpable nodal metastases are evident. Although subset analysis of the recently published data from the Intergroup trial has been interpreted to show that, for a subset of patients, there is a survival advantage to ELND, when reasonable statistical principles are applied to these subset analyses, the differences are not statistically significant. An earlier World Health Organization study, a Mayo Clinic study, and this Intergroup study provide corroborative evidence against a survival advantage to ELND over delayed selective lymphadenectomy in patients with isolated

nodal metastases. The morbidity of lymphadenectomy is significant, especially for inguinal nodes, and general anesthesia or spinal anesthesia is required.

Sentinel lymph node biopsy techniques have been developed in the past several years, based on initial work by Donald Morton. Dr. Morton has demonstrated convincingly that the node (or nodes) draining a primary tumor site can, in most cases, be identified either by using a vital blue dye or a technetium-labeled sulfur colloid injected into the skin, which is taken up into the lymphatics. Furthermore, it is evident that the negative predictive value of a negative sentinel node biopsy approaches 100% and that the sensitivity of sentinel node biopsy exceeds the sensitivity of standard complete node dissections because the pathologist can examine the sentinel nodes more carefully, by serial sectioning, than is practical for an entire node dissection.

The advantage of sentinel node biopsies is that reliable staging information can be obtained with minimal morbidity, using a technique that requires only local anesthesia and that can be performed at the time of wide local excision. This procedure can generally be performed on an outpatient basis. If metastatic melanoma is found in the nodal basin, then a complete node dissection can be scheduled electively. The finding of a positive sentinel node upstages a patient's classification to stage III, making the patient eligible for adjuvant therapy with high-dose alpha-interferon or for inclusion in experimental tumor vaccine protocols. It is reasonable to consider sentinel node biopsy in patients with melanomas greater than 1 to 1.5 mm thick. Most surgeons are using technetium-labeled sulfur colloid to identify the draining nodal basin and to localize the sentinel nodes preoperatively. A hand-held gamma camera then can be used intraoperatively to localize the sentinel nodes definitively before and after excision. Simultaneous injection of vital blue dye can further confirm the identity of radiolabeled nodes as sentinel; some surgeons use both techniques together.

SUMMARY

The management of melanoma can be handled on an ambulatory basis for most procedures, from initial diagnosis by biopsy of a suspicious lesion, to wide excision and sentinel node biopsy. Keys to optimal management include early diagnosis, aggressive resection of the primary lesion with attention to the orientation of the incision, and complete staging of patients with intermediate and thick melanomas by sentinel node biopsy, when appropriate.

Selected Readings

1. Balch CM, Houghton AN, Milton GW, Sober AJ, Soong S-J, eds. Cutaneous Melanoma. 2nd ed. Philadelphia: JB Lippincott, 1992.
2. Balch CM, Soong S-J, Bartolucci AA, et al. Efficacy of an elective regional lymph node dissection of 1 to 4 mm thick melanomas for patients 60 years of age and younger. Ann Surg 1996;224:255–266.
3. Breslow A. Thickness, cross sectional areas and depth of invasion in the prognosis of cutaneous melanoma. Ann Surg 1970;172:902–908.
4. Clark WHJ, From L, Bernadino EA, et al. The histogenesis and biologic behavior of primary human malignant melanoma of the skin. Cancer Res 1969;29:705–726.
5. Kirkwood JM, Strawderman MH, Ernstoff MS, et al. Interferon alfa-2b adjuvant therapy of high-risk resected cutaneous melanoma: the Eastern Cooperative Oncology Group Trial EST 1684. J Clin Oncol 1996;14:7–17.
6. Morton DL, Wen DR, Wong JH, et al. Technical details of intraoperative lymphatic mapping for early stage melanoma. Arch Surg 1992;127:392–399.
7. Reintgen D, Cruse CW, Wells K, et al. The orderly progression of melanoma nodal metastases. Ann Surg 1994;220:759–767.
8. Rhodes AR. Public education and cancer of the skin. What do people need to know about melanoma and nonmelanoma skin cancer? Cancer 1995;75:613–636.
9. Sim FH, Taylor WF, Pritchard DJ, et al. Lymphadenectomy in the management of stage I malignant melanoma: a prospective randomized study. Mayo Clinic Proc 1986;61:697–705.
10. Slingluff CL Jr. Tumor antigens and tumor vaccines: peptides as immunogens. Semin Surg Oncol 1996;12:446–453.
11. Slingluff CL Jr, Stidham KR, Ricci WM, et al. Surgical management of regional lymph nodes in patients with melanoma. Experience with 4682 patients. Ann Surg 1994;219:120–130.
12. Veronesi U, Adamus J, Bandiera DC, et al. Delayed regional lymph node dissection in stage I melanoma of the skin of the lower extremities. Cancer 1982;49:2420–2430.
13. Veronesi U, Cascinelli N. Narrow excision (1-cm margin). A safe procedure for thin cutaneous melanoma. Arch Surg 1991;126:438–441.

Chapter 37

Perianal Disease

Paul C. Shellito

A complete evaluation of any patient with an anorectal lesion includes four separate maneuvers: careful anal inspection, digital rectal examination, anoscopy, and sigmoidoscopy (preferably flexible). If colonic disease is possible, barium enema radiography or colonoscopy should be added. The best anoscope is a smooth, tapered cylinder (nondisposable), absent a portion of its distal circumference ("Vernon David" type). The anal canal is closed by surrounding sphincter musculature; therefore, to examine it properly, the sphincters must be held open by the anoscope so that a given quadrant of the canal is exposed in the cutaway portion of the instrument (Fig. 37–1). If pain or stenosis precludes anal manipulation, examination under anesthesia may be necessary. Lidocaine ointment may be used to make office examination of a painful anus possible. Unsuspected fistulas, inflammatory bowel disease, and cancer must not be overlooked before treatment starts. Similarly, it is important not to miss infection with human immunodeficiency virus (HIV) or other sexually transmitted diseases (STDs), because treatment is consequently greatly influenced. The likelihood of mismanagement is minimized by obtaining a thoughtful history, having a high index of suspicion (especially for "atypical lesions" and for homosexuals), obtaining serologic tests when appropriate, and obtaining biopsy or culture of suspicious lesions. In general, because of high failure and complication rates, all but palliative anorectal surgery should be avoided in patients with inflammatory bowel disease and in those who are immu-

nosuppressed, granulocytopenic, or infected with HIV. Nevertheless, HIV-positive patients may benefit greatly if biopsy or culture reveals a specific treatable infectious cause for an anorectal problem.

Much anorectal surgery can be done in the outpatient setting. In the operating room, the best exposure is obtained with the patient in the prone jack-knife position with the buttocks

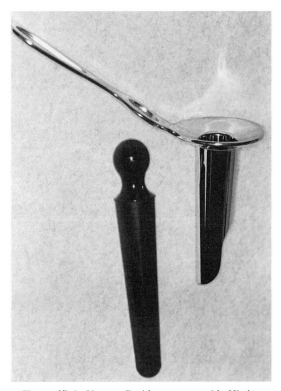

Figure 37–1. Vernon David anoscope with Hirshman handle.

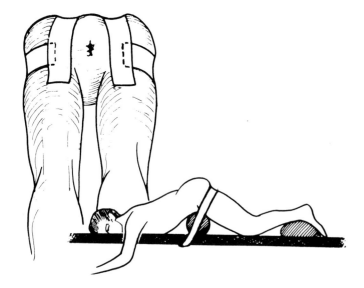

Figure 37–2. Prone jack-knife position. (From Goldberg SM, Gordon PH, Nivatvongs S. Essentials of Anorectal Surgery. Philadelphia: JB Lippincott, 1980:81.)

taped apart (Fig. 37–2). However, in an office setting, patients feel more comfortable in a lateral posture, with the buttocks extending slightly beyond the edge of the examining table (Fig. 37–3). A headlight greatly aids the surgeon in anorectal examination and surgery. Local anesthesia is often effective for routine anorectal surgery. By starting above the dentate line and progressing slowly caudally with submucosal injections, the surgeon can place the anesthetic nearly painlessly. Even when spinal or general anesthesia is used, it is worthwhile to inject bupivacaine (Marcaine) around the anus. This reduces pain immediately after surgery and eases the patient's trip home that day. Good quality operating anoscopes are invaluable for anorectal surgery. At least a bivalve speculum (Pratt), a hemicylindrical anoscope (Ferguson), and a large cylindrical scope with one quadrant missing (Fansler) should be available. When perioperative fluids are sharply limited, urinary retention after sur-

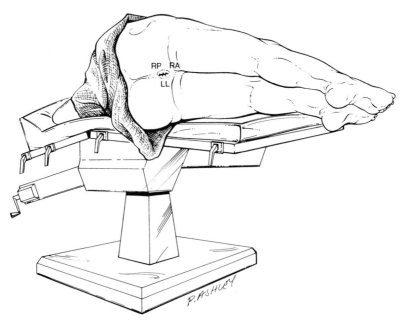

Figure 37–3. Lateral position. RP = right posterior; RA = right anterior; LL = left lateral. (From Mazier WP. Surgery of the Colon, Rectum and Anus. Philadelphia: WB Saunders, 1995:234.)

gery is minimized. Postoperatively, no more than analgesics, frequent warm perineal baths, and stool softeners (psyllium powder) is required. Anal packing and dilatations are painful and unnecessary. Follow-up evaluation is best done in 3 to 4 weeks, by which time healing is sufficient to allow repeat anal examination.

ANAL FISSURE AND STENOSIS

Anal fissures are small superficial longitudinal splits or ulcerations in the anoderm. (The anoderm is the sensitive thin squamous epithelium that lines the anal canal between the dentate line and the anal verge, and it is devoid of sweat glands and hair follicles.) Fissures are associated with a high internal sphincter tone (or at least sphincter spasm with defecation), which may arise from a diet low in fiber. The tight sphincter causes a relative anal stenosis such that bowel movements ultimately split open the anoderm. Most often, fissures are located in the midline posteriorly,

although they are occasionally anterior, especially in women. The external sphincter, which lies immediately outside the internal sphincter, is arrayed in loops or slings, which are weakest anteriorly and posteriorly. Relative lack of support there probably accounts for the location of typical fissures. Alternatively, the pathophysiologic characteristics of fissures may be ischemic ulcers induced by the tight internal sphincter. When a fissure persists, it gradually acquires signs of chronicity: induration, deepening, and undermining of the fissure edges, visible white transverse internal sphincter muscle fibers at its base, a hypertrophic anal papilla at the dentate line proximally (which may be large enough to mimic a polyp, except that it is covered by anoderm, not mucosa), and a distal tag of edematous skin and scar tissue (the misnamed "sentinel pile") (Fig. 37–4).

Fissures cause pain and bleeding with bowel movements. The diagnosis is made simply by careful and gentle inspection with the patient's buttocks spread apart, sometimes with the help of local anesthetic ointment. Besides fissures, the causes of acute anal pain

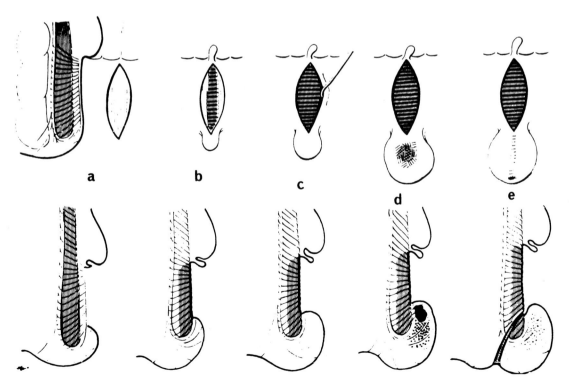

Figure 37–4. Anatomic changes that take place as an acute anal fissure becomes chronic. (From Notaras MJ. Anal fissure. In: Rob C, Smith R, eds. Operative Surgery. 3rd ed. London: Butterworths, 1977:355.)

are perianal abscess (which may be elusive if it is only intersphincteric), thrombosed external hemorrhoid, and occasionally an anal foreign body (which might be an unsuspected swallowed chicken or fish bone). These are usually readily distinguishable from fissures upon examination. However, other uncommon conditions such as inflammatory bowel disease, leukemia, syphilitic chancre, tuberculosis, herpes simplex, HIV infection, or cancer may cause anal fissures or ulcers. Because these should be treated nonoperatively when possible, it is important to differentiate them from "typical" fissures. The important clues to the uncommon conditions are fissures that are lateral, multiple, or unusually deep or broad based. Anal ulcers associated with acquired immunodeficiency syndrome (AIDS) may also be accompanied by a weak sphincter tone.

Some idiopathic fissures may heal with nonoperative therapy. Bulk stool softeners and frequent warm sitz baths are all that are required. Ointments, creams, and suppositories give additional symptomatic relief. The indication for surgery is a recurrent or persistent fissure that, despite medical treatment, causes symptoms severe enough to distress the patient. Because fissures are associated with a tight internal sphincter, surgical treatment dilates or divides this muscle. Afterward, the sphincter pressure returns to normal. Fissurectomy with posterior internal sphincterotomy, anal dilatation, and lateral internal sphincterotomy have been advocated. The first may result in a prolonged healing time and sometimes fecal soiling caused by a "keyhole deformity." Anal dilatation is acceptable, but disrupting the internal sphincter by tearing is less attractive than careful incision. Lateral internal sphincterotomy probably gives the lowest complication and recurrence rates, and is the preferred treatment.

Lateral internal sphincterotomy may be done using either an open or closed ("subcutaneous") technique. In both, the internal sphincter is divided between the level of the dentate line and the anal verge. The dentate line is readily seen. The lower end of the internal sphincter, which lies at the anal verge, may be palpated when the sphincter is gently held on stretch with an open operating anoscope. (The "intersphincteric groove" is the palpable depression between the caudal ends of the two sphincters; the external sphincter edge lies just external and slightly inferior to that of the internal sphincter.) For an open sphincterotomy, a 1.5- to 2.0-cm longitudinal incision is made between the dentate line and the anal verge with an anal speculum in place. Under direct vision, the surgeon slowly divides the white fibers of the internal sphincter using multiple light strokes of a small (number 15) knife blade. Because the dentate line is the midpoint of the anal canal, a 50% internal sphincterotomy is the result. After hemostasis, the anoderm is closed longitudinally with a fine absorbable suture (Fig. 37–5). The open technique provides clear exposure of the anatomy, especially for novices. The closed technique has the advantage of a somewhat smaller wound, but the disadvantage of a relatively blind procedure. With an anal speculum providing slight stretch on the sphincters, an index finger is placed in the anal canal, palpating the inner aspect of the internal sphincter. A tiny knife (a cataract knife or number 11 blade) is then inserted along the plane between the two sphincters via a small stab wound at the intersphincteric groove. The blade is directed medially, and the lower half of the internal sphincter is slowly divided, guided by the palpating finger. The anoderm of the lower anal canal is not opened, and the small stab wound is closed with one or two absorbable sutures (Fig. 37–6).

Alternatively, a slightly larger wound at the anal verge may be created, big enough to insert the tip of fine blunt-tipped scissors. The anoderm is elevated from the underlying internal sphincter up to the level of the dentate line, and the intersphincteric plane is similarly dissected. The internal sphincter is then divided with the scissors (in this situation, there is at least a partial view of the anatomy), and the small wound is closed. For any type of lateral internal sphincterotomy, the fissure itself need not be disturbed, although a large hypertrophic anal papilla or distal skin tag should be excised. Also, edges of a fibrotic fissure may be conservatively debrided and the fissure loosely closed, although that is of secondary importance.

Lateral internal sphincterotomy cures the anal fissure in approximately 95% of cases. Nevertheless, up to 15% of patients are left

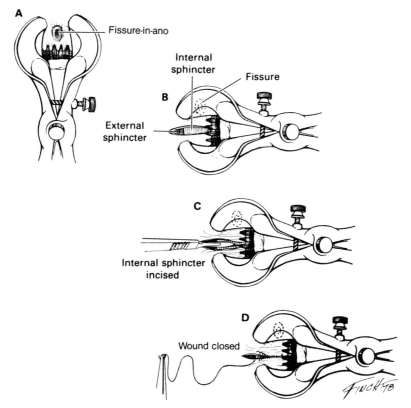

Figure 37–5. Open lateral internal sphincterotomy. (From Goldberg SM, Gordon PH, Nivatvongs S. Essentials of Anorectal Surgery. Philadelphia: JB Lippincott, 1980:95.)

Figure 37–6. Closed lateral internal sphincterotomy. (From Gingold BS. Simple in-office sphincterotomy with partial fissurectomy for chronic anal fissure. Surg Gynecol Obstet 1987;165:47. By permission of Surgery, Gynecology and Obstetrics, now known as the Journal of the American College of Surgeons.)

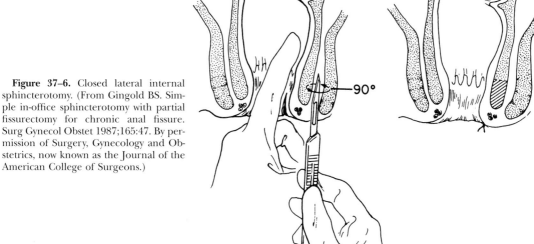

with a minor continence defect. Therefore, caution should be used when surgery is considered for patients susceptible to incontinence, such as elderly patients or those with chronic loose stools. Recurrent or persistent fissures are sometimes due to a misdiagnosed ulcer or an inadequate sphincterotomy. Anal manometry may be useful then to assess whether anal canal pressure is still elevated. In selected patients, a second lateral internal sphincterotomy on the opposite side may be done.

Management of anal stenosis is based on its cause. If a patient has not had previous anal surgery, the narrowing is usually caused by a tight internal sphincter (often in association with a fissure), probably from a lifetime of insufficient dietary fiber or perhaps mineral oil overuse. Internal sphincterotomy is likely to be curative. On the other hand, if the patient has had previous surgery and there is anal scar tissue present, then flap anoplasty may be required for relief. Y-V anoplasties and sliding island flap anoplasties are applicable and may be performed bilaterally if necessary. Anal stenosis associated with Crohn's disease is probably best managed by gentle dilatation only and may need to be done periodically.

ANORECTAL ABSCESS

Idiopathic anorectal abscesses start in a deep crypt gland at the dentate line. These glands can extend down through the internal sphincter muscle to the space between the internal and external sphincters. Thus, an intersphincteric abscess results, which is the initiating event for almost all perianal abscesses.

From there, the sepsis most often follows an intersphincteric path inferiorly to form a perianal abscess, or, less often, a transsphincteric route to give rise to an ischiorectal or postanal space abscess. In a horseshoe abscess, the sepsis spreads first through the posterior midline of the anal canal, to the deep postanal space. From there the infection may extend laterally to one or both ischiorectal spaces. The deep postanal space is located between the coccyx posteriorly, the anal canal anteriorly, the anococcygeal raphe and superficial external sphincter inferiorly, and the levator muscles superiorly. Rarely, an abscess may spread superiorly to form a supralevator abscess (Fig. 37–7).

The presentation of an abscess is usually clear, with swelling, redness, tenderness, fluctuance, and sometimes fever. Occasionally, there is only swelling and pain, without obvious fluctuance or even redness, but a collection of pus is nevertheless almost always present. Deep ischiorectal abscesses may produce nothing more than fever and vague pain (worse with sitting). Rarely, a small intersphincteric abscess may be a source of puzzling anal pain, because little may be present on examination other than point tenderness at the anal verge in one quadrant. As discussed for fissures, the differential diagnosis of acute anal pain includes abscesses, fissures, thrombosed external hemorrhoids, and anal foreign bodies. Perianal tenderness, induration, and erythema in granulocytopenic patients do not always indicate a frank underlying abscess, because there might not be a sufficient quantity of white blood cells to generate pus.

Prompt surgical drainage is indicated when-

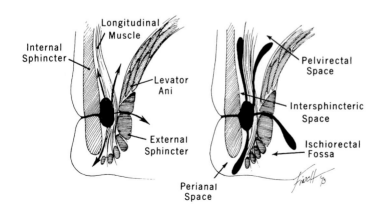

Figure 37–7. Pathways of extension of anorectal abscesses. (From Schwartz S. Principles of Surgery. New York: McGraw-Hill, 1974:1154.)

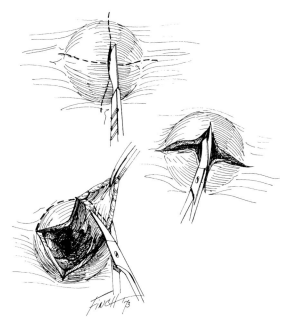

Figure 37–8. Cruciate incision for drainage of a perianal abscess. (From Schwartz S. Principles of Surgery. New York: McGraw-Hill, 1974:1154.)

ever a perianal abscess is found. Swelling and pain around the anus should be treated by lancing the lesion, even if fluctuance is not obvious, except in immunocompromised patients. Initial large-bore needle aspiration may pinpoint the location of an uncertain abscess. Usually under local anesthesia, a cruciate incision is made directly over the most superficial part of the abscess. Once the pus is released, excision of a small disc of overlying skin (by snipping off the four corners of the cruciate incision) ensures adequate and lasting drainage (Fig. 37–8).

General anesthesia may be needed in some cases to evaluate and drain large, deep, or complex abscesses. Because some abscesses do not invariably lead to a persistent anal fistula later, routine examination under anesthesia and division of the fistula at the time of abscess drainage are not ordinarily needed. Such actions only risk unnecessary sphincter damage. Unless surrounding cellulitis is present, antibiotics are not required after incision and drainage in immunocompetent patients. Perianal inflammation in granulocytopenic patients should be managed initially with broad-spectrum intravenous antibiotics, sitz baths, and treatment of the underlying hematologic dis-

order. Definite fluctuance should be present before proceeding to incision and drainage in these patients.

Unusual and complicated abscesses require special attention, usually after careful examination with the patient under general anesthesia. A postanal space abscess may be reached by a posterior midline incision between the anal verge and the tip of the coccyx, and by spreading the underlying fibers of the superficial external sphincter (which are mostly longitudinal in this location). A posterior midline internal sphincterotomy may be added to unroof the associated responsible crypt gland. Ischiorectal extensions of the abscess (horseshoe abscess) are best drained by lateral overlying counter incisions, perhaps with placement of latex rubber (Penrose) drains between the midline and lateral openings, temporarily tied in place (Fig. 37–9).

It is important to be certain of the origin of a supralevator abscess before carrying out drainage. An intersphincteric abscess with a high supralevator extension should be drained endorectally, not percutaneously, or else a difficult suprasphincteric fistula will ensue. Conversely, an ischiorectal (transsphincteric) abscess with a supralevator extension must be drained percutaneously, not transanally, or an extrasphincteric fistula may follow (Fig. 37–10).

FISTULA IN ANO

Because most anal fistulas result from drained abscesses, their genesis is also in the crypt glands of the dentate line. The fistula track is the remnant of the sometimes circuitous path that the abscess once took between the dentate line and the perineum. Often, the tract between the anal canal and perineum follows a more or less straight radial course, especially for anterior fistulas. A horseshoe abscess or fistula (as discussed above) results when a posterior midline crypt abscess extends through the internal and external sphincters into the deep postanal space, and then spreads laterally into the right or left ischiorectal fossa. Anal fistulas present as a draining, slightly tender small perianal sinus. The patient usually recalls an initiating perianal abscess. Once

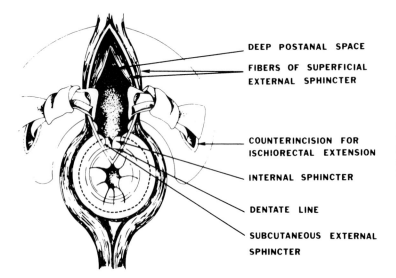

DEEP POSTANAL SPACE

FIBERS OF SUPERFICIAL
EXTERNAL SPHINCTER

COUNTERINCISION FOR
ISCHIORECTAL EXTENSION

INTERNAL SPHINCTER

DENTATE LINE

SUBCUTANEOUS EXTERNAL
SPHINCTER

Figure 37–9. Drainage of a horseshoe abscess. (From Held D, Khubchandani I, Sheets J, et al. Management of anorectal horseshoe abscess and fistula. Dis Colon Rectum 1986;29:793–797.)

established, the fistula is unlikely to heal permanently without surgery. Nevertheless, the skin over the external orifice sometimes temporarily heals over until the underlying sepsis erupts again, resulting in intermittent swelling and discomfort, followed by purulent drainage. The differential diagnosis includes draining Bartholin's abscesses or perianal furuncles, low pilonidal sinuses, and perianal hidradenitis suppurativa.

Surgery is indicated for any bothersome anal fistula; the procedure depends on the anatomy of the track. Fistulas are best categorized as intersphincteric, transsphincteric, suprasphincteric, and extrasphincteric (Fig. 37–

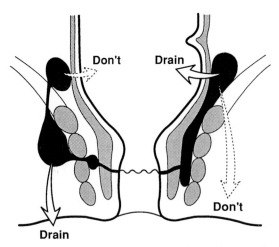

Figure 37–10. Correct drainage of supralevator abscesses. (From Beck D, Wexner S. Fundamentals of Anorectal Surgery. New York: McGraw-Hill, 1992:135.)

11). The first type is by far the most common. Simple fistulotomy and marsupialization, which divides the internal sphincter, is curative and safe. After laying open the fistula over a probe, granulation tissue is curetted out of the track, and the anoderm and perianal skin are sutured down to the underlying cut edge of the fibrous track with absorbable suture to decrease the size of the wound and discourage secondary hemorrhage. Other fistula types require careful assessment under anesthesia before deciding about surgery. A preoperative transanal ultrasound or even nuclear magnetic resonance imaging may help define the anatomy in complex cases.

In the operating room, *dilute* methylene blue solution injected into the track via a Mark's needle inserted into the external fistula orifice can be helpful; it identifies the internal opening at the dentate line, and preferentially stains granulation tissue, making the track easier to follow during fistulotomy. Excision of the fibrous track is rarely necessary for any fistula and only risks excessive sphincter damage. With any type of fistula, connecting blind tracts or cavities must be meticulously identified and opened. If at the time of surgery the internal opening cannot be found, only the known portion of the tract should be unroofed, and further search postponed until a later time (when it may become more obvious). When a transsphincteric or suprasphincteric fistula is found, the encompassed external sphincter muscle should be managed

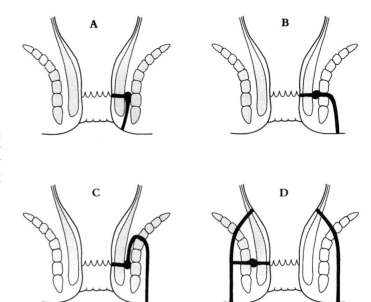

Figure 37-11. Types of anal fistulas: (A) intersphincteric, (B) transsphincteric, (C) suprasphincteric, and (D) extrasphincteric. (From Beck D, Wexner S. Fundamentals of Anorectal Surgery. New York: McGraw-Hill, 1992:135.)

cautiously. Major incontinence always follows division of the puborectalis muscle (anorectal ring). Division of a portion of the external sphincter leads to an unpredictable degree of incontinence. In general, the older the patient and the more muscle divided, the greater the loss of control. Anterior fistulas in women are also risky, because of the thin perineal body between anus and vagina.

Whenever there is doubt about whether a fistulotomy will lead to substantial incontinence, the safest course is to place a seton. For the seton operation, anoderm and internal sphincter are divided over the fistula, and lateral subcutaneous tracks are opened up. The heavy silk seton thread is then placed slightly snugly around the remaining isolated external sphincter muscle (Fig. 37-12). The seton promotes drainage and shrinkage of the fistula track. Also, the surrounding fibrous reaction that it stimulates prevents gaping of the sphincter after a staged completion fistulotomy 1 to 3 months later (after the first wound has healed in around the silk seton). This minimizes the likelihood of an eventual wide sphincter defect (Fig. 37-13). Some surgeons prefer to tighten the seton periodically in the office, thus slowly cutting through the encompassed tissue, but this is inconvenient and usually quite painful. Setons are appropriate for

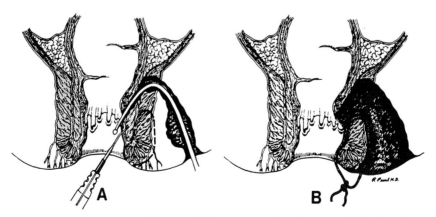

Figure 37-12. Seton treatment of deep anal fistulas. (A) Probe passed through fistula. (B) Division of internal sphincter, anoderm, and lateral subcutaneous tract; seton placed around remaining intact external sphincter. (From Pearl RK, Andrews JR, Orsay CP, et al. Role of the seton in the management of anorectal fistulas. Dis Colon Rectum 1993;36:574.)

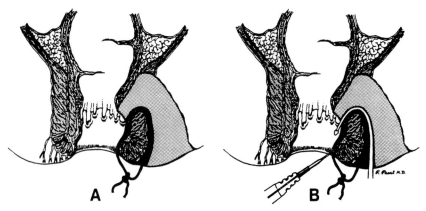

Figure 37–13. Seton treatment of deep anal fistulas (6–8 weeks later). **(A)** Previous partial fistulotomy wound has healed around the seton. **(B)** Completion fistulotomy with division of the encompassed external sphincter and removal of the seton. (From Pearl RK, Andrews JR, Orsay CP, et al. Role of the seton in the management of anorectal fistulas. Dis Colon Rectum 1993;36:574.)

many transsphincteric and all suprasphincteric fistulas.

Another attractive option for treatment of deep fistulas is endoanal flap closure of the internal fistula orifice, with laying open of only the track outside the sphincter. In this operation, a superiorly based trapezoidal or U-shaped flap is created, with its tip slightly caudal to the internal fistula orifice. The flap thickness consists of rectal mucosa, submucosa, and internal sphincter muscle, and the base should be about twice the width of the tip. After the flap is elevated, the tip containing the internal fistula opening is trimmed off. The underlying deep tissue (external sphincter) is closed with a few long-term absorbable sutures, thus occluding the track. The flap is then advanced downward and sutured over this closure with interrupted fine long-term absorbable stitches (Fig. 37–14). Finally, for complex or recurrent fistulas, autologous fibrin glue application offers a chance for cure. Horseshoe fistulas can be managed either by staged division with a seton or by posterior sphincterotomy to open the deep postanal space, with simple curettage of the lateral tracks. Increasingly, horseshoe fistulas are being managed by endoanal flap closure also. Low rectovaginal fistulas originating from trauma, childbirth, or infection can be well treated by transanal flap closure without colostomy. The vaginal end of the fistula (the lower pressure side) is left open for drainage. De-

pending on the cause, an extrasphincteric fistula requires a more radical approach. As opposed to the other fistula varieties, it does not begin at the dentate line. When it comes from diseased bowel in the pelvis (e.g., diverticulitis, inflammatory bowel disease), resection of the abnormal intestine is usually curative. For the rare persistent iatrogenic or traumatic extrasphincteric fistula, curettage of the track and construction of a temporary diverting colostomy may be necessary. Anal fistulas recur because of inadequate drainage of the originating anal gland, associated abscesses, or ramifying blind tracts. Alternatively, the explanation may be an unsuspected and unusual cause such as cancer, a foreign body, inflammatory bowel disease, tuberculosis, actinomycosis, or HIV infection. Major and persistent incontinence after a fistulotomy (or any localized anal trauma) is best managed by overlapping sphincteroplasty. Six to 12 months should elapse before sphincteroplasty is contemplated, however, to allow maturation of fibrosis and because incontinence sometimes resolves with time alone.

Anorectal fistulas associated with Crohn's disease have an especially high rate of recurrence or persistence. There is often active disease elsewhere in the gastrointestinal tract, especially proctitis. In approximately 10% of cases, anorectal abnormalities are the first manifestation of Crohn's disease. Incontinence may result from repeated anal surgery in these patients. Nevertheless, superficial abscesses and fistulas may be dealt with in the usual way (perhaps with concomitant oral metronidazole). If there is no associated proctocolitis, success rates are reasonable, but not as good as in normal patients. Endoanal flap closure, with or without colostomy, is another option for treatment of deeper fistulas in these patients (including rectovaginal fistulas), especially if the rectal mucosa appears uninflamed. Deep or complex symptomatic fistulas may be simply palliated by placement of a loose permanent seton to maintain drainage. Again, occasionally fibrin glue may help. Proctectomy is sometimes the only recourse for symptomatic extrasphincteric fistulas associated with Crohn's disease, or for any patient with severe perianal Crohn's disease (multiple or

deep fistulas, recurrent strictures, recurrent rectovaginal fistulas), but the necessity for this is unusual.

CONDYLOMATA ACUMINATUM

Anal condylomata acuminatum (venereal or genital warts) are caused by a human papilloma virus (HPV), which seems to thrive in the warm and moist perineum. Most often, it is spread by sexual contact (frequently in homosexual men), but, occasionally, patients acquire it by close nonsexual contact from unknown sources. Condylomata are often multiple (anal and genital), cover wide areas of perineal skin, and may extend into the anal canal. The warts almost always lie caudal to

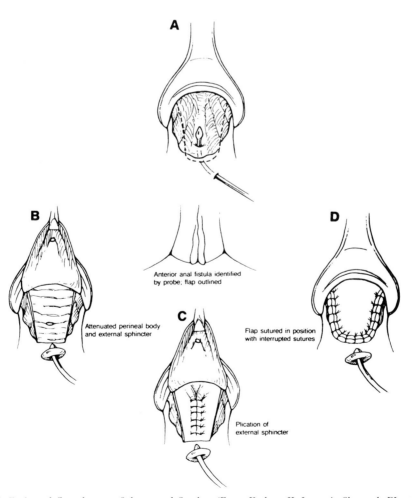

Figure 37–14. Endoanal flap closure of deep anal fistulas. (From Kodner IJ, Jazor A, Shemesh EI, et al. Endorectal advancement flap repair of rectovaginal and other complicated anorectal fistulas. Surgery 1993;114:685.)

the dentate line, except in immunodeficient patients. The fleshy cauliflower or frond-like appearance of these large or small lesions is typical, but the differential diagnosis also includes condyloma latum (secondary syphilis) and especially squamous cell carcinoma. Thus, biopsy samples should be obtained before treatment (especially because podophyllin alters cellular morphology), and, occasionally, darkfield examination should be performed for spirochetes. HPV infection (especially types 16 and 18) is also associated with anal squamous cell carcinoma in situ (CIS) or anal intraepithelial neoplasia, as well as invasive anal cancer.

Anal condylomata are difficult to treat because of their high recurrence rate. It is not likely that the virus is ever completely eradicated, despite elimination of the macroscopic warts. Recurrences may occur from reinfection from others, autoinoculation from overlooked lesions, or reactivation of endogenous latent viruses. Thus, successful therapy requires repeated follow-up visits and attention to contacts. Careful anoscopy is important; otherwise lesions within the anal canal can may be missed. Repeated topical applications in the office of Bichloroacetic Acid, trichloroacetic acid, or podophyllin can be used on limited and relatively small warts. Extensive disease, however, requires excision and cauterization (electrocautery or laser) under anesthesia, with follow-up chemical treatment of residual lesions. Excision and cauterization should be applied as carefully as possible only to the warts, sparing the intervening segments of normal anoderm to minimize the risk of later anal stenosis. Intralesional or intra-anal injections of alpha-interferon, especially in conjunction with excision and cauterization, may be helpful for difficult cases. HIV-positive patients respond particularly poorly to treatment, probably because of the associated immunodeficiency. Furthermore, except in healthy-appearing patients early in the course of their disease, excision and cauterization is often followed by chronically unhealed wounds. Giant condyloma acuminatum (Buschke-Löwenstein's tumor) contains invasive squamous cell carcinoma in approximately 50% of cases, so early and radical excision is recommended. If the lesion is extensive or recurrent, or if invasive cancer is found, abdominoperineal resection may be necessary, or perhaps radiation and chemotherapy.

BOWEN'S DISEASE

Perianal Bowen's disease is a slowly growing intraepithelial neoplasm (squamous cell CIS). The pathogenesis is unknown but may in many cases be associated with HPV infection. The disease progresses to frank invasive squamous cell carcinoma in approximately 5% of cases.

The lesion is more common in women than men and most often afflicts patients in their 40s and 50s. The abnormal epithelium may be small, inconspicuous, and asymptomatic, such that it is sometimes discovered accidentally after unrelated anorectal surgery such as hemorrhoidectomy. On the other hand, there may be small or large areas of epidermis with irregular, erythematous, scaly plaques. Symptoms, if any, are nonspecific—itching, discomfort, burning, and occasionally bleeding. The differential diagnosis includes condyloma acuminatum, anal skin tags or external hemorrhoids, fungal infections, psoriasis, contact dermatitis (or any other dermatitis), Paget's disease, squamous cell carcinoma, and downward spread of rectal cancer. Because signs and symptoms are so nonspecific, the diagnosis is frequently delayed; it is wise to obtain a biopsy sample of any unusual or persistent anal skin lesion. Furthermore, Bowen's disease may be associated with CIS or invasive carcinoma of the vulva or cervix, especially if there is coexisting HPV infection or condylomata acuminatum. Otherwise, there is no increased risk of internal malignancy in these patients.

Surgery is indicated for Bowen's disease because there is risk of progression to cancer. Full-thickness wide local excision of the abnormal epithelium is carried out, with primary closure, split-thickness skin grafting, or even secondary closure. Nevertheless, control of the lesion may be difficult because the neoplastic epithelium may extend well beyond the gross margins of abnormal-appearing skin. Thus, it is appropriate to "map" the anal epithelium at the commencement of the operation by taking multiple biopsy samples for frozen section pathologic analysis. Biopsy samples are taken 1 cm from the edge of the lesion and from four quadrants in the anal canal (just below the dentate line), anal margin, and perianal skin. Margins of the excised tissue are also evaluated to ensure complete removal. Full excision and coverage is difficult when the area of Bowen's disease is large. Some authors have taken a more conservative approach by removing gross disease only, and following the patient closely thereafter. Recurrence is always a potential problem after excision of Bowen's disease; even after meticulous resection, the disease reappears in at least 5% of patients. Careful long-term follow-up is essential.

PAGET'S DISEASE

Perianal Paget's disease is a rare and poorly understood intraepithelial adenocarcinoma. The extramammary variety can occur wherever apocrine glands are located. It is a slowly growing malignancy that may remain localized for years, but may also become invasive and lethal. The pathogenesis is unclear, but there are probably two overlapping varieties. The first is an initially benign form (but with a great tendency to recur locally), which arises either from primitive multipotential cells in the epidermis or from apocrine glands. The second type is a less common malignant lesion, which arises from direct intraepithelial "pagetoid" extension of an underlying anorectal adenocarcinoma. Histologically, Paget's disease is characterized by large, irregular, pale "Paget's cells," with a high mucin content, which spread widely through the epidermis and adnexa. Twenty percent to 40% of patients with Paget's disease present with invasive cancer, and, in another 20% of all patients, it develops during later follow-up.

Extramammary Paget's disease occurs most commonly in patients in their 60s and 70s, and affects both sexes equally. It can occur in the perianal area or on the genitalia; in women, the vulva is the most common site. The lesion is a scaly, erythematous, indurated plaque, which may be moist, or occasionally ulcerated. As in Bowen's disease, symptoms are either absent or nonspecific, so diagnosis is often late. Again, biopsy should always be per-formed for any unusual or persistent perianal lesion. The differential diagnosis is the same as for Bowen's disease. Concomitant visceral carcinomas are more common in these patients than in the general population and include cancer of the ovary, colon, prostate, and especially rectum.

Because of its invasive potential, Paget's disease should be excised whenever it is diagnosed. If there is no apparent associated invasive adenocarcinoma, careful mapping and wide local excision are carried out as for Bowen's disease. The lesion may be multifocal and frequently extends beyond the grossly apparent margins, making successful one-stage removal difficult. If there is an adjacent invasive cancer, it is treated accordingly (usually abdominoperineal resection), but the prognosis is poor. Without associated invasive cancer, the prognosis is good, but recurrences are common (20%–60% of cases). Again, careful long-term follow-up is indicated.

PRURITUS ANI

Pruritus ani is a common and bothersome condition that has many causes. The anal area is predisposed to itching because the epithelium there is normally very sensitive. Accumulated moisture (perspiration or mucous discharge) and fecal soiling can initiate irritation, which is made worse by friction between the buttocks during walking or working, or by overzealous rubbing with toilet paper after bowel movements. Perianal skin irritation leads to itching, which, when scratched, gives rise to the "itch–scratch" cycle of ongoing irritation and itching. Obesity can exacerbate the condition, because the anal area holds perspiration more readily and cleaning is more difficult. Diarrhea from any cause also worsens pruritus ani, because moisture, soiling, and the frequency of anal wiping is increased.

The differential diagnosis includes many possibilities, and the more common ones are enumerated here. The intergluteal cleft and genital area are early sites for psoriasis, which may not resemble psoriasis elsewhere. Candidiasis may occur, especially if the patient is taking antibiotics or if the perineal area is chronically moist from frequent baths. Contact dermatitis may result from lotions or dyes and fragrances in soaps or toilet paper. Antibiotic ointment and anesthetic ointment are particularly common causes of allergic dermatitis. Pinworm infection (*Enterobius vermicularis*) is seen in children but is rare in adults. Erythrasma is caused by *Corynebacterium minutissimum.* Condyloma acuminatum, Bowen's disease, and Paget's disease may cause pruritus ani. Sometimes hemorrhoids, anal fistulas, and fissures contribute to itching, probably from discharge of mucus or pus and from slight fecal soiling. Most often, however, no specific and convincing cause can be found.

The diagnostic evaluation includes a careful history, touching on the possibilities previously listed. A thorough anorectal examination ensures that any anatomic abnormalities are found. In the early stages, nonspecific pruritus ani may be accompanied by acute inflammation and superficial excoriation of the perianal skin. In the chronic stage, the skin becomes thickened, with coarse folds radiating out from the anus. Whenever pruritus ani persists, despite treatment, and especially if there is an abnormal area of skin visible, a biopsy should be performed. Laboratory tests are rarely helpful in the assessment of pruritus ani. Occasionally, skin fluorescence under an ultraviolet (Wood's) light reveals erythrasma or a "tape test" demonstrates pinworm eggs (clear tape applied to the perianal skin in the morning and later examined under a microscope).

The treatment of pruritus ani is usually nonsurgical. Nevertheless, warts, fissures, fistulas, and sizeable hemorrhoids can be operated on if present. If a specific infestation or infection can be identified, it is treated accordingly. Most cases are managed with anal hygiene measures that keep the anal area clean and dry. Warm sitz baths are recommended, especially after bowel movements. Witch hazel perineal pads, diaper wipes, or simply cotton pads moistened with warm water can alternatively be used after bowel movements. Colored or perfumed toilet paper and soaps should be avoided. After baths or use of moist wipes, the perineum should be carefully dried by patting (not wiping) with a tissue or use of a blow drier. Reaccumulation of moisture can be avoided by wearing loose, 100% cotton underwear, applying cornstarch (not irritating talcum) to the area, or tucking a small ball of cotton next to the anal orifice and keeping it there during the day. Sometimes elimination of caffeine, beer, tomatoes, and spicy food helps. In general, creams, ointments, and suppositories are not useful, and they occasionally make the problem worse by inducing contact dermatitis. Although steroid creams halt acute itching, chronic use can cause epidermal atrophy and increased susceptibility to irritation. If the patient must use a cream, a neutral agent such as Balneol Perianal Cleansing lotion or A and D ointment is acceptable, but only if used with the other measures to keep the anus clean and dry. The patient should be encouraged not to scratch, which perpetuates the cycle of ongoing irritation and itching.

HOMOSEXUALS, SEXUALLY TRANSMITTED DISEASES, AND ANORECTAL DISEASES

Any "typical" anorectal disorder (described previously) may occur in homosexuals, but men or women who engage in anoreceptive intercourse are also at risk for numerous STDs, which may in turn produce anorectal disease. Furthermore, opportunistic infections and even neoplasms affecting the anorectum often develop in patients infected with HIV. When a homosexual or HIV-positive patient has an anal complaint, the lesion may appear unusual, and the differential diagnosis includes many possibilities. Sorting out the cause can be difficult. This is especially true because symptoms are typically nonspecific (e.g., anal pain, discharge, bleeding, diarrhea). Also,

Table 37–1. Causes of Anal Ulcers in Homosexual Patients

Herpes simplex virus (most common)
Syphilitic chancre
Cytomegalovirus
Herpes zoster
Lymphogranuloma venereum (*Chlamydia trachomatis*)
Chancroid (*Haemophilus ducreyi*)
Donovanosis (granuloma inguinale caused by *Calymmatobacterium granulomatis*)
Neoplasms
Idiopathic cause

Table 37–2. Causes of Anorectal Masses in Homosexual Patients

Condyloma acuminatum (most common)
Kaposi's sarcoma (most common malignancy)
Lymphoma
Abscess (common bacterial, mycobacterium, gonorrhea)
Squamous cell carcinoma
Donovanosis (granuloma inguinale)
Molluscum contagiosum (caused by a pox virus)

Table 37–3. Causes of Proctitis and Colitis in Homosexual Patients

Common bacterial (e.g., *Shigella, Salmonella*)
Campylobacter
Cytomegalovirus
Gonorrhea
Amebiasis
Clostridium difficile
Cryptosporidium (a protozoan)
Herpes simplex virus
Lymphogranuloma venereum (may be associated with a stricture)
Mycobacterium avium-intracellulare complex

multiple STDs may occur simultaneously. Tactful questions about sexual practice are important; the patient may not spontaneously disclose homosexuality or a history of anoreceptive intercourse.

When the diagnosis is difficult, it is useful to categorize the observed lesions as an anal ulcer/fissure, mass, or proctitis according to the findings on physical examination (inspection, digital examination, anoscopy, sigmoidoscopy). Besides "typical" anal fissure, the causes of anal *ulcers* in homosexuals include those listed in Table 37–1. Up to one half of anal ulcers in AIDS patients have no identifiable cause. Typical benign anal fissures should be differentiated from idiopathic AIDS ulcerations as well as from ulcerations due to a specific infection or neoplasm. Benign fissures are painful, small, located anteriorly or posteriorly between the dentate line and anal verge, and associated with a hypertonic anal sphincter. Idiopathic AIDS ulcerations are usually in the posterior midline and are also painful, but they are more proximal in the anal canal (at the dentate line), larger, and deeper than common fissures. They penetrate through the internal sphincter (often into the deep postanal space), have overhanging edges, and are associated with a lax sphincter (Figs. 37–15 and 37–16).

The causes of anorectal *masses* in homosexuals include those listed in Table 37–2.

Causes of *proctitis* and *colitis* in homosexuals are listed in Table 37–3. When evaluating a particular patient with an unusual lesion, the following simple approach usually produces the diagnosis:

Biopsy any mass, ulcer, or abscess wall (for pathologic study and culture)

Culture swab any ulcer or anal discharge (for virus, gonorrhea, chlamydia, *Haemophilus ducreyi,* and perform dark field examination for spirochetes)

Figure 37–15. Clinical differences between a typical anal fissure *(right)* and an idiopathic AIDS ulcer *(left).* (From Viamonte M, Dailey TH, Gottesman L. Ulcerative disease of the anorectum in the HIV-positive patient. Dis Colon Rectum 1993;36:804.)

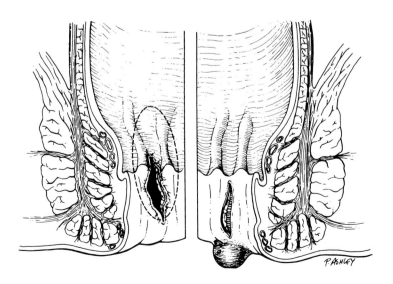

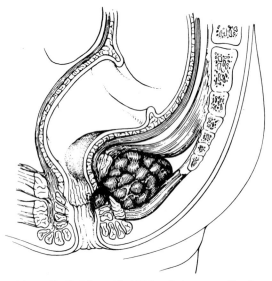

Figure 37–16. Idiopathic AIDS anal ulcer extending into the deep postanal space. (From Viamonte M, Dailey TH, Gottesman L. Ulcerative disease of the anorectum in the HIV-positive patient. Dis Colon Rectum 1993;36:804.)

Sigmoidoscopy and *rectal biopsy* (for proctitis or stricture for pathologic study and culture)

Stool tests for proctitis (for routine culture and sensitivity, ova and parasites, *Clostridium difficile,* and mycobacterium)

Serologic tests (for syphilis, chlamydia, and HIV)

The treatment of an anorectal lesion in a homosexual or HIV-positive patient depends on the cause. STDs should be treated medically when possible. Anorectal surgery in AIDS patients should be conservative, because healing tends to be prolonged and never occurs in approximately half of cases. In general, the more advanced the HIV disease and the more complex the anorectal lesion, the less likely healing is to occur. However, this is unpredictable for any individual patient. Generally, healthy, well-nourished ambulatory HIV-positive patients with relatively simple lesions do well after surgery, but "chronically ill" patients with advanced AIDS or those with deep or extensive anorectal lesions do not. CD4 counts do not seem to improve predictability of outcome over general clinical impression of the patient. Although a surgical wound may not heal, judicious surgery may still be helpful in terms of symptom relief. Abscesses should be drained. Simple, superficial fistulas in healthy patients may be opened, but complex or deep fistulas are best left alone or treated with only a chronic indwelling noncutting seton to maintain drainage. Venereal warts may be excised or fulgurated, unless the patient is extremely ill or has extensive lesions. "Typical" anal fissures in healthy patients can be treated with lateral internal sphincterotomy unless the patient has chronic diarrhea (which risks disabling incontinence). Although idiopathic AIDS ulcerations rarely heal after surgery, conservative debridement to allow easy drainage of feces and pus may alleviate the pain. Hemorrhoids should in general be treated nonoperatively in AIDS patients. A patient complaining of "hemorrhoids" may actually have an STD or a neoplasm.

Selected Readings

1. Abel ME, Chiu YSY, Russell TR, et al. Autologous fibrin glue in the treatment of rectovaginal and complex fistulas. Dis Colon Rectum 1993;36:447–449.
2. Beck DE, Fazio VW. Perianal Paget's disease. Dis Colon Rectum 1987;30:263–266.
3. Beck DE, Fazio VW, Jagelman DG, et al. Perianal Bowen's disease. Dis Colon Rectum 1988;31:419–422.
4. Berardi RS, Lee S, Chen HP. Perianal extramammary Paget's disease (review). Surg Gynecol Obstet 1988;167:359–366.
5. Burke EC, Orloff SL, Freise CE, et al. Wound healing after anorectal surgery in human immunodeficiency virus infected patients. Arch Surg 1991;126:1267–1271.
6. Caplin DA, Kodner IJ. Repair of anal stricture and mucosal ectropion by simple flap procedures. Dis Colon Rectum 1986;29:92–94.
7. Christensen MA, Pitsch RM, Cali RL, et al. "House" advancement pedicle flap for anal stenosis. Dis Colon Rectum 1992;35:201–203.
8. Chu QD, Vezeridis MP, Libbey NP, et al. Giant condyloma acuminatum (Buschke-Löwenstein tumor) of the anorectal and perianal regions. Dis Colon Rectum 1994;37:950–957.
9. Fleshner PR, Freilich MI. Adjuvant interferon for anal condyloma: a prospective randomized trial. Dis Colon Rectum 1994;37:155–159.
10. Friedman AE, Eron LJ, Conant M, et al. Natural interferon alpha for treatment of condylomata acuminata. JAMA 1988;259:533–538.
11. Held D, Khubchandani I, Sheets J, et al. Management of anorectal horseshoe abscess and fistula. Dis Colon Rectum 1986;29:793–797.
12. Jensen SL, Sjolin KE, Shokouh-Amiri MH, et al. Paget's disease of the anal margin. Br J Surg 1988;75:1089–1092.
13. Kodner IJ, Mazor A, Shemesh EI, et al. Endorectal advancement flap repair of rectovaginal and other complicated anorectal fistulas. Surgery 1993;114:682–690.

14. Lewis TH, Corman ML, Prager ED, et al. Long term results of open and closed sphincterotomy for anal fissure. Dis Colon Rectum 1988;31:368–371.

15. Luchtefeld MA. Perianal condylomata acuminata (review). Surg Clin North Am 1994;74:1327–1338.

16. Milsom JW, Mazier WP. Classification and management of postsurgical anal stenosis. Surg Gynecol Obstet 1986;163:60–64.

17. Modesto VL, Gottesman L. Sexually transmitted diseases and anal manifestations of AIDS (review). Surg Clin North Am 1994;74:1433–1464.

18. Noffsinger A, Witte D, Fenoglio-Preiser CM. The relationship of human papillomaviruses to anorectal neoplasia. Cancer 1992;70:1276–1287.

19. Pearl RK, Andrews JR, Orsay CP, et al. Role of the seton in the management of anorectal fistulas. Dis Colon Rectum 1993;36:573–579.

20. Petros JG, Bradley TM. Factors influencing postoperative urinary retention in patients undergoing surgery for benign anorectal disease. Am J Surg 1990;159:374–376.

21. Schouten WR, van Vroonhoven TJMV. Treatment of anorectal abscess with or without primary fistulectomy: results of a prospective randomized trial. Dis Colon Rectum 1991;34:60–63.

22. Seow-Choen F, Nicholls RJ. Anal fistula (review). Br J Surg 1992;79:197–205.

23. Smith LE, Henrichs D, McCullah RD. Prospective studies on the etiology and treatment of pruritus ani. Dis Colon Rectum 1982;25:358–363.

24. Standards Task Force, American Society of Colon and Rectal Surgeons. Practice parameters for the management of anal fissure. Dis Colon Rectum 1992;35:206–207.

25. Sullivan ES, Garnjobst WM. Pruritus ani: a practical approach. Surg Clin North Am 1978;58:505–512.

26. Ustynoski K, Rosen L, Stasik J, et al. Horseshoe abscess fistula: seton treatment. Dis Colon Rectum 1990;33:602–605.

27. van Tets WF, Kuijpers HC. Continence disorders after anal fistulotomy. Dis Colon Rectum 1994;37:1194–1197.

28. Walker WA, Rothenberger DA, Goldberg SM. Morbidity of internal sphincterotomy for anal fissure and stenosis. Dis Colon Rectum 1985;28:832–835.

29. Wedell J, Meier zu Eissen P, Banzhaf G, et al. Sliding flap advancement for the treatment of high level fistulae. Br J Surg 1987;74:390–391.

30. Williams JG, MacLeod CA, Rothenberger DA, et al. Seton treatment of high anal fistulae. Br J Surg 1991;78:1159–1161.

31. Williams JG, Rothenberger DA, Nemer FD, et al. Fistula in ano in Crohn's disease: results of aggressive surgical treatment. Dis Colon Rectum 1991;34:378–384.

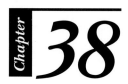
38

Hemorrhoids

Eugene Foley

Like other anorectal procedures, most hemorrhoid surgery can be easily and efficiently accomplished in the ambulatory setting, particularly because of the rapid technologic expansion that has provided a number of ambulatory approaches to hemorrhoidal disease. These approaches limit the number of patients requiring formal three-quadrant surgical hemorrhoidectomy to a small minority undergoing hemorrhoidal surgery. Additionally, like many other traditionally inpatient procedures, there has been a trend for even surgical hemorrhoidectomy to be done increasingly in the ambulatory setting. This chapter defines and classifies the spectrum of hemorrhoidal disease, discusses the indications for surgical therapy, reviews the applicability and results of the presently available outpatient surgical techniques, and identifies the limits of ambulatory surgery in the treatment of hemorrhoidal disease.

PREOPERATIVE EVALUATION

In initially evaluating hemorrhoidal disease, it is crucial to specifically define and classify the nature of the disease, because this classification substantially influences the type of treatment that is applied. Hemorrhoids can be anatomically categorized into internal or external hemorrhoids, on the basis of their relationship to the dentate line. Internal hemorrhoids are mucosally lined, submucosal venous plexuses that emanate above the dentate line, whereas external hemorrhoids are covered by anoderm or perianal skin. Additionally, some hemorrhoids are best classified as combined, having

both an internal and external component. This distinction can often be made by history. Painless bleeding and prolapse are the hallmark symptoms of internal hemorrhoids, and skin tags, perianal irritation, and acute thrombosis are the major symptoms related to external hemorrhoids. Internal hemorrhoids are additionally stratified into four grades, with grade 1 being nonprolapsing, grade 2 being intermittently prolapsing but spontaneously reducing, grade 3 being intermittently prolapsing and requiring manual reduction, and grade 4 being continuously prolapsing hemorrhoids that are irreducible. To determine applicability of treatment options, hemorrhoids must be classified by the aforementioned system.

It is axiomatic that a full differential diagnosis of anorectal disease should be considered at the initial evaluation. Even though the chief complaint of anorectal disease is often "hemorrhoids," it is equally true that a large number of these patients suffer from pruritus ani, fistulous disease, and anal fissures. These common anorectal problems are often readily definable by physical examination and anoscopy. The differentiation of prolapsing hemorrhoids from mucosal or full-thickness rectal prolapse may be more difficult. In general, prolapsing hemorrhoids and rectal prolapse may be differentiated by careful consideration of the orientation of mucosal folds in the prolapsing tissue. The folds in prolapsing hemorrhoids are aligned radially, whereas the mucosal folds of a rectal prolapse are concentric. Additionally, the diagnosis of a prolapsed hypertrophied anal papilla or distal rectal adenoma or carcinoma should be considered in the evaluation of prolapsing anal tissue.

The possibility of carcinoma should always be considered in evaluating the "bleeding hemorrhoid." This necessitates at least a proctosigmoidoscopic examination for all patients at the initial evaluation, and, for patients selected on the basis of symptoms, age, and other risk factors, a full colorectal evaluation with colonoscopy or flexible sigmoidoscopy and barium enema. A proctosigmoidoscopic examination for the younger patient also helps protect against the possibility of ill-advised hemorrhoidal surgery in the setting of active proctitis or Crohn's disease. These considerations, in addition to lighted office anoscopy to fully classify the hemorrhoidal disease, are the basis of the preoperative workup for hemorrhoidal surgery.

Although there are many different techniques of anorectal examination, my preference is to position the patient kneeling on an elevated proctoscopy table after a Fleet enema is given. After a digital rectal examination and proctoscopy, a lighted anoscope is passed into the anal canal. The patient is asked to "bear down," allowing identification and quantification of the amount of internal hemorrhoidal prolapse. Care is taken to examine the three common regions of hemorrhoidal disease: the left lateral, right posterior, and right anterior quadrants.

THERAPY

The single goal of the treatment of hemorrhoidal disease is to ameliorate specific symptoms. Even large hemorrhoids that are minimally bothersome to a patient require no specific therapy. Additionally, many minor hemorrhoidal symptoms such as minor bleeding may be adequately controlled nonoperatively. Irregular bowel habits, with either constipation or diarrhea, can substantially increase the symptoms of bleeding, discomfort, and prolapse. The use of a high-fiber diet has been shown to significantly reduce the amount of pain and bleeding associated with hemorrhoidal disease. Additionally, control of diarrhea with antidiarrheal preparations may be of benefit to some patients. Warm bath soaks may

be helpful to decrease the perineal discomfort associated with hemorrhoidal disease. Conversely, the use of perianal creams or suppositories has never been conclusively shown to improve the symptoms of hemorrhoids, despite the extent of their marketing.

In summary, minor symptoms related to hemorrhoids can be adequately treated with the addition of a fiber supplement and increased dietary water consumption to control constipation (or, conversely, antidiarrheal medicines) and warm bath soaks. Failure of these approaches to control symptoms or the presence of more severe symptoms leads a patient or physician to consider an operative approach.

INTERNAL HEMORRHOIDS

Although internal hemorrhoids have traditionally been treated with formal surgical excision, a number of less invasive techniques have been popularized over the past several decades to treat the bleeding and prolapse of internal hemorrhoids in the ambulatory setting. The following discussion is a brief review of each technique, its efficacy, and its applicability.

Rubber Band Ligation

Rubber band ligation of internal hemorrhoids was initially described by Blaisdell in 1958 and was later refined by Baron. It has become by far the most popular nonexcisional form of treatment for symptomatic internal hemorrhoids, and it can be easily and rapidly performed in the office setting. Most grade 1 to 3 internal hemorrhoids may be treated by banding.

After a Fleet enema, the patient is placed in the left lateral or kneeling position (my preference) on a proctoscopy table. The internal hemorrhoidal plexuses are visualized with an anoscope and drawn into the hemorrhoidal bander with an Allis clamp. The ligator is fired, placing a tight rubber band around the base of the hemorrhoid. A suction ligator can be used that brings the hemorrhoidal tissue into the bander automatically, obviating the need for the somewhat cumbersome Allis clamp.

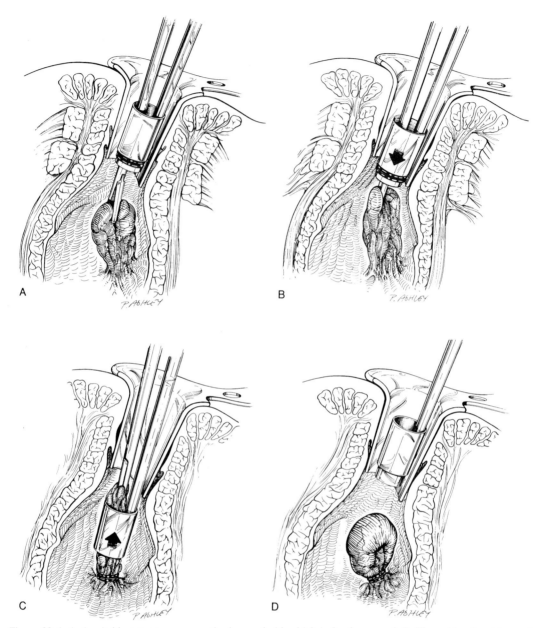

Figure 38–1. A, A suitable retractor exposes the hemorrhoid, which is firmly grasped. **B,** The rubber band is carefully "eased" toward the hemorrhoid while traction is exerted on it. **C,** One or two bands are placed at the base. **D,** Satisfactory placement of the band causes no pain. (From Mazier P. Surgery of the Colon, Rectum, and Anus. Philadelphia: WB Saunders, 1995.)

Care must be taken to band only hemorrhoidal tissue above the dentate line, proximal to the area of somatic sensation (Fig. 38–1). Some authors describe injecting several milliters of 0.25% bupivacaine just below the band to limit postoperative discomfort. There is some controversy as to how many quadrants can be treated at a single session. I treat a single hemorrhoid at the first session. If the first application proceeded without significant discomfort, I band the remaining quadrants 3 to 4 weeks later.

Following banding, many patients experience some minor discomfort, usually a perianal "pressure sensation" secondary to sphincter spasm. A mild analgesic, fiber supplementation, and warm bath soaks are prescribed for all patients following the procedure. Acute pain upon application of the band denotes a position too close to the dentate line, and immediate band removal is indicated. In approximately 7 to 10 days, the banded hemorrhoid sloughs off. Some patients report some anal bleeding at this time, although this is usually self-limited. Overall, in appropriately selected patients, rubber band ligation is efficacious, with 80% to 90% of patients experiencing complete or greatly improved symptomatic relief.

Internal hemorrhoidal banding is a safe technique. The most common complication is postprocedure pain, estimated to occur in 5% to 10% of cases. Significant delayed hemorrhage at the time of hemorrhoidal sloughing (1–2 weeks) is infrequent, occurring in approximately 1% of cases. This complication may require intraoperative suturing for control. Additionally, a small number of patients (2%–3%) may experience thrombosis of external hemorrhoids distal to the banded hemorrhoid. The most feared complication of rubber band ligation, however, is *postbanding pelvic cellulitis*. Initially reported by O'Hara in 1980, this syndrome is characterized by severe perianal pain, urinary retention, fever, and progressive, life-threatening sepsis. Several authors have described this syndrome, but the overall number and rates of reported cases remain small, with perhaps 10 cases being reported in tens of thousands of procedures. However, patients should be educated to report such symptoms, and early aggressive treatment with broad-spectrum antibiotics and operative debridement should be undertaken. The cause of this condition remains unknown, although it is presumed to represent widespread anaerobic sepsis. There has been some speculation that undiagnosed human immunodeficiency virus (HIV) infection may play a role, although this remains unproven.

There are some anatomic limitations for rubber band ligation. Because the band must be placed proximal to the dentate line, this technique is not applicable to external or combined hemorrhoids. Additionally, the presence of grade 4 internal hemorrhoids significantly reduces the efficacy of the technique, when compared with its use on grades 1 to 3 hemorrhoids. A further disadvantage is the common need for sequential procedures, especially if treating three-quadrant disease.

Despite these limitations, rubber band ligation remains a popular, cost-effective, and efficacious way to treat small to moderately sized symptomatic internal hemorrhoids in the ambulatory setting.

Sclerotherapy

Smaller internal hemorrhoids (grades 1 and 2) can also be treated with sclerotherapy. As in other areas of the body, the technique involves the injection of a sclerosing agent, most commonly 5% phenol and oil or sodium morrhuate. After preparation of the patient with a Fleet enema, the hemorrhoidal plexuses are visualized with an anoscope. Approximately 3 to 5 mL of sclerosant are injected into the submucosal plane at the apex of the hemorrhoid. The sclerosant should not be injected intravascularly. A submucosal weal indicates an appropriately placed injection. The use of an angled injection needle improves visualization during the procedure. All hemorrhoidal plexuses can be treated in a single session. There is some controversy regarding the need or efficacy of repeated interval injections. Some authors have recommended repeating injections as needed at 6- to 8-week intervals, whereas others prefer switching to a different modality for persistent or recurrent disease to avoid anal stenosis with repeat injections. A single prospective trial comparing single session injections versus multiple sessions showed no improved efficacy with multiple session therapy.

Possible complications of sclerotherapy include postprocedure pain and discomfort, mucosal sloughing, abscess formation, and anal stricture. The more serious complications appear quite rarely. Sclerotherapy is 60% to 80% effective in substantially reducing the symptoms from grade 1 or 2 internal hemorrhoids. The technique should not be used for larger internal hemorrhoids or for combined or external hemorrhoids. Although not universally documented, it is widely believed that sclerotherapy is somewhat less effective than rubber band ligation. This fact, in addition to more complicated office equipment management and the restriction of this treatment to smaller hemorrhoids, may be the basis for the lack of popularity of this technique in the United States.

Infrared Coagulation

In 1979, Neiger and coworkers described a new technique for the treatment of small (grades 1 and 2) internal hemorrhoids. An infrared photocoagulator produces infrared radiation focused by a photoconductor, which is converted to heat when it contacts tissue. Its destructive capabilities are regulated by alterations in both energy intensity and duration. Normally, a pulse of 1 to 1.5 seconds is delivered approximately three to five times to each hemorrhoidal plexus, with the amount of treatment based on visual inspection of the coagulant during treatment. Treatments can be repeated at 2- to 3-week intervals.

Large reported series have documented that infrared coagulation is easy to apply and is strikingly free of significant complications. Additionally, efficacy comparable to rubber band ligation or sclerotherapy has been documented by prospective trials. The potential disadvantages of infrared coagulation appear to be its limited application to grade 1 or smaller grade 2 internal hemorrhoids, the expense of the equipment when compared to rubber band ligation, and the reported need for a higher number of treatment sessions to achieve adequate symptom control when compared with rubber band ligation or sclerotherapy.

Other Nonexcisional Approaches

A number of additional approaches to the outpatient treatment of hemorrhoids have been described, including cryotherapy, direct current therapy, and bipolar diathermy. Similar to the techniques described previously, each of these techniques involves localized tissue destruction with resulting inflammation and subsequent fibrosis, ablating the hemorrhoidal plexuses. Cryotherapy destroys the tissue through the sequence of rapid deep freezing and rewarming, via the application of liquid nitrous oxide or a liquid nitrogen probe. Although initially heralded as a means of painless hemorrhoidectomy, follow-up trials have noted a high degree of wound healing problems and prolonged anal drainage. These findings, in addition to the expense of equipment, have generally tempered the recent enthusiasm for this technique in comparison to rubber band ligation or infrared coagulation.

The use of bipolar diathermy (Bicap) and direct current (ultroid) therapy has been described in more limited studies. Bipolar coagulation involves the applications of electric current and subsequent heat between two electrodes at the tip of a hand-held applicator. Visible coagulum is noted and the entire hemorrhoid is coagulated. Theoretically, this involves a more superficial burn than that achieved during monopolar coagulation. In direct current therapy, a grounding pad is placed on a patient's thigh and an electric current is passed via a hand-held probe through the hemorrhoid. The current is increased to a maximal tolerable threshold and treatment usually takes about 10 minutes. Both techniques often require several treatments. Although both techniques have been shown to be moderately effective, the long duration of therapy necessary for direct current therapy seems to make this impractical. Additionally, the ease, safety, and efficacy of rubber band ligation, infrared coagulation, and sclerotherapy have prevented these techniques from being widely used.

Comment

The large number of different available techniques and the numerous, sometimes conflicting, reports comparing these techniques make it difficult to establish the best ambulatory treatment for grades 1 to 3 internal hemorrhoids. The overall approach to this common clinical problem is often quite varied, even among physicians who are experienced and successful in this field. It probably becomes most important for physicians treating symptomatic internal hemorrhoids in the office setting to develop an individualized, logical approach based on current information and personal experience. Most physicians in the United States prefer rubber band ligation, infrared coagulation, sclerotherapy, or some combination of these techniques. Overall, there is greater enthusiasm for these modalities than for cryotherapy, bipolar diathermy, and direct current coagulation based on the advantage of these techniques in efficacy, ease of application, and relative safety.

I favor rubber band ligation over infrared coagulation and sclerotherapy. I believe that most patients with symptomatic internal hemorrhoids less than grade 4 or large grade 3 receive effective and economic treatment with rubber band ligation without the cumbersome aspects of sclerotherapy injections or the cost of infrared coagulation. Additionally, I believe that rubber band ligation is applicable to a larger range of hemorrhoid presentations, being more effective than infrared coagulation or sclerotherapy for the larger grade 2 and grade 3 hemorrhoids. The only disadvantage of rubber band ligation is for smaller symptomatic grade 1 hemorrhoids, which are often difficult to band. In this minority of cases, I rely on infrared coagulation with acceptable results. With this approach, I have not needed to use sclerotherapy. Patients whose symptoms have been uncontrollable with rubber band ligation or infrared coagulation, have large grade 3 or grade 4 internal hemorrhoids, or have a significant external component, undergo formal surgical hemorrhoidectomy.

SURGICAL HEMORRHOIDECTOMY

Surgical hemorrhoidectomy has traditionally been done in the inpatient setting, requiring 3 to 4 days of hospitalization. Like many procedures in the present climate of cost containment, the need for prolonged hospitalization has come under increasing scrutiny. In one large-volume colorectal clinic, approximately 90% of patients can be discharged within 23 hours after surgical hemorrhoidectomy, and many can be discharged within several hours. This experience supports the position that the most elective hemorrhoidectomies can be done in the ambulatory setting, saving a hospital admission for the emergent treatment of gangrenous strangulated hemor-

rhoids or the treatment of early postoperative complications of hemorrhoidectomy.

There are many techniques described for surgical hemorrhoidectomy. I favor the commonly used closed, or Ferguson, hemorrhoidectomy (Fig. 38–2). After receiving two Fleet enemas preoperatively, the patient is placed in the prone jackknife position (which I prefer over the traditional Sims position). The buttocks are taped apart. In many cases, hemorrhoidectomy can be done under local anesthesia with mild intravenous sedation, especially in patients requiring a single-quadrant excision. For patients with extensive hemorrhoids requiring three-quadrant excision or for especially muscular or obese patients, I find a spinal or general anesthesia preferable. The anal canal is inspected after insertion of a medium-sized Hill-Ferguson anal retractor, and the extent of hemorrhoidectomy is preoperatively planned. Even with general or regional anesthesia, a 0.25% bupivacaine solution with 1:200,000 epinephrine is injected into the submucosal space at each plexus to be excised for improved hemostasis and postoperative analgesia. A 3-0 chromic suture is used to ligate the proximal pedicle and is left in place. This ligation is done above the anorectal ring to prevent postoperative anal stenosis at the level of the pedicles, especially when excising three quadrants. A number 15 blade is used to incise the distal plexus at the perianal skin. The distal aspect of the incision is taken well out onto the perianal skin to avoid a distal dog ear, the source of postoperative skin tags. The anoderm and mucosa are then excised along each side of the plexus in the direction of the pedicle, with care taken to avoid excess anoderm excision. The underlying internal sphincter fibers are identified beneath the hemorrhoid and preserved by retraction in the lateral direction. The hemorrhoid is excised just distal to the pedicle ligature, the pedicle is re-suture ligated, and then the incision is completely closed by running the pedicle chromic suture distally toward the perianal skin. Care is taken to avoid excessive tension on this closure. The remaining quadrants are then excised in similar fashion. The ability to pass a medium-sized Hill-Ferguson retractor into the anus upon completion of the procedure protects against postoperative stenosis.

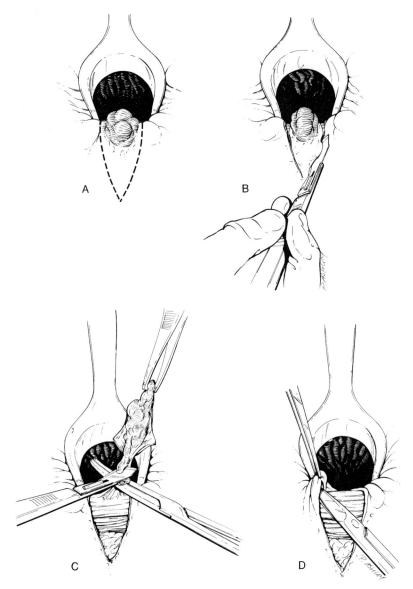

Figure 38–2. The Ferguson closed hemorrhoidectomy. **A,** The amount of tissue to be excised is outlined. **B,** The hemorrhoidal complex is incised to the level of the subjuvant muscle and superiorly to the anorectal ring. **C,** Hemorrhoidal tissue is excised and the pedicle secured. **D,** Anoderm and perianal skin are sharply undermined and accessory hemorrhoidal tissue is excised.

Postoperatively, the patient is given narcotic analgesic by mouth, stool softeners, and a fiber supplement. Additionally, I ask each patient to soak in a warm tub 3 to 4 times a day to help relieve sphincter spasm. As discussed, most patients may be discharged following surgery, saving admission for those patients with poorly controlled postoperative pain or concern regarding the presence of early postoperative complications.

The most common complication following surgical hemorrhoidectomy is urinary retention. Perhaps the single most important feature preventing this complication is perioperative restriction of fluid. A randomized study has shown that perioperative intravenous fluid and postoperative oral fluid restrictions can reduce the rate of cases of postoperative urinary retention requiring catheterization to 3% to 5%. Such alterations in practice can dramatically reduce the number of patients requiring hospitalization following hemorrhoidectomy.

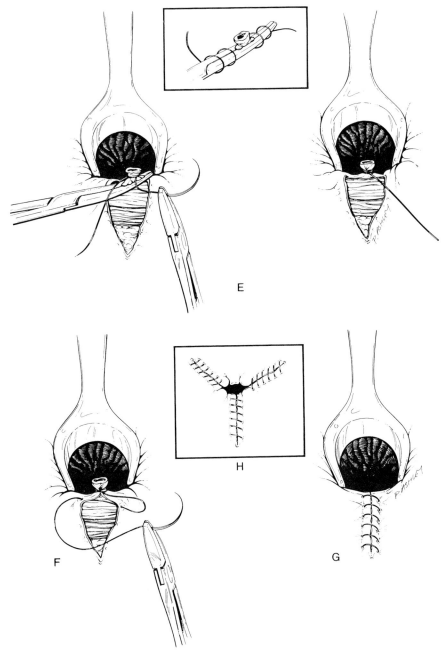

Figure 38–2 *Continued.* **E,** The hemorrhoidal pedicle is secured with a suture if necessary. **F,** A running suture closes the wounds. **G,** The wound is secured without excessive tension. **H,** The sutured wounds are properly separated. (From Mazier P. Surgery of the Colon, Rectum, and Anus. Philadelphia: WB Saunders, 1995.)

Early bleeding in the immediate postoperative period is unusual and, in almost all cases, is secondary to inadequate ligation of the pedicles. With care taken to do this appropriately, the incidence of this complication should be extremely low, and monitoring for early bleeding should not be a clear reason to prevent hemorrhoidectomy from being done in the ambulatory setting. Pain and fecal impaction in the early postoperative period can usually be controlled or prevented by the aforementioned bowel regimen on an outpatient basis. The most feared long-term complication of hemorrhoidectomy is anal stenosis, a preventable complication when proper care is taken to avoid excessive anoderm resection at the primary surgery. With proper technique, the rate of this complication should be less than 1%. Depending on its severity, anal stenosis may require further surgery with anoplasty.

A number of other techniques have been used for surgical hemorrhoidectomy, including open hemorrhoidectomy, Parks hemorrhoidectomy, and the Whitehead procedure. All have their proponents, although patient selection, perioperative care, and the relationship to the applicability in the outpatient setting are all similar to the closed Ferguson approach. Selection of which surgical approach is used remains an individual preference.

Another technique is "laser hemorrhoidectomy." Several randomized trials have shown no benefit in using the laser to excise hemorrhoids when compared to "cold knife" procedures in terms of postoperative pain, urinary retention, blood loss, or the need for hospitalization. Without more conclusive evidence of some advantage, it seems unlikely that this more expensive technique should displace more traditional approaches.

Several large retrospective questionnaire studies have been done, each of which suggests that surgical hemorrhoidectomy satisfactorily relieves preoperative symptoms in greater than 90% of patients. The need for additional surgery for recurrent or persistent disease is low, occurring in less than 5% of patients.

Traditionally, three-quadrant surgical hemorrhoidectomy has been an inpatient procedure, but there is a growing trend to do the procedure in the ambulatory setting. Adherence to the surgical details discussed as well as the perioperative management regarding pain control and fluid restriction have allowed many centers to provide this care routinely in the ambulatory setting. Such an approach will be increasingly mandated by the growing cost containment forces. In view of these recently published experiences, it seems reasonable to reserve inpatient therapy for the minority of patients who experience poorly controlled postoperative pain, urinary retention, or bleeding. Additionally, patients undergoing emergency surgery for gangrenous strangu-lated hemorrhoids may require routine inpatient observation for a short period.

EXTERNAL HEMORRHOIDS

Acute Thrombosis

A common complication of external hemorrhoids is acute thrombosis. This invariably presents as an acute, tender perianal lump. The patient may have had a previous history of similar difficulties or other symptoms related to hemorrhoids. The treatment of this condition depends on the duration of symptoms at the time of presentation. Because the natural history of acutely thrombosed external hemorrhoids is for the pain to diminish after 48 to 72 hours, if a patient is seen after this time, then treatment should be nonoperative, using analgesics, bath soaks 3 to 4 times a day, and stool softeners. If the patient is seen within 48 to 72 hours of the initiation of symptoms, then a simple excision can be performed to attain more rapid pain resolution. This is a procedure that almost always can be done in the office setting. The skin around the thrombosed hemorrhoid is anesthetized with a mixture of 0.5% lidocaine, 0.25% bupivacaine, and 1:200,000 epinephrine. I favor excision of the hemorrhoid rather than simple incision, the latter carrying an unacceptable early recurrence rate. The postprocedure management is the same as described previously, with analgesics, bath soaks, and stool softeners. Patients should undergo proctosigmoidoscopic examination at the follow-up visit to rule out a precipitating underlying anorectal disorder such as distal rectal carcinoma.

External Hemorrhoidal Skin Tags

The other common symptom of external hemorrhoids are external hemorrhoidal skin tags. Depending on the size, these can often be excised locally in the office setting under local anesthesia. More extensive external hemorrhoids and those associated with internal hemorrhoids should be treated by formal surgical hemorrhoidectomy. Because of the somatic sensation of the perianal skin in the region of the external hemorrhoids, other nonexcisional forms of treatment such as rubber band ligation, sclerotherapy, and infrared coagulation are unacceptable for the treatment of external hemorrhoids.

CONCLUSION

Most symptoms from hemorrhoidal disease can be successfully treated in the ambulatory setting. Acutely thrombosed external hemorrhoids and external hemorrhoidal skin tags can be easily excised in the office setting under local anesthesia. Additionally, grades 1 to 3 internal hemorrhoids can effectively be treated in the office setting by one of several effective techniques such as rubber band ligation, infrared coagulation, or sclerotherapy. Finally, for the small percentage of patients with hemorrhoids that are poorly controlled or too large for other techniques, elective multiple quadrant surgical hemorrhoidectomy can be safely completed in the ambulatory setting with adherence to meticulous technique and appropriate perioperative care.

Selected Readings

1. Ambrose NS, Hanes MM, Alexander-Williams J, et al. Prospective randomized comparison of photocoagulation and rubber band ligation in treatment of haemorrhoids. BMJ 1983;286:1389–1391.
2. Ambrose WS, Morris D, Alexander-Williams J, et al. A randomized trial of photocoagulation or injectional sclerotherapy for the treatment of first and second degree hemorrhoids. Dis Colon Rectum 1985; 28:238–240.
3. Bailey HR, Ferguson JAC. Prevention of urinary retention by fluid restriction following anorectal operation. Dis Colon Rectum 1976;19:250–252.
4. Barron J. Office ligation treatment of hemorrhoids. Dis Colon Rectum 1963;6:109–113.
5. Corman ML. Colon and Rectal Surgery. Philadelphia: JB Lippincott, 1993.
6. Gordon PH, Nivatrongs S, eds. Principles and Practice of Surgery for the Colon, Rectum, and Anus. St. Louis: Quality Medical Publishing, 1992.
7. Leicester RJ, Nicholls RJ, Chir M, et al. Infrared coagulation: a new treatment for hemorrhoids. Dis Colon Rectum 1981;24:602–605.
8. Mazier WP. Hemorrhoids, fissures, and pruritus ani. Surg Clin North Am 1994;74:1277–1292.
9. Medwell SJ, Friend W. Outpatient anorectal surgery. Dis Colon Rectum 1979;22:480–482.
10. Oh C. One thousand cyrohemorrhoidectomies: an overview. Dis Colon Rectum 1981;24:613–617.
11. Russell TR, Donohue JH. Hemorrhoidal banding: a warning. Dis Colon Rectum 1985;28:291–293.
12. Smith L. Ambulatory surgery for anorectal diseases. South Med J 1986;79:163–166.
13. Smith LE, Goodrean JJ, Fouty WJ. Operative hemorrhoidectomy versus cryodestruction. Dis Colon Rectum 1979;22:10–16.
14. Sonagore A, Mazier WP, Luchtefeld MA, et al. Treatment of advanced hemorrhoidal disease: a prospective, randomized comparison of cold scalpel vs contact Nd:Yag laser. Dis Colon Rectum 1993;36:1042–1049.
15. Steinberg DM, Liegois H, Alexander-Williams J. Long-term review of the results of rubber band ligation of hemorrhoids. Br J Surg 1975;62:144–146.

Chapter 39

Pilonidal Cysts and Sinuses

Joseph Minasi • John S. Minasi

HISTORICAL NOTES

In 1833, H. Mayo described the case of a young woman affected with a hair-containing sinus in the sacrococcygeal area. In 1847, Anderson reported "the extraction of hair from an ulcer," and subsequent authors described similar findings. The anatomic factor was thought to be the justification for a congenital origin. The sinus was lined with squamous epithelium and frequently contained hair. The term "pilonidal" for cyst and sinus was introduced by R. Hodges in 1880 from the Latin *pilus*, or hair, and *nidus*, or nest. In 1946, this subject was brought to controversial consideration by Patey and Scarff. They favored the theory of an acquired origin rather than the congenital one. The pilonidal sinus was mostly present in young men and women with relatively large, deep-clefted buttocks. The growth of the buttocks creates a distention of the follicle that allows the introduction of hair (Fig. 39–1).

In 1983, J. Bascom introduced his interpretation of the evolution of pilonidal disease and described the stages of development from the normal follicle to the infected cyst and sinus.

Pilonidal disease is not limited to the postanal area between the nates. It has been described and treated in other areas, especially in the hands, mostly in the interdigital webs. The umbilicus, axilla, feet, clitoris, and periareolar area of the breast have also been found to be affected. Repetitive trauma from saddles (e.g., horse, bicycle) predisposes a person to this condition. Among military personnel moving about in vehicles with a hard seat, it was commonly referred to as "jeep disease."

A professional cause can be justified. Barbers, wool and mattress workers, and fur handlers have been affected. An acquired etiology for this disease is demonstrated by the fact that grass and hair of a color different from that of the patient have been reported. The congenital contribution in some patients cannot entirely be discarded. A malformation of the development of the neuroenteric canal over the sacrococcygeal area may lead to the formation of a sinus lined with skin. No skin appendages have been described. The hair,

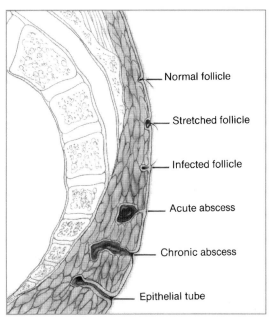

Figure 39–1. Pathogenesis of pilonidal abscess and sinus. (From Nivatvongs S. Pilonidal disease. In: Gordon P, Nivatvongs S, eds. Principles and Practices of Surgery of the Colon, Rectum, and Anus. St Louis: Quality Medical Publishing, 1992:269.)

when present, is a contribution from the outside (Fig. 39–2).

PATHOLOGY

The area in which this abnormality occurs is naturally septic. In affected persons, the sinus is subject to repeated infections from an early age. Males are affected more often than females at a ratio of approximately 5:1. Women may be affected at an earlier age because the deposition of fat in buttocks goes along with pubertal changes. The continuous trauma of a minor malformation may lead to the development of a cyst. This always starts at the end of a sinus. The subsequent infection favors the formation of other sinuses, which discharge the purulent material formed within. The pilonidal sinus is always superficial to the postsacral fascia and, when isolated, is found in the midline approximately 5 cm above the anal border.

Patients have swelling, pain, and purulent discharge when an acute infection develops. The spontaneous resolution of the acute stage leaves a draining sinus. Repeated acute episodes widen the extension of the cyst. Other sinuses may open to the surface. If a sinus extends toward the anal canal, a communicat-

ing fistula may form. The acute episode is followed by remission if the purulent material is spontaneously discharged. The remission can last for a long time. However, it is rare for the acute episode not to recur.

CLINICAL FINDINGS

Patients with pilonidal disease may complain of spontaneous discharge from the area between the buttocks. The discharge is purulent and occasionally is accompanied by moderate bleeding. Prolonged sitting on a bouncy means of locomotion may be the precipitating cause. If the abscess is covered by a thick skin, it rarely opens spontaneously early in the process; it enlarges cephalad. The extension is tortuous; when it reaches the epidermis, a new discharging sinus ensues. The chronic abscess favors the formation of a flat epithelial lining that covers the sinus and extends to the cavity. The newly formed cyst is an indolent process with moderate discharge and may last for a long time.

The responsible organisms are *Staphylococcus aureus*, *Streptococcus viridans*, *Bacteroides* species, and intestinal coliforms. The gastrointestinal organisms are responsible for suprainfections.

Most (>90%) sinus tracts run cephalad,

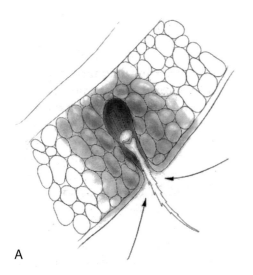
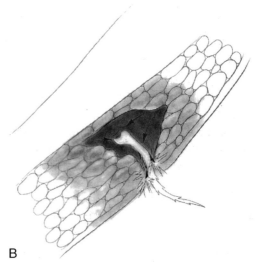

A

B

Figure 39–2. Ingestion of hair by a chronic pilonidal abscess cavity. Scales of hair direct the inward movement of hair. Motion causes movement in the cavity. **(A)** standing; **(B)** sitting. (From Nivatvongs S. Pilonidal disease. In: Gordon P, Nivatvongs S, eds. Principles and Practices of Surgery of the Colon, Rectum, and Anus. St Louis: Quality Medical Publishing, 1992:269.)

whereas a small number (<10%) extend caudally. The differential diagnosis should include fistula-in-ano, hidradenitis suppurativa, and any furuncle of the skin. Less common diagnoses to consider include specific granulomas such as syphilitic or tuberculous ones, osteomyelitis with multiple draining sinuses, and actinomycosis of the sacral region.

TREATMENT

The treatment of pilonidal disease varies according to the stage at which the patient seeks medical attention. The treatment options are nonoperative management, conservative excision, incision and drainage, incision and marsupialization, wide local excision with or without primary closure, and excision and reconstruction (e.g., cleft closure, Z-plasty, Karydakis advancing flap procedure, musculocutaneous rotation flaps).

Nonoperative Management

If an acute episode with abscess formation was never experienced, the conservative approach is indicated, that is, daily scrupulous toilet, removal of hair and debris protruding from the opening of the sinus, application of mild antiseptic, and application of a dry dressing between the nates if they touch the midline. This is the military approach. With periodic examination of the sacrococcygeal area to ensure patient compliance and with reeducation, this modality carries a high success rate with minimal disability.

Sclerotherapy, although not popular, is also an effective nonoperative management. Debridement of loose hairs is performed (as is curettage of the sinus) and then 80% phenol is applied to obliterate the epithelium. It is necessary to protect the skin from the sclerosant. The injection can be repeated every 4 to 6 weeks as necessary.

Consecutive Excision

Excision of the midline pits and thorough cleansing of the hair and debris from the ab-

scess cavity is a minimally invasive technique appropriate for small wounds. Healing is usually complete within 3 weeks. Longitudinal incisions can be made off the midline to avoid prolonged healing from excessive friction. The wound may be closed primarily or packed open.

Incision and Drainage

Any pilonidal abscess should have incision and drainage as the necessary operative management. The abscess is usually lateral on either side and cephalad. Because of poor healing of the intergluteal cleft, creation of a midline wound should be avoided; if it is necessary, it should be made small. A longitudinal incision is made lateral to the midline and deepened into the abscess cavity. Hair must be removed if present. The patient must clean the area at least daily in the shower or tub. Hairs around the area should be shaved or treated with depilatory weekly until the wound has completely healed. Antibiotics are not indicated except when accompanied by cellulitis or in the immunocompromised patient. Incision and drainage alone may be curative in 60% of patients (Fig. 39–3).

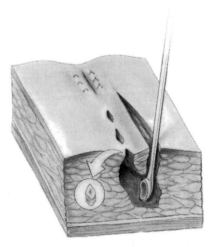

Figure 39–3. Lateral incision to the abscess cavity. Granulated tissues are scraped with a curette. (From Nivatvongs S. Pilonidal disease. In: Gordon P, Nivatvongs S, eds. Principles and Practices of Surgery of the Colon, Rectum, and Anus. St Louis: Quality Medical Publishing, 1992:272.)

Incision and Marsupialization

In incision and marsupialization (Fig. 39–4), the sinus tracts are probed to evaluate their extension and direction. The skin is then incised longitudinally and laterally to unroof the cyst. The deep cyst wall is curetted clean of hair and debris. The redundant skin edges are excised and the wound saucerized. The margins should then be rounded. An oval wound with the long axis along the midline of the sacrococcygeal area is formed. The fibrous tissue is sewn to the edges of the wound. This technique minimizes the wound by 50% to 60%. It also prevents premature closure of the wound. The area must be cleaned and packed daily, requiring 6 to 8 weeks to heal in most cases.

Wide Local Excision With or Without Primary Closure

In wide local excision, en bloc excision of the sinus tracts with a 5-mm margin of normal tissue is carried down to the sacrococcygeal fascia. If no overwhelming tension exists, the wound can be closed primarily, which may shorten healing time. If tension exists, the wound may be packed open or the edges can be approximated to the sacrococcygeal fascia

to decrease wound size. The wound is then packed. Dehiscences of primary closures may be packed open with only a moderate increase in healing time. There is no advantage to wide excision over marsupialization except for small cysts that can be closed primarily.

Excision and Reconstruction

The problem of delayed healing from midline wounds is addressed with the reconstructive procedures. The procedures are reserved for the chronic, recurrent sinus. These procedures generally involve flap mobilization, closed suction drainage, and strict limitations on patient activity. Z-plasty, Karydakis advancing flap procedure, and musculocutaneous rotation flaps are not appropriate outpatient procedures but are considered for difficult cysts and in the rare cases of carcinoma arising in a chronic pilonidal sinus.

The cleft closure as described by Bascom is a reconstructive procedure that requires closed suction drainage, but it has been carried out successfully in outpatient settings (Fig. 39–5). With the buttocks pressed together, the contact lines are marked with ink. Then the cheeks are taped apart. The sinuses are excised to one side of the apex of the marked line. A dermal flap is mobilized to the other

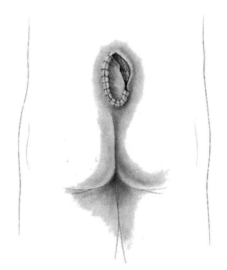

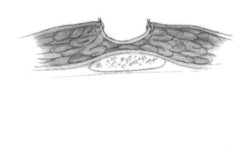

Figure 39–4. Marsupialization. Fibrotic wall at the base of the wound is sutured to the edges of the skin all around with continuous absorbable suture. (From Nivatvongs S. Pilonidal disease. In: Gordon P, Nivatvongs S, eds. Principles and Practices of Surgery of the Colon, Rectum, and Anus. St Louis: Quality Medical Publishing, 1992:273.)

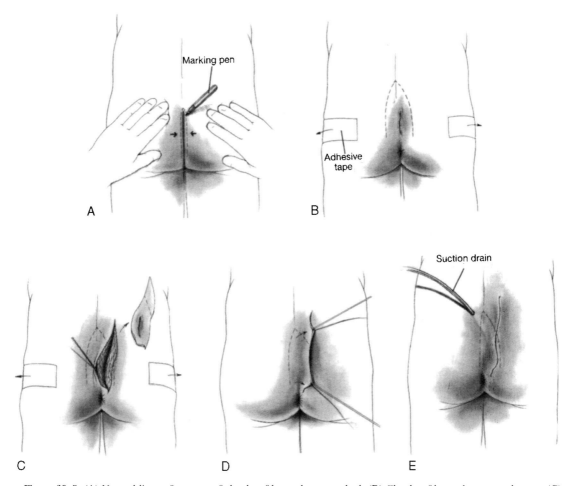

Figure 39–5. (A) Natural lines of contact of cheeks of buttock are marked. **(B)** Cheeks of buttock are taped apart. **(C)** Unhealed wound is excised in a triangular shape. **(D)** After skin flap is raised out to marked line, tapes are released. Skin flap is positioned to overlap edges of wound on opposite side. Excess skin is excised. Closed suction drain is placed in subcutaneous tissue, which is closed with 3-0 chromic catgut. **(E)** Skin is closed with subcuticular 4-0 polydioxanone suture. (From Nivatvongs S. Pilonidal disease. In: Gordon P, Nivatvongs S, eds. Principles and Practices of Surgery of the Colon, Rectum, and Anus. St Louis: Quality Medical Publishing, 1992:278.)

line, then the tapes are released. Excess skin is tailored and the edges approximated after placement of a closed suction drain. The closure uses deep absorbable suture and subcuticular skin closure. The drain is removed after 4 days. Normal activity is resumed after drain removal.

ANESTHETIC CONSIDERATIONS

Simple incision and drainage and small procedures in cooperative patients may be handled with infiltration of local anesthetics. More involved procedures may require the addition of sedating agents, such as midazolam or pro-

pofol. The use of regional or general anesthesia is used frequently and does not preclude outpatient surgery.

POSTOPERATIVE CONSIDERATIONS

Immediate postoperative care after discharge emphasizes pain control, avoidance of constipation, wound care and hygiene, and activity restriction. Pain is often moderately severe but can usually be controlled with oral narcotics; stool softeners are used to avoid difficulty in defecation. If the wound is open, narcotics may be necessary for longer periods until the granulating wound ceases to be painful during dressing changes. It is often difficult for the patient to do all wound care; therefore, a care giver must be instructed in the proper technique for wet to dry dressing for open wounds. A Water-Pik and hand-held shower are excellent tools for hygiene. Strenuous activity should be restricted for several weeks. External nylon sutures in primary closures should be left for 14 to 21 days as necessary. Weekly to every other week office visits are necessary to monitor adequacy of wound care, assessment of healing, and removal of surrounding hair growth until healing is complete.

RECURRENCES

Recurrences are seen in 20% to 40% of patients overall. They should be treated with the same principles in mind. Recurrence alone does not warrant radical reconstructive procedures.

Selected Readings

1. Bascom J. Pilonidal sinus. In Fazio V, ed. Current Therapy in Colon and Rectal Surgery. Toronto: BC Decker, 1990:32–39.
2. Kronborg O, Christensen K, Zimmerman-Nielsen C. Chronic pilonidal disease: A randomized trial with a complete 3-year follow-up. Br J Surg 1985;72:303–304.
3. Nivatvongs S. Pilonidal disease. In: Gordon P, Nivatvongs S, eds. Principles and Practices of Surgery of the Colon, Rectum, and Anus. St Louis: Quality Medical Publishing, 1992:267–279.
4. Patey DH, Scarff RW. Pathology of postanal pilonidal sinus: Its bearing on treatment. Lancet 1946;2:484.
5. Sohn N, Weinstein W. Sacrococcygeal pilonidal sinus. In Cameron J, ed. Current Surgical Therapy. St Louis: Mosby, 1995:250–253.
6. Sola J, Rothenberger DA. Chronic pilonidal disease. An assessment of 150 cases. Dis Colon Rectum 1990;33:758–761.
7. Wexner S, Binderow, S. Pilonidal disease, presacral cysts and tumors, and pelvic and perianal pain. In: Zuidema G, ed. Shackelford's Surgery of the Alimentary Tract. Philadelphia: WB Saunders, 1996:432–449.

Transanal Excision: Traditional Approach

James O. Keck • *Patricia L. Roberts*

Transanal excision is generally performed for benign tumors of the lower rectum. While surgical removal of these lesions is generally straightforward when they are small, sessile rectal tumors can also be extensive, occupying a large portion of the rectum. Working within the confines of the anal canal to remove them may challenge the skills of the most experienced surgeon. However, successful transanal excision obviates the need for open surgery, and patients usually experience minimal morbidity afterward. This makes transanal excision one of the most satisfying surgical procedures and makes it ideal for performance in an ambulatory setting.

INDICATIONS

The most common indication for transanal excision is for the removal of villous adenomas or tubulovillous adenomas of the rectum. Smaller pedunculated adenomas of the rectum are generally removed by snaring or "hot biopsy" during either proctoscopy or flexible endoscopy procedures. However, larger pedunculated lesions may also require formal transanal excision.

Transanal excision can almost always be performed for adenomas situated in the distal third of the rectum. This is true even for lesions that occupy most of all of the circumference of the rectum. Villous tumors that start in the distal third but extend into the middle third of the rectum can also usually be excised

by one of the techniques described in this chapter. Adenomas in the middle third of the rectum and those that extend even higher present particular difficulties. However, the mobility of the rectal mucosa on the rectal wall and of the rectal wall itself may be such that transanal excision is possible. See Chapter 40 for an alternative approach to tumors in the middle third of the rectum. In general, extensive lesions of the upper rectum or rectal lesions that extend up into the sigmoid colon are best managed by anterior resection or colo-anal anastomosis.

The role of transanal excision in the management of invasive rectal carcinoma is controversial. In patients with known liver metastases, palliative transanal surgery is often indicated for low rectal cancers. This may take the form of excision, electrocautery, or laser ablation. In this situation, the aim of surgery is to avoid local complications of the cancer, especially pain, bleeding, and obstruction, without the need for a colostomy. Similarly, such local treatment may be indicated in patients who are extremely frail or medically unfit for rectal resection.

Although abdominoperineal resection has traditionally been considered the "gold standard" treatment for distal rectal cancer, transanal full-thickness excision with the intention of cure may be used for selected lesions. In general, this approach should be reserved for tumors that are small, superficial, and well or moderately well differentiated, and do not show evidence of venous or lymphatic invasion. Even in these favorable circumstances, as many as 10% of patients have lymph node metastases and, therefore, are not cured by transanal excision. More recently, it has been suggested that radiotherapy, given preoperatively or postoperatively, may improve the results of local excision for rectal cancer.

This chapter focuses on the role of transanal excision for benign rectal lesions with special attention to villous adenomas of the rectum, which are the most common lesions removed by this method.

PATHOPHYSIOLOGY

Tubular adenomas, tubulovillous adenomas, and villous adenomas are precancerous lesions; removal of these lesions decreases the risk of development of colorectal cancer. Adenomas are thought to arise from a combination of genetic, environmental, and dietary factors; they are common, occurring in up to 30% of the population older than age 40 years. There is a wealth of evidence supporting the adenoma–carcinoma sequence, and most colorectal cancers arise from preexisting adenomas; de novo cancer is rare.

Through the molecular biologic work of Vogelstein and others, a multistep theory of genetic alterations leading to the development of carcinoma has been elaborated. Indeed, both adenomas and carcinomas share genetic traits, including *ras* gene mutations and allelic loss of chromosome 5 and chromosome 18. A series of genetic changes occurs that becomes more prevalent as the polyp becomes larger. With increasing size there is an increasing change of malignancy, although there is no linear relationship between the size of a villous adenoma and the presence of cancer. On occasion, villous adenomas may be quite large and still be benign. Invasive cancer, which may occur in 4.2% to 52% of lesions, is, however, more likely in a villous adenoma than in a tubular adenoma. This may be related to the larger surface area of a villous adenoma compared with a comparable tubular adenoma. The presence of ulceration and induration are better predictors of malignant invasion than the size of a villous adenoma.

In series of neoplastic polyps, villous adenomas comprise 10% to 20% with approximately 75% occurring in the rectum. Villous adenomas may be associated with diarrhea, hypokalemia, and fluid secretion. This constellation of findings has been termed the McKittrick-Wheelock syndrome. It has been postulated that this fluid secretion occurs in response to secretion of prostaglandin E_2, which is produced by the tumor.

SURGICAL TECHNIQUE

A number of techniques are available for the transanal removal of rectal adenomas depending on their size and position. Variations on traditional transanal excision include snaring and fulguration, and rectal mucosectomy. In general, the preoperative preparation and assessment and the postoperative care are similar for all these approaches.

Preoperative Preparation

Before operation, the patient undergoes a standard history and physical examination, and appropriate laboratory and radiographic tests are obtained. Colonoscopy should be performed to exclude synchronous neoplastic lesions, which occur in 40% to 50% of patients with a rectal adenoma.

On the day before surgery, a clear liquid diet is advised and patients undergo mechanical bowel preparation with either a polyethylene glycol–based lavage solution or oral sodium phosphate solution. Bowel preparation can be undertaken safely and effectively on an outpatient basis in most cases. Patients who cannot tolerate outpatient preparation for a variety of reasons such as nausea, vomiting, and dehydration are admitted to the hospital for bowel preparation. Prophylactic intravenous antibiotics are given within 1 hour of surgery and two doses are given postoperatively. Our preference is a second generation cephalosporin.

Intraoperative Considerations

Transanal excision may be performed under a regional or general anesthetic. Depending

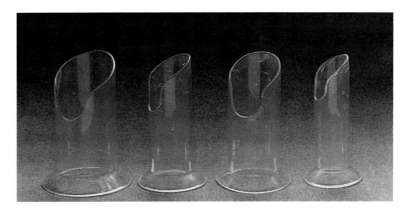

Figure 40–1. Ferguson plastic anoscopes are useful for transanal excision. They are available in graduated lengths and diameters.

on the location of the lesion, the patient is placed in the prone jack-knife position or lithotomy position. The prone position allows blood to fall away from the operative field with gravity and allows for more effective surgical assistance. Lithotomy position is preferred for posterior lesions and the prone jack-knife position for anterior lesions.

Exposure of the lesion is key to the performance of the procedure. To facilitate exposure, the operating surgeon wears a headlight. A variety of retractors, instruments, and anoscopes should be available in the operating room and, in different circumstances, each of them may be useful. These retractors include a Pratt bivalve speculum, a Parks' self-retaining retractor, Hill-Ferguson retractors, Ferguson plastic anoscopes (Fig. 40–1), a small Deaver retractor, and a dinner fork (Fig. 40–2). If

rectal mucosectomy is performed, the Lone Star retractor (Lone Star Medical Products, Houston, TX) is particularly useful. A solution of saline containing 1:200,000 epinephrine is infiltrated and helps reduce operative bleeding as well as elevate the lesion from the underlying muscle.

Allis forceps are used to grasp the distal end of the partially mobilized rectal mucosa during transanal excision. For rectal mucosectomy, it is necessary to have at least a dozen such forceps. Stay sutures are also useful to provide traction on the mucosa at or above the upper limit of the tumor, and polyglycolic acid or chromic catgut sutures are suitable for this. Traction on these sutures is helpful in exposing the lesion; the lesion tends to retract with progressive dissection. Similar sutures can be used to close or marsupialize defects in the

Figure 40–2. Various instruments are helpful for transanal excision. A sterilized dinner fork aids in the dissection by pushing the lesion away from the underlying rectal wall. Upward traction on the villous adenoma with the use of a sterilized dinner fork (**A**) aids in the dissection with the Metzenbaum scissors (**B**). (Courtesy of Lahey Clinic, Burlington, MA.)

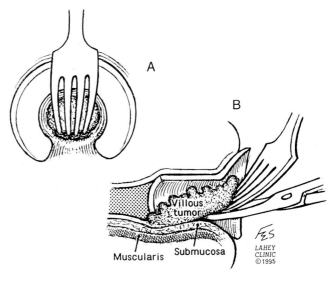

rectal mucosa. The defect is closed in either a longitudinal or transverse fashion depending on the size and configuration of the lesion. For large lesions, an attempt is made to close the defect transversely so the lumen of the rectum is not compromised. The tails of the sutures are left long in case there is bleeding and it is necessary to return to the operative field. A double-action needle holder is useful, particularly for placement of sutures in the mid or upper rectum.

Because of the high incidence of focal carcinoma in sessile rectal tumors, it is helpful for the pathologist to receive an oriented, pinned-out specimen. Fine sutures can be used to fix the specimen to paper or cardboard, which is then marked to show which edges are distal and proximal, left and right, or anterior and posterior as appropriate. Such orientation is invaluable when it is necessary to reexcise the tumor bed in patients who are found to have superficial cancers or tumor margins that are not clear.

Specific techniques of transanal excision, snaring and fulguration, and rectal mucosectomy are described in the following section:

Transanal Excision

Transanal excision is the preferred approach for most sessile rectal tumors. Using a self-retaining retractor, such as the Parks' retractor, the entire lesion is visualized and a solution of saline with 1:200,000 epinephrine is infiltrated into the submucosal plane. It may be necessary to withdraw and replace the retractor a number of times to infiltrate the entire lesion if it is large.

Dissection generally begins below the lesion and a 1-cm margin should be included with the operative specimen. Dissection can proceed with the scissors, although we prefer using the electrocautery with the spatula blade. Meticulous use of electrocautery minimizes bleeding and prevents the operative field from filling with blood. A flap of tumor-bearing mucosa is thus raised, and the lower end of this can be grasped with Allis clamps for traction. Once again, the orientation of the retractor may need to be changed from time to time to accommodate larger lesions. Occasionally, self-retaining anal retractors prevent the dissected

flap of rectal mucosa from prolapsing out of the anal canal. In this case, after commencing the dissection, it may be helpful to withdraw the retractor and use a hand-held retractor, such as the Hill-Ferguson or small Deaver. Ferguson plastic anoscopes also allow smaller lesions to prolapse into the operative field. Stay sutures placed at or just above the upper extent of the tumor are helpful for traction during dissection.

When a level has been reached 1 cm above the tumor, the flap is divided and the specimen is removed and immediately pinned out and oriented. At this stage, the resultant defect is inspected for bleeding and the cautery used to achieve hemostasis. The defect may be left open to heal by secondary intention, which is safe, especially in the distal extraperitoneal rectum. Alternatively, a running suture can be used to partially or completely close the defect. This approach is preferred because it results in more secure hemostasis.

Lesions that begin well above the dentate line can be removed by raising a flap of normal mucosa below the tumor and using this to pull the lesion down. This flap should begin at the dentate line and be developed in a manner similar to the performance of a standard hemorrhoidectomy. If the resultant defect is to be closed, it may be done either longitudinally or transversely depending on the size of the defect.

Occasionally, it is useful to prolapse a smaller lesion right out of the anal canal and to remove it by creating a false pedicle. This pedicle can be suture ligated or even stapled using a linear stapler. Laparoscopic stapling devices may similarly be used in the lower rectum using an anal retractor.

When transanal excision has been completed, it is essential to demonstrate that the lumen of the rectum has not been greatly compromised or that the walls of the rectum have not been sewn to each other. This is easily accomplished with a rigid proctoscope.

Snaring and Fulguration

Snaring and fulguration are performed less often than is formal transanal excision. It may occasionally be useful for sessile lesions that have a polypoid exophytic component and for

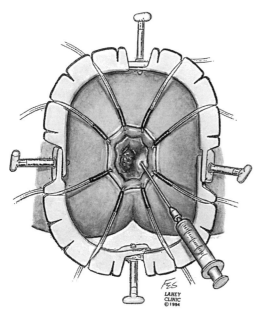

Figure 40–3. The Lone Star retractor (Lone Star Medical Products, Houston, Texas) provides excellent exposure of the anal canal and lower rectum. A saline solution with 1:200,000 epinephrine is injected into the submucosal plane to facilitate the dissection and aid in hemostasis. (Courtesy of Lahey Clinic, Burlington, MA.)

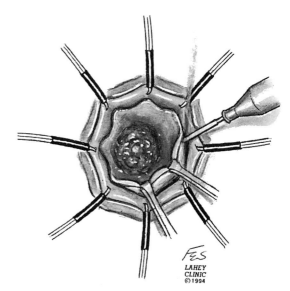

Figure 40–4. An incision is made with the Bovie cautery distal to the lesion and continued circumferentially. (Courtesy of Lahey Clinic, Burlington, MA.)

lesions that begin in the mid and upper rectum. It may also be indicated for tumor recurrence after transanal excision.

Infiltration with saline and 1:200,000 epinephrine is performed. A wire loop snare is used to shave off the more exophytic portions of the lesion. A needle point cautery is then used systematically to extirpate the base and the sessile components of the lesion. A curette is used to scrape away coagulated tumor to reveal any residual adenoma. Material for pathologic inspection is collected in a piecemeal fashion. A major disadvantage of this technique is that it does not allow for accurate pathologic staging.

Rectal Mucosectomy

The management of large or circumferential villous tumors of the rectum can be especially difficult. Sir Alan Parks described removing all of the lower rectal mucosa in strips in patients with circumferential lesions. Rectal mucosectomy, a technique adapted from restorative proctocolectomy for ulcerative colitis or familial adenomatous polyposis, is similar except that the mucosa is removed as a contin-

uous sleeve. It is somewhat analogous to the Delorme operation for rectal prolapse.

The performance of rectal mucosectomy is facilitated by the use of a Lone Star retractor (Lone Star Medical Products, Houston, TX) (Figs. 40–3 through 40–8). This provides exposure by effacement of the anal canal with mini-

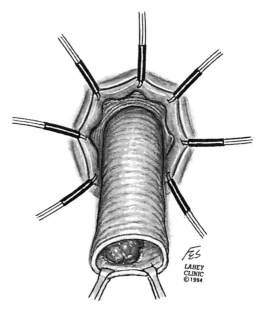

Figure 40–5. A circumferential dissection is carried out to at least 1 cm above the upper extent of the tumor. (Courtesy of Lahey Clinic, Burlington, MA.)

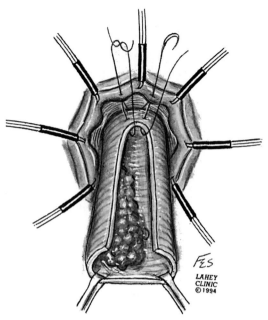

Figure 40–6. The rectal mucosal tube is split and anchoring sutures are placed between the proximal rectal mucosa and the dentate line to prevent retraction of the proximal mucosa. (Courtesy of Lahey Clinic, Burlington, MA.)

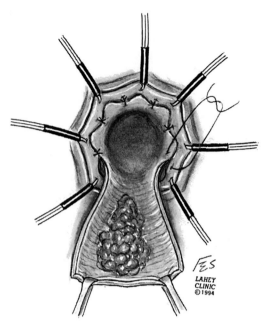

Figure 40–7. The anastomosis is carried out with absorbable interrupted sutures. (Courtesy of Lahey Clinic, Burlington, MA.)

mal dilatation and is less likely to injure the anal canal than two Gelpi retractors placed at right angles. Once again, a dilute solution of epinephrine is injected into the submucosal plane circumferentially, beginning at the dentate line.

A circumferential incision is made and the cut edge grasped with Allis clamps. Dissection may be difficult in the upper anal canal, particularly in heavy individuals, but it gets easier once the submucosa of the rectum is entered. In this plane, the dissection may be advanced by gently pushing a piece of gauze proximally. When a point has been reached with at least a 1-cm margin above the tumor, the sleeve of mucosa is bivalved, preferably away from the tumor, and partially divided. Polyglycolic acid or chromic catgut sutures are placed between the proximal rectal mucosa and the dentate line, and a circular anastomosis is made as the mucosa above the tumor is progressively divided. A rigid proctoscope is used to ensure patency of the lumen.

Postoperative Care

Most patients can be safely discharged home after transanal excision, although patients in

whom a large rectal defect has been created usually require admission to the hospital for 1 to 2 days after surgery. Patients who are discharged on the day of the procedure should be warned to watch for bleeding, fever, or undue pain. Mild analgesia is prescribed. Bulk-forming agents should be taken for several weeks after surgery. Sitz baths are helpful in

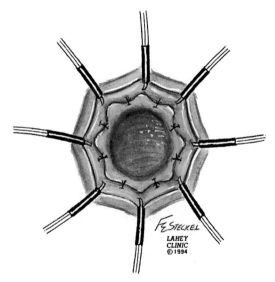

Figure 40–8. The completed anastomosis. (Courtesy of Lahey Clinic, Burlington, MA.)

the immediate postoperative period. A printed instruction sheet is helpful.

COMPLICATIONS

The main complications that may occur after transanal excision are bleeding, stenosis, incontinence, and perforation.

Bleeding may occur immediately after surgery (primary hemorrhage) or may be delayed for 7 to 10 days (secondary hemorrhage). Primary hemorrhage is a failure of adequate hemostasis, and secondary hemorrhage may occur with separation of the eschar (in the case of fulguration) or dissolution of sutures (in the case of transanal excision or mucosal proctectomy). Significant bleeding occurred in 8.5% of 122 patients undergoing transanal excision in a series from the Ferguson Clinic, Grand Rapids, MI. Similarly, in a series from the Lahey Clinic, Burlington, MA, the incidence of bleeding was 12% after transanal excision and 9% after snaring and fulguration. Significant postoperative bleeding was not seen in 12 patients who underwent rectal mucosectomy. Primary closure of rectal defects probably reduces the incidence of primary hemorrhage after transanal excision and it may prevent secondary hemorrhage. Patients who undergo transanal excision in an ambulatory setting must be aware of the risk of postoperative bleeding and must know how to seek medical attention if bleeding occurs. Patients who experience significant bleeding require readmission and resuscitation; many patients must return to the operating room for control of bleeding with cautery or with oversewing of blood vessels. For patients with massive hemorrhage, insertion of a large Foley catheter into the distal rectum with inflation of the balloon may tamponade the bleeding and help stabilize the patient while the operating team is assembled.

Incontinence is uncommon after transanal excision. Transient incontinence was seen in 9% and persistent incontinence in 4% of patients undergoing transanal excision or snaring and fulguration in the Lahey Clinic series. This incidence of incontinence is not surprising given the advanced age of many of the patients in the series and given the recognized

problem of leakage following rectal mucosectomy for ulcerative colitis. The alternative to rectal mucosectomy for patients with giant rectal villous tumors may be abdominoperineal resection or colon-anal anastomosis. Rectal stenosis is also an uncommon complication of transanal excision, although occasional cases occur. Rectal perforation following transanal excision is usually of the extraperitoneal rectum. It occurs with pain and fever, without peritonitis; most cases resolve with therapy of intravenous antibiotics.

RESULTS

Transanal excision relieves the symptoms caused by benign rectal tumors and prevents the development of cancer in most cases. However, both tumor persistence and tumor recurrence may occur after transanal excision. A useful definition of tumor persistence is the presence of tumor at the same site as the index lesion within 6 months of surgery, whereas tumor recurrence is defined as the presence of tumor in the same location more than 6 months postoperatively, after an apparent disease-free interval.

In the Ferguson Clinic series, the rates of tumor persistence and recurrence were 27% and 30%, respectively. In some patients, persistence or recurrence is due to an inadequate initial operation. However, it may also be possible that, with large villous adenomas of the rectum, the entire rectal mucosa undergoes a field change and is biologically unstable. This concept is supported by results from the Lahey Clinic, where rates of both tumor persistence and recurrence were significantly lower after rectal mucosectomy compared with transanal excision or snaring and fulguration. Snaring and fulguration was associated with a particularly high rate of tumor persistence (44%).

The incidence of invasive carcinoma in villous adenomas of the rectum has been estimated as 20% overall, although this rate increases with the size of the lesion. Data from the Cleveland Clinic, Cleveland, OH, showed an incidence of invasive cancer of 10% in a large series of villous and tubulovillous lesions of the colon and rectum. However, for lesions larger than 4 cm in diameter, the incidence increased to 32%. In the Lahey Clinic series, the incidence of invasive cancer was 10% despite a mean tumor diameter of 5.1 cm. The reason for this lower than expected incidence of cancer is uncertain, although it may be significant that 40% of the tumors were found incidentally, often in the course of screening for colorectal cancer.

FOLLOW-UP

In view of the high risk of tumor persistence and recurrence, close follow-up of patients who have undergone transanal excision is necessary. The rectum should be visualized by rigid proctoscopy or flexible sigmoidoscopy every 3 months for the first year after transanal excision and then every 6 months for the next year. Complete colonoscopy should be performed a year after transanal excision and then every 3 years if results are normal.

SUMMARY

Transanal excision is a challenging but rewarding procedure that can oftentimes be performed in an ambulatory setting. It is indicated for the surgical removal of villous adenomas and tubulovillous lesions of the distal and mid rectum. Along with traditional transanal excision, other transanal surgical approaches, such as snaring and fulguration, and rectal mucosectomy, are occasionally useful.

Complications of transanal excision are unusual, although patients should be aware of the risk of postoperative bleeding. Persistence or recurrence of rectal villous adenomas is common after transanal excision, possibly because of a field change in the rectum, and close follow-up is essential.

Selected Readings

1. Galandiuk S, Fazio VW, Jagelman DG, et al. Villous and tubulovillous adenomas of the colon and rectum: A retrospective review, 1964–1985. Am J Surg 1987;153:41–47.
2. Groff W, Rubin RJ, Salvati EP, et al. A method of management of a circumferential villous tumor of the rectum. Dis Colon Rectum 1981;24:151–154.
3. Keck JO, Schoetz DJ Jr, Roberts PL, et al. Rectal mucosectomy in the treatment of giant rectal villous tumors. Dis Colon Rectum 1995;38:233–238.
4. Nivatvongs S, Balcos EG, Schottler JL, et al. Surgical management of large villous tumors of the rectum. Dis Colon Rectum 1973;16:508–514.
5. Parks AG, Stuart AE. The management of villous tumours of the large bowel. Br J Surg 1973;60:688–695.
6. Pello MJ. Transanal excision of large sessile villous adenomas using an endorectal traction flap. Surg Gynecol Obstet 1987;164:281.
7. Roberts PL, Schoetz DJ Jr, Murray JJ, et al. Use of a new retractor to facilitate mucosal proctectomy. Dis Colon Rectum 1990;33:1063–1064.
8. Sakamoto GD, MacKeigan JM, Senagore AJ. Transanal excision of large, rectal villous adenomas. Dis Colon Rectum 1991;34:880–885.
9. Taylor EW, Thompson H, Oates GD, et al. Limitations of biopsy in preoperative assessment of villous papilloma. Dis Colon Rectum 1981;24:259.
10. Thomson JP. Treatment of sessile villous and tubulovillous adenomas of the rectum: Experience of St. Mark's Hospital, 1963–1972. Dis Colon Rectum 1977;20:467–472.

ENDOSCOPIC SURGERY

Transanal Excision: Endoscopic Microsurgical Technique

Bruce A. Orkin

Transanal endoscopic microsurgery (TEM) is a fairly new method of minimally invasive surgery that allows surgical access to the mid and upper rectum. Using specially designed equipment and techniques, lesions of the rectum may be excised and other procedures may be performed at levels not previously accessible. The rectum is dilated with carbon dioxide, and the stereoscopic magnified optical system and special long instruments permit operative maneuvers such as grasping, cutting, cautery, and suturing. There are major advantages associated with this approach, including little postoperative pain, limited hospitalization, unrestricted mobility, little morbidity, and rapid return to normal activities. This method was developed by Gerhart Buess and colleagues in Germany during the early 1980s, and they have continued to champion its use. Although the technique has been used fairly extensively in Europe, its acceptance has been slow in North America, primarily because of the prohibitive initial cost of the equipment and the limited number of patients for whom it is appropriate.

INDICATIONS

Transanal excision of polyps and small carcinomas of the rectum is currently standard practice. Transanal excision of pedunculated lesions is easily accomplished using endoscopic snare techniques via either a standard rigid proctoscope or a flexible endoscope. When the lesion is sessile and is located in the low rectum (within 6–8 cm of the anal verge), surgical excision may be performed using a variety of operating anoscopes and specula. Above the 8 to 10 cm mark, sessile adenomas have been excised endoscopically with snares in a piecemeal manner and have been fulgurated with electrocautery. These methods are a poor substitute for controlled and complete excision with a clear margin because of the risk of cutting across an unrecognized malignant focus and the risk of recurrence. In addition, a complete specimen is not available for pathologic examination and determination of margins and depth of penetration of occult malignancies. Other alternatives are major resective procedures via either the abdominal or posterior parasacral approach. These operations carry much higher morbidity and mortality rates.

Transanal endoscopic microsurgery is an ideal method of excising sessile adenomas that are beyond the reach of standard transanal techniques. Even quite large or circumferential adenomas may be approached when the surgeon has gained experience. TEM is also extremely helpful in those patients who have had endoscopic removal of a polyp that is shown to have a focus of carcinoma on pathologic examination. Pedunculated lesions without a clear margin or with invasion into the stalk are well treated by disc excision of the polypectomy site and pathologic examination for residual carcinoma. Sessile lesions may be treated for cure if the malignant process is limited to the mucosa.

Early invasive adenocarcinomas may be treated by local excision with a high cure rate if the lesion is limited to the submucosa (stage T1, TNM classification system). Less than 10% of these lesions are associated with lymph node metastases. If the lesion extends into or through the muscularis propria (stage T2, T3), the risks of local recurrence, lymph node metastases, and distant spread increase dramatically. Selection of patients for local treatment of rectal carcinoma is based on the patient's risk of recurrence and on overall considerations such as operative risk and known metastases. Specific tumor criteria are size less than 3 cm, circumference less than one third of the rectal lumen, exophytic morphology, well or moderately well differentiated histology, mobility (if the lesion is within the reach of a palpating digit), and technical accessibility. Endorectal ultrasound is the best method of determining depth of invasion; this is an indispensable adjunct to clinical evaluation. It may also be used effectively for follow-up of patients to detect early local recurrence. Endorectal ultrasound is more than 90% accurate in the determination of depth of tumor invasion. It is less useful for identifying lymph node metastases (up to 75% accurate).

Patients being considered for local treatment of a known rectal carcinoma are preoperatively staged with proctoscopy to clearly localize the lesion and to obtain biopsy specimens, colonoscopy to clear the colon of synchronous lesions, endorectal ultrasound, and chest radiography. I usually obtain a computed tomography (CT) scan of the abdomen to check the liver for metastases, but this is generally a low-yield study. Patients whose condition is staged T1, N0, M0 (i.e., invasion into the submucosa and without lymph node or distant metastases) are candidates for TEM excision for cure.

Occasionally, patients with more advanced lesions may be considered for TEM excision. Very elderly and high-risk patients with T2 lesions may be candidates if they and their families understand the relative risks of recurrence and operative morbidity. Patients with larger lesions who have known metastases may

be treated for palliation as long as complete excision of the primary tumor is possible. Partial excision is of limited value in the absence of obstruction. TEM may be used to treat stenoses due to carcinoma by local excision or with laser vaporization and debulking.

Additional indications for TEM include excision of other rectal lesions such as carcinoids and excision of persistent solitary rectal ulcers if rectal prolapse is not the cause. Although Professor Buess has advocated transrectal, presacral rectopexy for rectal prolapse, my experience has been poor with this approach, so I prefer other techniques. Postoperative strictures may be approached using TEM and a stricturoplasty technique. Rectal bleeding from unresectable tumors or due to radiation changes may also be treated this way.

Transanal endoscopic microsurgery is a new technique that is difficult to learn and difficult to perform. The system is complicated and expensive, and a trained operating room staff is necessary. Surgeons who learn this technique must go through an intensive training course, usually followed by further practice on inanimate and animal models and then by proctored cases.

PREPARATION AND CONVERSION

Patients undergoing TEM are prepared as for any major resective procedure. Most surgeons use a combination of mechanical bowel preparation with either polyethylene glycol lavage solutions or laxatives and enemas, along with oral and intravenous antibiotics. This bowel preparation may be performed at home by most patients. Currently, more than 90% of patients undergoing elective colorectal procedures at my institution are prepared at home and come to the operating suite the morning of their surgery.

Obtaining an informed consent is very important in these patients. The advantages and disadvantages of this technique should be explained in detail. When operation is for a malignancy, the risk of missed lymph node metastases must be discussed and the patient must be willing to take this risk. All patients must give consent for conversion to an open, trans-

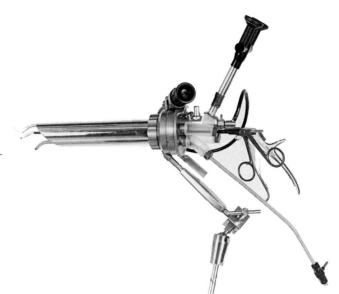

Figure 41–1. The transanal endoscopic microsurgical set with instruments in place.

abdominal resection because this may be necessary if the procedure is not completed using TEM. Conversion may be necessary if the operating scope does not reach above the lesion because of bowel angulation, narrowing of the lumen, or curvature of the sacrum. Entry into the peritoneal cavity is a relative indication for conversion because some of these defects may be closed transluminally with minimal spillage.

TECHNICAL CONSIDERATIONS

The equipment necessary for transanal endoscopic microsurgery include the TEM set (Fig. 41–1), the TEM instruments, the combination endosurgical unit, and a standard electrocautery unit. A video monitor or a video tape machine may also be desirable.

The TEM operating set is centered around the "basic element." This is a unit with two locking collars to hold the operating rectoscope and the faceplate along with a handle (Fig. 41–2). The operating rectoscopes are 4 cm in diameter and measure either 12 or 20 cm in greatest length. Each is beveled at the distal end and comes with an appropriately sized obturator used for insertion of the scope into the rectum (Fig. 41–3). There are two faceplates (the adaptor and the working insert). One is a simple closed plate with a viewing window and a light source adaptor used

for initial positioning of the rectoscope. The second has five ports: one for the optical system and four for instrument insertion. Each rectoscope and faceplate fit snugly into the basic element and are locked in place when in

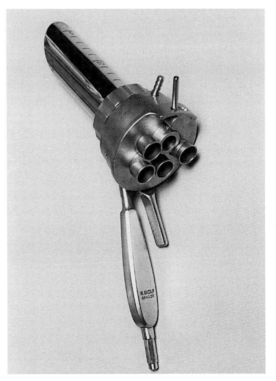

Figure 41–2. The basic element with rectoscope and operating faceplate attached.

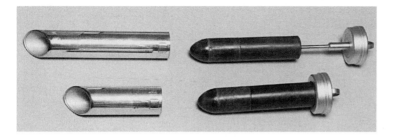

Figure 41–3. The 12- and 20-cm operating rectoscopes and their obturators.

use. The optical system is composed of a stereo telescope with binocular eyepieces (Fig. 41–4). The view at the distal end of the system is angled down at about 45°. The image is magnified six times. The stereo telescope has additional channels that are used for insufflation of carbon dioxide, for irrigation of the viewing port, and for the light source. A central channel is used for a second viewing scope that may be attached to a video monitor. The entire assembly is anchored to the operating table using a U-shaped support arm. This comes with a standard clamp that attaches to most operating tables and a Martin universal joint system. The arm attaches to the TEM system by clamping of the handle of the basic element. The Martin arm is then loosened to position the scope and tightened to immobilize the setup. The Martin arm makes it easy to adjust the position of the rectoscope, which must be moved frequently during the procedure.

A specially designed set of instruments is an integral part of the system (Fig. 41–5). Most are angled down at the working end to approximate the viewing angle. Instruments include straight and angled needle holders and right- and left-angled forceps. Straight right- and left-curved scissors and a high-frequency electrocautery "knife" are also available. Perhaps the

most unique instrument is the suture clip forceps. Because it is nearly impossible to tie sutures in this closed system, silver clips are used to anchor the sutures. These are similar to the lead weights used on fishing lines in that they are split down the middle and are crimped to close tightly on a suture. There is also a specially angled, insulated suction–cautery probe for use by the assistant. Laparoscopic instruments may be substituted for some of those in the TEM set. In particular, a disposable cautery scissors may be used in place of both the high-frequency knife and the TEM scissors.

A combination endosurgical unit completes the system. This box incorporates the carbon dioxide insufflation and pressure control systems and the irrigation and low-pressure suction systems (Fig. 41–6). Low-pressure suction is necessary to avoid loss of the insufflation pressure and rectal distention.

Usually, TEM is performed under a general anesthetic because of the prolonged and absolute immobility required of the patient. Rarely, regional anesthesia and sedation may be used. No local anesthetics are necessary, although a local anesthetic with a known dilution of epinephrine may be used for dissection plane injection. A urinary catheter is generally placed, especially when anterior lesions are to

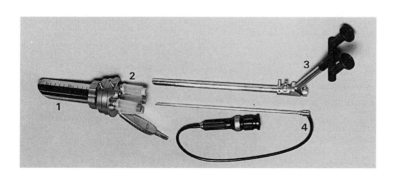

Figure 41–4. The optical system: *(1)* The 12-cm operating rectoscope. *(2)* The sleeves and caps attached to the operating faceplate ports. *(3)* The stereo telescope with binocular eyepieces. *(4)* The monocular eyepiece, which may be used for the assistant or may be attached to the video system.

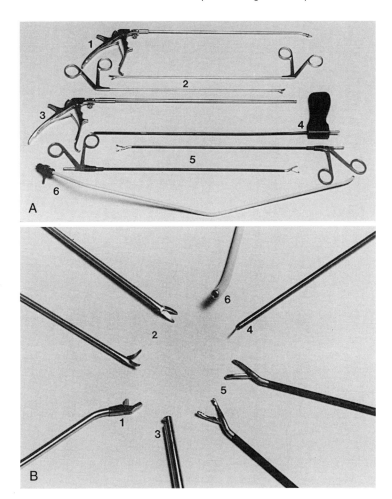

Figure 41–5. Transanal endoscopic microsurgical instruments. **(A)** Full view. **(B)** Detail of instrument heads. *(1)* Needle holder. *(2)* Right and left curved scissors. *(3)* Silver clip applier. *(4)* High-frequency electrocautery knife. *(5)* Right and left curved grasping forceps. *(6)* Angled suction and cautery probe.

be excised. The anesthesiologist should administer a minimal volume of fluid to prevent urinary retention in patients who are to be discharged home postoperatively. Usually, very little blood is lost and no major planes are opened, so fluid loss is minimal. Intravenous antibiotics are given after the induction of anesthesia.

The lesion to be removed must be positioned dependently so that the surgeon may look down on it. This means that the surgeon must determine the correct orientation of the lesion preoperatively so that the operating room personnel are prepared to correctly position the patient. Rigid proctoscopy before surgery is necessary because it is the best determinant of accessibility for TEM, and flexible endoscopy cannot correctly identify the orientation of the lesion. Posterior lesions are the easiest to view and excise and are the best to start on when learning the technique. For

posterior lesions, the patient is placed in the lithotomy position with the mid sacrum resting on a pad on the edge of the operating table and the perineum positioned well over the edge. Lateral lesions are approached with the patient in the lateral decubitus position. The legs are positioned at 90° out on a lateral table or arm board with pads between them. Again the perineum must be well out over the edge of the table. The support/Martin arm is attached to the table on the side opposite the legs.

Anterior lesions are the most difficult to access because of the curve of the anterior rectum and are the most hazardous because of the proximity of the vagina and the peritoneal cavity in the cul-de-sac. It is also most difficult to position the patient for excision of an anterior lesion because the surgeon must sit in between the patient's legs. A standard jackknife position cannot be used. The patient is initially placed on the table in the prone posi-

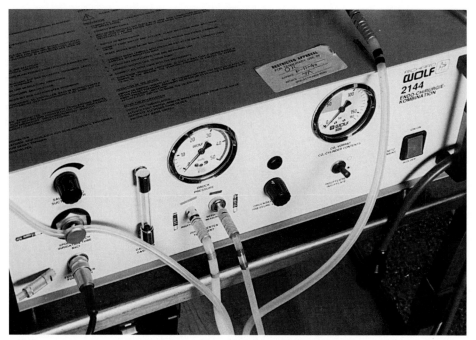

Figure 41–6. The combination endosurgical unit, which includes the carbon dioxide insufflation and pressure control systems and the irrigation and low-pressure suction systems.

tion over longitudinal chest rolls and a transverse hip roll. The feet of the table are then slowly lowered all the way down with assistants holding the patient's legs. The legs are bent 90° at the hips and at the knees and are supported in place with lithotomy stirrups projecting horizontally from the operating table. Pads are placed between the anterior thighs and the operating table. The operator sits on a stool between the patient's legs. It is important to protect the patient's extremities during positioning and during the procedure.

THE PROCEDURE

The procedure is begun by visualizing the lesion with a rigid proctoscope to confirm its position and to assess the completeness of the bowel preparation. The rectum is irrigated with saline and povidone–iodine. A vaginal preparation is performed in women, the perineum is cleansed, and the patient is draped. The appropriate rectoscope is seated and locked in the collar of the basic element. The anal canal is gently dilated digitally. Some authors have stated that an internal sphincterotomy is occasionally used to allow for place-

ment of the scope, but I have not found this to be necessary. The lubricated scope is inserted into the low rectum through the anal canal with the obturator in place. The obturator is immediately removed and all further advancement is performed under direct vision. The viewing faceplate is attached along with the light cord and an insufflation bulb. The rectoscope is advanced and positioned over the lesion. The viewing faceplate is then replaced with the operating faceplate. The optical system is inserted through the faceplate and locked in place. The various lines for carbon dioxide insufflation, monitoring of rectal pressure, and providing light, suction, irrigation, and electrocautery are attached. The instrument ports are sealed with plastic caps and the rectum is insufflated with carbon dioxide to a pressure of 15 mm Hg. All ports must be kept sealed to maintain rectal insufflation. Each port has a plastic sleeve and cap. The caps may be closed or may contain holes sized to fit the various instruments. Each time an instrument is changed, the port must be occluded by squeezing the plastic sleeve. This minimizes the loss of carbon dioxide. Figure 41–7 shows the instruments in place relative to a patient with a posterior lesion.

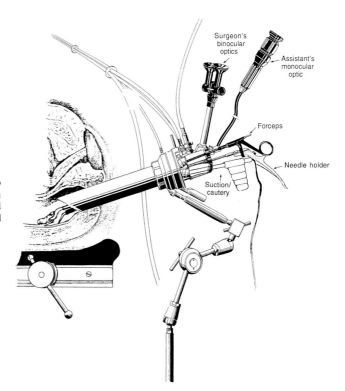

Figure 41–7. Instruments in place relative to a patient with a posterior lesion. (From Orkin BA: Treatment of rectal cancer. In Berk DE and Wexner SD (eds): Fundamentals of anorectal surgery. New York, McGraw-Hill, 1992, p. 297.)

The limits of the resection are marked with electrocautery of the mucosa before any other manipulation takes place (Fig. 41–8). Because the edges of the lesion and other landmarks may become obscured during the course of the dissection, it is easy to get too close or too far away unless there are clear lines to follow. A margin of at least 1 cm is desirable. Some surgeons inject a solution of epinephrine (either 1:100,000 or 1:200,000 in saline) in the submucosal or deep planes to reduce bleeding. A long retractable needle instrument is used for this purpose.

The dissection begins at the right lateral edge and proceeds to the left. The lesion may be removed in the submucosal plane or by transecting the full thickness of the bowel wall and staying in the perirectal fat. The submucosal plane is acceptable for benign lesions; however, all malignancies must be removed with a full thickness of the bowel wall. In practice, most excisions are performed into the fat. All bleeding must be controlled immediately or the operative field becomes obscured. Most bleeding vessels may be controlled with the electrocautery, either by direct application of the cautery tip or by grabbing the bleeding

site with the insulated forceps and cauterizing via the forceps. These forceps may be attached directly to the cautery current. The specimen is handled only by the normal margin; the operator should avoid grasping the neoplastic tissue with the forceps because it tends to bleed and tear, risking implantation of cells into the dissection plane. The operating site must be kept in the lower one half of the visual field so that the angle of the instruments does not run into the optical channel as it runs down the superior side of the rectoscope. In addition, the immediate operative site should be somewhat to the right to allow the specimen to be pulled to the left. The surgeon grasps and retracts the specimen with the forceps in the left hand and cuts and coagulates with the knife or cautery scissors in the right hand (Fig. 41–9). The rectoscope must be repositioned every few minutes to maintain the proper field. The stereo telescope also may be moved in and out or rotated slightly to improve the view.

Once the specimen has been completely excised, it should be firmly grasped by a forceps along the margin at a known side to keep it oriented. The faceplate is then removed with

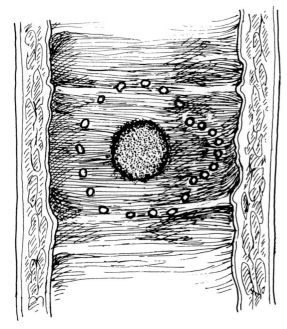

Figure 41–8. The limits of the resection are marked with a margin of at least 1 cm using the electrocautery. This is done before any other manipulation so that the edges of the lesion and other landmarks will be clearly visible throughout the course of the dissection. (From Smith LE: Transanal endoscopic microsurgery for rectal neoplasms. Gastrointest Endosc Clin North Am 1993; 3:336.)

the forceps in place so that the specimen may be removed from the rectoscope. The insufflator is turned off and a moist sponge is placed through the scope into the defect in the rectal wall. The specimen is then carefully pinned out on a cork board with orienting marks for the pathologist (Fig. 41–10). The specimen is handed directly to the pathologist who examines it for clear margins. Any areas that are suspect are submitted for immediate frozen pathologic examination to ensure complete excision. In the case of a close or positive margin, additional tissue may be removed from the correct side with this careful approach to the margins. The sponge is removed and the field is irrigated through the open rectoscope.

The operating faceplate is reattached to the basic element and the rectum is insufflated. The defect appears much larger than the originally marked resection margins because the elastic tissues of the rectal wall pull it apart once the specimen is removed. Some surgeons

think that these defects may be left open which is true when the excision has been performed entirely in the submucosal plane. However, most TEM surgeons close the defect with sutures. This is often the most difficult part of the procedure. Again, the process begins at the right edge and proceeds to the left. Occasionally, the defect may be closed longitudinally and beginning superiorly if it is not very wide and is in a broad part of the rectal lumen. Because this increases the likelihood of lumenal stenosis, most defects are closed in the transverse direction.

A standard, absorbable monofilament 3-0 suture is used. A silver clip is placed 4 to 6 cm from the needle and the suture is trimmed. The needle driver with the suture is inserted into the rectum along with a forceps. The first bite is taken through the right lateral side of the defect from the lumenal side into the deep fat. The edges are then approximated in a running over-and-over manner, beginning in the fat and proceeding out through the upper edge of the mucosa and then going from the lower mucosal surface into the exposed fat (Fig. 41–11). All bites are full thickness. The needle should be kept pointing to the left while the tissue is brought down over it with

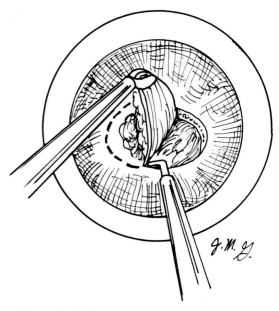

Figure 41–9. The surgeon works from right to left, grasping and retracting the specimen with the forceps in the left hand and cutting and coagulating with the knife or cautery scissors in the right hand.

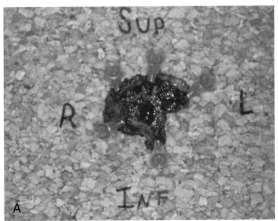 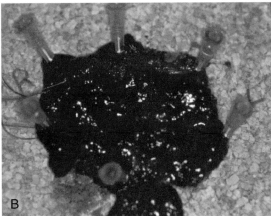

Figure 41–10. The specimen is pinned out on a cork board with orienting marks for the pathologist. **(A)** A 2- by 3-cm villous adenoma. **(B)** A 6- by 8-cm villous adenoma.

the forceps. The closure is completed by crimping the suture with another silver clip. The suture needs to be pulled tightly before placement of the clip so that the edges of the wound do not separate once tension is released. Larger defects may require two or three sutures to complete the closure. The faceplate is removed and the rectum is irri-

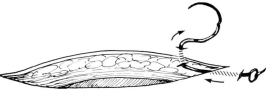

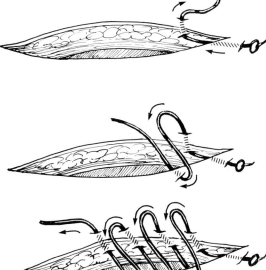

Figure 41–11. Edges are approximated in a running over-and-over manner, taking full-thickness bites and starting at the right. (From Smith LE: Transanal endoscopic microsurgery for rectal neoplasms. Gastrointest Endosc Clin North Am 1993;3:336.)

gated. The operating rectoscope is removed. If there is any question, patency of the lumen is tested by proctoscopy. At times, the faceplate may be removed for direct visualization and manipulation.

POSTOPERATIVE MANAGEMENT

Postoperatively, the patient may be discharged home after the anesthetic has worn off if the lesion was small or if the dissection was clearly in the submucosal plane. Postoperative antibiotics are not necessary, although some surgeons recommend several doses. A mildly to moderately strong pain medication is prescribed; narcotics are avoided because of their constipating effects. Bowel management is crucial after these procedures to avoid complications. All discharged patients are placed on a high-fiber diet, a fiber supplement, 6 to 8 glasses of fluids per day, and a stool softener, all beginning the day after surgery. The patient is told what signs of complications to look for, including large amounts of blood per rectum, increasing pain or fever, and chills and sweats. Urinary retention is a significant problem in these patients. If they are unable to urinate within 8 to 12 hours of discharge, patients should go to the emergency room for catheterization. Some passage of blood is expected, but, if patients pass a large amount of blood, they should go to the emergency room. A clinic visit is scheduled for 3 weeks after surgery.

When lesions are larger or there are any other medical concerns, the patient is kept overnight in the hospital. Patients undergoing excision of large lesions are constipated for 2 days with loperamide and codeine. After the second postoperative day, these medications are stopped and patients are started on the bowel management program described previously. They are discharged the next day if they have tolerated a regular diet and have had a bowel movement. Patients who do not have a bowel movement within 2 days of starting the bowel management program take 30 mL of milk of magnesia. Constipation and impaction must be avoided.

Patients are followed up every 3 months with proctoscopy. Any suspicious lesions are biopsied. Colonoscopy is performed after 1 year to look for metachronous lesions and is performed as indicated thereafter based on findings. Patients who undergo excision of malignancies have a carcinoembryonic antigen (CEA) level drawn every 3 months and undergo endorectal ultrasound to identify local recurrences. They also have a chest radiograph obtained once each year.

RESULTS

This discussion of the results of TEM is based on the work of Professor Buess and his colleagues in Tubingen, Germany, and on our experience at the George Washington University and elsewhere in the United States. The German group operated on 356 patients, the last 274 of whom were entered into a prospective follow-up program. My colleagues and I recently reviewed the U. S. experience of six surgeons who performed 130 procedures; all patients were evaluated and have been followed up prospectively. In our series, 81 patients were operated on for adenomas, 48 for carcinomas, and 16 for other indications including rectal prolapse, carcinoids, rectal stricture, and solitary rectal ulcer syndrome. The lower edge of 50% of these lesions was greater than 8 cm from the anal verge. Adenomas averaged 4 cm in greatest diameter whereas carcinomas averaged less than 3 cm in diame-

ter. Operative time averaged approximately 2 hours and estimated blood loss was less than 100 mL. Procedures for carcinoma typically take less time and less blood is lost because they tend to be smaller in size. The procedure was converted to an open operation in 9 of 130 (7%) patients, usually because the upper portion of the lesion could not be reached with the operating rectoscope. Hospital stay averaged less than 1 day when the procedure was completed transanally.

Overall, patients do well after successful TEM. Most have little pain if the lesion was located in the mid or upper rectum. To date, there has been only one mortality reported, and that was a patient of Professor Buess who suffered a pulmonary embolism.

Complications specific to the procedure included hemorrhage, peritoneal perforation, infection, suture line dehiscence, stenosis, rectovaginal fistula, and incontinence. In Professor Buess' report on 310 patients, 5% sustained complications. Two patients required anterior resection for extended peritoneal perforation, suture lines underwent dehiscence in five patients, and fistulas developed in another five. Hemorrhage necessitating reoperation occurred in two patients, and symptomatic stenosis developed in one patient. In 74 patients operated on for carcinoma, major complications occurred in 9%, including two rectovaginal fistulas and two suture line dehiscences. Two of these patients required a temporary diverting colostomy. In our series, four (3%) patients suffered intraoperative complications, 11 (8%) had early postoperative problems, and four (3%) had later difficulties. In our series, there were no infectious complications, although there were several episodes of significant bleeding. No fistulas developed in our patients. Transient fecal soiling may occur due to anal dilation; however, only one patient in our series has persistent soiling. One other patient underwent treatment with biofeedback and is currently continent.

The rectal lumen may be occluded by suturing when a large rectal lesion is removed. This may be avoided by careful suturing and proctoscopic examination at the conclusion of the procedure. Late stenosis may also occur if a large lesion was removed. This is generally amenable to dilation. In our series, a stricture developed in one patient after removal of a 6-by 8-cm villous adenoma of the mid rectum. This responded well to proctoscopic dilation and as of this writing the patient remains asymptomatic 60 months later.

Sessile adenomas are extremely well treated by TEM with recurrence rates of 3.5%. Most of these lesions may be retreated locally with snare excision, electrocautery, or reexcision. In one of our patients, a recurrence of his villous adenoma developed 10 months after initial TEM. On biopsy, there was a focus of intramucosal carcinoma, so he underwent a radical low anterior resection; there was no residual carcinoma in the small villous lesion remaining in the specimen.

Results after excision of early rectal carcinomas have also been good. Professor Buess recently reported his group's experience with 74 patients undergoing TEM excision for carcinoma since 1983. There were no mortalities and 9% of patients had a major complication. These were thought to be related to large excisions with tension on the suture line, resulting in suture line dehiscence in two patients and rectovaginal fistulas in another two. Of the 29 patients with a T1 lesion, only one (3%) has recurrence. On reexamination of this specimen, there was some question about the completeness of the removal of this lesion, raising the possibility that it may represent persistence of the tumor rather than true recurrence. Their patients with T2 and T3 lesions have had much higher recurrence rates, so they currently recommend either radical surgery or the addition of radiation and chemotherapy for this group. In the U. S. series, 42 patients were operated on for carcinoma with completion of the TEM procedure. One of 24 (4%) patients with a T1 lesion had recurrence, whereas 47% of 15 patients with T2 lesions and all three patients with T3 lesions had recurrences. Therefore, I strongly advocate radical resection for all patients with T2 or T3 lesions who can tolerate the procedure.

If this is not possible or acceptable, then full-dose combination radiation and chemotherapy is an alternative.

SUMMARY

The technique of TEM allows surgeons controlled access to the mid and upper rectum. The advantages of minimally invasive surgery in the rectum are significant, with little pain and rapid recovery while the morbidity rate is acceptably small. The TEM method requires a great deal of practice, the procedure may be tedious and time-consuming, and the equipment is expensive. Furthermore, there are relatively few patients who are candidates for the procedure. For now, it will be performed primarily in major centers with a large referral base and by surgeons with a special interest. It is clear that TEM is one of the new methods of minimally invasive surgery that will encourage the movement of surgical procedures into the outpatient setting.

Selected Readings

1. Buess G. Review: Transanal endoscopic microsurgery (TEM). J R Coll Surg Edinb 1993;38(4):239–245.
2. Buess G, Mentges B, Manncke K, Starlinger M, Becker HD. Minimal invasive surgery in the local treatment of rectal cancer. Int J Colorect Dis 1991;6:77–81.
3. Buess G, Mentges B, Manncke K, Starlinger M, Becker HD. Technique and results of transanal endoscopic microsurgery in early rectal cancer. Am J Surg 1992;163:63–70.
4. Orkin BA. Local treatment of rectal neoplasms. In: Mazier WP, Levien DH, Luchtefeld MA, Senagore A, eds. Surgery of the Colon, Rectum and Anus. Philadelphia: WB Saunders, 1994.
5. Saclarides TJ, Smith L, Ko ST, Orkin B, Buess G. Transanal endoscopic microsurgery. Dis Colon Rectum 1992;35(12):1183–1191.
6. Smith LE. Transanal endoscopic microsurgery for rectal neoplasms. Gastrointest Endosc Clin North Am 1993;3(2):329–341.
7. Smith LE, Ko ST, Saclarides T, Caushaj PF, Orkin BA, Khanduja K. Transanal endoscopic microsurgery—USA registry results. Abstract accepted for presentation at the 1995 American Society of Colon and Rectal Surgeons meeting, Montreal.

Chapter 42

Special Considerations for Therapeutic Lower Endoscopy

Richard L. Whelan • John Morgan Cosgrove
Shawn Garber

The term *endoscopy* is derived from the Greek "endo" (within) and "skopeo" (to examine); however, its use is restricted to the employment of an instrument to examine the interior of body cavities. The first attempts to visualize the interior of the intestine were by Hippocrates. He used a speculum for examining the anorectum, especially in cases of hemorrhoids and fistulas. The first gastroscope was introduced by Kussmaul in 1868. Use of the instrument was first demonstrated in a professional sword swallower. However, insufficient illumination made these first attempts at gastroscopy of no practical value.

The major advance in the efficacy of endoscopy was the introduction of optical lenses. In 1879, Nitze, in association with an optician, Beneche from Berlin, and an instrument maker, Leiter from Vienna, made the first cystoscope. Illumination was supplied with an electrically heated platinum wire, which needed a constant stream of water for cooling. Nitze later designed a gastroscope with similar properties, but the instrument never gained acceptance.

In 1932, the first semiflexible gastroscope was introduced by Rudolph Schindler in collaboration with Wolf, an optical physicist. The instrument was built by Lang, who in 1917 had noted that an image could be transmitted through a curved tube by a series of thick convex lenses as long as the curvature was not too great. Practical success with fiberoptics was not achieved until the 1950s with the work of Hopkins and Kapany. Basil Hirschowitz at the University of Michigan developed the first fiberoptic gastroscope, which was manufactured in 1958.

Endoscopy was revolutionized by fiberoptics. Fiberoptic instruments have not only reduced the danger of endoscopy and increased the surface area available for viewing but have also expanded the field of gastrointestinal endoscopy from one of limited therapeutic benefit to one of sophisticated therapeutic intervention. In the hands of the skillful endoscopist, present-day fiberscopes allow diagnostic and therapeutic intervention that was unthinkable even to the most imaginative minds of Schindler's era. William Wolff and Hiromi Shinya at Beth Israel Hospital in New York helped to develop and popularize colonoscopic polypectomy in 1973. They published a series of more than 1600 polypectomies performed without a complication.

New techniques involve the use of tiny cameras at the distal end of the endoscopic instrument, transmitting digitized images to a video screen. Such "video endoscopy" provides an outstanding image. The merger of fiberoptic and computer technology led to the development of video imaging. In 1982, Welch Allyn, Inc., placed a computer chip called a *charged coupled device* (CCD) at the end of a gastroscope. This electronic sensor transmits the image to a video processor, which transmits the image to a video monitor.

The availability of high-quality flexible endoscopes has greatly facilitated the development of lower gastrointestinal endoscopy. Colonoscopy has come to replace surgery for the treatment of many colonic lesions.

INSTRUMENTS

The components essential for performing ambulatory diagnostic and therapeutic colonoscopy include flexible endoscopes, 60 to 185 cm long. They contain fine coated glass fibers, a suction channel, an air and irrigation channel, and a biopsy channel through which a snare or biopsy forceps may be placed. The tip of the instrument is maneuvered in two directions by a dial control on the scope. The instrument is attached to a light source. The colonoscope is also attached to an irrigating fluid reservoir and suction unit. Direct visualization is achieved through the scope, by placement of a video camera on the main body of the scope, or by placement of cameras at the tip of the scope and transmitting digitized images to a video screen.

ENDOSCOPY UNIT

Hospital Endoscopy Unit

The ultimate goal of an endoscopy unit is to function independently with its own trained staff. Endoscopy is still performed in some hospitals in surgical operating rooms or radiology departments. However, in most hospitals endoscopic procedures are performed in a single endoscopy suite where both gastroenterologists and surgeons share space. The endoscopy unit should be equipped with adequate facilities and personnel to safely perform diagnostic and therapeutic endoscopic procedures. Recommended facilities for a fully equipped endoscopy unit are listed in Table 42–1.

Personnel

Properly trained personnel are essential to the safe and efficient performance of endoscopic procedures. The examination room nurse is most important in ensuring that the patient is properly monitored and tolerates the procedure. The nurse monitors the

Table 42–1. Facility Requirements for an Endoscopy Unit

Scheduling and secretarial office
Holding room
Recovery room—monitored setting
Patient waiting room
Examination rooms
Instrument room (optional)
Physician's consultation room
Bathrooms
Dictation or computer transcription room (optional)
Dressing room
Fluoroscopy room

patient's oxygen saturation as well as pulse and blood pressure during the procedure. Other responsibilities include starting intravenous access, setting up the room, checking the instruments, positioning the patient, cleaning the instruments after each procedure, drawing up and recording all medications used, setting up cautery equipment, operating biopsy forceps and polypectomy snares, and fixing specimens in formalin and labeling them. The nurse may also assist in abdominal manipulation during the procedure.

Other personnel who are available in hospital-based endoscopy units but who may not be available or needed in an office setting include a circulating nurse and an endoscopy assistant. The circulating nurse may be in charge of equipment, snares, forceps, and instruments during complicated therapeutic procedures. The endoscopy assistant, who may be a resident or fellow in training, is involved with assisting in the actual performance of the procedure.

Recovery room nurses monitor vital signs after procedures and determine when a patient is awake and able to ambulate. The nurse can also review discharge instructions with the patient.

OFFICE ENDOSCOPY

Many endoscopic procedures may be done in a properly equipped private office. The decision to perform endoscopy in an office is influenced by the patient's age, general medical condition, and diagnosis. Elderly patients with multiple medical problems and known polyps or large polyps are best examined in a hospital setting.

Conscious Sedation

During flexible colonoscopy, the diagnostic and therapeutic results, as well as patient acceptance and comfort can be modified and improved by adequate sedation. Conscious sedation refers to the state that allows a patient to tolerate unpleasant procedures while maintaining adequate cardiorespiratory function and the ability to respond purposefully to verbal command or active stimulation. Patients undergoing conscious sedation must be closely monitored.

The most frequently used sedative regimen is a combination of an intravenous narcotic and a benzodiazepine. The safety, reproducibility, and effectiveness of intravenous combined narcotic and benzodiazepine sedation is well documented. The combination of narcotic and benzodiazepine agents provides a safe method of sedation, producing an anxiety-free, amnesic, somnolent state coupled with reversible respiratory depression. In adults, the dosage of meperidine and diazepam is consistent throughout age groups (meperidine 0.75 mg/kg; diazepam 0.12 mg/kg). Because of drug synergism, the overall total dosage is decreased, which provides safe buffer with regard to respiratory depression and allows the endoscopist a means of reversal with naloxone if oversedation occurs.

Patient Preparation

It is important that patients fully understand what the endoscopic procedure entails and what they are likely to experience. A well-informed patient is more likely to be cooperative and helpful during the examination. The risks, potential benefits, and complications should be reviewed with the patient, if possible, well in advance of the procedure. Written consent must also be obtained. Recommendations concerning patient bowel preparation follow.

Flexible Sigmoidoscopy

Bowel preparation for flexible sigmoidoscopy varies from endoscopist to endoscopist. A single Phospho-Soda enema given immediately before the examination requires that a staff be willing to perform bowel preparations in the endoscopy suite and that there be adequate space and facilities. Some clinicians believe that two Fleet enemas given on the day of the examination suffice. Although the latter prep is adequate for some patients, in most, the bowel is not well prepped beyond the 20 cm level. Two to three 1-quart tap water enemas (one the night before and two the morning of the examination) allow a 60-cm examination in most patients. This preparation is not popular with most patients because it can be cumbersome and difficult to carry out alone. We recommend 8 to 10 ounces of magnesium citrate be taken early the evening before the examination, followed by two Fleet enemas the morning of the examination. This provides an adequate preparation for most patients.

Recommendations vary in terms of dietary restriction as well. Some clinicians do not restrict the diet at all; we recommend a low-residue light dinner the evening before and fluids only for breakfast the day of the procedure.

Colonoscopy

Adequate bowel preparation is crucial to complete colonoscopy. Because of the great variability in colonic motility among patients, preparation results vary greatly. Some patients require a longer and more exhaustive preparation than others. Currently, the polyethylene glycol (PEG) electrolyte mixtures and Phospho-Soda preparations are the most widely used in the United States. Various standard bowel preparations are as follows:

1. Retrograde preparation: Although rarely used, repeated "high colonic enemas" (1–3 L) until clear satisfactorily clean out most patients with a nonredundant colon. This can be a lengthy and laborious process and is not popular with patients. Large-volume enemas are difficult to self-administer and therefore are not a good option for those who live alone.

2. Purgatives and enemas: Castor oil (30–50 mL), senna (140 mg of sennosides), magnesium citrate (usually two 10-ounce bottles over a 2-day period), or bisacodyl (pills or supposi-

tory) can be combined with saline or tap water enemas given several hours before the examination until clear. The purgatives may cause abdominal cramps.

3. Saline or balanced electrolyte lavage: The administration of 3 to 4 L of 0.9% saline or a balanced electrolyte solution via oral ingestion or nasogastric tube is an effective preparation. A significant amount of sodium, chloride, and water is absorbed by the gut and can cause problems for patients with congestive heart failure or renal failure. Since the introduction of the PEG-containing preparations, saline lavage has been rarely used.

4. PEG balanced electrolyte solutions: These preparations were formulated to avoid the problems posed by the saline lavage preps. Sodium sulfate was substituted for sodium chloride to minimize the absorption of sodium. Alone, the sodium sulfate solution would be hypotonic and would result in net water absorption. PEG is added to make the solution isosmotic. Minimal net absorption of fluid and electrolytes results from this prep. This is one of the most widely used methods of colonic preparation.

It is recommended that 4 L of PEG/electrolyte solution be ingested over a 2- to 3-hour period. Although it is well tolerated by most patients, nausea and vomiting develop in some or they are unable to complete the preparation. For this reason, some advise giving a prokinetic agent such as metoclopramide (10 mg) or domperidone (10 mg) 30 to 60 minutes before starting the preparation.

5. Sodium phosphate preparation. Fleet oral Phospho-Soda prep has become popular in the past few years. Two doses of the solution are ingested; the first dose is taken in the morning the day before the examination and the second dose in the late afternoon. After each dose, the patient drinks eight glasses of water or a clear liquid. Several studies have shown that Phospho-Soda provides as good a preparation as and is better tolerated than the PEG solutions. However, significant dehydration can result, which poses a difficulty for heart and renal failure patients. Therefore, this prep is not advised for these patient groups.

Dietary recommendations during bowel preparation vary, but most clinicians advise restriction of the diet to a low-residue or, preferably, a liquid diet for the 24 hours before examination. Severely constipated patients may require a 48-hour period of restriction to liquids. Similarly, these patients often require additional laxatives, enemas, or PEG solution to obtain thorough bowel preparation.

INDICATIONS FOR AND TECHNIQUE OF COLONOSCOPY AND COLONOSCOPIC POLYPECTOMY

Indications

There are many indications for colonoscopy (Table 42–2). The most common one is probably unexplained rectal bleeding. Patients found to have occult blood on repeated stool guaiac testing require examination. Abdominal pain or persistent diarrhea are also common indications. The finding of an adenoma on flexible sigmoidoscopy is, for most gastroenterologists and surgical endoscopists, an indication for colonoscopy. All patients found to have a cancer should have a complete colonic examination to rule out a synchronous lesion. Synchronous cancers are found in 3% to 4% of these patients, while adenomas are found in 30% to 40%. Patients with a personal history of colon or rectal cancer require periodic

Table 42–2. Indications for Colonoscopy

Unexplained rectal bleeding
Guaiac-positive stool
Unexplained abdominal pain
Change in bowel habits
Persistent diarrhea
Colon carcinoma (for clearance of rest of colon)
Surveillance following resection of colon carcinoma
Adenoma found on flexible sigmoidoscopy or barium enema
Past history of adenoma
Chronic ulcerative colitis
Crohn's disease
Contrast enema finding
Nondiagnostic contrast enema
Family history of colon cancer
Personal or family history of familial polyposis
Radiation colitis
Ischemic colitis
History of stricture

examinations to rule out metachronous polyps and cancers. A patient with a first-degree family history of colon cancer should undergo periodic colonoscopic examinations. However, there is disagreement regarding when to begin these examinations and how often they should be repeated.

Surveillance should probably begin in the 30s in those individuals with a family history of colon cancer occurring in siblings or parents in their 30s, 40s, and 50s (cancer family syndrome). These surveillance examinations should be repeated every 3 to 5 years. Patients with first-degree relatives found to have a cancer at an older age should probably have surveillance examinations at about 40, to be repeated every 3 to 5 years. Those with ulcerative colitis or familial polyposis are at very high risk for development of cancer and warrant more frequent examinations. Patients with Crohn's disease and ischemic or radiation colitis also require intermittent examinations. Some clinicians recommend that women with a personal history of breast cancer undergo periodic examination because there is evidence to suggest that they are at higher risk for cancer development. Intraoperative colonoscopy is indicated when trying to localize a nonpalpable polyp, cancer, or source of acute gastrointestinal bleeding.

How often should colonoscopy be repeated in patients with a history of adenomas? For many years, it was thought that all such patients deserved lifetime periodic colonoscopic surveillance. Recently, investigators have suggested that patients with a history of a single adenoma of the sigmoid or rectum may not require such follow-up. The proper interval between examinations is also controversial. Yearly colonoscopy was commonly performed for polyp patients in the 1970s and early 1980s. It has since been realized that it takes at least 1 to 3 years for polyps to form. Currently, most clinicians advise follow-up colonoscopy every 2 to 5 years. It is very important that the colon be thoroughly "cleared" before such a schedule is implemented. Many researchers agree that patients with more than four adenomas on the index examination should have a repeat examination 1 year later because there is considerable chance that other polyps were missed on the initial study.

Colonoscopy Technique

Most endoscopists practice a one-person technique wherein both insertion of the scope and manipulation of the controls on the head of the scope are carried out by one individual. The following comments pertain to one-person technique. The head of the scope (with the deflection wheels) is held by the left hand while the right hand manipulates the shaft of the scope. We recommend holding the head of the scope between the palm of the hand and the third, fourth, and fifth fingers. The thumb manipulates the two deflection wheels while the index finger controls the air–water and suction buttons.

The examination is begun with the patient in the left lateral decubitus position, except in the intraoperative setting where the patient is in the modified lithotomy or modified Sims' position. The scope is inserted only after a digital examination of the anorectum has been completed. One of the most important principles of endoscopy is that, with few exceptions, the scope is advanced only when the lumen and path of the colon are clearly visualized.

The endoscopist has a limited number of maneuvers that can be used to safely advance the scope when performing colonoscopy: (1) advancement and withdrawal of the scope, (2) torquing of the scope either clockwise or counterclockwise, (3) deflection of the scope tip, (4) application of pressure to the abdomen during advancement, (5) change of position of the patient, (6) insufflation and suction, and (7) use of a stent. The proficient endoscopist uses all these tools to carry out the examination quickly, safely, thoroughly, and as painlessly as possible.

Much of the difficulty encountered during colonoscopy results because the sigmoid and transverse segments of the colon are mobile (not fixed) and lengthy. The sharp angulation of the bowel at the flexures may also cause problems. Inserting a flexible scope through the nonfixed segments is analogous to pushing a piece of al dente spaghetti through a long piece of cooked macaroni. The shaft of the scope tends to buckle and bend as it is pushed into the colon (Fig. 42–1). This is especially likely to occur when it is necessary to keep the tip of the scope significantly deflected to see

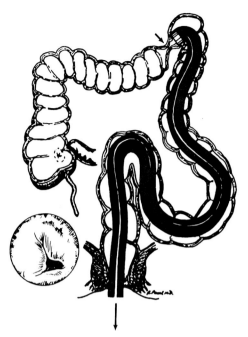

Figure 42–1. Due to the mobile nature of the sigmoid colon, a large loop may form in the colonoscope as advancement past the splenic flexure is attempted. Further advancement of the scope only serves to enlarge the loop. (From Prasad ML, Pearl RK. Colonoscopy. In Pearl RK, ed. Gastrointestinal Endoscopy for Surgeons. Boston: Little, Brown, 1984, p 104.)

the lumen and advance the scope. The shape of the inserted part of the scope at such times resembles a cane, with the tip and end of the scope being the crooked handle. At such times, attempts at further insertion often result in a bowing out of the shaft of the scope while the scope tip either remains in place or moves backward (the curved handle of the cane gets bigger). The insertion force in this instance is not transmitted to the tip of the scope but to the curved part of the shaft. Further insertion in this instance may result in the formation of a "loop." The forces generating the loop may result in the scope tip moving backward, which is known as paradoxical motion. The endoscopist then needs to push more and more scope into the patient to move the scope tip ahead even a short distance. This is termed loss of "one to one motion" (one inch of scope pushed in the anus results in the scope tip moving one inch forward).

When a loop is developed or is forming, the endoscopist has five choices. The *first* is to have an assistant apply pressure to the abdominal wall over the loop to prevent the loop from growing and allow the tip to progress forward. Abdominal pressure can be applied either generically to where the loop is thought to be or by carefully palpating the abdomen for the loop itself. The *second* method is to reduce the loop by withdrawing the scope until one to one motion is regained (Fig. 42–2) and then to reinsert using a different strategy (e.g., insert with torque, apply abdominal pressure, or change the patient's position and attempt further insertion). *Third*, gravity may be used to help straighten a loop or alter the insertion dynamics so that forward movement of the scope may occur. All four possible positions (supine, prone, and left and right lateral decubitus) may be helpful and should be tried. The *fourth* and least desirable option is to simply keep pushing the scope to "push through the loop." In some instances, after the loop has developed to a crucial point, the tip may begin moving forward. The *fifth* choice is to

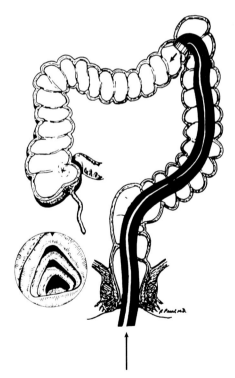

Figure 42–2. One technique of overcoming a sigmoid loop is to apply suction to the bowel wall to create a fixed point at the tip of the scope, then withdraw the scope to straighten it and remove the loop. Advancement into the transverse colon is then often possible. (From Prasad ML, Pearl RK. Colonoscopy. In Pearl RK, ed. Gastrointestinal Endoscopy for Surgeons. Boston: Little, Brown, 1984, p 105.)

withdraw the scope entirely and then repeat the examination with a stent in place. The stent is a stiff hollow tube through which the scope is placed. Under fluoroscopic guidance, when the scope is in the sigmoid and not looped, the stent device is advanced into the patient; this prevents a sigmoid loop from forming. If inserted improperly, it can tear or perforate the bowel. Most endoscopists do not use stents.

An important basic principle of colonoscopic technique is that it is always safer to insert the scope with the shortest possible length of scope inside the patient. This means insertion without loops. At times, after other options have failed, it is necessary to push through a loop or insert carefully while the loop is compressed externally. Once the scope is well past the difficult area, an attempt should be made to straighten the scope (reduce the loop). Applying clockwise torque while withdrawing the scope often prevents the tip from moving backward and may result in forward motion of the tip even though the scope is being pulled out. Another method is to "hook" a haustra or a bend in the colon during withdrawal. This may also prevent loss of ground. The endoscopist should always be aware of how much scope is in the patient and should strive to minimize the amount of scope inserted.

The rectosigmoid and sigmoid colon can be difficult to negotiate. There is a strong tendency for loops to form in this segment, the most common being the alpha loop. This can usually be avoided by inserting the scope while placing clockwise torque on the shaft. Once an alpha loop is formed, the best way to reduce it without losing too much ground is to withdraw the scope while placing clockwise torque on the shaft. Applying pressure to the left lower quadrant or suprapubic area can limit the formation of a sigmoid loop and facilitate further movement of the scope tip.

Maneuvers that may help in getting past the splenic flexure are to (1) place the patient in the supine or right lateral decubitus position, (2) make sure that the scope is straight (without loops) before attempting the flexure, (3) apply clockwise torque, (4) have the patient take a deep inspiration (which pushes the diaphragm down). A long and redundant transverse colon can also be difficult to intubate.

Abdominal pressure directed at preventing bowing of the transverse colon into the lower abdomen may help passage through the transverse colon. Compression directed at preventing sigmoid loop formation may still be helpful in decompressing the right colon onto the scope. Placing the patient in the right lateral decubitus position can facilitate right colon intubation. There is often a U-shaped loop in the transverse colon when the hepatic flexure is reached. Withdrawal with either left or right torque often results in the scope tip moving quickly into the proximal right colon. If possible, the ileum should be intubated. If an attempt is always made to enter the valve, the endoscopist will become proficient at this maneuver.

Confirmation of full colonic insertion can be done in a number of ways. Intubation of the ileum is the most reliable method. Fluoroscopy can confirm that the scope is in the right lower quadrant; however, that does not always mean that the caput has been reached. Visualization of the confluence of the taenia, the appendiceal orifice, and the ileocecal valve, although less reliable than ileal intubation, can also be used to confirm completion of the examination. Transillumination of the scope light through the right lower quadrant is also helpful but can be misleading if the scope tip is actually in a redundant transverse loop that is in the right lower quadrant. Following the path of the transilluminated light while withdrawing the scope can confirm that the scope was in fact in the right colon. The light should travel from the right lower to the right upper quadrant on withdrawal. If it moves directly to the left side, the farthest point of insertion was probably the mid or distal transverse colon. Pressing in on the right lower abdominal wall may compress the insufflated cecum, which supports the idea that the right colon has been intubated. Usually the detailed examination is carried out on withdrawal of the scope. Care should be taken to suction each segment after the examination of that area is completed.

Polypectomy

Polyps less than 0.5 cm can usually be destroyed via multiple cold biopsies. Alternatively, "hot" biopsies can be taken with an

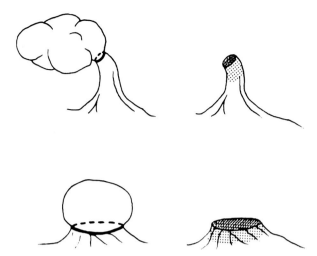

Figure 42–3. Technique of polypectomy for a pedunculated polyp. The polypectomy snare is tightened at the point of smallest diameter of the stalk, then electrocautery is applied. Spread of tissue injury due to the cautery is shown by the stippled area. (From Prasad ML, Pearl RK. Colonoscopy. In Pearl RK, ed. Gastrointestinal Endoscopy for Surgeons. Boston: Little, Brown, 1984, p 111.)

insulated biopsy forceps through which monopolar current is run. This obtains a biopsy and also fulgurates a small surrounding area. A snare can be used to encircle and remove these small lesions but is not necessary. It can also be difficult to recover the small polyps that have been snared. Alternatively, the tip of the snare can be used as a fulguration tool and the small polyp simply destroyed without taking a sample. Because the majority of 2- to 5-mm colonic polyps are adenomas, destroying such polyps is recommended.

Pedunculated polyps are best removed using a polypectomy snare. Both monopolar and bipolar snares are available. Monopolar snares are more commonly used in most endoscopy suites in the United States. A grounding plate is needed when using a monopolar cautery unit. The opened snare should be maneuvered over the top of and around the polyp. The snare is then slowly closed. Ideally, the narrowest part of the stalk should be snared (Fig. 42–3). Next, the polyp should be manipulated by pushing in and pulling back on the snare tubing. This allows the endoscopist to view the polyp and snare from different angles. The positioning of the snare can be checked in this way. Most endoscopists prefer a low-power coagulation setting for polypectomy (15 to 25 W). As the current is run through the snare, the assistant holding the snare handle slowly closes the snare, which slowly cuts through the polyp. This should be done over 15 to 30 seconds. It is thought that swelling of the heated tissue within the compressing snare is an important factor in maintaining hemostasis after polypectomy. Blanching or whitening of the tissue near the stalk is usually a sign that sufficient cautery has been applied. The snared polyp should be held away from the wall of the well-insufflated bowel before the current is applied. Many clinicians routinely "jiggle" the shaft of the snare while applying current (Fig. 42–4). This serves to vary the

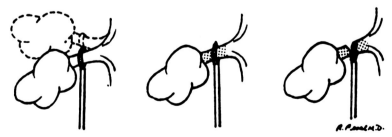

Figure 42–4. During polypectomy, moving the snare can minimize the likelihood of the polyp's having prolonged contact with the wall of the adjacent bowel and transmitting an electrical injury to it. (From Prasad ML, Pearl RK. Colonoscopy. In Pearl RK, ed. Gastrointestinal Endoscopy for Surgeons. Boston: Little, Brown, 1984, p 115.)

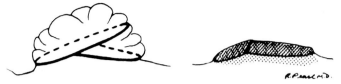

Figure 42–5. Technique of polypectomy for a large sessile polyp. Removal of the polyp in a piecemeal fashion is the safest approach. Stippling represents the extent of electrocautery injury. (From Prasad ML, Pearl RK. Colonoscopy. In Pearl RK, ed. Gastrointestinal Endoscopy for Surgeons. Boston: Little, Brown, 1984, p 111.)

position of the polyp and prevent serious injury to the surrounding bowel wall, which may be in contact with the side of the snare that cannot be seen by the endoscopist.

The severed polyp may adhere to the base after the snare has been fully closed. The snare can be reopened to verify that the wire has gone through the stalk. Once complete division has been confirmed, the closed snare should be withdrawn back into the scope. The polyp can then be pushed off the base with the scope or the closed snare. The polyp base and the immediate area should be carefully inspected to be sure that hemostasis has been obtained and that no significant injury to the surrounding wall has occurred. Small polyps that are snared can often be suctioned through the working channel into a trap. Retrieval of larger polyps can present a problem. Wire baskets can be used to entrap the polyp. In some cases it may be possible to remove several polyps at a time. Most often, however, it is necessary to remove the scope fully to bring the specimen out.

Small and moderate-sized sessile polyps can usually be snared without undue difficulty. By tenting the snared polyp into the lumen, a narrow pseudostalk can usually be made. Care should be taken not to include too much of the wall in the snare because a perforation or full-thickness burn may result. Large sessile polyps are the most difficult to excise. If the endoscopist is comfortable with it, careful piecemeal excision can be attempted (Fig. 42–5). The precise location of the snare should be ascertained before the current is applied. The snare should be closed slowly when larger pieces of tissue are being removed. Some polyps may be best removed during the course of several different examinations 3 to 4 weeks apart. Follow-up colonoscopy to reexamine the site of any lesion that was removed in piecemeal fashion is necessary. If the endoscopist's impression is that a sessile lesion is most likely malignant, no attempts at removal should be made.

Selected Readings

1. American Society of Anesthesiologists Guidelines for Sedation and Analgesia by Non-Anesthesiologists. Park Ridge, IL: American Society of Anesthesiologists, 1993.
2. Andrus C, Dean P, Prosky J. Evaluation of safe, effective, intravenous sedation for utilization in endoscopic procedures. Surg Endosc 1990;4:179–183.
3. Church JM. Endoscopy of the Colon, Rectum, and Anus. New York: Igaku-Shoin, 1995.
4. Cotton PB, Williams CB. Practical Gastrointestinal Endoscopy. 3rd ed. Oxford: Blackwell Scientific, 1990.
5. Hirschowitz BI. A personal history of the fiberscope. Gastroenterology 1979;76:864–869.
6. Marks J. History of endoscopic surgery in minimal invasive surgery. In: Andrus C, Cosgrove J, Longo W, eds. Principles and Outcomes. Reading, UK, Harwood Academic Publishers, 1997.
7. Sivak MV Jr, ed. Gastroenterologic Endoscopy. Philadelphia: WB Saunders, 1987.
8. Wolff WI. Colonoscopy and endoscopic polypectomy. N Y J Med 1973:73:641–642.

Chapter 43

Special Considerations for Therapeutic Upper Endoscopy

Peter B. Kelsey

Three decades of technologic development have propelled the field of gastrointestinal endoscopy from an era of limited and rigid observation to an era in which flexible endoscopes fitted with video chip cameras permit the delivery of a wide variety of interventional tools to apply to clinical emergencies. Effective use of these techniques has resulted in marked improvement in patient management, decreased mortality and morbidity, decreased lengths of hospital stay, and decreased costs. In this chapter, specific clinical emergencies and the therapeutic techniques used to approach these emergencies are discussed. The most common emergency requiring therapeutic intervention is gastrointestinal bleeding. Cholangitis and gallstone pancreatitis are also addressed.

GASTROINTESTINAL BLEEDING

Much has been written about the management of gastrointestinal bleeding. Whereas several excellent studies and reviews discuss the variety of interventional modalities, little has been written about the steps that lead to the application of these tools. This is crucial because in practice more errors are probably made because of lack of attentiveness to the fundamentals than are made through faulty application of the appropriate technique. At my institution, in which there is a large referral population, approximately 50% of missed or delayed diagnoses result from misinterpretation of tests that were already performed. Therefore, in the workup of gastrointestinal bleeding, we emphasize the following steps. First and most important is source identification. Source identification refers to the precise localization of the bleeding source. In the case of esophageal varices, we seek the precise site of origin of the bleeding. In the patient with multiple jejunal or cecal arteriovenous malformations (AVMs), we seek the lesion that is most likely responsible for the bleeding. Proper source identification not only helps in the selection of the specific therapy most likely to effect hemostasis but also ensures the best clinical outcome and decreases the use of resources. After site identification, the therapeutic modality is chosen and applied.

Source Identification

Typically, a patient with high-volume gastrointestinal bleeding is seen in the emergency department or in the inpatient setting with hemodynamic instability, usually associated with either hematemesis or melena. There may be a nasogastric tube aspirate that confirms the upper source. There may be a history of predisposing conditions, such as the use of ulcerogenic medications, portal hypertension, or a history of prior ulcer disease. The initial upper endoscopic view identifies patients in whom no blood is seen in the upper gastrointestinal tract and those in whom recent or new blood is seen.

In patients in whom there is no evidence of recent bleeding, the upper endoscopy examination should be performed by visual passage of the scope through the upper hypopharynx. This allows for aspiration of debris from the oral pharynx as well as examination of the hypopharynx for either fresh blood or lesions. Squamous cell carcinoma or lymphoma in the hypopharynx is missed by the technique of manual scope passage. Once the scope is positioned in the upper esophagus, it should then be slowly advanced through the length of the esophagus, with careful observation in a circumferential manner.

Probably the most commonly missed lesions in the esophagus are those located in the upper third or varices that are transiently decompressed and thus flattened. In the acute setting of hypotension, varices may collapse. Often by repeated insufflation and aspiration in the esophageal lumen, the investigator can develop a sense of whether subtle varices are present. Contact injury due to medications such as doxycycline, quinidine, and nonsteroidal anti-inflammatory drugs may occur anywhere along the esophagus, but this lesion, when present in the upper third as with other subtle superficial injury, can be missed.

Before the scope passage from the esophagus to the stomach, the gastroesophageal (GE) junction should be carefully examined for Mallory-Weiss tears and ulcerations. Mallory-Weiss type injury may occur during the endoscopy itself, either as a consequence of retching or forceful passage of the scope through a tight, nonrelaxed lower esophageal sphincter (LES). Thus it is crucial early on in the examination to know whether this lesion is present. Once the scope is in the stomach, the endoscopist needs to look for the presence of a giant hiatal hernia, which may be difficult to detect if it is very large. A cough or some other Valsalva maneuver and the resulting diaphragmatic contraction create an impression on the gastric lumen in the area of the hiatus. This is the area where linear ulcerations may be found. These lesions probably result from repeated trauma as the stomach rolls in and out of the hiatus. Even though these lesions rarely cause high-volume bleeding that results in hypotension, they can result in significant chronic iron deficiency and anemia, most commonly in elderly persons.

Once the esophageal lumen and GE junction have been carefully examined, the scope is gently passed into the stomach and air is insufflated into the stomach before being aspirated. All aspiration at this point should be done under direct visualization in order to minimize the possibility of inducing suction injury to the gastric epithelium. Such injury generates lesions that are often indistinguishable from the subtle vascular lesions of the stomach. As the upper part of the stomach is examined, any lesions that are visualized should be documented photographically. Having this photographic documentation may become invaluable if detection of a bleeding site is not accomplished. If the patient then requires a repeat examination in 2 weeks' time and the same lesions are seen, these lesions then become more viable candidates as a potential bleeding source.

The gastric cardia and body is carefully examined, and the scope is gently passed down through the length of the stomach along the greater curvature to the area of the antrum. The observation of several contraction waves as they roll through the antrum is helpful to visualize certain areas of the epithelium that may be otherwise difficult to see. Again, this area may be photographed. At this point, the scope is retroflexed to look at the incisura. The areas most difficult to view during upper endoscopy are those relating to the area of the incisura and to the greater curvature behind the endoscope in the upper body of the stomach while the scope is retroflexed.

When the scope is initially retroflexed in the antrum, it should be gently swept, using a torquing motion, back and forth across the incisura until the incisura is entirely visualized, both from the retrograde and the antegrade directions. The scope is gently pulled back in the retrograde position into the upper body of the stomach. The scope can be torqued to allow a full 360° view of the entire cardia and upper body of the stomach. If no lesions are identified, the scope is returned to the antegrade position and passed down again to the area of the pylorus.

The scope is next gently passed through the pylorus but is immediately pulled back to avoid trauma to the opposing duodenal cap wall. The tip of the endoscope should peek into the duodenal cap before further examination of the duodenum occurs. The endoscopist should make every effort to view the entire cap before proceeding. Once the cap is cleared, the scope is then passed, under direct vision as much as possible, through the duodenal sweep and into the duodenum itself. Visualization of the duodenal sweep is often the most difficult part of the examination. This may require several pushes and pull-backs through this area to adequately visualize each fold. An effort should be made to observe the ampulla to see whether fresh bile is present. The observation of fresh bile reduces, but does not eliminate, the possibility of hemobilia.

Once the first pass of the scope has been completed and the area is found to be unremarkable, the scope is then returned into the body of the stomach for a more careful examination. The scope is deflected in the retrograde manner and pulled back up into the upper body of the stomach. Using either a closed biopsy forceps or some other smooth-tipped probe, individual gastric rugae are carefully examined. The endoscopist looks specifically for a Dieulafoy ulcer. This lesion usually is found in the cardia but may be found anywhere in the gastrointestinal tract. It is often subtle, with a 1- to 2-mm depression, and occasionally a central clot or brown spot.

If no bleeding site has been located, the endoscopist may then return the scope into the duodenum and administer intravenous glucagon (1 mg) to the patient. Glucagon causes relaxation of the stomach and duodenum. As a result, the endoscopist can pull through the duodenal sweep with greater ease to look at the duodenal folds and cap. If no lesion is seen, the final option for the endoscopist is to remove the upper endoscope and pass a side-viewing scope. The side-viewing scope allows for better viewing of the cardia and duodenal cap. Within the rim of the pylorus inside the duodenal cap, small ulcers and, rarely, tumors (e.g., islet cell tumors) can remain hidden from the view of a forward-viewing scope. With the side-viewing scope passed to the ampulla, there is a better view of this area and the duodenal sweep. The endoscopist should be experienced with the safe passage

of a side-viewing scope before attempting this portion of the examination.

If, during this examination, one or more lesions are seen that arouse suspicion of being a bleeding source, provocative stimulation may be indicated. Large ulcers with overlying clots or posterior duodenal ulcers with overlying clots are obvious sources of recent bleeding; dislodgment of these clots is contraindicated due to the high potential for vigorous bleeding. If a suspicious lesion is seen, and is not obviously bleeding, it may be appropriate to use either a blunt end of a biopsy forceps, a cytology brush, or a water jet to dislodge or aggravate the lesion. If the lesion is caused by scope trauma or is an insignificant vascular malformation, no significant bleeding erupts. If, however, the trivial lesion begins to bleed briskly, then it is a strong candidate as the source of bleeding. The inexperienced interventional endoscopist may have reservations about aggravating such lesions. However, without stimulation of these lesions to make them bleed, the causative role of a lesion cannot be properly verified. In addition, if high-volume bleeding is provoked, appropriate therapy can be applied and the effectiveness of the therapy evaluated.

Should no bleeding source be identified despite this extensive effort, the clinical course of the case would dictate the selection and timing of a future workup. Enteroscopy, colonoscopy, angiography, and other tools might then be used in evaluating the condition.

The initial endoscopic examination may reveal large quantities of blood without an immediately obvious source. In this situation, patient safety may become a primary issue in terms of aspiration. In general, patients who are seen in the emergency department with variceal bleeding seem to be the population at greatest risk for aspiration during interventional endoscopy. This is probably due to the combination of an altered mental status due to encephalopathy and the continued outpouring of fresh blood into the esophageal lumen. The endoscopist may decide to intubate the patient after the scope has been swiftly passed into the esophagus. If no varices are seen but the stomach is full of blood, a careful but aggressive attempt may be made to evacuate the stomach without intubation. It might be prudent in these situations to minimize the use of conscious sedation so that the patient's gag and coughing reflexes are not entirely suppressed. If active variceal bleeding is identified and the risk of aspiration is enhanced because of an altered mental status, elective intubation is likely to reduce the morbidity associated with the procedure. Having the patient intubated also provides for a more controlled situation for the endoscopist to successfully deploy the appropriate therapy.

Whether the patient is intubated or not, the scope is passed through the hypopharynx under direct vision so that the hypopharynx can be aspirated and carefully inspected. Once the scope is passed into the esophagus, any food, debris, clot, or blood should be aspirated. In rare situations, the endoscopist views a long cord of fully clotted blood. Long smooth ropelike cords of clotted blood in the gastrointestinal lumen result from very rapid bleeding that suddenly fills an entire luminal space and then congeals as a smooth cast of that lumen. This situation most frequently occurs with large artery–enteric fistulas. If a clotted cast of the esophagus is encountered and the patient has a history of an aortic root graft, the examination should be terminated and the vascular surgical team consulted. Further evaluation might include a computed tomography (CT) scan, an angiogram, or emergency surgery.

The situation frequently arises wherein a large clot is found in the fundus but no bleeding site is immediately apparent. Before beginning the laborious task of clot evacuation from the stomach, the endoscopist may choose to quickly and gingerly pass the scope above the sea of clot, along the lesser curve and into the antrum, which is often above the meniscus of blood if the patient is lying in a left lateral decubitus position. This allows visualization of the pylorus. The direction of blood flow through the pylorus should be observed. The scope is then quickly passed into the duodenal cap and sweep. If blood is seen pouring from a lesion in the duodenum, the endoscopist must then decide whether the patient is at risk for aspiration of the large gastric clot as the duodenal lesion is approached. If no lesion is seen in the duodenal sweep or antrum, the scope is removed back to the clot in the stomach. At this point, the clot must be removed.

The need for accurate source identification cannot be overstated. If no source is identified, a large clot in the stomach is not removed, and no therapy is performed at that time, there is a very high likelihood of rebleeding from the same source within the next few days. This results in delay of therapy, increased cost of care, and possibly increased morbidity. It is therefore important both for the patient and for resource utilization to invest the time and skill on the first examination to completely evacuate the gastric clot. The preferred method for doing this is with a large-channel therapeutic upper endoscope. The standard diagnostic endoscopes have a channel of insufficient caliber for clot aspiration. In a patient with relatively fresh upper gastrointestinal bleeding, the therapeutic endoscopes can often, when used appropriately, evacuate 1 to 2 L of formed clot from the stomach within a period of 10 to 15 minutes. Another option is the passage of a large gastric tube. These tubes are more effective at removing large volumes of clot. The disadvantage of using these tubes is that often patients are bleeding from sensitive upper gastrointestinal tract lesions, which might be further injured by the blind passage of large tubes. Also, these large gastric lavage tubes generate so many mucosal artifacts that they may further obscure the field and render it impossible to identify subtle lesions (e.g., a Dieulafoy ulcer).

The technique of effective clot aspiration using a large-bore endoscope may include two approaches. In the first approach, the scope tip is used to aspirate individual chunks of clot by flicking the tip of the scope in and out of the clot, allowing the suction to clear the channel of clot before the scope is returned to the area. This also manually breaks up the clot. In the second approach, a large rope of clot may be partially suctioned into the scope and removed entirely by removing the scope from the patient. Every effort should be made to completely evacuate the stomach of all clot. Not only does this facilitate a diagnosis but it also eliminates a large blood load from the gastrointestinal tract. Leaving the stomach empty of blood at the conclusion of the procedure allows for accurate identification of re-bleeding via nasogastric suctioning.

Once the stomach is completely evacuated of clot, the same methodical search can be undertaken as described previously. When esophageal varices are obvious, it is crucial to identify the exact site of bleeding. A single band, well placed over this site, may be sufficient to terminate an event of variceal bleeding. However, six or seven bands placed adjacent to the actual bleeding site may be of only transient benefit, and rebleeding could occur within the ensuing 48 hours, necessitating a second examination. When a lesion is suspected of being the source of bleeding but no actual bleeding is present, provocative stimulation may be indicated. In most cases, the patient is more likely to suffer increased morbidity from inaccurate or ineffective bleeding source identification than any adverse outcome related to the dislodgment of suspicious clots. This type of provocative bleeding stimulation applies throughout the gastrointestinal tract, except when there is a high suspicion of an aortic–enteric fistula or an ulcer exists with a visible vessel. Often in the evaluation of chronic gastrointestinal bleeding sources, duodenal or upper jejunal telangiectasias are identified on standard endoscopy or enteroscopy. To verify that these lesions are reasonable candidates for the source of bleeding, their surface can be scratched. If rapid bleeding does not occur, the endoscopist should look elsewhere.

Selection and Application of Interventional Technique

Once the source of bleeding has been accurately identified, the selection of the appropriate interventional technique is fairly straightforward. Source identification is of utmost importance because of the wide variety of techniques that are available to manage acute gastrointestinal bleeding.

Esophageal Varices

If the exact bleeding site from an esophageal varix is identified, the accurately deployed variceal band is the single most effective tech-nique in achieving immediate hemostasis. Random placement of six or seven bands without specific identification of the site of variceal rupture frequently results in recurrent bleeding within 48 to 72 hours, necessitating a second examination. Therefore, most experienced interventional endoscopists choose endoscopic variceal ligation as the primary modality for the management of acute esophageal varices.

Technique. Once the index bleeding site has been determined, its location is noted. As the scope is then slowly withdrawn, additional sites to be banded are noted by the distance from the incisors and wall orientation (i.e., 40 cm at 9 o'clock, 38 cm at 3 o'clock, and so on). This is important because once the banding apparatus is fitted to the endoscope, the range of view becomes so narrowed that landmarks are less readily identifiable. The endoscopist must maintain absolute consistency in scope and hand position to minimize the variation of the orientation of the esophagus to the scope. Once the sites to be banded are identified, the scope is removed. Use of overtubes increases the speed and safety of band ligation. The newer designs greatly reduce the risk of esophageal injury during placement. I place these overtubes over a Maloney dilator. The overtube is held in place by the nursing assistant once the dilator is removed. The nursing assistant must maintain control of the overtube, and suction must be readily available. The endoscope, with the variceal band apparatus in position, is maneuvered down through the overtube and into the esophagus. Again, the endoscopist identifies the site to be banded with the aid of the previously determined coordinates. The most distal band is placed first. A freshly banded varix will fully occupy the esophageal lumen. Attempting scope passage beyond this area risks dislodgment of the band.

Once the varix is identified, the scope tip is deflected in that direction. The suction button is gently depressed to slowly pull the varix into the banding cylinder (Fig. 43–1). Too rapid depression of the suction channel often results in an unroofing and tearing of the esophageal varix. Once the varix is aspirated into the cylinder of the ligation device, the cylinder is nudged forward 1 to 2 mm and the triggering

A

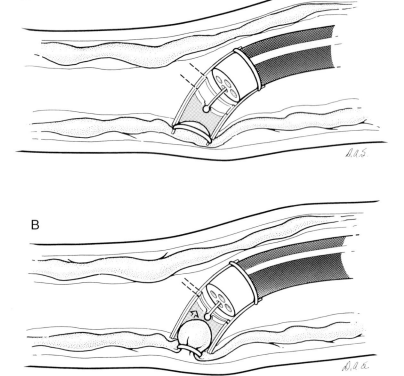

B

Figure 43–1. (A) Endoscopic variceal rubber band ligation. The ligating device is attached to the tip of the therapeutic endoscope. The varix is identified and suction is applied, pulling the varix into the cup of the ligating device. **(B)** Once the varix is suctioned into the cup of the ligator, the trigger is pulled and the rubber band is released to ligate the base of the varix. (From Ponsky JL. Atlas of Surgical Endoscopy. St. Louis: Mosby–Year Book, 1992:34–35.)

fishing line is pulled, thus deploying the band. At this point, the suction button is released. The air button can be depressed to blow the banded varix out of the cylinder, and the scope is removed. The scope is cleaned off, a new band is loaded, and the scope is repositioned to the next set of coordinates. Rapid, multifire banding systems eliminate the need to remove the scope between individual band placements. An attempt should be made, particularly on the first session of variceal banding, to place the bands as close together as possible. This allows for multiple band deployment. Ideally, in a patient with more than four varices, I prefer to deploy five to 10 bands during the first session. In general, the more bands placed during the first session, the fewer sessions are needed to achieve complete variceal obliteration.

In patients who have had a history of sclerotherapy, particular difficulties may be encountered. Patients may have a very fibrotic esophageal wall but may still have areas in which large varices percolate in and out of the lumi-

nal surface. In these patients, band deployment may not be either possible or effective because the esophageal mucosa may not be pliant or supple enough, due to the sclerotherapy-induced fibrosis, to be sucked into the banding cylinder. Often the banding cylinder prematurely deploys as the endoscopist tries to aspirate mucosa into the cylinder. In these situations, other sites may have to be selected, and the endoscopist may resort to the use of conventional sclerotherapy. Sclerotherapy as the primary modality for management of esophageal varices has not been used at my institution for more than 5 years due to the improved efficacy of esophageal banding.

Once effective hemostasis is achieved, attention should be directed toward minimizing fluid resuscitation so as not to overdistend splanchnic blood flow. By this time, the patient should have been fully resuscitated and the use of octreotide considered. At my institution, banding is often repeated in 7 to 14 days and at intervals thereafter until obliteration of varices is achieved.

Ulcers, Telangiectases, and Miscellaneous

Aside from esophageal variceal bleeding, the remaining lesions of the stomach and duodenum that can contribute to high-volume gastrointestinal bleeding can often be grouped together in terms of therapeutic options and techniques used. Again, site identification is crucial to success. At my institution, a combination of injection sclerotherapy and some form of thermal device is used in treating a typical gastric ulcer or Dieulafoy ulcer (Fig. 43–2). It is often useful to inject an area with 1/10,000 epinephrine, with a standard sclerotherapy needle. We might choose a four-quadrant injection of 0.5 to 2 ml solution (Fig. 43–3). This raises a bleb circumferentially that blanches the mucosa. This alone often achieves temporary, if not permanent, hemostasis for

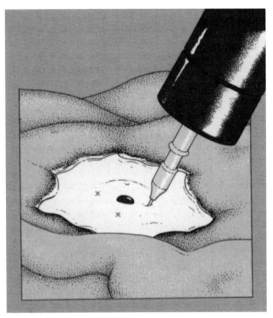

Figure 43–3. Injection technique for peptic ulcer bleeding. Injection is carried out with the same needle used for sclerotherapy. A 98 percent ethanol solution is used for injection, with 0.1 to 0.2 ml increments being used in four quadrants, 1 to 2 mm from the vessel. (From Fleischer D. Therapy for gastrointestinal bleeding. In: Waye J, Geenen J, Fleischer D, eds. Techniques in Therapeutic Endoscopy. 1987, Gower Medical Publishing. By permission of Mosby International.)

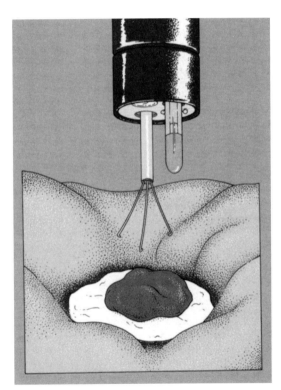

Figure 43–2. A double channel therapeutic endoscope is helpful for both removing the clot overlying an ulcer crater and being able to then immediately deliver hemostatic treatment with heater probe, injection, or cautery through the other channel. (From Fleischer D. Therapy for gastrointestinal bleeding. In: Waye J, Geenen J, Fleischer D, eds. Techniques in Therapeutic Endoscopy. 1987, Gower Medical Publishing. By permission of Mosby International.)

many of these lesions. Once this is performed, either a bicap probe or a heater probe is the tool of choice. We prefer to deploy the thermal device directly onto the bleeding source (Fig. 43–4). One theoretic advantage of using a bicap device is that there may be less penetrating tissue necrosis, thus lessening the likelihood of transmural injury and perforation. The thermal device should be applied firmly against the lesion to collapse the feeding vessel and seal it shut. This often requires multiple 1- to 2-second pulses. The pulse width and the selected level of energy should be sufficient to produce a white halo of thermal blanching around the tip of the probe. The tissue surface adjacent to the probe may actually boil and smoke during the brief application of current. The tip of the thermal probe should be clean to minimize the peeling of the thermal rind and thus reexposure of the bleeding vessel. A thermal probe may be applied two or three times or more to achieve the desired hemostatic effect. If the four-quadrant epinephrine injections are deployed within 1 cm of the

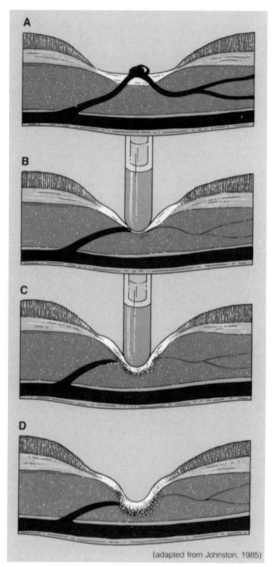

Figure 43–4. Coaptive coagulation. (**A**) A visible vessel is seen in the ulcer base. (**B**) The coagulation device is applied to the center of the vessel. (**C**) Once positioned properly, thermal energy is delivered to coagulate the vessel. (**D**) After probe removal, a white burn mark is seen where the probe had been applied. (From Fleischer D. Therapy for Gastrointestinal Bleeding. In: Waye J, Geenen J, Fleischer D, eds. Techniques in Therapeutic Endoscopy. 1987, Gower Medical Publishing. By permission of Mosby International.)

duodenal cap, one should be concerned with both the risk of perforation and the proximity of the ulcer to a major branch of the gastroduodenal artery. High-volume bleeding from this area, in my experience, is likely to necessitate some other form of intervention owing to the large size of the feeding arterial vessel. In Dieulafoy ulcers, combined injection sclerotherapy and thermal cautery techniques have been shown to be successful, but these lesions still have the propensity for high-volume rebleeding. In such a situation, we might use the banding ligation technique in which the Dieulafoy lesion is aspirated into the banding cylinder and the band deployed around the entire lesion.

Lower Gastrointestinal Bleeding

Site identification is just as crucial for the lower intestine, even though it is more difficult. First, if the site of bleeding can be localized to a specific region of the colon or a specific diverticula, a conservative approach might be selected. If the patient requires surgical intervention, the appropriate area could be managed. At my institution, high-volume gastrointestinal bleeding from diverticulosis has not occurred much more commonly on the right than the left. Therefore, a blind right hemicolectomy for diverticular bleeding is not appropriate. We find that colonoscopy during an acute gastrointestinal bleed of unknown source can be quite helpful. Our technique involves the rapid instillation of GoLYTELY into the gastrointestinal tract for lavage. We may often assist the patient in this effort by placing a nasogastric tube and then pushing 500 mL of GoLYTELY every 15 to 20 minutes, aspirating between each application. In most situations, the scope can be passed by an experienced individual without high risk. By creating a steady downstream flow of effluent of stool and GoLYTELY, the most upstream portion of red blood may be identified. High-volume bleeding from hemorrhoids or sigmoid diverticula can result in retrograde passage of blood into the cecum. In the unprepared bowel, it might be impossible to determine the site of bleeding. If, however, a GoLYTELY-induced catharsis occurs, ongoing bleeding is more easily identified. Furthermore, the

bleeding site and adequate technique can be used to deliver thermal injury directly to the bleeding site, hemostasis will almost certainly be achieved.

Several lesions and locations deserve special attention. Whenever a deep ulcer is encountered on the medial posterior surface of the skilled endoscopist can, in more than 90% of individuals, intubate the terminal ileum. In so doing, that individual can observe the ileal effluent for blood. This step is crucial in determining whether the workup for the bleeding source will be continued in the colon or in the upper small bowel.

The lesions most likely to be identified as bleeding sources in the colon are diverticula, angiodysplasia, cancers, and inflammatory bowel disease. From an endoscopic standpoint, no effective hemostatic technique is as yet available to manage diverticular bleeding. Likewise, high-volume bleeding from a Crohn's erosion or a malignancy is still best handled surgically. The lesions of angiodysplasia can be managed effectively by using a bicap technique. Because these lesions most frequently occur in the cecum and right colon, and often require repeated thermal applications in a single session, many operators prefer the use of a bicap device. This device allows for less tissue penetration and, theoretically, reduces the likelihood of full-thickness injury and perforation. In this technique, the bicap probe is applied directly to the center of the angiodysplastic lesion. Sufficient thermal delivery is applied so that a blanching halo appears around the periphery of the contact area. This may be safely performed two or three times over a 5- to 10-minute period. The area is observed until complete hemostasis is achieved. If these lesions stop bleeding with this therapy, it is unusual for them to recur as important bleeding sources.

For further details regarding the diagnosis and treatment of lower gastrointestinal bleeding and lesions, the reader is referred to Chapter 42.

INTERVENTIONAL BILIARY AND PANCREATIC ENDOSCOPY

Emergent therapeutic endoscopy is also used in the management of acute biliary and pancreatic emergencies. These emergencies most commonly are ascending cholangitis with biliary obstruction or gallstone pancreatitis. From the standpoint of the endoscopic technique, the management of these two conditions is similar. Our approach to both acute

bacterial ascending cholangitis and gallstone pancreatitis is one of immediate endoscopic intervention. Several recent reports have unequivocally demonstrated that the endoscopic transpapillary management of cholangitis is the most effective technique, resulting in decreased mortality and use of hospital resources. Because it has been shown that urgent endoscopic intervention in patients presenting with cholangitis is not deleterious, we recommend intervention within 24 hours of presentation. The optimal management options for acute gallstone pancreatitis are less clear. Endoscopy is helpful when choledocholithiasis and continued biliary obstruction are possibly contributing to ongoing worsening of the pancreatitis. Mild cases of gallstone pancreatitis do not require endoscopic intervention. In this chapter, the endoscopic approach to these two patient groups is considered.

Often patients seen in the emergency room have an abrupt onset of pain. They may be febrile, hypotensive, and require fluid resuscitation. Clinical shock may be present; this condition may require pressor support in addition to antibiotics and oxygen. Occasionally, patients have outright respiratory failure and require intubation. In these situations, a rapid response by the intensive care team is required to stabilize the patient and allow transfer to the appropriate fluoroscopic facility. We have, in certain desperate situations, provided drainage in the emergency room in the absence of fluoroscopy. In most cases, however, the patient can be transported, if necessary, while being given pressors and on a ventilator, to a fluoroscopy unit. The patients are prepared while they are in the prone position. A bite block is inserted into their mouths. A side-viewing endoscope is passed directly through the hypopharynx into the stomach. When food debris is in the stomach, this represents the threat of aspiration in a nonintubated individual. Care must be taken not to overdistend the stomach with air during scope passage into the duodenum. Once the scope is passed into the duodenum and the ampulla is identified, a rapid assessment can be made to choose the most appropriate endoscopic retrograde cholangiopancreatography (ERCP) tool. Unless a stone is actually crowning at the ampullary orifice, we almost always choose to cannu-

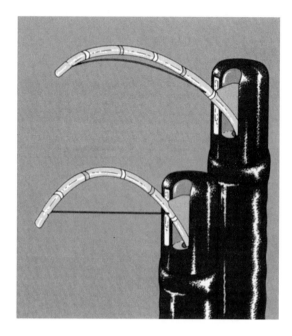

Figure 43–5. Lateral-viewing endoscopes with a regular papillotome protruding from the working channel. The pull type papillotome assumes a bow shape when traction is applied on its handle. A fully bowed position is appropriate for performing papillotomy. (From Venu RP, Geenen JE. Endoscopic sphincterotomy. In: Waye J, Geenen J, Fleischer D, eds. Techniques in Therapeutic Endoscopy. 1987, Gower Medical Publishing. By permission of Mosby International.)

late the papilla with a papillotome (Fig. 43–5). If there is no evidence of a coagulopathy, a papillotomy is usually performed. In patients who are septic with evidence of hyperbilirubinemia, it is preferable to cannulate the common bile duct with a guide wire through a papillotome. Once the biliary tree is cannulated with a wire, the papillotome can then be advanced over the wire into the biliary tree, and, before any injection is made, as much bile as possible is aspirated. This can be sent for culture. More importantly, however, aspira-

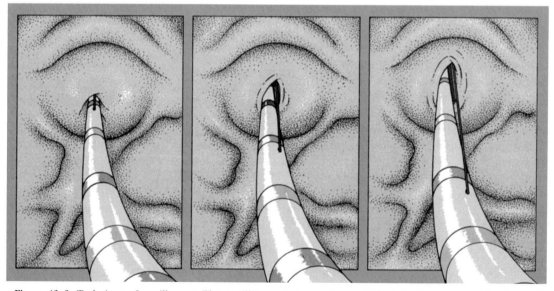

Figure 43–6. Technique of papillotomy. The papillotome is inserted completely into the common bile duct. After aspiration of bile, gentle injection of contrast confirms papillotome position. In order to remain within the intramural segment of the common bile duct, the papillotome is then retracted into the duodenum until the wire becomes visible. As the wire is seen, it is tightened to the flexed position. About half the wire should be visible outside the papilla. Energy for papillotomy is then applied through the wire. (From Venu RP, Geenen JE. Endoscopic sphincterotomy. In: Waye J, Geenen J, Fleischer D, eds. Techniques in Therapeutic Endoscopy. 1987, Gower Medical Publishing. By permission of Mosby International.)

tion of bile from the previously obstructed biliary system lessens the likelihood of high-grade bacteremia that will occur if a contrast injection is made into this closed space. The biliary system may be emptied by aspirating through the papillotome as much as possible before any injection. Once aspiration is achieved, contrast medium is gently instilled into the biliary tree, using only as much as is needed to determine the nature of the biliary obstruction and the presence of stones. If stones are identified, then it is determined whether they can be easily removed at that time.

For inpatients who are very ill with sepsis and coagulopathy and in whom there is concern about the ability to remove stones either because of their size or number, it is preferable to simply place a nasobiliary tube across the ampulla. This can be left high in the biliary tree. The advantage of using a nasobiliary tube is that drainage can be easily observed over the next several days and bedside cholangiograms can be obtained with little difficulty. The disadvantages of this approach relate to the need for a second procedure to clear the duct and the risk of nasobiliary tube dislodgment.

An indwelling stent may be selected instead of a nasobiliary tube. However, there are disadvantages to this choice. Stent clogging may not become apparent until the patient becomes septic, and the patient must have an additional procedure to remove the stent and indwelling stones. Furthermore, there is no way to monitor the patient for adequate biliary drainage during the recuperative period, such as is possible with a nasobiliary catheter.

If the patient does not have coagulation problems and if the ducts are well visualized during ERCP, it may be preferable to do a generous papillotomy and remove all of the stones that are seen at the time of the initial presentation (Fig. 43–6). This is the case for gallstone pancreatitis. In this situation, the papillotome is introduced into the biliary tree. The technique of guide wire cannulation of the biliary tree eliminates the risk of further pancreatic injury by repeated and undesired pancreatic duct injections. The biliary tree should be decompressed first before a contrast injection is performed. If the patient's history

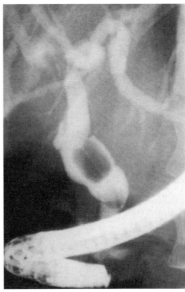

Figure 43–7. Radiographic picture of common bile duct stone extraction using a balloon catheter. The balloon is fully inflated and appears as the dark oval located above the stone, which is the rounded filling defect located below the balloon. The bile duct is dilated. Sweeping the balloon down the bile duct will allow extraction of stones such as this once an adequate papillotomy has been performed. (From Venu RP, Geenen JE. Endoscopic sphincterotomy. In: Waye J, Geenen J, Fleischer D, eds. Techniques in Therapeutic Endoscopy. 1987, Gower Medical Publishing. By permission of Mosby International.)

is very compatible with choledocholithiasis-induced pancreatitis, the decision to perform a papillotomy may be made in advance of the cholangiogram. If so, only a small amount of contrast medium may be needed to demonstrate the absence of large stones. A papillotomy is then performed and an inflated stone balloon is pulled back through the duct (Fig. 43–7). It may not be necessary to aggressively repeat the cholangiogram after balloon passage if it can be demonstrated that there are no filling defects larger than the diameter of a balloon pulled through the papillotomy. Any smaller stones should pass without incident.

Selected Readings

1. Cotton PB, Williams CB. Therapeutic upper endoscopy. Practical Gastrointestinal Endoscopy. 3rd ed. Cambridge, MA: Blackwell Scientific, 1990:56–84.
2. Brady PG. Endoscopic removal of foreign bodies. In: Silvis SE, ed. Therapeutic Gastrointestinal Endoscopy. 2nd ed. New York: Igaku-Shoin, 1990:42–97.
3. Sivak MV Jr, Blue MG. Endoscopic sclerotherapy of

esophageal varices. In: Silvis SE, ed. Therapeutic Gastrointestinal Endoscopy. 2nd ed. New York: Igaku-Shoin, 1990:42–97.

4. Chung SCS, Leung JWC, Leong HT, et al. Adding a sclerosant to endoscopic epinephrine injection in actively bleeding ulcers: A randomized trial. Gastrointest Endosc 1993;39:611–615.

5. Ponsky JL. Atlas of Surgical Endoscopy. St. Louis: Mosby–Year Book, 1992.

6. Fleischer D. Therapy for gastrointestinal bleeding. In: Waye J, Geenen J, Fleischer D, eds. Techniques in Therapeutic Endoscopy. Philadelphia: WB Saunders, 1987:1.1–1.21.

7. Waye JD. Esophageal variceal sclerotherapy. In: Waye J, Geenen J, Fleischer D, eds. Techniques in Therapeutic Endoscopy. Philadelphia: WB Saunders, 1987:2.1–2.13.

8. Mamel JJ, Weiss D, Pouagare M, Nord HJ. Endoscopic suction removal of food boluses from the upper gastrointestinal tract using Stiegmann-Goff friction-fit adaptor: An improved method for removal of food impactions. Gastrointest Endosc 1995;41:593–596.

9. Lee LG, Lieberman DA. Complications related to endoscopic hemostasis techniques. Gastrointest Endosc Clin North Am 1996;6:305–321.

10. Talbot-Stern JK. Gastrointestinal bleeding. Emerg Med Clin North Am 1996;14:173–184.

11. Gupta PK, Fleischer D. Nonvariceal upper gastrointestinal bleeding. Med Clin North Am 1993;77:973–992.

12. Laine L, Stein C, Sharma V. Randomized comparison of ligation versus ligation plus sclerotherapy in patients with bleeding esophageal varices. Gastroenterology 1996;11;529–533.

13. Saeed ZA, Stiegmann GV, Ramirez FC, Reveille RM, et al. Endoscopic variceal ligation is superior to combined ligation and sclerotherapy for esophageal varices: A multicenter prospective randomized trial. Hepatology 1997;25:71–74.

Chapter 44

Special Considerations for Bronchoscopy

Cameron D. Wright

Chevalier Jackson founded modern bronchoscopy, and the same type of rigid open-tube bronchoscope that was used then is still used today. Shigeto Ikeda developed the flexible fiberoptic bronchoscope in 1964 and revolutionized the field of endoscopy. Bronchoscopy, once performed only by surgeons in the operating room, is currently performed by a variety of physicians in the intensive care unit, hospital ward, outpatient surgery unit, and endoscopy suite.

INDICATIONS

Indications for bronchoscopy are broad. The common indications are listed in Table 44–1. Investigation and management of lung cancer is the most common indication for diagnostic bronchoscopy. Bronchoscopy has many therapeutic uses, which are also listed in Table 44–1. Because bronchoscopy is quite safe, there are few absolute contraindications. These include lack of informed consent and inability to adequately oxygenate the patient during the procedure. Relative contraindications are listed in Table 44–2. The risk–benefit ratio should always be judged in these situations to determine whether the small risk of bronchoscopy is acceptable. For example, if a patient has an obstructing, nonresectable tracheal tumor, rigid bronchoscopy (rather than flexible fiberoptic bronchoscopy) with core-out or laser ablation is indicated. Alternatively, bronchoscopy would be beneficial in a

patient with an obstructed bronchus from a mucous plug, even if that patient has had a recent myocardial infarction. Uncooperative patients should have general anesthesia rather than local anesthesia. Bleeding after biopsy is more common in patients with uremia (platelet dysfunction), pulmonary hypertension, and any coagulopathy. These conditions should be corrected before the procedure is undertaken.

Table 44–1. Indications for Bronchoscopy

Diagnostic uses
  Evaluation of lung lesions of unknown etiology on chest radiograph
  Hemoptysis
  Unexplained cough
  Localized wheeze or stridor
  Localization of origin of positive sputum cytology
  Unexplained vocal cord paralysis, phrenic nerve paralysis, superior vena cava syndrome, chylothorax, pleural effusion
  Staging of lung cancer
  Acquisition of bacteriologic samples
  Acquisition of diagnostic material from patients with diffuse or focal lung disease
  Assessment of airway patency
  Evaluation of tracheostomy or endotracheal tube problems
  Trauma with suspected tracheal or bronchial tear
  Suspected impending or frank tracheoesophageal fistula
  Smoke or noxious fume inhalation
  Aspiration of gastric contents
Therapeutic uses
  Aspiration of blood or mucous plugs
  Removal of foreign bodies
  Dilation of airway strictures
  Removal of airway tumors by core-out, forceps, or laser
  Placement of difficult intubation
  Placement of airway stent
  Control of massive hemoptysis
  Placement of brachytherapy catheter

Table 44–2. Relative Contraindications to Bronchoscopy

Recent myocardial infarction
Unstable angina
Acute arrhythmias
Hypoxemia
Tracheal obstruction
Uncontrolled asthma
Respiratory insufficiency
Uncooperative patient
Uremia
Pulmonary hypertension
Coagulopathy

FACILITIES

Bronchoscopy is commonly performed in the operating room, outpatient surgery unit, hospital ward, intensive care unit, or endoscopy suite. It is ideally done in a dedicated endoscopy room that contains all necessary equipment and supplies. The room should be large enough to accommodate a portable or permanent fluoroscopy unit. When bedside procedures are necessary, a bronchoscopy cart can be readily made to hold a bronchoscope light source and necessary supplies and accessories for use in the ward and intensive care unit.

Endoscopy suites, often shared with gastrointestinal endoscopists, offer the optimal environment for outpatient bronchoscopy. Dedicated endoscopy rooms with all the necessary equipment can be used in a much more efficient (and less costly) manner than an operating room environment. In addition, specialized endoscopy nurses or technicians can not only facilitate performance of the procedure but also reduce breakage and maintenance costs of the expensive equipment.

Essential equipment, whatever the setting of the procedure, includes two suction lines (one for the bronchoscope and one for oral suctioning) and one oxygen line, because all patients should have supplemental oxygen during bronchoscopy. Monitoring equipment should include a pulse oximeter, an automatic blood pressure device, and an electrocardiographic monitor.

PREPARATION OF THE PATIENT

A brief history and physical directed at the presenting pulmonary problem and the car-

diac system should be recorded. A history of any bleeding disorders (e.g., easy bruising; excessive bleeding after cuts, dental procedures, or minor surgery) is, in general, a much better screen of the coagulation system than laboratory tests. The procedure should be carefully explained to the patient and informed consent should be obtained. Cooperation and mutually satisfactory completion of the procedure is enhanced if the patient is adequately educated about the procedure and the necessity for compliance with all requests during the procedure itself. If general anesthesia is to be used, the patient should not eat 8 hours before the procedure. If local anesthesia is to be used, clear liquids can be taken until 4 hours before the procedure. A chest radiograph is the only test that is absolutely necessary before outpatient diagnostic bronchoscopy, but, if biopsy is planned, a complete blood count, prothrombin time, partial thromboplastin time, and platelet count is prudent. Patients with valvular heart disease should have prophylactic antibiotics if biopsy or rigid bronchoscopy is to be performed. Intravenous access should be secured.

An oxygen saturation monitor should be attached and monitored. The patient should also be monitored with an automatic blood pressure cuff and an electrocardiograph monitor. Oxygen should be administered during and after the procedure until the patient's saturation returns to baseline. Bronchoscopy commonly causes a decline in P_{0_2} of 20 mm Hg, which declines even further with prolonged suctioning, bleeding after biopsy, or bronchoalveolar lavage.

RIGID BRONCHOSCOPY

The relative advantages and disadvantages of rigid bronchoscopy are listed in Table 44–3. Even though it is possible to do rigid bronchoscopy under local anesthesia in a cooperative patient, it is difficult and unpleasant. General anesthesia is therefore used, creating a relative disadvantage of rigid bronchoscopy compared with flexible bronchoscopy. Limited visibility beyond the lobar orifices limits rigid bronchoscopy to work in the trachea and main bronchi. The key advantages are absolute con-

Table 44–3. Relative Advantages of Rigid Versus Flexible Bronchoscopy

Rigid		Flexible	
Pro	**Con**	**Pro**	**Con**
Enables performance of large biopsy	General anesthesia is used	Uses local anesthesia	Small biopsy only is available
Controls airway	Peripheral capability is limited	Enables complete examination	Small-bore suction only is used
Enables large-bore suction	It is difficult to learn	Provides distal visibility	Maintenance is troublesome
Removes foreign body		Enables performance while patient is on a ventilator	
Controls massive hemoptysis			
Removes tracheal obstruction			
Dilates strictures			
Enables laser ablation of tumors			
Pediatric use			

trol of the airway and the potential to perform numerous therapeutic maneuvers.

A typical rigid bronchoscope is shown in Figure 44–1 and consists of a polished hollow stainless steel tube (standard adult sizes are 7, 8, and 9 mm) with an accompanying glass rod light carrier within the wall of the broncho-scope. A glass-ended eyepiece may be fitted into the end of the bronchoscope so standard ventilation through a side arm may be carried out. Jet ventilation using the Venturi effect may also be used. Large suction tubes or bi-opsy forceps may be passed down the broncho-scope. Optical quality telescopes (0°, 30°, 90°) greatly enhance the quality of the view ob-tained. Pediatric-size rigid bronchoscopes allow examination of children.

FLEXIBLE BRONCHOSCOPY

The relative advantages and disadvantages of flexible bronchoscopy are listed in Table

44–3. Flexible bronchoscopy can be easily per-formed in most patients with local anesthesia, a key advantage. The flexible distal tip of the flexible bronchoscope allows very peripheral portions of the airway to be visualized and sampled. This is a distinct advantage over rigid bronchoscopy. Because the working channel is small (standard 2.2 mm), however, the suction and biopsy capabilities are less than that of the rigid bronchoscope. Maintenance of the flexible bronchoscope is exacting due to the delicate nature of the plastic-covered fiberop-tic bundles. Sterilization is commonly per-formed by short-term immersion in commer-cially available disinfectant solutions such as Cidex 7 or Sporicidin. Flexible bronchoscopes can also be sterilized by gassing with ethylene oxide but the time required (usually 12 hours) is not practical.

A typical adult flexible bronchoscope is shown in Figure 44–2. This illustrates the ex-tensive flexibility of the distal tip of the bron-choscope. Three sizes of flexible scopes are

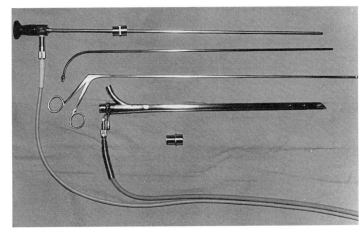

Figure 44–1. Standard adult rigid bron-choscope with light cable, straight biopsy forceps, suction, eyepiece, and optical telescope with light cable.

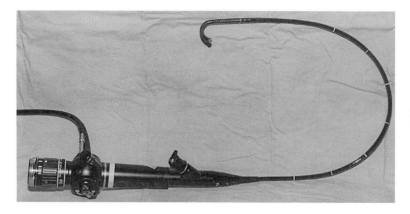

Figure 44–2. Standard adult flexible bronchoscope demonstrating flexibility of the distal tip.

commonly available: pediatric (3.5 mm scope diameter, 1.2 mm working channel), small adult (4.9 mm diameter, 2.2 mm channel), and standard adult (5.9 mm diameter, 2.2–2.8 mm channel). Video bronchoscopes, state-of-the-art technology, have high-resolution monochrome charged coupled device (CCD) chips, which have superior optics and are a great improvement for teaching over the old teaching head attachment. In addition, digital photographs as well as video cassettes can be made of the examination, facilitating documentation and communication of the findings of the procedure. The working channel (usually 2.2 mm) can accommodate biopsy forceps (smooth, clam-like, alligator type, spear type), brushes, and hollow aspiration needles. Figure 44–3 demonstrates the relative sizes of the working instruments of a rigid bronchoscope (suction, foreign body forceps, large cup biopsy forceps) and flexible bronchoscope (biopsy forceps, brush). Overall, the flexible bronchoscope is the superior diagnostic instrument and is the one most commonly used, especially in the outpatient setting.

SEDATION AND ANESTHESIA

Appropriate premedication can produce sedation, relief of anxiety, retrograde amnesia, and an antitussive effect, and it can help dry secretions. Whether it is effective or helpful in bronchoscopy is undetermined. Diazepam (2–5 mg) or midazolam (0.5–2.5 mg) is usually titrated in small intravenous doses to provide

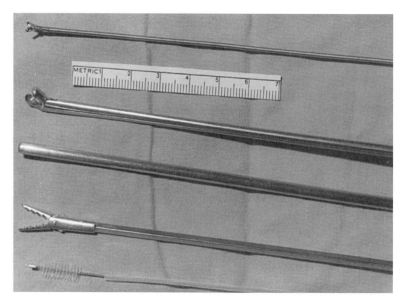

Figure 44–3. Working instruments for use in rigid and flexible bronchoscopy. From top to bottom: flexible biopsy forceps, rigid biopsy forceps, rigid suction, rigid alligator foreign body forceps, and flexible brush. Note the difference in size in rigid suction versus flexible biopsy forceps.

sedation, relieve anxiety, and induce anesthesia with minimal risk of respiratory depression. Meperidine (10–25 mg) or fentanyl (25–50 µg) can also be titrated in small intravenous doses to enhance sedation and reduce coughing. Atropine (0.4–0.8 mg intramuscularly) is sometimes used to promote drying of secretions. Patient safety is enhanced if small doses of sedation are given, followed by evaluation of the effects on the patient before larger amounts are administered. An informed, cooperative patient is the safest candidate for bronchoscopy.

Lidocaine is commonly used for local anesthesia because tetracaine has been associated with an excessive incidence of cardiovascular collapse. Lidocaine has a half-life of approximately 90 minutes, and the total dose should be kept at less than 400 to 500 mg per the usual 70-kg adult. Patients are instructed to gargle with small amounts of 4% lidocaine, which they then expectorate. A 1% spray is then administered with an atomizer to the hypopharynx and larynx. By touching the back of the pharynx with the tip of the atomizer, the physician can determine the degree of anesthesia reached and guide administration. The nose should be anesthetized as well if this route for insertion is chosen. Nasal mucous membranes can be shrunk with topical dilute cocaine or phenylephrine if necessary. The vocal cords and upper trachea are anesthetized with small amounts (2–5 mL) of lidocaine administered through the bronchoscope before the procedure is begun. Additional lidocaine is administered as necessary down the working channel as the procedure is performed.

TECHNIQUE OF BRONCHOSCOPY

Rigid Bronchoscopy

After satisfactory induction of general anesthesia with the patient in the supine position, the larynx and vocal cords are first visualized. To facilitate introduction of the instrument, the patient's head should be in the classic sniffing position, which also facilitates laryngoscopy and placement of an endotracheal tube. By elevating just the tip of the epiglottis with the tip of the bronchoscope, the physician can obtain an excellent view of the entire glottis. The instrument is rotated 90° to facilitate passage through the vocal cords, and then careful inspection of the trachea and main bronchi is performed. The optical telescopes should be used to obtain a magnified view. The 0° telescope is appropriate for the trachea, main bronchi, and lower lobes, whereas the 90° telescope is appropriate for the right and left upper lobar orifices. A flexible bronchoscope can readily be passed through the rigid bronchoscope to visualize the more peripheral bronchi if necessary. Thick secretions can be suctioned and large biopsy samples can be obtained with either straight or angled cut biopsy forceps.

Flexible Bronchoscopy

Fiberoptic bronchoscopy can be performed through either the nose or mouth. Passage through the nose readily guides the endoscopist immediately to the glottis, facilitating easy placement of the bronchoscope into the trachea. However, passage through the nose is uncomfortable for many patients and is not always possible. In addition, the need for multiple specimens may necessitate the removal and reinsertion of the bronchoscope, which can become quite unpleasant. Alternatively, with a bite block in place, the instrument may readily be inserted through the mouth. Introduction of the instrument into the glottis can be facilitated by temporarily withdrawing the patient's tongue out of the patient's mouth. The larynx and vocal cords should be inspected and vocal cord mobility should be assessed. The trachea and carina followed by the main bronchi and lobar orifices should then be assessed. Figure 44–4 shows the usual bronchoscopic anatomy as visualized from the viewpoint of standing at the patient's head. The main carina should be assessed for sharpness and mobility. Widening or fixation of the carina suggests pathologic involvement of the subcarinal nodes. The secondary carinas should be examined in this manner as well. The mucosa throughout the tracheobronchial tree should be carefully inspected for areas of

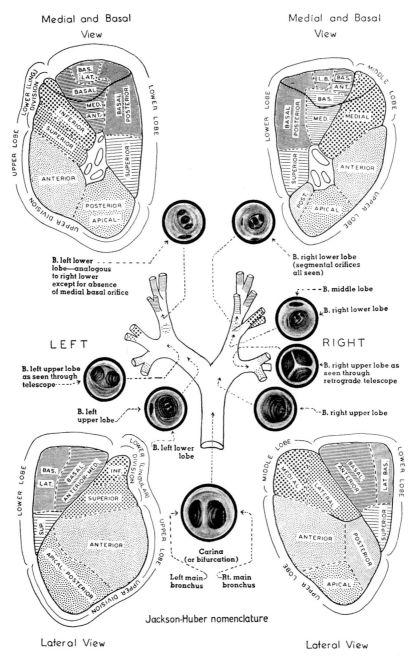

Figure 44–4. Illustration demonstrating the bronchopulmonary segments and the lobar and segmental branches tree. The tree is shown "upside down" because this is the same view seen by the endoscopist. (From Jackson C, Jackson CL. Bronchoscopy. Philadelphia: WB Saunders, 1950.)

bronchitis, submucosal edema, and tumor. All lobar and segmental bronchi should be carefully examined, with particular attention given to the area where the chest radiograph is abnormal. Secretions should be collected for appropriate testing. Endobronchial tumors and extrinsic bronchial compression are common findings associated with carcinoma of the lung. Biopsies are performed in areas of endobronchial lesions or where tumor is suspected in the submucosa of the bronchus. Bleeding can be controlled with wedging of the bronchoscope in the segmental bronchus, irrigation with saline, or instillation of topical dilute epinephrine. Several biopsy samples should be obtained because the diagnostic yield increases with the increasing number of specimens. Cytologic brushings should be performed after biopsy of suspicious lesions as well. Brushings should be quickly smeared onto a glass slide and then immediately immersed in 95% ethanol to prevent drying.

Transbronchial needle biopsy can be used to sample mediastinal nodes and submucosal central mass lesions. Cytologic specimens can be obtained of lesions that were previously not diagnosable. Sheathed needles are passed through the working channel of the bronchoscope and advanced into the suspicious area. The physician must be careful of the mediastinal structures so that vascular structures are not sampled. The needle is inserted into the lesion, which is gently aspirated. The needle is then withdrawn and saline is used to flush the needle to obtain a cytologic specimen.

In immunocompromised hosts, bronchoalveolar lavage is especially useful to diagnose opportunistic infections such as *Pneumocystis carinii* pneumonia. It is performed by wedging a tip of the bronchoscope in a small, subsegmental bronchus, instilling a large volume of sterile saline (100–300 mL), and collecting the return (usually 50%). This method of lavage samples the most distal portions of the airway as well as the alveoli, thus complementing ordinary bronchoscopic examinations.

Transbronchial lung biopsy can be performed of peripheral lesions if visible under fluoroscopy or of diffuse pulmonary infiltrates when diagnosing interstitial processes. When peripheral lesions are biopsied, not only should the biopsy forceps be superimposed over the lesion but the lesion should also move when the forceps are closed to confirm proper placement of the forceps. Fluoroscopy is usually used when transbronchial lung biopsy is performed for diffuse lung disease and to avoid biopsy of subpleural areas, which could lead to pneumothorax.

COMPLICATIONS

Complications of bronchoscopy are infrequent (Table 44–4). Complications are more

Table 44–4. Complications of Bronchoscopy

Anesthesia related
  Reactions to local anesthetic (cardiovascular collapse, seizures)
  Adverse effects of sedation (cardiovascular collapse, respiratory depression, aspiration)
  General anesthesia complications
Procedure related
  Laryngospasm
  Bronchospasm
  Respiratory depression
  Pneumothorax
  Hemorrhage
  Arrhythmia
  Myocardial infarction
  Fever
  Infiltrate
  Pneumonia
  Bacteremia
  Hypoxemia
  Air embolism
  Death (.01%)

frequent with rigid bronchoscopy than with flexible bronchoscopy. In part, this represents the use of general anesthesia but also is due to the possibility of trauma from a large straight tube inserted in a curved body orifice. The most common complications of flexible bronchoscopy are those related to sedation and local anesthesia. Cautious titration of sedation and avoidance of toxic doses of lidocaine are important. Pneumothorax is usually only seen after transbronchial biopsy and its incidence can be reduced if fluoroscopy is used and if the biopsy sample is not obtained if the patient experiences pain during the biopsy. Major hemorrhage is also usually only seen after transbronchial lung biopsy and is best avoided by not performing the biopsy in patients with pulmonary hypertension and coagulation disorders. Death is rare after bronchoscopy and is usually due to underlying cardiopulmonary disease.

Suggested Readings

1. Gal AA, Klatt EL, Koss MN, et al. The effectiveness of bronchoscopy in the diagnosis of *Pneumocystis carinii* and cytomegalovirus pulmonary infections in acquired immunodeficiency syndrome. Arch Pathol Lab Med 1987;111:238.
2. Jackson C, Jackson CL. Bronchoesophagology. Philadelphia: WB Saunders, 1990.

3. Sokolowski RW, Burgher LW, Jones FL, et al. Guidelines for fiberoptic bronchoscopy in adults. Ann Rev Respir Dis 1987;136:1066.

4. Stradling P. Diagnostic Bronchoscopy. 5th ed. New York: Churchill Livingstone, 1986.

5. Surratt PM, Smiddy JF, Gruber B. Death and complications associated with fiberoptic bronchoscopy. Chest 1976;69:747.

6. Wang KP. Flexible transbronchial needle aspiration biopsy for histologic specimens. Chest 1986;88:860.

Special Considerations for Pediatric Endoscopy

Bradley M. Rodgers • Osbert Blow

ENDOSCOPY OF THE UPPER GASTROINTESTINAL TRACT

The first inspection of the upper esophagus was performed by Bozzini in 1809 by placing a mirror in the throat. Fifty years elapsed before further contributions to the development of esophagoscopy were made by investigators such as Voltolini, Bevan, Semeleder, Stoerk, and Mackenzie. Waldenburg's telescopic esophagoscope was used to make the first endoscopic diagnosis of a pulsion (Zenker's) diverticulum in 1868. Professor Kussmaul of Freiburg is credited with the development of the science of esophagoscopy. Using an endoscope designed by Desormeaux to examine the urethra and bladder and with the help of a professional sword-swallowing "volunteer," he demonstrated that, with correct positioning of the subject's head and neck, examination of the entire esophagus was possible with a rigid instrument.

The fundamental operative principles of rigid (or hollow tube) esophagoscopy have remained essentially the same since Kussmaul's first treatise on endoscopy in 1870. The introduction of the Hopkins rod–lens telescope and the miniaturization of endoscopic instruments by Berci greatly advanced the field of pediatric endoscopy. Further advances with the technical development of the pediatric flexible endoscope have greatly increased the application of diagnostic pediatric endoscopy, and endoscopy is recognized as an indispensable tool in both the diagnosis and management of many gastrointestinal disorders in children. The field of pediatric endoscopy currently involves many specialty areas and a team approach is essential to the successful outcome of any endoscopic procedure.

EQUIPMENT

The development of rigid instruments with an optical lens system and flexible fiberoptic endoscopes that can be externally manipulated have greatly enhanced the capability of gastrointestinal endoscopy in the pediatric patient. Each type of instrument has its strengths and limitations. The newer flexible fiberoptic esophagogastroduodenoscopes are significantly smaller and provide excellent optical capabilities. They are equipped with suction, insufflation, irrigation, and instrument channels. All of these functions can be performed during continuous viewing. These endoscopes can generally be used without general anesthesia. They are essential for examination of the stomach and duodenum. Many procedures formerly requiring hollow-tube esophagoscopy (evaluation of esophageal inflammation and bleeding and variceal sclerotherapy) can be performed with flexible instruments in children. The management of foreign bodies and strictures remains an indication for rigid esophagoscopy, however.

Technologic advancements in both fiberoptics and miniaturization have led to the development of more sophisticated pediatric flexible endoscopes. Soon after its development, flexible endoscopy was considered a diagnostic tool with limited therapeutic ability. Currently, the flexible endoscope is not only useful in the diagnosis of many gastrointestinal disease states but also in their treatment. Flexible endoscopes are excellent instruments for the diagnosis and treatment of many upper gastrointestinal disorders in infants weighing 1500 to 2500 g. Most modern pediatric flexible endoscopes have outer diameters ranging between 6.4 and 7.9 mm. As a general guideline, any scope with an outer diameter of less than 10 mm is suitable for use in infants younger than 2 years old. Preterm and low–birth-weight children between 6 months and 3 years of age can undergo endoscopy with a fiberoptic bronchoscope that has a diameter as small as 3.5 mm. The use of larger instruments with diameters greater than 10 mm provides better visualization in children older than 10 years of age. The flexibility of these scopes makes endoscopy relatively safe in less experienced hands but does not eliminate the need for meticulous technique, especially in visualizing the lumen at all times as the scope is advanced. There is no substitute for a rigid scope for a child with a foreign body or massive bleeding, but the flexible scope can readily be used in the management of esophageal varices and gastric polyps. Another advantage of the flexible scope is that endoscopy may be performed with conscious sedation, whereas rigid upper gastrointestinal endoscopy requires the use of general anesthesia.

The Hopkins-Storz rod–lens systems of rigid esophagoscopes are available in lengths of 20 and 30 cm and vary in outer diameter from 4.8 to 8.2 mm. All but the smallest infant can tolerate a size 4 scope (outer diameter of 6.7 mm, length 30 cm). Size 3 to 6 scopes can be used in larger children (Fig. 45–1). Although smaller instruments have been designed for use in newborns, optical forceps are more easily managed in the size 4 and 5 scopes. The instrument channel can accommodate a large number 7 French flexible suction catheter, Fogarty balloon catheters, and a wide variety of forceps (e.g., alligator, grasping, toothed-grasping, circular cup biopsy, and punch biopsy).

Colonoscopes specifically designed for use in the pediatric population are thicker than upper gastrointestinal endoscopes and have an external diameter of approximately 1 cm. The colonoscope typically consists of a hand-held control unit with an eyepiece attached to a flexible shaft with a maneuverable tip. The flexible shaft contains discrete fiber bundles. Each bundle contains thousands of fine glass fibers, each approximately 10 microns in diameter. Cold light, delivered from an external light source, is transmitted by internal reflection through each fiber. Image distortion secondary to diffusion of light is prevented by coating each fiber with glass of a lower optical density. The faint grid that is occasionally superimposed on the final image is the manifestation of the difference between the external and internal character of each individual glass fiber. Channels for air insufflation, irrigation, suction, and biopsy are contained within the shaft. The tip of the colonoscope is versatile and can be directed more than 180° in either axis, permitting retroflexion when needed. Gentle torquing of the shaft provides additional rotation. This combination of features is controlled by the operator using the T-configured control unit. The fiberoptic shaft aligned with the eyepiece makes up the long axis of the T. The light source and the air and water supply are connected to the unit at the base of the T. At the center of the T lies the biopsy channel, air and irrigation button, suction knob, and the two dials for vertical and horizontal direction of the tip channel (Fig. 45–2). All of these features make the fiberoptic colonoscope an extremely flexible device that can negotiate virtually any configuration of the large intestine while transmitting a clear and accurate image to the operator.

INDICATIONS AND CONTRAINDICATIONS TO UPPER AND LOWER GASTROINTESTINAL ENDOSCOPY

The indications for pediatric upper intestinal endoscopy can be divided into four basic conditions, including accidental ingestion of foreign body or caustic material, gastroesophageal reflux, bleeding (hematemesis or me-

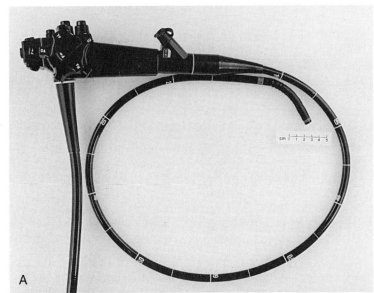

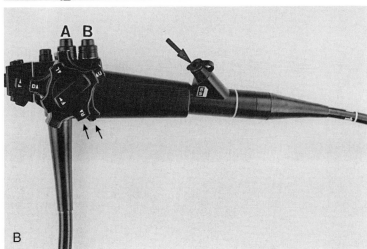

Figure 45–1. (**A**) Flexible gastroscope. The tip of this instrument has 4-way deflection for ease of passage. (**B**) Flexible gastroscope controls. Deflection of the tip is controlled by two large knobs *(small arrows)*. Suction (**A**) and irrigation-air insufflation (**B**) are controlled by buttons in the handle. Biopsy forceps and brushes may be passed through a side channel *(large arrow).*

lena), and abdominal pain (Table 45–1). These indications mostly support diagnostic endoscopy. Therapeutic procedures have been reported with increasing frequency. Some procedures, like sclerotherapy, have received wide acceptance as an alternative to shunt surgery for the treatment of variceal bleeding in children. Others like photocoagulation and thermocoagulation have been rarely documented in infants and children, primarily because of limitations of the instruments.

Recurrent abdominal pain is the most frequent complaint for which upper intestinal endoscopy is performed in the pediatric patient. Approximately 10% of children have abdominal pain, and most of these patients have no

somatic cause for their symptoms. Endoscopy is useful in the diagnosis of organic causes for abdominal pain. Indiscriminate use of this technique will result in a high percentage of negative examinations. A careful history and physical examination can significantly reduce the number of negative studies. Children who consistently localize their pain to the right upper quadrant or epigastrium and who have associated weight loss, nausea, vomiting, diarrhea, or occult blood and nondiagnostic plain and fluoroscopic radiographic studies should undergo upper endoscopy. Gross findings should not be overinterpreted and should always be confirmed histologically.

Upper gastrointestinal bleeding is the second

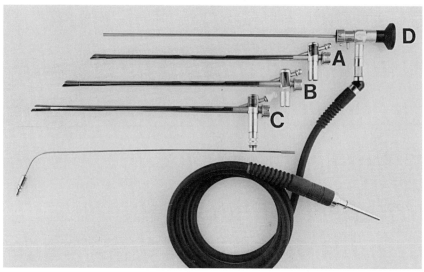

Figure 45–2. Rod-Lens rigid esophagoscopes. Illustrated are the 4.0 (**A**), 5.0 (**B**), and 6.0 × 30 cm (**C**) endoscopes. The Hopkins Rod-Lens telescope (**D**) passes through all of these instruments, providing a magnified image.

most common indication for performing upper endoscopy in a pediatric patient. Emergent endoscopy is almost never indicated in the pediatric population. Establishing venous access for volume replacement is the single most important therapeutic step in the management of these patients. Once the patient is adequately stabilized, attention can then be focused toward preparation for transfer to a center specializing in the care of the pediatric patient. If transfer is not possible or if the anticipated delay is to be longer than 24 hours, the patient may be prepared for endoscopy.

Careful examination of the nares should always precede any endoscopic examination to rule out epistaxis. The stomach should be lavaged until the returned fluid is clear. Most causes of bleeding can be controlled using conservative measures, allowing for a more

controlled study with a much higher yield of useful information. A diagnosis is established by endoscopy in nearly 80% to 95% of cases, a record that is superior to radiographic studies. Gastritis and gastric ulcers are the most common causes for upper gastrointestinal bleeding in infants, whereas duodenal ulcers and esophageal varices predominate in children and adolescents.

Gastroesophageal reflux or other symptoms of esophagitis such as dysphagia and odynophagia may be indications for upper endoscopy in children. In at least 10% of cases, patients with these complaints may have early evidence of esophageal strictures that can be diagnosed. Radiographic studies are useful in these patients and should be a prerequisite to the examination. If achalasia is suspected, features on the esophagogram are usually diagnostic, and endoscopy is rarely needed to provide further information.

Ingestion of foreign bodies and caustic agents is the fourth most common indication for endoscopy in children. The placement of safety caps on medications and household products has greatly reduced the frequency of ingestion of such substances in the United States. Physical findings including free burns on the lips, buccal mucosa, or pharynx are seldom reliable indicators of esophageal and gastric injury. Any child suspected of caustic substance inges-

Table 45–1. Indications for Upper Gastrointestinal Endoscopy

Recurrent abdominal pain
Bleeding
Gastroesophageal reflux
Esophageal stricture
Retained foreign body
Caustic ingestion
Other
Mass lesion on radiograph
Sclerotherapy
Placement of gastrostomy tube

tion should undergo endoscopy to examine the esophageal and gastric mucosa for the presence of superficial or deep burns or necrosis. The basic object of endoscopy in these patients is to determine whether the esophagus or stomach has been burned at all and whether the patient will require intensive treatment. Either rigid or flexible instruments may be used, although, for suspected esophageal injury (alkali ingestion), the rigid instrument may be safer. As a general principle, the endoscope should be passed only as far as the first definite sign of injury beyond the cricopharyngeal sphincter. If the flexible endoscope is used, it should not be passed blindly through the cricopharyngeal area. Air should be carefully insufflated to avoid distention and possible rupture of the injured esophagus. Edema is a sign of early damage. White or gray eschars are typically seen where the mucosa has been damaged more deeply by the caustic agent. Stricture is considered a late sign of caustic substance ingestion. Liquid caustics cause more damage than solid agents. Acids usually result in coagulative necrosis of the mucosal lining of the stomach, whereas alkalis damage the esophagus.

There are other diagnostic and therapeutic indications for upper intestinal endoscopy in children (see Table 45–1), such as pancreatic and biliary conditions, sclerotherapy, and percutaneous endoscopic gastrostomy.

The indications for colonoscopy are listed in Table 45–2. Although barium enema is of diagnostic value in a large number of cases of lower intestinal conditions, it is not as accurate as colonoscopy. Flexible colonoscopy is useful both as a diagnostic and therapeutic tool. The

most common indication for colonoscopy in the pediatric population is rectal bleeding. Polyps are frequently responsible for the bleeding seen in these patients. Polyps can be visualized and removed during the same procedure with colonoscopy. Other causes of lower intestinal bleeding that are readily diagnosed by colonoscopy include nodular lymphoid hyperplasia and vascular lesions. Vascular lesions are seen more commonly in older children and adults than in infants and younger children. Nevertheless, benign angiodysplastic lesions are readily treated endoscopically by electrocautery. Syndromes that are associated with intestinal malformations and rectal bleeding include blue rubber bleb syndrome, CREST syndrome (sclerodactyly and telangiectasia), Maffucci's syndrome (dyschondroplasia), Rendu-Osler-Weber syndrome, Turner's syndrome, and pseudoxanthoma elasticum.

Flexible colonoscopy does not replace careful inspection and palpation of the anus to rule out a local condition, such as anal fissure. Similarly, the workup of rectal bleeding does not start with lower endoscopy, especially in infants and young children. Upper gastrointestinal disease is frequently the cause of rectal bleeding in this age group. It should always be considered before searching for a lower intestinal cause. The ability to differentiate focal from inflammatory processes is what may make colonoscopy the initial diagnostic procedure of choice in patients with acute or chronic mild to moderate rectal bleeding. Severe bleeding (blood loss greater than 0.1 mL per minute) may warrant the use of radionuclide scanning. Colonoscopy should not be performed if radionuclide scanning is being considered because the reactive hyperemia that occurs after colonoscopy may complicate the interpretation of the results of the scan.

Diarrhea of more than 1 week's duration may warrant colonoscopy. Stool should be examined for bacteria and parasites, and a *Clostridium difficile* toxin assay should be performed in any child with chronic diarrhea. Polymorphonuclear leukocytes seen on microscopic examination of a stool sample makes an inflammatory process a more likely cause of rectal bleeding than a polyp. A negative microbiologic examination does not rule out an infectious cause. Symptoms and radio-

Table 45–2. Indications for Lower Gastrointestinal Endoscopy

Bleeding
Inflammatory bowel disease
Diarrhea of unclear cause
Recurrent abdominal pain
Evaluation of radiographic abnormality
Cancer surveillance in high-risk patients
Therapeutic intervention
  Polypectomy
  Removal of foreign body
  Treatment of bleeding
  Decompression of volvulus
  Balloon dilation of stricture

graphic findings of inflammatory bowel disease can be mimicked by infectious colitis caused by such pathogens as *Salmonella*, *Shigella*, and *Escherichia coli*, among others. Most patients with infectious colitis have spontaneous resolution of their symptoms. Persistent symptoms merit a repeat colonoscopy to exclude chronic inflammatory bowel disease. Allergic (noninfectious) colitis should be considered in any infant younger than 1 year of age with rectal bleeding and watery or mucousy diarrhea. Symptoms resolve only when the offending antigen is removed from the patient's diet. Barium enema frequently cannot detect the superficial patchy areas of mucosal inflammation seen by colonoscopy in these patients. A biopsy is necessary to confirm the diagnosis of allergic colitis.

The cause of chronic abdominal pain is often elusive and not usually solved by colonoscopy. Occasionally, colonoscopy differentiates between an abnormality of the terminal ileum and nodular hyperplasia in children with right-sided abdominal pain. Colonoscopy results are frequently normal; nevertheless, they provide reassurance to anxious parents. Colonoscopy is also useful as a screening method for family members of high-risk patients with polyposis syndrome or as a means to confirm radiographic findings.

Shock, acute massive intestinal hemorrhage, perforated hollow viscus, acute severe colitis, intestinal obstruction, recent surgical anastomosis, and cervical spine injury are absolute contraindications to pediatric gastrointestinal endoscopy. A combative patient who cannot be adequately sedated is also considered a contraindication to flexible endoscopy. Inadequate sedation or preparation accounts for the majority of incomplete examinations. Personnel who lack experience in sedating infants and children are strongly encouraged to seek the expertise of their anesthesiologist and perform endoscopy with general anesthesia. A relative contraindication to endoscopy, but an absolute contraindication to biopsy, is a severe coagulopathy. Correction of the coagulopathy should be completed before elective and semielective endoscopy is performed. Neither endotracheal intubation nor tracheostomy should be viewed as contraindications to endoscopy. Infants and children with congenital heart disease or prosthetic devices (e.g., valves, central lines, ventriculoperitoneal shunts) may safely undergo endoscopy, but the use of prophylactic antibiotics is recommended.

PREPARATION FOR UPPER AND LOWER GASTROINTESTINAL ENDOSCOPY

The preoperative evaluation of an infant or child for upper gastrointestinal endoscopy includes a thorough history from the parents and the patient when possible. Keeping terminology at a basic level and using descriptions and comparisons can be helpful, especially during the patient interview. Radiographic studies may be helpful in the workup of many types of gastrointestinal complaints. The conventional radiographs of the chest and abdomen are an important part of the initial evaluation and their value is frequently unappreciated. Plain radiographs are quick and inexpensive, and, if not diagnostic, can provide important clues to establishing the diagnosis. Findings on plain radiographs can provide helpful information in planning an upper gastrointestinal series.

Upper gastrointestinal series with barium contrast (or a water-soluble low-osmolar nonionic medium) is a safe and effective way to evaluate the pediatric patient with upper gastrointestinal symptoms. The upper gastrointestinal series is particularly useful in limiting the differential diagnosis of other conditions that resemble gastroesophageal reflux. The major limitation of radiographic studies is in the diagnosis of mucosal disease of the upper gastrointestinal tract. Therefore, endoscopy should be considered an essential part of the evaluation of many gastrointestinal diseases in children. Laboratory tests are of little use unless a specific concern arises such as coagulopathy or blood loss. Lastly, it has been shown that, when possible, parent and patient education enhances the endoscopic experience for the patient, the family, and the health care team (Table 45–3).

The single most important part of patient preparation is ensuring that the stomach is empty before endoscopy. *The Manual of Gastro-*

Table 45–3. Preparation for Upper Gastrointestinal Endoscopy

History (parents and patient)
Physical examination
Plain radiographs
Upper gastrointestinal series (barium or non-ionic contrast)
Laboratory tests (not usually indicated)
  Prothrombin and partial thromboplastin time (if coagulopathy is suspected and biopsy is planned)
NPO
  Younger than 4 months: clear liquids up to 2 hours before endoscopy
  Older than 4 months: clear liquids up to 3 hours before endoscopy
Parent and patient education

NPO = nothing by mouth.

intestinal Procedures Pediatric Supplement recommends giving nothing by mouth (NPO) for 4 hours before performing upper gastrointestinal endoscopy in patients younger than 4 years old. This interval does not lead to dehydration, but does ensure that the stomach is empty for the procedure. Similar recommendations have been made by the American Academy of Pediatrics Committee on Drugs.

There is no ideal regimen for preparing patients for lower intestinal endoscopy. We follow the protocol outlined in Table 45–4. The use of carbohydrate-based bowel preparations such as mannitol have been associated with bowel explosion during electrocautery. Colonic lavage solutions containing large macromolecules like polyethylene glycol that are not absorbed by the small intestine are excellent

Table 45–4. Preparation for Lower Gastrointestinal Endoscopy

History (parents and patient)
Physical examination
Plain radiographs
Laboratory tests (not usually indicated)
  Prothrombin and partial thromboplastin time (if coagulopathy is suspected and biopsy is planned)
Bowel preparation
  GoLYTELY 40 mL/kg 12 hours before procedure
NPO
  Older than 4 months: clear liquids up to 2 hours before colonoscopy
  Younger than 4 months: clear liquids up to 3 hours before colonoscopy
Parent and patient education

NPO = nothing by mouth.

osmotic agents that induce diarrhea. They are safe and eliminate the need for dietary restriction, laxatives, or enemas. The risk of dehydration is minimal in children older than age 5. Children younger than 5 years of age may experience dehydration with a vigorous mechanical preparation and they should receive intravenous fluids before endoscopy. The preparation must be tailored to the patient's limitations. Some children may be unable to drink large volumes and therefore require placement of a nasogastric tube to administer the bowel preparation solution. Other children may have colostomies or enterostomies and may require a limited preparation. Enemas and suppositories should generally be avoided because they can cause hyperemia, edema, petechiae, mucus depletion, and nonspecific inflammatory changes that may confuse the findings at colonoscopy. Although adequate bowel preparation is crucial to the success of any colonoscopy, compliance is equally important to the success of the procedure. Anxiety in older children can be decreased by introducing them to the endoscopy suite, personnel, and technique before the actual procedure is to begin. The child and the parents should be given ample opportunity to ask questions about the procedure.

TECHNIQUE

Rigid Esophagoscopy

Whereas flexible endoscopy can be performed with the patient sedated or anesthetized, rigid esophagoscopy requires the use of general anesthesia. Once the patient is adequately anesthetized and the security of the airway is confirmed, a sandbag or towel roll is placed under the patient's shoulders to extend the neck. The compressibility of the child's trachea makes intubation extremely important to the success of the endoscopy and safety of the patient. The head can then be moved passively during esophagoscopy. Although it is not necessary to have an assistant hold the head, it is desirable to have an assistant who is familiar with the instruments.

The endoscopist retracts the upper alveolar

ridge or upper teeth with the fingers of the nondominant hand. The distal end of the esophagoscope is steadied between the thumb and forefinger of the same hand. The proximal end of the esophagoscope is controlled with the dominant hand (like holding a pen or pencil). The assistant may need to rotate the head posteriorly to facilitate passage of the scope in a near vertical direction, along the right lateral border of the tongue. The tongue is displaced to the left as the scope is advanced lateral to the epiglottis into the right piriform sinus. The larynx is elevated with the tip of the scope and the cricopharyngeal sphincter is visualized. The scope is rocked anteriorly to open the sphincter and is gently insinuated through the sphincter into the upper esophagus.

To prevent perforation, the lumen of the esophagus must always be kept in view as the endoscope is advanced through the esophagus. Perforation is most likely to occur at the level of cricopharyngeus muscle. The child's small laryngeal and hypopharyngeal anatomy and the contraction of the cricopharyngeus sphincter can make the procedure challenging. Placement of a soft suction catheter through the esophagoscope and into the upper esophagus can be helpful. Alternatively, elevation of the larynx with a laryngoscope allows passage of the scope just behind the arytenoids into the esophagus. Direct visualization of the lumen is essential to a successful procedure. The lower esophageal sphincter (LES) and gastric rugae mark the distal limits of examination.

Flexible Esophagogastroduodenoscopy

The method of flexible endoscopy is similar to that of rigid esophagoscopy with certain key exceptions. These include the type of anesthesia used, the way in which the patient is positioned, and the needed expertise of the support staff.

The age of the patient, the rapidity of the examination, and the complexity of the treatment proposed determine the choice of anesthetic to be used. We believe that neonates, toddlers, and even some preteens and teenagers should undergo esophagogastroduodenoscopy under general anesthesia. Maximal control of the airway is thereby achieved, thus reducing the potential risk of aspiration. Furthermore, toddlers and children can have significant fears of the procedure, making the overall experience much less satisfying for the patient, the family, and the health care team. Advocates of the use of monitored conscious sedation for endoscopic procedures insist on the availability of a highly trained and specialized supportive staff, skilled in the care of children. The general surgeon attempting to perform the occasional upper gastrointestinal endoscopy on a child is strongly advised to do so under general anesthesia unless access to a center staffed with personnel trained in pediatric procedures is available. Pediatric endoscopy should not be considered a routine function of emergency medical personnel.

Flexible endoscopy in the patient under conscious sedation requires successful preoperative and postoperative teaching, adequate space, an excellent monitoring system, and prearranged anesthesia backup. An assistant is needed to administer sedatives and to continually observe the patient's vital signs (i.e., core temperature, heart rate, blood pressure, oxygen saturation). A nearby recovery area should be staffed with personnel specially trained in the care of the pediatric patient. The technique for performing rigid esophagoscopy can be applied to flexible upper endoscopy when performed under general anesthesia. However, the flexible scope also permits inspection of the stomach and duodenum.

Once adequate sedation is achieved with midazolam, fentanyl, or meperidine hydrochloride (Demerol) in age-appropriate doses, the patient is placed in the left lateral decubitus position. This position not only offers protection to the airway in case vomiting occurs but also facilitates the passage of the scope. The patient is encouraged to swallow while the scope is advanced into the upper esophagus. As with rigid endoscopy, care must be taken to avoid high esophageal perforation. Maintaining the esophageal lumen in view at all times minimizes the risk of such complications. A preliminary inspection of the esophagus is made as the scope is advanced toward the stomach. The gastroesophageal junction is carefully examined for any evidence of inflammation, hiatal hernia, or stricture. The stomach is insufflated sufficiently to permit adequate viewing, but overdistention should be avoided during the examination. All fluid should be aspirated at this time. Gastric folds should be flattened by insufflation and the fundus and antrum carefully inspected by forward viewing. Inspection of the cardia is best accomplished by retroflexion of the endoscope. After a systematic inspection of the stomach, the duodenum is entered, if possible, to complete the procedure. Once the scope is through the pyloric channel it can be passed into the duodenal bulb and turned clockwise (to the patient's right) into the second portion of the duodenum. Excess air is removed as the scope is withdrawn. The esophagus can be carefully examined on withdrawal, with little additional insufflation.

Areas of concern can be photographed, facilitating communication between the primary care physician and the pediatric specialist physician or surgeon, depending on the pathologic condition identified. Gross appearance is a poor predictor of histologic change in the upper gastrointestinal tract and abnormal-appearing areas should be biopsied.

Flexible Colonoscopy

When performing flexible colonoscopy, the endoscopist and assistant should wear protective clothing. Adequate sedation of the patient is achieved with midazolam, fentanyl, or Demerol in age-appropriate doses, and the patient is placed in the left lateral decubitus position with the knees flexed. This position not only offers protection to the airway in case vomiting occurs but also facilitates passage of the scope. Careful inspection and palpation of the perianal region and anus should precede the endoscopic procedure. The digital rectal examination assesses adequacy of the preparation and sedation. Lubrication with lidocaine (Xylocaine) jelly can provide additional patient comfort. The lubricated tip of the colonoscope is inserted with the examiner's index finger controlling the tip. Small puffs of air

are insufflated to identify the lumen of the rectum. Maintaining the intestinal lumen in view at all times minimizes the risk of complications. Stool residue present in the rectum or sigmoid colon does not indicate an inadequate preparation in that the remainder of the colon may be clean.

Negotiating the scope around the bends of the colon is singularly the most challenging aspect of lower intestinal endoscopy. The rectosigmoid junction is the first in the series of bends in the mobile sigmoid colon. Keeping the lumen in view is critical to the safe passage of the colonoscope beyond a bend. The direction of the lumen may be indicated by the direction of the mucosal blood vessels or the shadowing below a mucosal fold. If the lumen is only partially seen or not seen at all, the endoscope is not advanced. The endoscope is pulled back and another direction is tried. Occasionally, the lumen cannot be seen in any direction and a gentle blind pass is necessary. Information acquired from the previous attempts dictates the most likely trajectory to follow. The vascular pattern of the mucosa should pass across the view as the tip slides over it. Blanching of mucosal blood vessels, resistance, and pain indicate excessive pressure on the bowel wall or mesentery. If any of these signs develop, the endoscope should be withdrawn and the intestinal lumen identified.

The novice endoscopist may be lured into simply advancing the endoscope as long as the lumen is in view. This tendency to advance down the lumen inevitably leads to loop formation as the bowel is stretched over the endoscope. Loops are a major annoyance during colonoscopy and can be minimized, even avoided, if a low volume of air is used and the endoscope is pulled back at regular intervals during the procedure. Loops are easily detected under fluoroscopy. Very few colonoscopies are performed under fluoroscopy, however. Therefore, signs of loop formation should be quickly recognized before the loop becomes large and painful to the patient. Loss of the one-to-one ratio of pushing and tip advancement is the hallmark sign of loop formation. As soon as this loss of push to advance ratio is altered, the endoscope should be withdrawn until the ratio is reestablished. Other measures that may be necessary to eliminate the loop include torquing the endoscope, aspirating air, and applying pressure to the abdominal wall.

Loops commonly encountered during endoscopy include the N and alpha loops in the sigmoid colon. The alpha loop is formed when the sigmoid colon is stretched and twists on its mesentery. This loop is not very painful to the patient and frequently allows easy passage of the endoscope into the descending colon. Once the tip is in the descending colon, the colonoscope should be withdrawn with a clockwise rotation until the one-to-one push–tip advancement ratio returns. The N loop is frequently uncomfortable for the patient. N loops should be converted to alpha loops whenever possible. Maneuvers to reduce loops should be discontinued if the patient complains of severe pain. Passage through the transverse colon can result in N loop formation in the sigmoid colon.

The splenic and hepatic flexures represent potential areas of difficulty. Negotiation of the colonoscope beyond these two points can be facilitated if the tip is not too tightly deflected, intraluminal air is kept to a minimum, and the colonoscope is withdrawn with a clockwise rotation around the flexure. Five percent of children have a reversed splenic flexure that may require more advanced endoscopic skill to overcome. The end of the line is reached when the interhaustral markings of the cecum are seen. Other cecal landmarks include the appendiceal orifice, and the ileocecal valve. Transillumination deep in the iliac fossa is a useful index that the tip of the colonoscope is in the cecum. Careful examination of the colon may begin as the colonoscope is slowly withdrawn. The entire circumference of the mucosa must be viewed to successfully complete the procedure.

Areas of concern can be photographed, as with upper endoscopy. All findings should be histologically confirmed with biopsy.

COMPLICATIONS OF UPPER AND LOWER GASTROINTESTINAL ENDOSCOPY

Complications of gastrointestinal endoscopy are uncommon, occurring in 1% to 2% of

Table 45–5. Complications of Gastrointestinal Endoscopy

Anesthetic complications
Respiratory depression
Aspiration
Allergy
Procedure complications
Mucosal tears
Tracheal compression
Respiratory embarrassment
Perforation
Phlebitis at intravenous catheter site
Bacteremia

pediatric patients (Table 45–5). Complications are most likely to occur in patients who are either too heavily sedated or undersedated. Respiratory compromise is usually avoided by careful monitoring with a pulse oximeter. Respiratory compromise should always be anticipated, and its reversal is easily managed with readily available naloxone. Undersedation and combativeness are the usual causes for complications related to the procedure itself. These include mucosal tears, perforation, loosened or broken teeth, bleeding at a biopsy site, and aspiration. Phlebitis at the intravenous catheter site is known to occur. Endoscopy is a safe procedure with minimal risks, which are exceedingly outweighed by its high diagnostic and even therapeutic yield.

Selected Readings

1. Ament ME, Vargas J. Fiberoptic upper intestinal endoscopy. In: Walker WA, Durie PR, Hamilton JR, Walker-Smith JA, Watkins JB, eds. Gastrointestinal Disease: Pathophysiology, Diagnosis, Management. Philadelphia: BC Decker, 1991.
2. Auringer ST, Sumner TE. Pediatric upper gastrointestinal tract. Radiol Clin North Am 1994;32:1051–1066.
3. Benjamin B. Atlas of paediatric endoscopy, upper respiratory tract and esophagus. London: Oxford University Press, 1981.
4. Bines JE, Winter HS. Lower endoscopy. In: Walker WA, Durie PR, Hamilton JR, Walker-Smith JA, Watkins JB, eds. Gastrointestinal Disease: Pathophysiology, Diagnosis, Management. Philadelphia: BC Decker, 1991.
5. Brown-Kelly HD. Origins of oesophagology. Proc R Soc Med 1969;62:781–786.
6. Cadranel S, Rodesch P. Fiberendoscopy of the upper gastrointestinal tract. In: Gans SL, ed. Pediatric Endoscopy. New York: Grune & Stratton, 1981.
7. Gans SL. Esophagoscopy. In: Gans SL, ed. Pediatric Endoscopy. New York: Grune & Stratton, 1981.
8. Gans SL. Principles of optics and illumination. In: Gans SL, ed. Pediatric Endoscopy. New York: Grune & Stratton, 1981.

9. Lahoti D, Broor SL. Corrosive injury to the upper gastrointestinal tract. Ind J Gastroenterol 1993; 12:135–141.

10. Ross AJ III, O'Neill JA Jr. Rigid esophagoscopy. In: Holcomb GW III, ed. Pediatric Endoscopic Surgery. Norwalk, CT: Appleton & Lange, 1994.

11. Walsh S. Oh no the patient is six not sixty!: The pediatric endoscopy patient. Gastroenterology Nursing 1995;18:57–61.

12. Williams CB, Cadranel S. Colonoscopy. In: Gans SL, ed. Pediatric Endoscopy. New York: Grune & Stratton, 1981.

13. Wyllie R, Kay MH. Gastrointestinal endoscopy in infants and children. Pediatr Rev 1993;14:352–359.

46

The Use of Lasers in Endoscopic Surgery

T. L. Trus • J. G. Hunter

LASER PHYSICS

Light amplification by stimulated emission radiation (LASER) technology has rapidly evolved since the early 1960s. Before attempting to use this technology in clinical practice, a person should have a basic understanding of its biophysical properties and limitations.

The characteristics of a particular laser beam depend on the active medium used to generate the beam as well as the amount of energy applied to the medium. The active medium can be a gas, liquid, or solid. The lasing medium is activated by the transfer of energy from an outside source (light or electrical spark) (Fig. 46–1). This results in elevating the valence of electrons within the medium to a higher, more unstable state. As these electrons return to a more stable state, a photon or light particle is released. When this photon encounters another excited electron, the result is a "stimulated" electron decay that releases a second photon in phase with the first (Fig. 46–2). These synchronized photons (parallel waves of identical wavelengths) encounter more excited electrons and the process continues to amplify. The product of this collision cascade is coherent light in which all photons are of the same wavelength, and all wavefronts are synchronized in time and space (Fig. 46–3).

Because the crests of all the light waves are in sync, they create a wave whose amplitude is the sum of the individual waves. As a result, laser light is able to heat tissue much more

than noncoherent light. The amount of energy delivered to the lasing medium and the type of lasing medium determine the number of unstable electrons and hence the number of photons generated.

To generate a laser beam, coherent light traveling in one direction must be selected out. Lasing cavities are designed to amplify photons generated along a certain axis by reflecting them at mirrors placed at either end of the cavity. A small portion of coherent light is released at one end of the cavity, thus forming the laser beam, which is subsequently focused through a crystal (see Fig. 46–1). Photons emitted in other directions are lost as

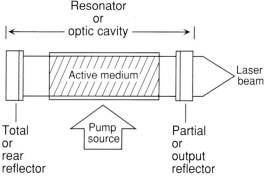

Figure 46–1. An external energy source is used to stimulate the lasing medium within an optical cavity. The cavity is bordered by a total reflecting surface at one end and a partial reflecting surface at the other. The latter allows passage of a small amount of energy to escape, thus forming the laser beam. (From Hunter JG, Sackier JM, eds. Minimally Invasive Surgery. New York, McGraw Hill, 1993.)

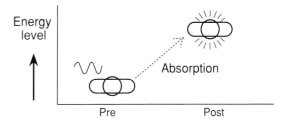

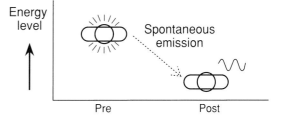

Figure 46–2. The absorption of energy raises an electron to an unstable state. As the electron returns to a stable ground state, a photon of light is released. The photon can encounter a second excited electron that "stimulates" a decay event. This results in the production of another photon, which is in phase with the first in both time and space. (From Hunter JG, Sackier JM, eds. Minimally Invasive Surgery. New York, McGraw Hill, 1993.)

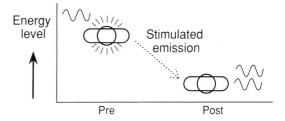

heat, which necessitates having extensive cooling systems of some laser units.

HARNESSING LASER ENERGY

Laser beams may be delivered as a continuous wave of energy or as pulsed energy. Continuous wave output is measured as a product of time and power. Pulsing is achieved by subjecting the lasing medium to large amounts of energy over short periods of time. Energy delivery is measured per pulse rather than as a function of time.

A laser beam is nothing more than focused coherent light. Focusing is achieved by lenses. The focal point of the beam has the highest concentration of photons and thus is capable

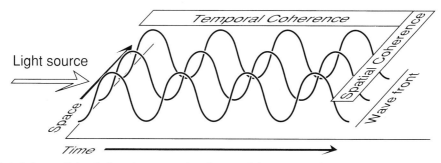

Figure 46–3. Coherent light of a laser beam contains photons of the same wavelength, synchronized in time and space. Because all wave crests are in phase, the power derived is the sum of each individual wave. (From Hunter JG, Sackier JM, eds. Minimally Invasive Surgery. New York, McGraw Hill, 1993.)

of rapid heat generation and tissue vaporization with little coagulation. Tissue beyond the focal point undergoes more gradual heating and superior coagulation. Laser light may also be delivered through quartz crystal fibers with the beam focused at the tip. The farther the tissue is placed from the fiber tip, the more divergent (and hence less powerful) the beam becomes. The problem of divergence can be alleviated by using fibers with contact tips. The contact tip absorbs the laser energy and converts it to heat.

TISSUE INTERACTION

Chromophores are present throughout tissue. Different chromophores absorb light of different wavelengths. Water, for example, has a high absorption in the ultraviolet and infrared portions of the spectrum. Tissue color is due to absorption of light in the visible spectrum. A red lesion, for example, absorbs light of a complementary color (green) and reflects red light, thus causing it to appear red in color. The advantage of this property is that a laser beam can be tailored (by choosing the appropriate lasing medium) to be absorbed by a lesion yet be reflected by surrounding tissue, thus minimizing "collateral" tissue damage.

Laser–tissue interaction can be photomechanical, photothermal, or photochemical. Most uses of lasers in medicine cause tissue injury by heating (i.e., photothermal). Pulsing parameters affect the type of laser–tissue interaction. A long low-power pulse causes a photo-

thermal interaction, spreading heat from the application point to surrounding tissue. Shortening the pulse time and increasing the power theoretically causes tissue ablation without significant thermal effects (i.e., photomechanical interaction). Conversely, a short-pulsed, low-power laser beam may act as a catalyst for a chemical reaction without appreciable thermal or mechanical tissue damage (i.e., photochemical interaction) (Fig. 46–4). The latter is the basic mechanism of photodynamic therapy discussed in subsequent paragraphs.

LAPAROSCOPIC LASER APPLICATIONS

Laser use in laparoscopy was first popularized by gynecologists. The advantage of selective absorption of laser light is clearly evident when treating red endometriosis lesions against a pale background. Argon lasers could be used to vaporize very thin layers of tissue in close proximity to vital structures, such as ureters, without damaging them.

General surgeons were first exposed to laser surgery in the dawn of laparoscopic cholecystectomy history. Early pioneers in this procedures in the United States were teams of general surgeons and gynecologists who were already facile in laser use. The benefits, cost effectiveness, and safety of lasers in laparoscopic cholecystectomy were soon questioned. An increasing shift toward electrocautery use in laparoscopic surgery was seen because it

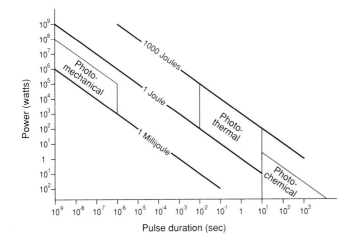

Figure 46–4. A variety of tissue effects can be obtained by varying the pulsing parameters of laser light. Short, high-power pulses result in photomechanical energy. Moderate-power pulses of somewhat longer duration result in photothermal energy. Long, low-power pulses result in energy that may be used to induce photochemical reactions. (From Hunter JG, Sackier JM, eds. Minimally Invasive Surgery. New York, McGraw Hill, 1993.)

was found to be faster, less expensive, and more hemostatic in more difficult cases.

Improvements in equipment coupled with increased experience in laparoscopic surgery have enabled surgeons to perform more difficult procedures such as laparoscopic common bile duct exploration. Occasionally, a large, impacted common bile duct stone can be particularly resistant to stone basket retrieval. Intraductal laser lithotripsy is particularly suited for this situation. Energy derived from a pulsed-dye laser is delivered through a flexible quartz fiber (320 or 550 μm) passed through a choledochoscope. The light energy delivered to the fiber tip against the stone wall is converted to acoustic energy, shattering the stone with very little effect on the surrounding soft tissue.

ENDOSCOPIC LASER APPLICATIONS IN THE UPPER GASTROINTESTINAL TRACT

Lasers have been used in numerous trials for the control of actively bleeding ulcers or ulcers with stigmata of recent hemorrhage. When using laser coagulation, care must be taken to avoid coagulating the ulcer crater itself because this may increase the risk of perforation or accelerate bleeding. Instead, the clinician should attempt to photocoagulate the ulcer rim, thus creating a rim of edema to tamponade the feeding vessel. Most studies have shown laser therapy to be more effective than no therapy but less effective than electrocautery contact devices in the control of upper gastrointestinal (GI) bleeding. The portability and relative inexpensiveness of electrocautery has resulted in its popularity as the preferred method of endoscopic control of upper GI bleeding in most centers.

Attempts at control of variceal hemorrhage using lasers have been relatively unsuccessful. More definitive treatment is required (e.g., banding, sclerotherapy) to avoid problems of rebleeding and possible accelerated bleeding seen in laser coagulation.

Ateriovenous Malformations

Argon lasers are particularly suited for arteriovenous malformation (AVM) coagulation because the depth of penetration is shallow and the selective absorption of hemoglobin is high. Thus, shallow photocoagulation of the lesion can be achieved, with minimal surrounding tissue damage. Numerous studies have demonstrated effective photocoagulation with laser therapy. Equivalent results have been achieved with less expensive, more portable electrocautery, limiting the widespread application of laser technology.

Endoscopic Laser Palliation of Esophageal Cancer

Several types of lasers have been used for tumor ablation, by far the most popular being the neodymium-yttrium aluminum garnet (Nd:YAG) laser. Ablation of obstructing esophageal cancer is most successful in short, straight segments of the esophagus containing an exophytic lesion. Long segments of tumor or segments containing a tracheoesophageal fistula are more successfully treated by stenting.

Laser ablation can be performed either antegrade or retrograde. The latter allows for more tissue ablation at one session because edema formation from laser ablation impedes endoscope passage to the distal tumor segment when the tumor is approached in an antegrade manner. Lower power settings (40–50 W) are more useful than high-power settings, because they ablate tissue as well as coagulate. High-power settings result in tissue vaporization associated with higher bleeding and perforation risks.

Results of Tumor Ablation

Laser ablation relieves upper GI obstruction in 97% of cases, but dysphagia is only relieved in 70% to 85% (most likely because of underlying motility disorders caused by tumor infiltration or laser injury). Unfortunately, dysphasia-free periods are brief, lasting only 3 to 6 weeks in most cases. An overall complication rate of 4.1% is reported. The perforation rate is approximately 2.1%. Hemorrhage or fistula formation occurs in less than 1% of cases.

Mortality rates of 1% are acceptable, particularly given the nature of the disease.

Photodynamic Therapy

Photodynamic therapy (PDT) uses the photochemical effects of low-power, long duration pulsing (e.g., 10^{-3} W for 10^{-3} seconds) of laser light to catalyze chemical reactions of photoactive drugs. Tumor-localizing agents such as hematoporphyrin derivative (HpD) or photofrin II are injected into patients and subsequently concentrate within the tumor. Light of a specific wavelength in the absorption spectrum of the drug is then used to initiate the release of oxygen free radicals, which destroy tumor cells without causing surrounding tissue

damage, because very little heat is generated from oxidative tissue injury (Fig. 46–5).

Photodynamic therapy is limited by the lack of light delivery to deeper tissues and the lack of HpD delivery to relatively ischemic regions within the tumor. These two problems limit the effectiveness of PDT to lesions confined to the mucosa and submucosa. The third problem with PDT is that of cutaneous dermatitis. HpD remains in the skin at high levels for several weeks after injection, forcing patients to remain in dim lighting for approximately 4 weeks after therapy to avoid activating the cutaneous HpD. Further research is required to develop sensitizers that are more specific or possess shorter half-lives and are activated by light of longer wavelengths to allow deeper tumor penetration.

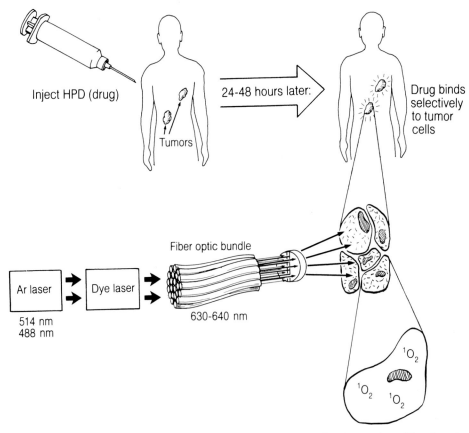

Figure 46–5. A photoactive drug is injected into the blood of a tumor-bearing patient. The drug is selectively concentrated in tumor cells over a 24- to 48-hour time period. Laser light of the appropriate wavelength is then used as a catalyst to stimulate oxidative, cytotoxic reactions within the tumor cells. (From Hunter JG, Sackier JM, eds. Minimally Invasive Surgery. New York, McGraw Hill, 1993.)

LASER APPLICATION IN THE LOWER GASTROINTESTINAL TRACT

Adenomatous Polyps

Laser destruction of adenomatous polyps has little use because the vaporization of the lesion destroys any chance of histologic examination. This is particularly worrisome in larger villous adenomas in which carcinoma may often be missed on simple biopsy. European series report 13% recurrence rates, with almost 6% of these being invasive carcinoma. There also exists a significant risk of perforation using a Nd:YAG laser. Therefore, laser ablation of adenomatous polyps should be reserved for patients with exceedingly high operative risk.

Palliation of Colorectal Cancer

European series have reported good success rates with Nd:YAG palliation of colorectal carcinoma. Most often, indications for treatment were abnormal discharge or obstruction. Symptom control was achieved in 85% of patients. Half the patients remained improved 6 months after treatment, and 25% remained so 1.5 years after treatment. Great care must be taken with lesions above the peritoneal reflection where perforation of an obstructed colon can be devastating.

SUMMARY

Laser applications for endoscopy or laparoscopy have undergone dramatic changes. Most applications, however, have proved to be no more effective than less expensive existing techniques. Many applications (e.g., tumor destruction) remain to be studied in randomized, controlled trials. New technology holds promise for tunable lasers for which the surgeon will be able to match the laser wavelengths for specific applications rather than matching an application to a specific wavelength of laser light.

Selected Readings

1. Birkett DH. Biliary laser lithotripsy. Surg Clin North Am 1992;72(3):641–654.
2. Brunetaud JM, Maunoury V, Cochelard D, et al. Endoscopic laser treatment for rectosigmoid villous adenoma. Gastroenterology 1989;97:272–277.
3. Cello JP, Grendell JH. Endoscopic laser treatment for gastrointestinal vascular ectasias. Ann Intern Med 1986;104:352.
4. Ell C, Demling L. Laser therapy of tumor stenoses in the upper gastrointestinal tract: An international inquiry. Lasers Surg Med 1987;7:491–494.
5. Fleischer D. Endoscopic Nd:YAG laser therapy for active esophageal variceal bleeding. Gastrointest Endosc 1985;31:4–9.
6. Goff JS. Bipolar electrocoagulation versus Nd:YAG laser photocoagulation for upper gastrointestinal bleeding lesions. Dig Dis Sci 1986;31:906–910.
7. Hunter JG. Laser or electrocautery for laparoscopic cholecystectomy? Am J Surg 1991;161:346–349.
8. Keye WR. Laparoscopic treatment of endometriosis. Obstet Gynecol Clin North Am 1989;69:157–166.
9. Krejs GF, Little KH, Westergaard H, et al. Laser photocoagulation for the treatment of acute peptic-ulcer bleeding. N Engl J Med 1987;316:1618–1621.
10. Lux G, Groitl H, Ell C. Tumor stenosis of the upper gastrointestinal tract: Therapeutic alternatives to laser therapy. Endoscopy 1986;18:37–43.
11. Straight RC. Photodynamic therapy in laser surgery and medicine. In: Dixon JA, ed. Surgical Applications of Lasers. 2nd ed. Chicago: Year-Book, 1987:310–349.
12. Vallon AG, Cotton PB, Laurence BH, et al. Randomized trial of endoscopic argon laser photocoagulation in bleeding peptic ulcers. Gut 1981:22:228–233.
13. Van Cutsem E, Boonen A, Geboes K, et al. Risk factors which determine the long-term outcome of neodymium-YAG laser palliation of colorectal carcinoma. Int J Colorectal Dis 1989;4:9–11.
14. Voyles CR, Meena AL, Petro AB, et al. Electrocautery is superior to laser for laparoscopic cholecystectomy. Am J Surg 1990;160:457.

PEDIATRIC SURGERY

47

Pediatric Hernias and Hydroceles

John H. T. Waldhausen

Inguinal hernia, hydrocele, and umbilical hernia are some of the most common congenital problems that surgeons see. The potential complications of these lesions require accurate diagnosis and timing of surgery. The surgical correction of these entities as well as orchiopexy for undescended testis can frequently be handled on an outpatient basis. This chapter discusses the diagnosis, indications, timing, and perioperative and operative care of these surgical conditions.

HERNIA AND HYDROCELE

Embryology and Pathogenesis

Congenital inguinal hernia and hydrocele occur due to the failure of the processus vaginalis to obliterate. Because of this, inguinal hernias in the pediatric age group are almost always indirect. The processus vaginalis forms during the third month in utero. The testis begins to descend in the seventh month, with a portion of the processus attached to it. The portion of the processus surrounding the testis becomes the tunica vaginilas, whereas the rest of the processus eventually obliterates. In up to 20% of adults, however, the processus vaginalis remains asymptomatically patent throughout life. It is this patency that predisposes a person to congenital inguinal hernia and hydocele and that sets these entities apart from adult inguinal hernias caused by fascial or muscular weakness. The type of repair needed for adult and congenital inguinal her-

nia is therefore also different. Because the testis descends in the retroperitoneum, the processus and therefore a hernia or hydrocele sac always lies anterior and medial to the spermatic cord structures. The difference between hernia and hydrocele is in the diameter and content of the sac (Fig. 47–1). The hydrocele contains only fluid when there is a narrow communication with the peritoneal cavity (communicating hydrocele), or it contains no fluid at all if the proximal processus has closed (noncommunicating hydrocele). A hernia sac is wide enough to potentially admit bowel or other intra-abdominal structures.

The exact cause of umbilical hernia is unknown. The midgut returns to the abdomen by the 10th gestational week, with each lateral body wall contracting and closing in the region of the umbilicus. Attached to this area are the umbilical vein, umbilical arteries, and the urachus. Incomplete fascial development, imperfect attachment of umbilical structures, or weakness in surrounding ligaments or fascial structures may predispose a person to this type of hernia.

Incidence

In the full-term infant, the incidence of congenital inguinal hernia is as much as 5%. This incidence decreases as the child gets older. The incidence is highest in the premature infant and increases with increasing prematurity. Males are more commonly affected than females (10:1), although girls are more likely to

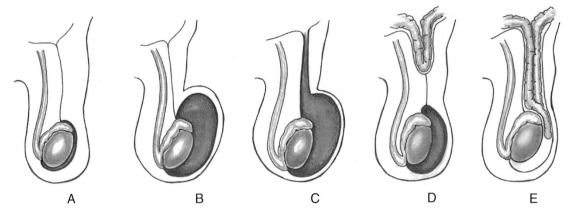

Figure 47–1. (A) Normal anatomy with obliterated processus vaginalis. **(B)** Noncommunicating hydrocele. **(C)** Communicating hydrocele. **(D)** Inguinal hernia. **(E)** Inguinoscrotal hernia.

develop incarceration and require an emergency operation. The greatest risk of incarceration occurs in the first 6 months of life, affecting 30% of term infants and as many as 60% of premature babies born with inguinal hernia. Congenital inguinal hernias are indirect because of the embryology involved. Direct and femoral hernias in children may be difficult to recognize and are rare (<1% of cases). Hydroceles also occur most often in younger children. The incidence of noncommunicating hydroceles in children older than 1 year is probably less than 1%. They are most frequent in male newborns and most resolve in the first 6 to 12 months of life.

Umbilical hernias are the most frequent type of hernia seen in children, being present in up to one of every six children. Black and low–birth-weight infants are affected most often. Most umbilical hernias close without treatment.

Most inguinal hernias in both male and female children occur on the right side (55%–70%). The incidence of bilateral hernias is controversial and has important implications regarding whether to explore the contralateral side. The possibility of a missed hernia, with the risks of incarceration or strangulation, must be weighed against use of a second anesthetic and the risk of injury to the vas and spermatic vessels during a negative exploration. Part of the controversy lies in defining what constitutes a positive contralateral exploration and whether finding a patent processus vaginalis is significant. A patent processus or an actual hernia has been reported in up to 85% of contralateral explorations in children younger than 2 months of age, with the rate decreasing to 11% after 1 year of age. In general, the incidence of bilateral inguinal hernia has been reported in up to 55% of low–birth-weight infants compared with a rate of 8% to 10% in term babies.

Associated Conditions

The following conditions are associated with an increased incidence of inguinal hernia: a positive family history (11.5%), undescended testis, ascites, hypospadias or epispadias, ventriculoperitoneal shunts, continuous ambulatory peritoneal dialysis, ambiguous genitalia, abdominal wall defects, and cystic fibrosis. In cystic fibrosis, it is not uncommon to find that the vas is absent at exploration. Connective tissue disorders such as Ehlers-Danlos syndrome and Hunter-Hurler syndrome also predispose a person to inguinal hernia. Children with ventriculoperitoneal shunts have a 16% incidence of previously unrecognized hernia, and 80% of these may be bilateral. Children with intersex problems may have inguinal hernias containing a gonad. In some cases, both ovaries and testes may be found at surgery. If possible, appropriate genetic evaluation and counseling should be done preoperatively because a gonadectomy, if indicated, can be done at the time of hernia repair. If both types of gonads are unsuspectedly encountered at operation, it is best to leave them in place until there is appropriate discussion with the parents, and genetic evaluation is performed.

Clinical Findings

Inguinal hernias and hydroceles usually present as a bulge anywhere from the internal ring to the scrotum. Other entities to consider are hydrocele, retractile or undescended testis, varicocele, and testicular tumor. In girls, the ovary frequently presents as a mass in the groin or labial fold within a hernia sac. Usually, the hernia reduces spontaneously or with gentle manipulation. The parents may give a history of recurrent groin swelling. Often, the bulge is only present with crying or straining, which increases intra-abdominal pressure. A silk glove sign may be present wherein the hernia sac is palpable over the cord structures as they cross the pubic tubercle. Not infrequently, a child has a seemingly positive history for inguinal hernia but no demonstrable lesion. In this situation, the clinician must judge the reliability of the history. If the hernia has been seen only by parents, a survey of pediatric surgeons showed that 55% of them would reevaluate the patient at a second visit; if the hernia was previously diagnosed by a physician, 65% of these surgeons would proceed with operation.

Hydroceles are either communicating or noncommunicating, depending on whether the narrow proximal portion of the processus vaginalis remains patent. Hydroceles may be present at birth or occur later in infancy and childhood. As with hernia, a communicating hydrocele may fluctuate in size, and fluid may be reducible into the peritoneal cavity. A noncommunicating hydrocele may be present within the scrotum or anywhere along the cord where the processus vaginalis exists. Typically, these lesions are stable in size, although some may grow slowly and, on occasion, become massive. A hydrocele can be transilluminated, indicating a sac full of fluid; however, in infants, any viscera within the scrotum may transilluminate, making diagnosis difficult. In general, with hydrocele, there is no palpable communication with the abdominal cavity. The cord is of normal size proximal to the hydrocele sac. Hernias often present with a thickening of the cord through the internal ring. On rectal examination, it may be possible to palpate the intestine going through the internal ring, diagnostic of a hernia. Rarely, if ever, is herniography indicated to make the diagnosis.

Incarcerated hernias occur as firm masses in the inguinal canal or scrotum. The mass may or may not be tender. Often, the initial complaint is fussiness, and the incarcerated hernia is discovered on subsequent examination. The diagnosis should always be considered in any infant or child with symptoms of small bowel obstruction. In boys, the hernia sac usually contains bowel; in girls, bowel, ovary, or fallopian tube is usually contained. Incarceration leads to strangulation with vascular compromise of the contents of the sac. Erythema and edema in the groin become increasingly prominent, and the child appears more systemically ill. Incarcerated hernias can be reduced between 75% and 96% of the time. If there is concern about strangulation, immediate operation is most prudent, even though the actual incidence of intestinal resection due to infarction is low (1.4%). In an infant's hernia, the internal and external rings almost overlap. Traction is first gently placed on the hernia sac to straighten the contents coming out of the canal. With the fingers of one hand, the surgeon forms a funnel around the internal ring; with the opposite hand, the surgeon pushes the contents back into the abdomen. While the child is kept calm or is sedated, elevation of the lower half of the patient's body may be useful. Sedation with midazolam, fentanyl, or chloral hydrate should be given only by physicians familiar with use of these medications in children and they should be monitored. Adequate equipment for resuscitation must be available because apnea may be easily induced in infants. Ice packs, although tolerated by some children, must be used with caution, and preferably not at all in an infant because of the risk of hypothermia.

Strangulation or incarceration is uncommon in umbilical hernias. Most often, until the age of 4 to 5 years, these hernias close spontaneously. Generally, these hernias are asymptomatic. Their physical appearance is often of greatest concern to the parents, particularly if the hernia is large and protuberant.

Surgery: Indications and Timing

All otherwise healthy full-term babies and older children are candidates for outpatient surgery. Premature babies, younger than 50 weeks' gestational age, should be operated on as inpatients because of the risk of postoperative apnea. Appropriate experience with pediatric anesthesia is essential, as are the availability of appropriate pediatric-sized instruments, monitoring, and the ability to admit the patient to the hospital if needed.

The timing of surgery depends on the patient's health and surgical condition. Otitis media and upper respiratory infections should delay surgery, and the hernia repair should not be performed in the presence of diaper rash. Inguinal hernias should, in general, be corrected once diagnosed. In patients who are candidates for outpatient surgery, growth of the child does not decrease the risks associated with surgery or anesthesia, assuming appropriately trained personnel are available. Delaying surgery does, however, increase the risk of incarceration and other complications.

As discussed, whether to perform bilateral exploration is controversial. As a general guideline, boys younger than 2 years old should have bilateral exploration as should girls younger than age 5 years. Communicating hydroceles should be regarded as hernias and should be repaired when diagnosed. Noncommunicating hydroceles in children younger than 1 year frequently resolve and may be observed, although the very large ones and those that are symptomatic (most often causing discomfort or fussiness) may require earlier operation. Needle aspiration is not indicated because it may be dangerous, and the hydrocele will probably recur. Noncommunicating hydroceles remaining or occurring in children older than 1 year of age should be repaired.

Incarcerated hernias, if nonreducible, need prompt surgery. If they are reduced, they should be repaired as soon as possible within the following few days, unless the viability of the reduced bowel is questionable. If so, prompt repair with examination for bloody or cloudy peritoneal fluid is most prudent. If these findings are present, an exploration for compromised bowel is warranted. Frequently, the incarcerated hernia reduces spontaneously when the patient is anesthetized. If a nonreducible, nontender incarcerated ovary is present, hernia repair may be scheduled electively within the following few days. If the incarcerated mass is tender, hernia repair must be done emergently. When strangulated bowel is present, patient resuscitation followed by immediate surgery is indicated. If a bowel resection is needed, it can be done through the herniotomy or via a second abdominal incision.

Umbilical hernias most often close spontaneously and can be observed with little risk until the patient is age 5 years. Those hernias that require surgery earlier are the large defects (greater than 2 cm) that are unlikely to close spontaneously and the hernias that are exceptionally protuberant.

Technique—Inguinal Hernia and Hydrocele

Anesthesia may be by general mask, endotracheal, or spinal technique. Further analgesia for postoperative discomfort may be by caudal block or by infiltration of the wound with local anesthetic, such as .25% Marcaine with epinephrine (1 ml/kg). Preoperative laboratory work is limited to a hematocrit. The temperature must be regulated in the operating room, and heating lamps and warm skin prep solutions should be used, especially for infants. The child is draped to include the lower abdomen and scrotum or labia in the field.

A transverse incision is made in a skin fold just above and lateral to the pubic tubercle extending 2 to 3 cm laterally, depending on the child's size (Fig. 47–2A). Scarpa's fascia, which can be quite prominent in the child, is incised with scissors. The fat beneath Scarpa's fascia helps to distinguish it from the external oblique muscle. The external oblique fascia and external ring are then exposed with blunt dissection. Exposure of the external ring is aided by dissecting the inguinal ligament and tracing it medially where the ring is found just lateral to the pubic tubercle. The external oblique fascia is then incised in the direction

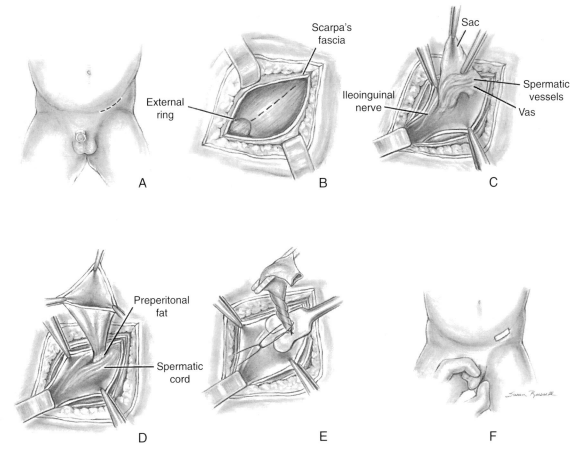

Figure 47–2. Inguinal hernia repair. **(A)** The incision for inguinal hernia or hydrocele is made just above and lateral to the pubic tubercle in a skin fold (*dotted line*). **(B)** Scarpa's fascia is opened and the external oblique and external ring are exposed. The external oblique fascia is opened along the dotted line. This incision may be carried through the ring or the ring may be left intact. Care is taken to avoid injury to the ileoinguinal nerve. **(C)** The cremasteric muscle fibers are split and the hernia sac grasped. The sac is then dissected free from the vas and cord vessels. The vessels are encountered first during dissection and the vas is encountered last. **(D)** The sac is clamped, divided, and dissected to the level of the internal ring where preperitoneal fat is seen. Before high ligation at the internal ring is performed, the sac is examined to ensure that it is empty. **(E)** The sac is twisted to keep abdominal contents out and the cord is protected while a high suture ligation is performed. Local anesthetic around the ileoinguinal nerve may be placed at this point. **(F)** Gentle traction is exerted on the testicle to pull it back into the scrotum and the cord structures into the inguinal canal. The incision is closed in layers.

of its fibers, either with a knife or scissors. This incision is carried through the external ring, although some surgeons prefer to leave the ring intact. Care must be taken to avoid injury to the ileoinguinal nerve; it is adherent to the cremasteric muscle fibers directly beneath the external oblique fascia (see Fig. 47–2*B*). Gentle blunt dissection under the lower flap of the cut external oblique fascia further exposes the cremasteric muscle and spermatic cord. The fibers of the cremaster are separated with a fine hemostat or forceps and the hernia sac can then be found anterior and slightly medial to the cord structures.

In some children, the sac can be extremely thin and friable. The sac may be grasped and then it and the attached cord structures are elevated to skin level. This allows better visualization for the subsequent dissection. However, because of concern for damage to the underlying transversalis fascia, some surgeons prefer not to lift the spermatic cord into the incision. Before beginning dissection of the sac, it is important to ensure that the cord is not twisted when raised to skin level. It is also easier to do this dissection if any bowel within the sac is reduced. When the hernia is separated from the cord structures, the sac is grasped with one smooth forceps, and another pair is used to dissect (see Fig. 47–2C). The vas and cord structures must not be grasped directly; they are very delicate and easily injured. Grasping the vas alone can cause permanent injury to the structure. Likewise, electrocautery must be used with caution near the cord, preferably not at all, because it is possible to cause thrombosis of the spermatic vessels via transmitted heat. Frequently, a small fat pad marks the initial plane of dissection between the sac and the cord. The loose areolar tissue around the vessels may be grasped and stripped from the sac, or the vessels and vas can be gently and bluntly pushed from the sac with the tip of the forceps. When dissection begins on the lateral portion of the sac, the cord vessels are encountered first. As the sac is rotated medially with dissection, the vas is encountered last. If the sac tears during dissection, it is essential to gain circumferential control, because tears can easily extend into the retroperitoneum. These become difficult to correct and, if not repaired adequately, can lead to recurrence.

Once the sac is dissected free, the proximal portion is clamped with a hemostat. With the vas and cord vessels out of the way, the sac is divided. Before performing high ligation, it is necessary for the surgeon to ensure that the sac is empty (see Fig. 47–2D). Approximately 21% of girls have the fallopian tube and ovary or uterus lying in the wall of the hernia; therefore, in girls, the sac is routinely opened for inspection. Although the distal sac may descend toward the scrotum or labia, it may be left in place. Some surgeons prefer to remove the distal sac, but, particularly in boys, this may increase the risk of hematoma or injury to the cord structures and testicles. In general, it is not necessary to pull the testicle into the incision unless there is an associated hydrocele around the testis. In this case, the hydrocele is opened anteriorly. Care must be taken to avoid injury to the vas because it may be circuitous and is prone to injury unless it is identified.

The divided hernia sac and cord are dissected free from each other to the level of the internal ring, where preperitoneal fat is noted. The sac is then twisted several times to keep abdominal contents out, and a high ligation is performed with nonabsorbable sutures (see

Fig. 47–2E). The cord must be protected during ligation of the sac so that the vas or vessels are not inadvertently pulled into the ligature. In general, nothing needs to be done to the internal ring unless a particularly large hernia caused it to dilate. Then, one or two sutures may be needed to narrow it around the cord. Reconstruction of the floor is not needed, except in the rare cases of direct hernia, in which case the area of the conjoined tendon may be sutured to the ileopubic tract. If a femoral hernia is repaired from an inguinal approach, a Cooper's ligament repair may be needed; however, these often can be repaired by a direct approach inferior to the inguinal ligament.

For sliding hernias, some surgeons may dissect the adherent contents free from the sac. Especially in infants, however, the sac may be quite thin and delicate, and it is probably safest to make no attempt at this dissection because it may injure the adherent structure or tear the sac. An incision is made in the sac on either side of the contained structure to just above the internal ring (Fig. 47–3A). This flap of tissue is then placed through the ring into the peritoneal cavity and a nonabsorbable purse-string suture is used to close the peritoneum (see Fig. 47–3B and C). In girls, the internal ring is then sutured closed.

When completing the hernia repair, gentle traction on the testis pulls it back into the scrotum and pulls the cord structures to the inguinal canal (see Fig. 47–2F). It is important to ensure that the testis is back within the scrotum, because it may become trapped within the inguinal canal after hernia repair if this is not done. If local analgesia for postoperative pain is to be used, the area around the ileoinguinal nerve as well as the wound edge can be infiltrated. The appropriate dose of the anesthetic must be used, because toxic levels are achieved much more quickly in children than in adults. The external oblique fascia is closed with reconstruction of the external ring, if needed. This and Scarpa's fascia are closed with absorbable sutures, such as those made of polyglycolic acid. The skin is then closed with fine subcuticular sutures, and a dressing of collodion, plastic film, or Steri-Strips is applied. Postoperative pain relief is usually satisfactory with acetaminophen as a suppository or elixir in infants, or acetamino-

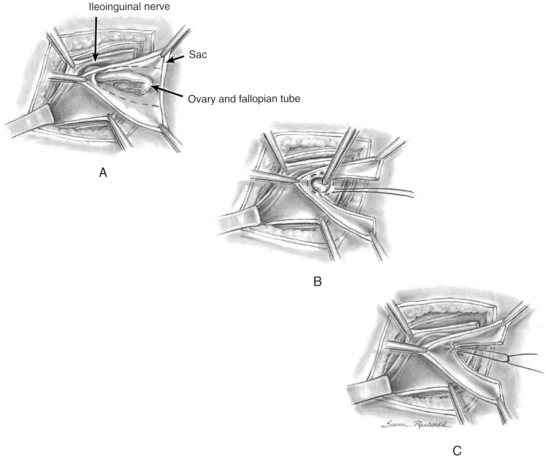

Figure 47–3. Sliding inguinal hernia. **(A)** After opening the sac, a sliding inguinal hernia is found with the ovary and fallopian tube in the posterior wall. An incision is made on either side of the ovary and fallopian tube to just above the internal ring (*dotted line*). **(B)** The flap of peritoneum containing the ovary and fallopian tube is placed within the abdominal cavity. A purse-string of nonabsorbable suture is placed circumferentially in the peritoneum just above the internal ring. **(C)** The purse-string is closed and the excess sac may be excised. In girls, the internal ring is sutured closed.

phen with codeine elixir (0.5–1.0 mg/kg codeine) in older children.

Technique—Umbilical Hernia

With the patient under general anesthesia, an incision is made within the fold of the inferior portion of the umbilicus (Fig. 47–4*A* and *B*). The incision should not extend past the umbilicus. Dissection is made down to the fascia and the sac is circumferentially dissected (see Fig. 47–4*C*). The sac may then be dissected from the umbilical skin and excised with fascial closure, or it may be evaginated into the peritoneal cavity without excision, followed by fascial closure (see Fig. 47–4*D*). Both methods work well with similar long-term results. The umbilical skin is tacked to the underlying fascia, and the incision is closed (see Fig. 47–4*E* and *F*). It is usually not necessary to excise any excess skin. A cotton ball or dental roll is placed within the umbilicus followed by application of a pressure dressing to prevent hematoma. This is left in place for 2 to 5 days.

Complications

The overall complication rate for pediatric inguinal herniorrhaphy is 2% or less, with an increase to 19% if it is performed after incarceration. Wound infection may occur in 1% to

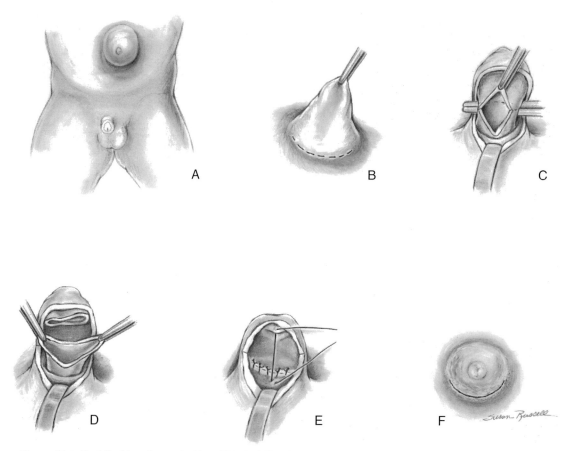

Figure 47–4. Umbilical hernia repair. (**A and B**) Umbilical hernia with infraumbilical skin crease incision. (**C**) The sac is circumferentially dissected and opened. (**D**) The fascial edges are exposed and the superior portion of the sac is dissected from the overlying skin. (**E**) The fascial defect is closed and the skin is tacked to the fascia. (**F**) Skin is closed with subcuticular suture, and a cotton ball and pressure dressing are placed.

2% of cases. The rate of recurrence is generally less than 1%. Risk factors for recurrence include the presence of ventriculoperitoneal shunts or peritoneal dialysis catheters, the presence of a sliding hernia, incarceration, and prematurity. Most often, recurrence is due to a missed tear in the sac. Although direct hernias are uncommon, they may occur after indirect repair, suggesting either a missed direct hernia or injury to the inguinal floor with mobilization of the cord.

Testicular atrophy can occur as a result of incarceration, secondary to compression of the spermatic vessels. It may also occur with injury to the spermatic vessels during operation. Even though the incidence of testicular atrophy is reported at 1%, it is probably less.

Injury to the vas can occur from direct division, from inadvertent ligation while tying off the sac, or during removal of a distal hernia

or hydrocele sac. The epididymis can also be cut during attempts to remove the distal sac. Heat injury from electrocautery as well as crushing injury from forceps can occur. The actual incidence of vas injury is unknown. If bilateral division occurs, the vas should be repaired using microscopic anastomotic technique by a surgeon skilled in this method. If a unilateral division is recognized, attempted repair is most prudent. Injury to the ileoinguinal nerve is uncommon with good surgical technique. Hematoma tends to be more prevalent after complete dissection of the distal sac. A rare complication that can occur months to years after herniotomy is a suture granuloma secondary to infection centered around a nonabsorbable suture used to close the hernia sac, usually a silk stitch. Incision and drainage with removal of the suture is the appropriate treatment.

Postoperative Care and Follow-up

Postoperative care is limited to keeping the incisions clean and dry. Collodion or plastic film dressing, particularly in infants, is usually adequate to provide a barrier between urine and stool, and the incision. There is little restriction of activity because this is difficult to enforce. Children are usually seen 1 to 2 weeks postoperatively for follow-up, although, because of the low incidence of problems found, this visit is as much for parental reassurance as it is for checking the patient.

ORCHIOPEXY

Embryology and Incidence

The testis begins descent into the inguinal canal at 28 weeks' gestation, the left testis preceding the right. It comes to rest in the scrotum in the eighth or ninth month of gestation. It is probable that adequate amounts of male hormones are needed for this to occur. The incidence of true undescended testis is, on average, 26.5% in the premature infant and 3.2% in the term baby, decreasing to 5.4% and 0.5%, respectively, at 1 year of age. A patent processus vaginalis or a true hernia is also present in more than 90% of the cases.

Associated Conditions

The workup and treatment for cryptorchidism depends on the physical examination and the presence of other anomalies. Generally, the criptorchid testis is unilateral and often palpable within the inguinal canal. In some cases, use of laparoscopy, ultrasound, computed tomography (CT), or hormonal therapy is useful as an adjunct in the workup and treatment for nonpalpable, unilateral, and bilateral undescended testes. There is an occasional association with congenital adrenal hyperplasia and the appearance of bilateral cryptorchidism as well as potential intersex anomalies in the cryptorchid patient with hypospadias. Cryptorchidism is associated with urinary tract anomalies, with an overall incidence of 10%. The incidence of upper urinary tract anomalies is greatest in patients with a family history of urinary tract malformations and in patients with multiple associated anomalies. Screening of these patients by ultrasound or intravenous pyelography (IVP) should be considered. There are also possible abnormalities of the vas and epididymis seen with cryptorchidism. This section discusses the palpable testis that cannot be manipulated into the scrotum. This includes the true undescended testis as well as the ectopic testis, which travels through the inguinal canal but is misdirected into the high suprapubic area or perineum.

Clinical Findings

In making the diagnosis, it is important to distinguish between the retractile and the true undescended testis. Retractile testes lie high in the scrotum or superficial inguinal pouch and can be manipulated into the scrotum. They do not require surgery. The child with true cryptorchidism has a flat, poorly developed scrotum on the ipsilateral side. The child should be examined in both the supine and upright positions. With warm hands, the inguinal canal is milked toward the scrotum. A similar examination should be performed with the child under anesthesia. If the testicle can be brought into the scrotum at either time, surgery is not indicated, because the testicle can be expected to descend on its own once puberty and adult levels of hormone are achieved.

Surgery: Indications and Timing

Most undescended testes descend on their own by the end of the child's first year of life. Observation until the child is 2 years of age is appropriate unless an associated hernia becomes symptomatic, requiring repair. The orchiopexy and hernia repair should then be performed together. Delay of surgery until the child is 2 years of age is preferable because of the delicacy of the infant's spermatic cord. Further delay incurs the risk of injury to the testis and is not warranted. In the postpubertal boy discovered to have cryptorchidism, the decision to perform orchiopexy or orchioectomy must be made. This is controversial, with advocates for both procedures, although the exact timing and age at which orchioectomy should be performed is also debated. Most pediatric surgeons, however, would advocate removal of the abdominally located testis and placement of a prosthesis in the postpubertal child, at least after he reaches age 16 years.

The child's parents must understand the goals and limitations of orchiopexy. The cryptorchid testis is more prone to trauma and torsion. Orchiopexy reduces these concerns. Because the scrotal and cremaster thermal regulatory machanism is absent, spermatogenesis may be altered in the cryptorchid testis because the testicle is subject to increased temperature. In addition, in boys with unilateral undescended testis, the contralateral scrotal testis may be abnormal, representing acquired disease. Testicular injury increases with duration and degree of undescent, although before the child's second or third birthday, this injury is probably minimal or nonexistent. Some studies show that fertility is improved after orchiopexy, but conclusive results are not available. The incidence of malignancy of the testis is approximately 0.0021% in the adult male population. This is increased 40 times in the cryptorchid population. Surgery does not decrease the incidence of malignancy but allows for earlier detection, because the testis can be more easily examined. An additional concern is physical appearance. This becomes more important as a child reaches school age and is subject to the scrutiny and possible ridicule by classmates. Orchiopexy is therefore best performed on preschoolers.

Technique

Orchiopexy is commonly done as an outpatient procedure using general anesthesia. Only standard orchiopexy is described here. An incision similar to that for inguinal hernia is made, although it is necessary to extend the incision more laterally for exposure. Scarpa's fascia is opened and the external oblique fascia is incised through the ring (Fig. 47–5A). Quite often, the testis is found within the canal or just at the internal ring. It is gently elevated into the incision and dissected free of the

remaining gubernaculum and surrounding adhesions (see Fig. 47–5B). The cremaster muscle is then mobilized from the cord, and the muscle fibers are divided. Associated hernias are in the usual anterior medial location and must be dissected free from the cord structures so that a high ligation may be performed (see Fig. 47–5C and D).

The greatest limiting factor in gaining adequate length on the cord is caused by the spermatic vessels. A narrow ribbon retractor is placed within the internal ring posterior to the hernia sac and peritoneum and is elevated to expose the retroperitoneal space. The internal ring may need to be opened superiorly to facilitate this exposure. The greatest point of attachment to the vessels is the lateral spermatic fascia proximal to the point where the vas diverges from the cord (see Fig. 47–5E). This fascia is divided, whereas much of the other surrounding loose tissue can be teased away from the vessels using gentle blunt dissection. This is performed up to the lower pole of the kidney. Usually, this provides adequate length. If further length is needed, the testis and cord structures can be transposed beneath the inferior epigastric vessels and fascia transversalis to create a more direct line between the abdomen and scrotum. This may be done by either dividing the vessels and fascia with resuture of the fascia over the cord or by drawing the testis and cord beneath these structures with a right angle clamp, exiting via a new opening near the pubic tubercle. In so doing, care must be taken to avoid injury to the peritoneum.

A tunnel is then made into the scrotum with a finger or ribbon retractor. This also enables the surgeon to stretch the scrotum to accommodate the testicle. A scrotal skin incision is made and a pouch created between the skin and dartos fascia by blunt dissection (see Fig. 47–5F). A hemostat placed through the scrotal incision is used to pierce the dartos fascia and create an opening through which the testis is drawn into the pouch. Care must be taken to avoid twisting the spermatic vessels at this stage. The opening in the dartos should be as small as possible so that the testis does not retract back through it into the inguinal canal. The tunica testis should be sutured to the dartos or the testis pexed to the septum to

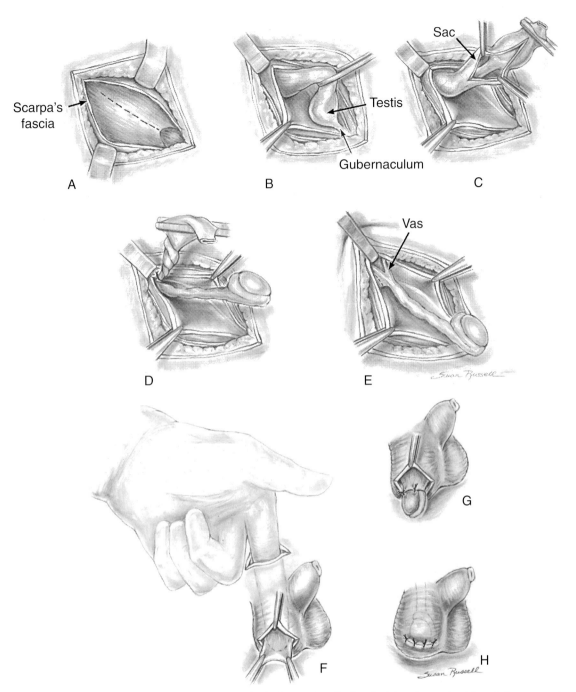

Figure 47–5. Orchiopexy. **(A)** An incision is made similar to that for inguinal hernia repair, although it may need lateral extension. Scarpa's fascia is opened and the external oblique fascia is incised through the external ring. **(B)** The testis is dissected from surrounding adhesions and the gubernaculum is divided. **(C and D)** There is often an associated hernia sac in the anteromedial position. This must be dissected from the cord vessels and vas and a high ligation performed. Cremasteric muscle fibers surrounding the cord structures are divided to help gain adequate cord length. **(E)** A ribbon retractor is placed in the internal ring to expose the retroperitoneum and lateral spermatic fascia. This fascia is cut (*dotted line*) and loose adhesions around the spermatic vessels are divided to gain further cord length. The vas diverges medially toward the pelvis. **(F)** A tunnel is made into the scrotum and a scrotal incision is made. A pouch is created between the skin and dartos fascia, and the fascia is incised. **(G)** The testis is pulled through the dartos fascia, and the fascia is sutured to the tunica testis. **(H)** The testis is placed into the dartos pouch, and the scrotal incision is closed with absorbable suture.

prevent torsion (see Fig. 47–5G). Some surgeons may further secure the testis by passing a suture through the distal tunica and then out of the scrotum beneath the incision, tying this to a button or dental roll. The scrotal incision is closed with chromic sutures to obviate the need for suture removal and is dressed with collodion (see Fig. 47–5H). The groin incision is closed as described for hernia repair.

Complications

The potential complications of orchiopexy are similar to those of inguinal hernia repair, with potential injury to the spermatic cord structures being the most significant. Injuries severe enough to compromise the gonad occur in less than 5% of cases. Retraction of the testis is uncommon. Testicular atrophy and subsequent decrease in function may be caused by vascular injury, either directly or secondary to excess tension when placing the testis into the scrotum. Adequate mobilization of the spermatic cord with dissection into the retroperitoneum is therefore necessary.

The parents and then the child, when he is old enough, should be told about the importance of regular testicular self-examination to detect early any malignancy that might occur.

Follow-up

A routine postoperative clinic visit is usual, with further visits scheduled as needed to ensure that the testis remains in the scrotum once the postoperative scrotal swelling resolves. The testes themselves may frequently swell, due to partial lymphatic and venous obstruction, but this usually resolves in 2 to 4 weeks. Long-term follow-up with testicular examination can usually be provided in the pediatrician's office.

As with hernia repair, there is little restriction of activity in younger children because such restriction cannot be enforced. Plastic film or collodion dressings keep the incision dry and separate the incision from urine and stool. Activity in older children is limited as comfort allows, although activity such as bike riding should be avoided for several weeks.

Selected Readings

1. Cox JA. Inguinal hernia of childhood. Surg Clin North Am 1985;65(5):1331–1342.
2. Fonkalsrud EW. Undescended testes. In: Welch KJ, Randolph JG, Ravitch MM, O'Neill JA, Rowe MI, eds. Pediatric Surgery. 4th ed. Chicago: Year Book Medical, 1986:793.
3. Grosfeld JL. Current concepts in inguinal hernia in infants and children. World J Surg 1989;13(5):506–515.
4. Moss RL, Hatch EI Jr. Inguinal hernia repair in early infancy. Am J Surg 1991;161(5):596–599.
5. Neblett WW III, Holcomb GW III. Umbilical and other abdominal wall hernias. In: Ashcroft KW, Holder TM, eds. Pediatric Surgery. 2nd ed. Philadelphia: WB Saunders, 1993:557.
6. Othersen HB Jr. The pediatric inguinal hernia. Surg Clin North Am 1993;73(4):853–859.
7. Rowe MI, Lloyd DA. Inguinal hernia. In: Welch KJ, Randolph JG, Ravitch MM, O'Neill JA, Rowe ME, eds. Pediatric Surgery. 4th ed. Chicago: Year Book Medical, 1986:779.
8. Sheldon CA. Undescended testis and testicular torsion. Surg Clin North Am 1985;65(5):1303–1330.
9. Skandalakis JE, Colborn GL, Androulakis JA, et al. Embryologic and anatomic basis of inguinal herniorrhaphy. Surg Clin North Am 1993;73(4):798–836.
10. Skinner MA, Grosfeld JL. Inguinal and umbilical hernia repair in infants and children. Surg Clin North Am 1993;73(3):438–448.
11. Weber TR, Tracy TF Jr. Groin hernias and hydroceles. In: Ashcraft KW, Holder TM, eds. Pediatric Surgery. 2nd ed. Philadelphia: WB Saunders, 1993:562.

Chapter 48

Special Considerations for Outpatient Pediatric Surgery

Eugene D. McGahren III

ENLARGED LYMPH NODES

General Considerations in Children

Enlarged lymph nodes are a common finding in infants and children. Usually, they represent a reaction to regional scratches or superficial infections. Enlarged nodes that require surgical intervention result from group A streptococcal or staphylococcal infections, nontuberculous mycobacterial infection, cat scratch disease or Hodgkin and non-Hodgkin lymphomas. Other causes of lymph node enlargement include fungal infections, tuberculosis, mononucleosis, taxoplasmosis, brucellosis, tularemia, or infection with cytomegalovirus, Epstein-Barr virus, or human immunodeficiency virus (HIV). Lymph nodes usually come to attention when they are visible or palpable in the cervical, supraclavicular, axillary, or inguinal regions. A careful history should be taken to investigate for fever, night sweats, weight loss, fatigue, exposure to cat or other animal scratches, exposure to individuals with bacterial or viral infections, erythema or drainage of the involved nodal area, and the time course for the enlargement of the node or nodes in question. Investigative studies may include a chest radiograph, a computed tomography (CT) scan of the chest or involved nodal area, a tuberculin skin test, skin or serology test for cat scratch disease, a monospot test, and a complete blood count, depending on the suspicions raised by the history and physical examination. This section addresses selected causes of lymph node enlargement that often lead to surgical intervention. General principles of lymph node excision are also addressed.

Suppurative Lymphadenitis

Suppurative lymphadenitis is usually caused by a primary infection from a group A streptococcal or staphylococcal species, or by secondary infection of an inflamed lymph node by these same organisms. Antecedent history may include a viral illness, pharyngitis, local trauma, or infection of the skin. Usually, involved nodes are single or closely approximated in the cervical region, although axillary and inguinal regions may be alternative sites of involvement. Symptoms and signs include fever, overlying erythema, and leukocytosis. Antibiotics may provide definitive treatment and prevent abscess formation. If abscess formation occurs, however, needle aspiration or formal incision and drainage combined with antibiotics result in a cure. If incision and drainage is necessary, the wound should be washed daily. In children, this is easily accomplished with a bath of hot, soapy water, with the skin edges of the wound teased open by the parent or caretaker. A gauze strip may then be placed in the wound to keep the skin open so that healing may occur from the inside. There is no need for aggressive or deep packing of the wound. Occasionally, a suppurative lymph node or nodes effectively encase a small abscess or otherwise remain enlarged after antibiotic treatment. In such cases, the persistent enlargement necessitates removal for cure or to rule out a malignancy.

Atypical Mycobacterial Lymphadenitis

Atypical mycobacterial lymphadenitis results from infection from nontuberculous (atypical) mycobacterial species. Even though there are 13 such strains, *Mycobacterium avium* accounts for 80% of clinical infections in children. *Mycobacterium kansasii* and *Mycobacterium scrofulaceum* account for virtually all of the rest. These bacteria live in soil. Children, typically aged 1 to 5 years, inoculate themselves by playing in contaminated soil or water and introducing the bacteria through their mouths. Constitutional symptoms are usually not present. Lymphadenitis is the most common manifestation of infection, primarily affecting superior cervical or submandibular nodes. Posterior cervical, auricular, axillary, or inguinal nodes may also be affected. In some instances, enlarged lymph nodes resolve spontaneously, but most progress to suppuration and subsequent chronic drainage, which can persist for months.

Exclusion of a tuberculous cause of the lymphadenitis may be necessary. Children with nontuberculous mycobacterial infections typically have anterior cervical node involvement, a normal chest radiograph, no history of exposure to individuals with tuberculosis, and a moderate response (3–15 mm) to a medium-strength tuberculin skin test. In contrast, children with nodal manifestation of tuberculous infection characteristically have posterior cervical node involvement, an abnormal chest radiograph, a history of exposure, and a strong response to a skin test.

Diagnosis and definitive treatment of nontuberculous mycobacterial lymphadenitis is accomplished by removal of involved nodes. Often, a collection of closely clustered nodes is present and it is necessary to remove all nodes that are visibly abnormal to avoid leaving any infection behind. If drainage has occurred before removal, it is best to delay surgery until healing is as complete as possible to optimize conditions for dissection and excision. Antituberculin medication is not needed with complete excision.

Cat Scratch Disease

Cat scratch disease is the most common cause of chronic lymphadenopathy in children. It commonly results from an infected scratch by a cat or kitten, but it may result from scratches from other animals as well. An incubation period of approximately 2 weeks precedes lymph node enlargement in the nodal region draining the scratched area. Usually, axillary nodes are involved because scratches tend to occur on the arms. However, epitrochlear, inguinal, cervical, and submandibular nodes are occasionally affected.

The nomenclature surrounding the offending infectious agent has been confusing. *Afipsia felis* was once thought to be the cause of cat scratch disease. More recently, *Rochalimea henselae* has been identified as the likely infectious agent. However, the name *Bartonella* now replaces the genus name *Rochalimea*.

Affected lymph nodes enlarge over a period of weeks before receding in size. Resolution of the enlargement usually takes 2 to 4 months, but may take longer. Overlying erythema may be present when nodes are at their largest, but cellulitis, suppuration, and drainage are relatively rare. Other clinical manifestations may include fever, fatigue, malaise, headache, or anorexia, but these are unusual in children.

Diagnosis is suggested by a history of a cat scratch or exposure to cats. Definitive diagnosis may be made by a positive skin test for cat scratch disease or by the presence of a serologic antibody to *Bartonella henselae*. If cat scratch disease is diagnosed, nodes may be allowed to regress spontaneously. In the absence of such information, however, other investigations may be necessary to rule out other causes of the lymphadenopathy. When the diagnosis is in doubt, removal of the affected node is necessary. Cat scratch disease may then be definitively diagnosed after histopathologic examination.

LYMPHOMA

The most significant concern raised by the presence of enlarged lymph nodes in a child is that of lymphoma. Both Hodgkin and non-Hodgkin lymphoma may present with enlarged lymph nodes in one or more locations.

These nodes tend to be firm, nontender, and discrete and may or may not be mobile. An affected child may be asymptomatic or may exhibit symptoms such as fever, weight loss, night sweats (the "B" symptoms of Hodgkin lymphoma), cough, abdominal pain, or superior vena cava syndrome. Children suspected of having Hodgkin or non-Hodgkin lymphoma require extensive imaging and blood workup, but the diagnosis hinges on examination of biopsied tissue, usually an excised lymph node.

Hodgkin lymphoma commonly presents with painless enlargement of lymph nodes in cervical, supraclavicular, axillary, or inguinal regions, with no obvious inciting cause. Such nodes are usually easily accessible, and an excised node serves as a superior pathologic specimen when compared to a needle-aspirated specimen. Non-Hodgkin lymphoma often involves symptoms that result from tumor involvement of chest, mediastinal, or abdominal structures. Easily accessible enlarged lymph nodes are not often present, but, when they are, they tend to occur in the head and neck region. Children with non-Hodgkin lymphoma sometimes suffer symptoms that require immediate attention with hospitalization and workup. However, if enlarged lymph nodes are the only manifestation of disease, diagnosis may be pursued on an outpatient basis while other potential causes of lymph node enlargement are being ruled out.

Surgical Considerations for Lymph Node Removal in Children

In children, lymph node removal for diagnosis or cure can usually be accomplished on an outpatient basis. In most cases, a general anesthetic is required. Occasionally, a discrete, solitary lymph node may be removed from a cooperative adolescent using sedation and local anesthetic. Depending on the location of the node, it is usually possible to identify a natural skin crease in which to make an incision. Careful dissection is necessary so as not to disrupt nodal tissue; this can be accomplished by manipulating perinodal tissue rather than the node itself for traction and exposure. Fine scissors and cautery are necessary for dissection, and any significant vascular

or lymphatic channels connected to the lymph node should be ligated to avoid hematoma or seroma formation.

If nodal enlargement is caused by an inflammatory or infectious process, it is necessary to remove any obviously involved nodes to provide definitive treatment if the infecting agent turns out to be nontuberculous mycobacteria. Dissection planes may be compromised and care must be taken to avoid injuring surrounding vessels and nerves. In some instances, treatment with antibiotics and, if necessary, drainage of an obvious fluctuant region may be required before surgery to minimize the inflammatory changes at surgery. If lymphoma is suspected, the removal of two or three of the largest nodes (if more than one is obvious) is sufficient to make the diagnosis.

In all cases, swabs and specimens should be sent for Gram stain, acid-fast stain, and aerobic and anaerobic bacterial, fungal, viral, and mycobacterial cultures. The pathologic specimen should be sent fresh so that appropriate processing may be done for tumor studies if indicated.

Primary wound closure can usually be accomplished. In small children, absorbable subcuticular sutures are used to avoid the trauma of subsequent removal of sutures. If concern for infection exists, a subcuticular monofilament suture may be preferable, because it may be removed early if infection ensues; otherwise, it allows excellent cosmetic results when removed at 5 to 10 days after a normal healing process. Clear adhesive strips are used to reinforce the wound.

LUMPS AND BUMPS

Sebaceous Cyst

Sebaceous glands occur in all regions of the body except the palms, soles, and dorsa of the feet. Each gland consists of a peripheral layer of flat cells and a central layer of lipidized cells. Lipidized cells disintegrate during their migration toward the central duct and form sebum. Sebum consists of cellular debris, triglycerides, phospholipids, and cholesterol. If a gland becomes occluded, a sebaceous cyst forms. These cysts tend to be firm, discrete,

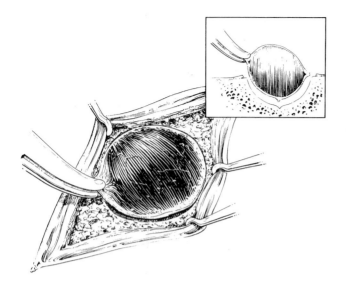

Figure 48–1. An epidermoid cyst positioned within the periosteum and causing an indentation of underlying bone. (From Dudley H, Carter DC, Russell RCE, Spitz L, Nixon HH. Rob and Smith's Operative Surgery, Pediatric Surgery. 4th ed. London: Butterworths, 1988.)

spherical lesions and may be adherent to overlying skin. In some cases, an area of pointing may be evident. Sebaceous cysts may become intermittently inflamed or infected, sometimes requiring antibiotic therapy or incision and drainage for relief of infection. If drained, however, the cysts will recur after drainage.

Definitive treatment requires excision of the cyst. An elliptical incision is made over the area of the cyst, incorporating the adherent or pointing area within the skin ellipse. The cyst is then carefully removed in its entirety by careful sharp dissection. Care should be taken to avoid rupture of the cyst because this increases the possibility of infection and increases the likelihood that cyst tissue will be left behind with subsequent regeneration of the cyst. A sebaceous cyst that is removed in its entirety should not recur.

Dermoid Cyst

Dermoid cysts are lined by epidermis and contain epidermal appendages such as keratin and hair. These cysts are caused by sequestration of epithelium along lines of embryonic fusion. Thus, they present as firm, round, sometimes movable masses at the corners of the eye, the midline of the nose, the lateral aspect of the eyebrow, over suture lines in the scalp, and in the midline and lateral aspects of the neck.

Like sebaceous cysts, dermoid cysts may be-

come inflamed or infected. An infected cyst should be treated with antibiotics or incised and drained. When discovered, a dermoid cyst should be removed. It tends to be deep-seated and may actually sit within the periosteum and cause an indentation of underlying bone (Fig. 48–1). Although it may be firmly adherent to underlying tissue, it is still amenable to complete dissection along a clean dissection plane. An encephalocele may present similarly to a cranial dermoid cyst; a CT scan of the head easily differentiates between these two lesions.

Thyroglossal Duct Cyst

During embryologic development, the thyroid gland tissue migrates from the foramen cecum to its normal resting position. Tissue remnants from this migration can form a thyroglossal duct cyst. The cyst and its associated duct consist of stratified squamous, or ciliated, pseudostratified columnar epithelium with associated mucus-secreting cells. The duct connects the cyst to the site of the foramen cecum at the base of the tongue. A thyroglossal duct cyst does not open to the skin, which helps to differentiate it from a branchial cleft remnant.

A thyroglossal duct cyst usually presents as a relatively discrete midline neck mass that moves up and down with swallowing. In some cases, the first manifestation of a cyst may be infection requiring antibiotics or drainage. When discovered, and after any active infection is resolved, the cyst should be removed. Consideration may be given to obtaining a thyroid scan to determine whether the cyst is actually aberrant thyroid tissue. If it is, then it may be the only thyroid tissue present. Even if the lesion is thyroid, however, it should still probably be removed because malignant degeneration of such tissue has been reported.

Cyst resection (Sistrunk procedure) begins with an elliptical incision around the cyst area. A wide dissection around the duct is then performed up to the hyoid bone. The middle third of the bone is resected with bone cutters, and dissection around the duct continues up to the base of the tongue. It is helpful for the anesthesiologist to press on the base of the tongue from inside the mouth to facilitate the final portion of the dissection. A suture ligature of absorbable suture is placed to close the duct at the underside of the tongue. The duct, cyst, and hyoid segment are removed in continuity (Fig. 48–2). The incision is closed in layers, and a subcuticular closure using absorbable suture may be performed. If any tissue is left behind, recurrent infection or cyst growth may occur, requiring re-excision. If the pathologic specimen reveals thyroid tissue, a thyroid scan is indicated to determine whether any normal thyroid gland exists. If it does not, thyroid supplementation is needed.

Hemangioma

Hemangiomas represent abnormal endothelial cell proliferation and may manifest in a variety of types, sizes and locations. They are the most common birth defect. The most common types of hemangiomas in children are juvenile hemangiomas. These include the strawberry mark, the strawberry capillary hemangioma, and the capillary-cavernous hemangioma. The strawberry mark is characterized by a pale halo surrounding a telengiectasia of 1 to 3.5 cm. It invariably resolves spontaneously. A strawberry capillary hemangioma is often not evident at birth, but manifests as a small red spot after a few weeks of life. It grows rapidly over the ensuing 3 to 12 months before resolving by age 1 to 4. The capillary-cavernous hemangioma is characterized by a large venous component and presents as a spongy, bluish lesion with an overlying capillary component. This lesion may resolve spontaneously, but is more likely to remain stable in size, or even grow. The presence of a cutaneous hemangioma in a child should always prompt questioning about airway difficulties, cardiopulmonary status, hepatomegaly, or easy bleeding because concurrent hemangiomas of the airway or the liver may cause such complications.

Hemangiomas amenable to outpatient surgery are those cutaneous hemangiomas that do not resolve by age 4, are complicated by ulceration, bleeding, or infection, or that cause an undesirable cosmetic appearance. A small hemangioma of this nature can usually be excised using an appropriately sized elliptical incision with primary closure. However, there should be no cosmetic or functional risk taken in removing hemangiomas because of their propensity for spontaneous resolution. If a hemangioma causes obstruction of vision, obstruction of a lumenal structure, thrombocytopenia, atypical growth of an organ, or cardiopulmonary decompensation from arteriovenous shunting, more extensive evaluation and therapy are necessary.

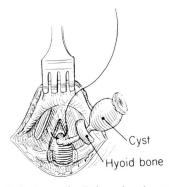

Figure 48–2. Removal of thyroglossal cyst and tract along with middle third of the hyoid bone (Sistrunk procedure). (From Rowe MI, O'Neill JA, Grosfeld JL, et al, eds. Essentials of Pediatric Surgery. St Louis: Mosby, 1995:330.)

Lymphangioma

Lymphangiomas result from lymphatic duct obstruction or malformation in utero. A lymphangioma that is primarily cystic is termed "cystic hygroma." These lesions are usually found in the cervical, axillary, mediastinal, or inguinal region. They may present as well-demarcated, isolated lesions or as infiltrative lesions with extensions that enwrap adjacent structures.

A lymphangioma is often obvious at birth as a visible prominence. However, it may go unnoticed until inflammation or infection causes acute swelling and possibly overlying cellulitis. Once a lymphangioma is identified, imaging studies such as ultrasound, CT, or magnetic resonance imaging (MRI) scanning should be obtained to evaluate the extent of the lesion. This is especially true if the lesion occurs in the neck because it may encircle vital structures and extend into the mediastinum.

In some cases, an isolated small lymphangioma is amenable to removal on an outpatient basis. Removal is accomplished by careful sharp and blunt dissection around the cystic structure. Care is taken to keep the lymphangioma intact so that the planes for dissection are more easily identified. Any lymphatic channels leading into the lesion should be ligated to prevent formation of a seroma. Definitive treatment of a lymphangioma requires complete excision. However, vital structures should *never* be sacrificed for the sake of removing all portions of a lymphangioma. Unexcised portions of a lymphangioma may cause regeneration of the lesion, although they occasionally obliterate. An extensive lymphangioma that appears amenable only to partial resection requires careful preoperative planning and hospital admission. Future repeat resections may be necessary, although sclerosing agents such as bleomycin or OK-432 may be of some help in the treatment of a large infiltrative lesion.

Branchial Cleft Remnants

The branchial arches represent embryologic centers of development of head and neck structures. Each arch is considered to have a cleft and a pouch. The first cleft forms the external auditory canal while the remaining clefts obliterate. The first pouch forms the eustachian tube, the middle ear cavity, and the mastoid air cells; the second pouch forms the palatine tonsils and supratonsillar fossa; the third pouch forms the inferior parathyroid

and thymus glands; and the fourth pouch forms the superior parathyroid glands. Cysts, sinuses, fistulas, and ectopic cartilage may persist as remnants of these arches, commonly termed "branchial cleft remnants."

Remnants of the second cleft are the most common. The external opening, if present, is located along the midanterior border of the sternocleidomastoid muscle. If the remnant exists as a true fistula, it courses upward between the external and internal carotid arteries, over the hypoglossal and glossopharyngeal nerves to the pharynx.

A remnant of the first cleft manifests as a skin dimple or ectopic cartilage anterior to the ear. The tract of this remnant passes in close proximity to the facial nerve on its course to the external auditory canal.

A third branchial cleft remnant presents externally just superior to the medial head of the clavicle. Its tract courses lateral to the bifurcation of the common carotid artery, superior to the spinal accessory nerve, and to the piriform fossa. Remnants of the first and third branchial cleft remnants are relatively rare.

A branchial cleft remnant usually presents as a skin dimple, draining area, or cyst in the area appropriate for the particular cleft. If the lesion is a true fistula of second or third cleft origin, then saliva or formula chronically drains from the external opening. Occasionally, infection is the presenting manifestation, dictating antibiotic therapy and possibly incision and drainage. Branchial cleft remnants do not resolve spontaneously and there may be a long-term risk of malignant change if the remnant is still present in adulthood. For all of these reasons, excision is recommended when a branchial remnant is discovered. Excision begins with an elliptical incision incorporating the external site. Dissection is then carried out along the tract, taking care to protect surrounding structures (Fig. 48–3). It is helpful to gently manipulate a small lacrimal duct probe into the dimple within the ellipse of skin and up the tract to more easily follow the course of the tract. Injection of dyes or methylene blue for this purpose results in diffuse staining and blurs dissection planes. Dissection is carried out until a blind ending sinus or cyst is encountered. If a fistula is present, dissection is carried as high as possi-

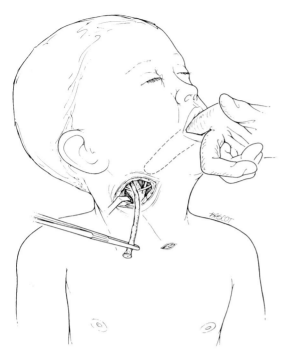

Figure 48–3. Excision of a second branchial cleft fistula. The anesthesiologist's finger facilitates the higher portion of the dissection by depressing the pharynx. (From Raffensperger JG. Congenital cysts and sinuses of the neck. In: Raffensperger JG, ed. Swenson's Pediatric Surgery. 5th ed. Norwalk, CT: Appleton & Lange, 1990.)

ble. A second or third counterincision made parallel and superior to the first may be required. In the case of second and third branchial remnants, the anesthesiologist may facilitate the higher portion of the dissection by depressing the tongue or pharynx with a finger. The superior portion of the fistula is suture ligated and the tract is then removed. Primary closure is then accomplished. Recurrence may occur if the remnant is not entirely resected. Excision of a branchial remnant may usually be accomplished on an outpatient basis; however, removal of a fistula or bilateral fistulas warrants consideration for hospital admission to ensure that swallowing and breathing are not compromised.

Torticollis

Torticollis represents fibrosis of the midportion of the sternocleidomastoid muscle. It usually presents in infants and may be secondary to a breech presentation or other difficulty in delivery. The infant's head is rotated away from the side of the lesion and toward the ipsilateral shoulder. The fibrosis is palpable as a mass at the midsternocleidomastoid muscle, which is frequently the reason why such infants are brought to attention. If torticollis is not addressed, asymmetry of the head and neck structures may ensue.

Most infants with torticollis do not require surgery. Massage of the fibrotic area, gentle rotation of the neck, and stimulation designed to cause the infant to turn its head toward the side of the torticollis allow resolution over a number of weeks. When torticollis does not respond to such treatment and asymmetry of head and neck structures is becoming evident, surgical intervention is warranted. This usually occurs at 6- to 12-months of age for an infant.

Surgical treatment involves resection of the middle third of the sternocleidomastoid muscle through a lateral supraclavicular incision. The muscle should not be reapproximated because new scarring and fibrosis may result. Physical therapy is undertaken postoperatively to ensure full range of motion of the neck. The remaining sternocleidomastoid muscle atrophies and any asymmetry resolves.

Gynecomastia

Gynecomastia represents enlargement of the breast tissue in males. Characteristically, this occurs in early adolescence and is transient in nature, lasting from a few months to 2 years. The pubertal boy has a gradual growth of tissue under his nipple with some mild tenderness. Attention should be paid to any evidence of nipple discharge or testicular abnormalities because these may represent the presence of a prolactinoma or a gonadal tumor. Also, ingestion of exogenous estrogens or steroids should be ruled out.

If gynecomastia causes undue discomfort, cosmetic abnormality, or emotional distress, removal of breast tissue may be warranted. This is accomplished through a 180° incision along the lower half of the areolar border. All breast tissue down to the pectoral fascia, including the axillary tail, is removed. Care should be taken to remove all breast tissue adherent to the nipple. Subcutaneous fat is

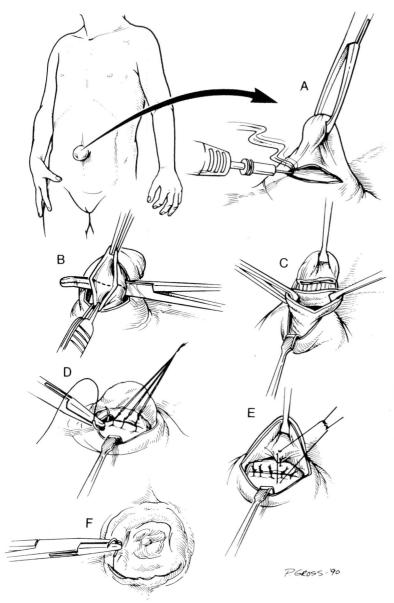

Figure 48–4. Technique for umbilical hernia repair: **A,** An infra-umbilical skin crease incision is made. **B,** The hernia sac is opened, leaving a portion of the sac attached to the umbilical skin. **C,** The umbilical sac is completely divided and excised to strong fascia. **D,** The fascial defect is closed in a transverse fashion with interrupted simple sutures. **E,** The remaining umbilical sac, which is attached to the umbilical skin, is secured to fascia with interrupted absorbable sutures. **F,** The skin is closed with a subcuticular suture. Pressure dressing is placed to prevent formation of a hematoma or seroma. (From Neblet WW III, Holcomb GW III. Umbilical and other abdominal wall hernias. In: Ashcraft KW, Holder TM, eds. Pediatric Surgery. 2nd ed. Philadelphia: WB Saunders, 1993:559.)

reapproximated under the nipple to avoid an indented appearance. A drain may be needed if the amount of tissue removed is substantial. The skin incision is closed in a subcuticular manner with fine absorbable suture.

If an obese male desires mastectomy for gynecomastia, it is first prudent to initiate a diet and exercise plan to accomplish weight loss. This may help resolve the gynecomastia. However, if mastectomy is still indicated, weight loss allows a better cosmetic result.

Prominent breast buds of prepubescent girls may be caused by a variety of factors, almost always benign, and cause should be sought through all nonsurgical avenues possible. Procedures done on the female breast bud in prepubescent girls may significantly compromise breast development later on.

UMBILICAL ANOMALIES

Umbilical Hernia

An umbilical hernia results from failure of the fascial ring to close around the umbilicus. It is a common lesion, with an incidence of approximately 5% in white infants and 30% to 35% in black infants. Umbilical hernias occur with equal frequency in boys and girls, but are seen with an increased frequency in premature infants, and in infants with Down syndrome, congenital hypothyroidism, mucopolysaccharidoses, and Beckwith-Wiedemann syndrome. Umbilical hernias are rarely symptomatic. The cosmetic appearance is usually the greatest concern. Most hernias close spontaneously by 5 years of age. Thus, observation is justified as long as a hernia is progressively getting smaller. Indications for surgery in children younger than 5 years of age include an unusually large protrusion of the skin resulting in excoriation, a fascial defect greater then 1.5 to 2 cm at 2 to 3 years of age, pain, incarceration, or strangulation of hernia contents. Occasionally, an older child or adolescent is seen with an umbilical hernia either found on a routine examination or because of umbilical pain caused by incarceration of preperitoneal fat. Repair should be undertaken in these children when the lesion is discovered.

An umbilical hernia is approached through an infraumbilical curvilinear incision (Fig. 48–4). Dissection is performed around the sac. The sac may be divided after making sure it is free of any bowel. The sac edges are excised to expose clean fascial edges. The fascia is then reapproximated transversely with interrupted sutures. Techniques accomplishing multiple fascial closure, such as the "vest-over-pants" technique, are not necessary. Excess sac tissue on the underside of the umbilical skin is excised. However, the sac tissue most adherent to the subdermis may be left behind to avoid damage to the skin and aid with umbilicoplasty. Strict hemostasis is accomplished to avoid hematoma formation. The underside of the skin is then secured down to the fascia. The subcutaneous layer is closed with interrupted absorbable suture and the skin is closed in subcuticular fashion with absorbable suture. A pressure dressing is left in place for 48 hours. Recurrences are rare and are due to inadequate technique, hematoma formation, or infection.

Umbilical Granulomas and Polyps

An umbilical granuloma is a persistent, friable portion of granulation tissue remaining

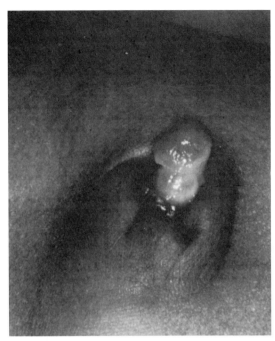

Figure 48–5. Demonstration of a patent urachus and bladder through injection of an umbilical sinus. (From Jona JZ. Umbilical anomalies. In: Raffensperger JG, Swenson's Pediatric Surgery. 5th ed. Norwalk, CT: Appleton & Lange, 1990.)

after sloughing of the umbilical cord. An umbilical polyp can look like a granuloma, but may also be a larger, cherry-red nodule (Fig. 48–5). A polyp represents a remnant of the vitelline duct and may contain ectopic gastric or small intestinal mucosa. Both lesions are characterized by a persistent serous drainage sometimes associated with surrounding erythema or frank cellulitis. An umbilical granuloma usually resolves with one or two applications of silver nitrate. If the lesion in question persists despite such treatment, however, it is probably a polyp. An umbilical exploration is thus warranted. Through an infraumbilical curvilinear incision, the umbilical stalk is dissected free and removed from the surrounding fascia. The fascia is closed as in an umbilical hernia repair. The stalk is removed in continuity with the involved umbilical skin. The skin may be closed from the underside with an absorbable suture and then secured to the fascia.

Urachal Duct Remnants

The urachal duct connects the umbilicus to the bladder during embryologic development.

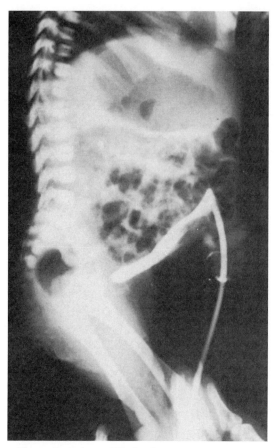

Figure 48–6. An umbilical polyp consisting of ileal mucosa. (From Jona JZ. Umbilical anomalies. In: Raffensperger JG, ed. Swenson's Pediatric Surgery. 5th ed. Norwalk, CT: Appleton & Lange, 1990.)

A remnant may exist as a cyst, a sinus, or a fistula. A urachal cyst presents as an enlarging or infected mass. Infection may proceed to abscess formation or frank peritonitis in the case of rupture. A cyst may present early in life or exist indolently for years before becoming symptomatic.

A urachal sinus usually presents with persistent drainage or infection. A fistula presents with persistent drainage of urine. Drainage may be voluminous if the infant or child suffers from any type of bladder outlet obstruction. In addition, the fistulous tract may allow bacteria into the bladder, resulting in urinary tract infections. In some cases, a fistula is actually discovered on a vesicoureterogram performed on a child for frequent urinary tract infections. Often, the diagnosis of a urachal remnant is apparent after a history and physi-

cal examination. However, the diagnosis may be confirmed by injecting radiographic contrast into the draining site (Fig. 48–6).

A urachal remnant may usually be removed electively. This is best approached through a curvilinear infraumbilical skin incision. A vertical incision in the fascia allows the best exposure of the remnant as well as access to the dome of the bladder. The entire remnant, including the involved umbilical skin should be removed. The opening, if any, at the dome of the bladder is closed with absorbable suture to avoid bladder stones that can result from nonabsorbable suture. Closure of the fascia and reapproximation of subcutaneous and cutaneous tissue is accomplished as described for umbilical hernias.

Omphalomesenteric Remnant

An omphalomesenteric remnant arises from the embryologic vitelline duct. It may manifest as a cyst, sinus, or fistula and often has a fistulous or atretic, band-like connection to the small intestine. An associated Meckel diverticulum may be present (Fig. 48–7). Enteric contents may drain through the umbilical lesion, and, occasionally, frank mucosal prolapse may occur. Rarely, bowel obstruction may result from volvulus around an intact tract. Outpatient surgery is limited to cysts and sinuses. Exploration is undertaken as described for the other umbilical anomalies in this section. The fascia may be opened either transversely or

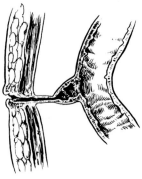

Figure 48–7. A patent omphalomesenteric duct with associated Meckel's diverticulum. (From Jona JZ. Umbilical anomalies. In: Raffensperger JG, ed. Swenson's Pediatric Surgery. 5th ed. Norwalk, CT: Appleton & Lange, 1990.)

vertically. If there is a patent tract to the bowel or a Meckel diverticulum, wedge resection with primary closure of the involved bowel is performed. This requires postoperative observation of the child in the hospital.

GENITOURINARY

Circumcision

Circumcision is often accomplished before a newborn infant's discharge to home. However, for various reasons, both medical and social, the decision to perform circumcision may be delayed. Still, most circumcisions are performed within the first few months of life, and can be accomplished as an outpatient procedure. The relative benefits of circumcision include a decreased incidence of urinary tract infections, phimosis, balanitis, and penile cancer. However, the decision to perform circumcision is still primarily a social or religious one and is usually left to the parents or caretakers.

Circumcision is accomplished by swaddling the infant on a papoose-type board. A penile block is performed using Xylocaine (1%) (0.5–1 mL) *without* epinephrine administered through a 25-gauge needle at the base of the dorsum of the penis (Fig. 48–8). The needle is inserted through Buck's fascia to the tunica albuginea and the anesthetic is injected over the dorsal nerve of the penis. In some instances, circumferential subcutaneous injection of anesthetic may be necessary, but this is done with extreme caution.

At our institution, we prefer to use a bell-type circumcision clamp (Fig. 48–9). This device provides an excellent cosmetic result and protects the glans from injury. The foreskin is retracted and the penis is prepped with Betadine. The foreskin is then brought back over the glans and stretched. A slit may be needed to accommodate placement of the bell. The clamp is applied and, after 3 minutes, the foreskin is removed sharply (Fig. 48–10). Cautery should *never* be used for resection of the foreskin. After removal of the bell, the penis is dressed with antibiotic ointment and a petroleum gauze. Traction on the foreskin should be avoided to prevent separation of the newly coapted layers of foreskin. Older infants may require suture reinforcement of the foreskin edges with 5–0 or 6–0 chromic suture.

Foreskin Adhesions

After circumcision, adhesion of foreskin to the glans may persist for a number of months. It ultimately resolves spontaneously. In certain instances, however, if adhesions persist, infection and pain may ensue. Gentle manual retraction of the foreskin is usually all that is needed to separate the adhesions. In the infant, this is accomplished without difficulty. In the toddler or young child, this may be too painful, and conscious sedation or general anesthesia is required. After the adhesions are separated, the parents or the child, if he is old enough to understand, are instructed to

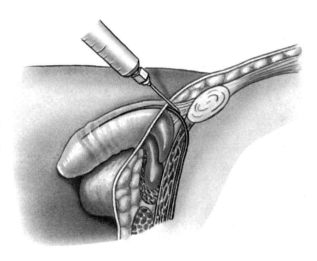

Figure 48–8. Technique for injection of local anesthetic for circumcision. (From Lohr JA, Howards SS, Rein MF. Urogenital Procedures. In: Lohr JA, Pediatric Outpatient Procedures. Philadelphia: JB Lippincott, 1991.)

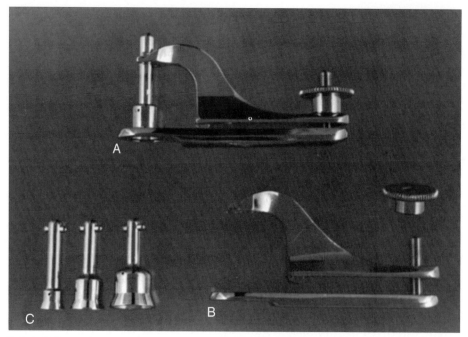

Figure 48–9. A, Bell-type circumcision clamp. **B,** Disassembled clamp. **C,** Bells of various sizes. (From Lohr JA, Howards SS, Rein MF. Urogenital Procedures. In Lohr JA, ed. Pediatric Outpatient Procedures, p. 159. Philadelphia, JB Lippincott Co., 1991.)

retract the foreskin regularly, especially during baths. This should prevent any recurrence.

Labial Adhesions

Labial adhesions are found in prepubescent girls aged 6 months to 6 years. The posterior one third to one half of the labia minora are fused. In some cases, a true skin bridge may be present. The cause is unclear, but adhesions may be due to a slight deficiency in estrogen production. Usually, the adhesions resolve as the girl matures and estrogen production increases. However, in some children, adhesions may cause urinary flow obstruction, stasis of urine in the vagina, obstruction of vaginal secretions, or undue anxiety for the parents or caretakers.

Adhesions may be treated by application of estrogen cream to the vaginal area twice a day for 2 weeks and at bedtime for 2 additional weeks. If this fails, an outpatient anesthetic can be planned for formal labial division. If no skin or mucosal bridge is present, the labia are separated using manual traction. If a bridge is present, separation is performed us-

ing scissors or a knife. The mucosal or skin edges are then approximated on each side using interrupted sutures of 6-0 chromic. Estrogen cream is then applied daily for 1 to 2 months. Good hygiene practices are stressed.

PERIANAL AND PERIRECTAL ABSCESS, FISTULA-IN-ANO

Perianal and perirectal infections are common in infants younger than 1 year old. A perianal abscess is usually caused by diaper rash, whereas a true perirectal abscess may represent a crypt abscess burrowing toward the skin. Both types of abscesses are similar in their appearance. An infant presents with redness, induration, and, in some instances, drainage of pus in the perianal region. Incision and drainage with antibiotic treatment for the surrounding cellulitis successfully treat approximately 50% of the lesions presenting in such a fashion. If drainage persists or infection recurs, however, a fistula is present. Any infection should be resolved before definitive treatment of a fistula-in-ano is undertaken.

At surgery, the infant is placed in the lithot-

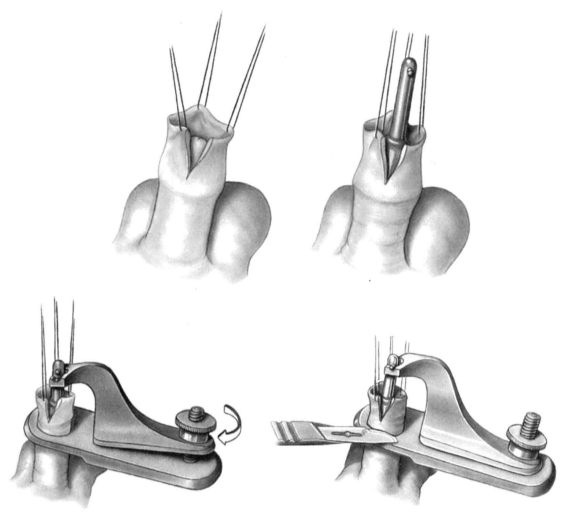

Figure 48–10. Technique for circumcision using the bell clamp. (From Lohr JA, Howards SS, Rein MF. Urogenital Procedures. In: Lohr JA, ed. Pediatric Outpatient Procedures. Philadelphia: JB Lippincott, 1991:159–161.)

omy position. The rectum is irrigated with dilute Betadine or neomycin solution. The anus is dilated with the surgeon's finger or a Hegar's dilator. A lacrimal duct probe is then placed into the external draining site and is gently passed until it emerges through an opening in a crypt along the dentate line. The fistula usually passes between the internal and external sphincters. The overlying skin, subcutaneous tissue, and muscle are divided with cautery. The base tissue of the fistula is then curettaged or cauterized. The wound is dressed with antibiotic ointment and petroleum gauze. The parents are instructed to clean the area two to three times a day, or after every bowel movement, with warm, soapy water, and to re-

apply the antibiotic ointment, until healing is complete. Continence is not affected.

A perirectal abscess and fistula-in-ano may be approached in a similar manner in the older child. In this age group, however, these conditions should raise the suspicion of inflammatory bowel disease, presence of a foreign body, or abuse.

INGROWN TOENAIL

An ingrown toenail is just as its name implies. This condition usually afflicts the great toe. A corner or edge of the nail curls in toward the surrounding skin and causes pain, erythema,

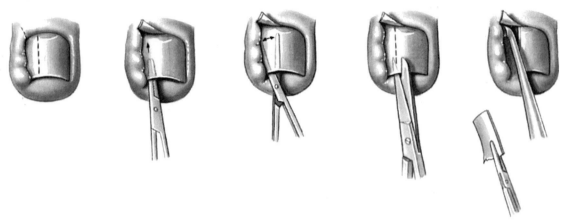

Figure 48–11. Technique for removal of ingrown portion of a toenail. (From McGahren ED, Rodgers BM: Minor pediatric surgical procedures. In: Lohr JA, ed. Pediatric Outpatient Procedures. Philadelphia: JB Lippincott, 1991:232.)

and, in some cases, infection. Initial therapy includes soaking the toe in hot, soapy water, teasing of the skin away from the nail, and antibiotics if infection is present. This condition rarely resolves without surgical intervention.

Surgical treatment can be accomplished in the office using 1% or 2% Xylocaine without epinephrine for a digital block of the great toe. In younger children, conscious sedation may be required as well. Once adequate anesthesia has been obtained, the nail is undermined along the affected side down to the base. Scissors are then used to cut and remove one third to one half of the nail on the symptomatic side (Fig. 48–11). The whole nail is removed if both sides are affected. Any granulation tissue along the adjoining skin is sharply excised. Curettage of the base and nail matrix prevents regrowth of the nail. However, most patients prefer to have the nail regrow, so this option should be discussed with the patient before the procedure. The nail bed is compressed until adequate hemostasis is obtained. Antibiotic ointment and petroleum gauze are placed on the nail bed, and the toe is loosely wrapped with gauze. The patient is instructed to wear a loose-fitting shoe, soak the toe two or three times a day in soapy water, redress the toe as before, and tease the lateral skin edges away from the nail bed as the nail regrows. The nail should also be trimmed straight across to prevent the corners from burrowing back into the skin. Despite these precautions, there is a significant incidence of recurrent ingrowth.

CENTRAL VENOUS ACCESS

The most common indications for central venous access in infants and children include need for parenteral nutrition, chemotherapy, or a prolonged course of antibiotics. Central catheters often remain in place for weeks to months, and their management is frequently done at home by trained parents or caretakers. Unless in-hospital therapy is required, catheter placement may be done as an outpatient procedure. Unlike in adults, general anesthesia is best used for infants and children in this setting.

In general, cuffed Silastic catheters are preferable for use in infants. Cuffed catheters or catheters with indwelling ports may be used for older children. Catheters are made in a variety of sizes starting at 2.5 French. The appropriate-sized catheter depends on the size of the child, but a rough guideline is 2.5 to 4.0 French for infants, 4.0 to 6.0 French for toddlers and school-aged children, and 9.0 French for adolescents. It is best to use the smallest catheter that meets the medical needs of the child to minimize the possibility of venous obstruction and subsequent thrombosis. Ports are also available in different sizes to accommodate patient size. Double lumen catheters and ports should be used only if specifically needed.

Most central catheters are placed so that the tip rests at the junction of the superior vena cava and the right atrium. In infants, access is best obtained via cutdown at the neck (Fig. 48–12). The right side is preferable because

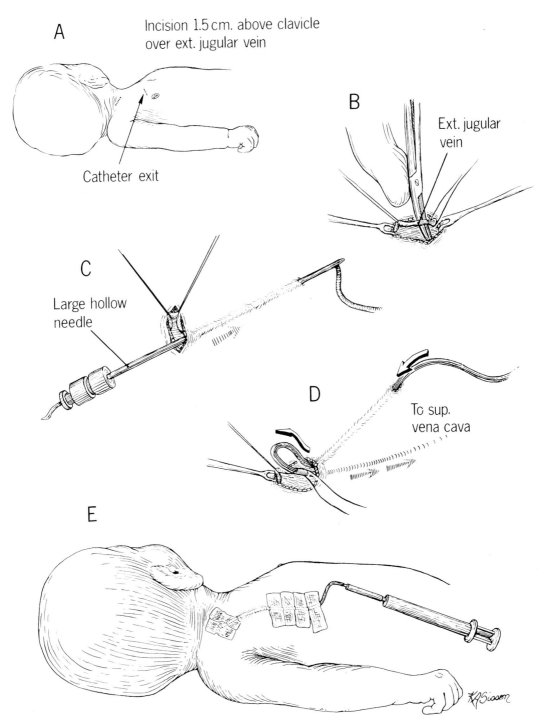

Figure 48–12. Technique for placement of a cuffed central venous catheter in an infant. **A,** The infant is positioned with shoulders elevated and neck extended. **B,** The external jugular vein is isolated. **C,** A large hollow needle is used as a tunneling device in this drawing. A hollow suction catheter, long clamp, or tendon passer is preferred to avoid penetration of the skin or chest by the needle. (From Luck SR. Vascular access. In: Raffensperger JG, ed. Swenson's Pediatric Surgery. 5th ed. Norwalk, CT: Appleton & Lange, 1990.)

the catheter takes a less tortuous course to its final position than it does from the left side, although either side may be used. An incision is made in a skin crease over the lower third of the sternocleidomastoid muscle. Identification of an access site is then made. The first preferred site is an external jugular vein. If this vein is prominent, it is isolated and ligated distally, with an untied suture placed around the proximal vein. Dissection of the vein proximally sometimes allows visualization of its junction with the subclavian vein. If a usable external jugular vein is absent, the sternocleidomastoid muscle is split along its fibers, and the internal jugular vein is isolated. It is best to search for a branch of the internal jugular vein, usually the facial, for actual venous access. If a branch is not of accessible size, the catheter is then best placed into the internal jugular vein through a small venotomy within a purse-string of fine nonabsorbable suture.

Once an appropriate vein site is chosen for access, the access device is placed. If a cuffed catheter is being used, a subcutaneous tunnel is made from the neck incision to an exit site in the mid upper chest. The tunnel is made using a long clamp, a suction catheter, or a tendon passer. Care is taken to avoid any proximity to the nipple in prepubescent girls because damage to the subareolar tissue may hamper breast development. The catheter is then grasped and passed back through the tunnel so that the cuff is seated 1 to 1.5 cm inside the exit site. The catheter is secured at the exit site with a 3–0 or 4–0 nylon suture. The catheter is cut to the appropriate length. The angle of Louis is a helpful landmark to estimate catheter length. The catheter is then placed into the selected vein. The proximal tie or purse-string is secured around the catheter. This securing tie should be snug enough to prevent bleeding, but not so tight that the catheter will not slide out at the time of removal. Absorbable suture is used to close muscle, subcutaneous tissue, and skin.

If a port is being used, exposure of the vein is accomplished as described. A transverse incision is then made in the upper mid-chest on the side being accessed. Dissection is carried down to but not through the pectoralis major fascia. A pocket that is large enough for the port is made at the fascial level. Four tacking sutures are preplaced, and the port is then secured into the pocket. The catheter is passed through the subcutaneous tunnel as described. The incision for the port is closed with absorbable sutures. Strict hemostasis should be accomplished before closure to avoid hematoma in the port pocket.

Rarely, central access may be required in an infant who has a nonpatent superior caval system. In these instances, the proximal saphenous vein may be accessed through a medial thigh incision just below the groin crease. The catheter is tunneled to an exit site on the lower lateral abdomen. The catheter tip should be positioned in the distal inferior vena cava. Some venous congestion is common in the leg but usually resolves when the catheter is removed.

In school-aged children and adolescents, venous access may be obtained via the subclavian vein using the Seldinger technique. The access needle is directed slightly more caphalad in the smaller child than in the adolescent or adult. The other principles of catheter or port placement have already been described.

Optimal positioning is done by placing a rolled towel under the patient's shoulders, turning the patient's head away from the side being accessed, and placing the patient in Trendelenburg position. A local anesthetic such as 1% or 2% Xylocaine or 0.25% to 0.5% bupivicaine is injected into the access area and subcutaneous tunnel to aid in postoperative comfort. Intraoperative fluoroscopy and a postprocedure chest radiograph should be used to confirm appropriate placement of the tip of the catheter. If the subclavian approach is used, the relatively stiff dilator and introducer should be placed under fluoroscopic guidance to avoid perforation of the superior vena cava or pericardium.

Cuffed catheters can be removed by introducing a clamp into the exit site and bluntly dissecting the cuff free. The cuff is grasped, and any fibrinous tissue proximal to the cuff is separated to allow withdrawal of the line. This procedure can be performed using local anesthesia and sedation, if needed, in infants and older cooperative children. Toddlers and young children usually require deep sedation or light general anesthesia. Removal of a port is a formal operative procedure. The previous incision is used. The port is dissected free and the anchoring sutures are cut. The port and catheter should then slide out easily. Any time the catheter does not slide out easily, a counterincision should be made over the point of resistance. This is usually where the catheter enters a vein or over an adherent cuff that is not reachable through the exit site.

Selected Readings

1. Aschcraft KW, Holder TM, ed. Pediatric Surgery. 2nd ed. Philadelphia: WB Saunders, 1993.
2. Behrman RE, Kliegman RM, Arvin AM, eds. Nelson Textbook of Pediatrics. 15th ed. Philadelphia: WB Saunders, 1996.
3. Dudley H, Carter DC, Russell RCG, Spitz L, Nixon HH, eds. Rob and Smith's Operative Surgery, Pediatric Surgery. 4th ed. London: Butterworths, 1988.
4. Glasson MJ, Taylor SF. Cervical, cervicomediastinal, and intrathoracic lymphangioma. Progr Pediatr Surg 1991:27:63–83.
5. Klein JD. Cat scratch disease. Pediatr Rev 1994;15(9): 348–353.
6. Kurtzberg J, Fraham ML. Non-Hodgkin's lymphoma. Pediatr Clin North Am 1991;38:443–456.
7. Lohr JA, ed. Pediatric Outpatient Procedures. New York: JB Lippincott, 1991.
8. Marcy SM. Infections of lymph nodes of the head and neck. Pediatr Infect Dis 1983;2(5):397–405.
9. Radkowski D, Arnold J, Healy GB, et al. Thyroglossal duct remnants. Arch Otolaryngol Head Neck Surg 1991;117:1378–1381.
10. Raffensperger JG, et al. Swenson's Pediatric Surgery. 5th ed. Norwalk, CT: Appleton & Lange, 1990.
11. Rowe MI, O'Neill JA, Grosfeld JL, Fonkalsrud EW, Coran AG, ed. Essentials of Pediatric Surgery. St Louis: Mosby, 1995.
12. Schoen EJ. The status of circumcision in newborns. N Engl J Med 1990;322:308–312.
13. Urba WJ, Longo DL. Hodgkin's disease. N Engl J Med 1992;326:678–687.
14. Welch KJ, Randolph JG, Ravitch MM, O'Neill JA, Rowe MI, eds. Pediatric Surgery. 4th ed. Chicago: Year Book Medical, 1986.
15. Whitman ED. Complications associated with the use of central venous access devices. Curr Prob Surg 1996;33(4):319–378.

Index

Note: Page numbers in *italics* refer to illustrations; page numbers
followed by t refer to tables.